Knee Ligaments
Structure, Function, Injury, and Repair

Knee Ligaments
Structure, Function, Injury, and Repair

Editors

Dale M. Daniel, M.D.
Associate Clinical Professor
Department of Orthopedic Surgery
University of California, San Diego, School of Medicine
La Jolla, California;
Staff Surgeon
Kaiser Permanente Medical Center
San Diego, California

Wayne H. Akeson, M.D.
Professor and Chairman
Department of Surgery
Division of Orthopedics and Rehabilitation
University of California, San Diego, School of Medicine
La Jolla, California

John J. O'Connor, B.E., M.A., Ph.D.
University Lecturer in Engineering Science
Department of Engineering Science
University of Oxford;
Fellow of St. Peter's College
Oxford, England

Raven Press 🖋 New York

Raven Press, 1185 Avenue of the Americas, New York, New York 10036

Made in the United States of America

Library of Congress Cataloging-in-Publication Data

Knee ligaments : structure, function, injury, and repair / editors,
  Dale M. Daniel, Wayne H. Akeson, John J. O'Connor.
      p. 576 cm.
    Includes bibliographical references.
    ISBN 0-88167-605-5
    1. Knee—Wounds and injuries. 2. Ligaments—Wounds and injuries.
3. Knee. 4. Ligaments. I. Daniel, Dale M., 1939–   . II. Akeson,
Wayne H., 1928–   . III. O'Connor, John J. (John Joseph), 1934–
    [DNLM: 1. Knee Joint. 2. Ligaments, Articular. WE 870 K675]
RD561.K577   1990
617.5′82′044—dc20
DNLM/DLC
for Library of Congress   90-8184
                                                              CIP

9 8 7 6 5 4 3 2 1

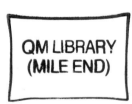

To those teams and especially to those residents, fellows, graduate students, therapists, and technicians whose creativity and energy turn ideas into experiments and theories that contribute to our understanding of knee ligaments

Preface

In 1938 Ivar Palmer published his classic thesis *On Injuries to the Ligaments of the Knee*. Palmer's observations were based on anatomical dissections and the correlation of the clinical examination with surgical pathology. Numerous clinicians following Palmer's lead have added to our knowledge of knee ligament function. In the early 1970s an increasing number of laboratory scientists began to study knee joint mechanics, ligament structure and function, and the response of ligaments to injury. In the past decade, there has been an explosion in knee ligament research. Clinicians have teamed with basic scientists, physiologists, chemists, and engineers. An increasing number of orthopedic residents have been given the opportunity to participate in laboratory research, and the development of orthopedic fellowship programs has provided additional clinicians with research background and capability. The ligament field is on the move. This volume is our effort to make a 1990 knee ligament "state of the union address."

The book is organized into five parts. Part I presents one surgeon's (author DMD) management of knee-ligament-injured patients. Part II reviews the normal ligament structure: anatomy, chemistry, and physiology. Part III explores ligament function. What are the material and structural properties of the ligaments? Do ligaments function as a sensory organ? How do they contribute to the passive and active stability of the joint? Can the muscles compensate for loss of ligament function? Part IV presents *in vivo* experiments on ligament injury and repair, including autograft remodeling. Considerations in choosing an animal model as well as in interpreting the results of animal research are discussed. Part V discusses the natural history of the ligament-injured knee, clinical measurement of knee stability, and the complications of ligament surgery. The volume concludes with a chapter on research design and statistical analysis of data.

The 1990s will bring significant advances in the care of knee-ligament-injured patients. Those advances will probably result from sound scientific investigations by M.D./Ph.D. research teams.

This volume will be of interest to the serious knee student, and to clinicians, therapists, and laboratory investigators. The text provides the reader with an understanding of knee ligament function which will allow improvement in knee ligament surgery and postoperative care.

Dale M. Daniel
Wayne H. Akeson
John J. O'Connor

Acknowledgments

The authors would like to thank the following associates, fellows, graduate students, residents, and research staff who have added to our understanding of the knee ligaments:

David Amiel: Mark Abel, Chip Billings, Clark Campbell, Albert Crenshaw, Babak Fazeli, Tom Ferro, Russ Foulk, Jan Friden, Mike Furniss, Alex Green, Fred L. Harwood, Ken Ishizue, Jeff Kleiner, Diana LeBow, Margot Leonard, Mike Mai, Thalia McKee-Woodburn, Rob Pedowitz, Steve Renzoni, Fran Shepherd, Dean Smith, Blake Thompson, Monica Wiig, and Abbe Zaro

Savio L-Y. Woo: Alan Balfour, Tracy Ballock, Michael Danto, Fred Field, Cyril Frank, Carol Frey, Jan Fronek, Mark Gomez, Scott Hacker, Scott Harris, J. Marcus Hollis, David Hawkins, Masahiro Inoue, Daniel Jacoby, Bryant Karras, Linda Kitabayashi, Edward Lee, Thay Lee, Hung-Chang Lin, Roger Lyon, Deidre MacKenna, James Marcin, Karen May, Erin McGurk-Burleson, Carlo Orlando, Robert Peterson, Mark Ritter, Richard Roux, Jeff Schultz, Terry Sites, Stephen To, Douglas Walker, Jack Wang, Jennifer Wayne, Jack Winters, and Eric Yam

Harry B. Skinner: Steven L. Buckley

Steven Paul Arnoczky: Julie Agel, Melissa Ashlock, Susan Cunningham, Alexander Joseph, Karen Kelsey, S. Jean Kilfoyle, John L. Marshall, John Matyas, Joseph Minei, Sylvester Oliver, Sten-Erik Olsson, Gary Peterson, Roy M. Rubin, Brian Saltzman, Guy B. Tarvin, William Thackery, Peter A. Torzilli, Philip B. Vasseur, Russell F. Warren, and Thomas L. Wickiewicz

John J. O'Connor: Staff of the Oxford University School of Engineering Science and the Nuffield Orthopaedic Centre, Oxford

Hans-Ulrich Stäubli: Lottie Applewhite, St. Birrer, R. Buchmann, and St. Sporri

Robert T. Burks: Roger Haut

Dale M. Daniel: David Anderson, Peter Barnett, James Blasingame, Samuel Blick, Cliff Colwell, Les Cooper, Scott Daniel, Timothy Donovan, Steve Erbey, David Faddis, David Flood, Louise Focht, Kim Foreman, Todd Krell, Chris Lafferty, James W. Lawler, Marmaduke Loke, Gary M. Losse, Larry Malcom, Peter Mandt, Emanuele Minardi, Dev Mishra, Beverly Morris, Wayne Mortensen, Tamara Mucha, John Murphy, T. Nessouli, Howard Peth, Daniel B. Robertson, G. Charles Roland, Lisa Schneider, Gregory H. Schwab, David Sutherland, Dick Watkins, Peter Woods, E. Paul Woodward, Marilyn Wyatt, and Nicholas Yaru

H. Paul Hirshman: Larry Brown, Clifford Colwell, Jr., Jan Fronek, and Alan Halling

Richard L. Lieber: Field Blenns, Basak Fazeli, Tom Ferro, Alex Green, Margot Leonard, Michael Mai, Thalia McKee-Woodburn, and Scott Shoemaker

The editors wish to thank Nancy Johnson, Jaime Davis, Robert Golden, and Nancy Kirkpatrick for their assistance in preparing and editing the manuscript and in the production of the book.

Contents

Contributors

Douglas J. Adams, MS *Biomechanics Research Engineer, Orthopedic Bioengineering Laboratory, Division of Orthopedic Surgery, University of California, San Diego, School of Medicine, La Jolla, California 92093*

Wayne H. Akeson, MD *Professor and Head, Department of Surgery, Division of Orthopedics and Rehabilitation, University of California, San Diego, School of Medicine, La Jolla, California 92093*

David Amiel, MD *Associate Adjunct Professor, Department of Surgery, Division of Orthopedics and Rehabilitation, University of California, San Diego, School of Medicine, La Jolla, California 92093*

Steven Paul Arnoczky, DVM, Dipl. ACVS *Director, Laboratory of Comparative Orthopedics, Hospital for Special Surgery, 535 East 70th Street, New York, New York 10021*

Robert L. Barrack, CDR, MC, USNR *Assistant Chairman, Department of Orthopaedic Surgery, U.S. Naval Hospital, 8750 Mountain Boulevard, Oakland, California 94627-5000, and Assistant Clinical Professor, Department of Orthopaedic Surgery, University of California, San Francisco, School of Medicine, San Francisco, California 94143*

Edmund Biden, PhD *Associate Professor, Department of Mechanical Engineering, University of New Brunswick, Fredericton, New Brunswick, Canada E3B 5A3*

E. Billings, Jr., MD *Orthopedic Surgery Resident, Department of Surgery, Division of Orthopedics and Rehabilitation, University of California, San Diego, School of Medicine, La Jolla, California 92093*

John Bradley, FRCS *Consultant Orthopaedic Surgeon, Department of Orthopaedic Surgery, Colchester General Hospital, Colchester C04 5JL, Essex, England*

Robert T. Burks, MD *Assistant Professor, Department of Orthopedic Surgery, Division of Sports Medicine, University of Utah Medical Center, Salt Lake City, Utah 84132*

J. J. Collins *Research Assistant, Orthopaedic Engineering Centre, Oxford University, Oxford OX3 7DL, England*

Dale M. Daniel, MD *Associate Clinical Professor, Department of Orthopedic Surgery, University of California, San Diego, School of Medicine, La Jolla, California 92037, and Staff Surgeon, Kaiser Permanente Medical Center, San Diego, California 92120*

David FitzPatrick, BA, BAI *Research Assistant, Department of Engineering Science, University of Oxford, Oxford OX1 3PJ, England*

John Goodfellow, MS, FRCS *Consultant Orthopaedic Surgeon, Nuffield Orthopaedic Centre, Oxford OX3 7LD, England*

H. Paul Hirshman, MD *Head, Section of Sports Medicine, Department of Orthopaedics, Scripps Clinic, La Jolla, California 92037*

Shuji Horibe, MD *Orthopedic Resident, Orthopedic Bioengineering Laboratory, University of California, San Diego, School of Medicine, La Jolla, California 92093*

Christopher Kershaw, FRCS *Senior Orthopaedic Registrar, Department of Orthopaedics, Leicester Royal Infirmary, Leicester LE1 5WW, England*

Scott Kuiper, MD *Orthopedic Surgery Resident, Department of Surgery, Division of Orthopedics and Rehabilitation, University of California, San Diego, School of Medicine, La Jolla, California 92093*

Michael K. Kwan, PhD *Assistant Professor of Surgery and Bioengineering, Orthopedic Bioengineering Laboratory, Division of Orthopedic Surgery, University of California, San Diego, School of Medicine, La Jolla, California 92093*

Richard L. Lieber, PhD *Assistant Professor, Department of Surgery, University of California, San Diego, School of Medicine, La Jolla, California 92093, and Division of Orthopedics and Rehabilitation, Veterans Administration Medical Center, La Jolla, California 92161*

Roger M. Lyon, MD *Orthopedic Resident, Orthopedic Bioengineering Laboratory, Division of Orthopedic Surgery, University of California, San Diego, School of Medicine, La Jolla, California 92093, and San Diego Veterans Administration Medical Center, La Jolla, California 92161*

Kenji Miyasaka, AB *Medical Student, University of California, San Diego, School of Medicine, La Jolla, California 92093*

Peter O. Newton, MD *Orthopedic Resident, Orthopedic Bioengineering Laboratory, Division of Orthopedic Surgery, University of California, San Diego, School of Medicine, La Jolla, California 92093, and San Diego Veterans Administration Medical Center, La Jolla, California 92161*

John O'Connor, BE, MA, PhD *University Lecturer in Engineering Science, Department of Engineering Science, University of Oxford, Oxford OX1 3PJ, and Fellow of St. Peter's College, Oxford OX2 2DL, England*

Karen J. Ohland, MS *Biomedical Engineer and Laboratory Manager, Orthopedic Bioengineering Laboratory, University of California, San Diego, School of Medicine, La Jolla, California 92093, and Veterans Administration Medical Center, La Jolla, California 92037*

Donald Resnick, MD *Professor, Department of Radiology, University of California, San Diego, School of Medicine, La Jolla, California 92093, and Chief, Radiology Service, San Diego Veterans Administration Medical Center, La Jolla, California 92037*

Alan Reznik, MD *New Haven Orthopedic Surgeons, P.C., 111 Park Street, New Haven, Connecticut 06511*

Barbara Riehl *Research Coordinator, Kaiser Permanente Medical Center, San Diego, California 92120*

Raymond A. Sachs, MD *Chief, Department of Orthopedics, Kaiser Permanente Medical Center, San Diego, California 92120*

David J. Sartoris, MD *Assistant Professor, Department of Radiology, University of California, San Diego, School of Medicine, La Jolla, California 92093, and Department of Radiology, San Diego Veterans Administration Medical Center, La Jolla, California 92037*

Jean P. Schils, MD *Osteoradiology Fellow, Department of Radiology, Cleveland Clinic Foundation, One Clinic Center, 9500 Euclid Avenue, Cleveland, Ohio 44195-5021, and Department of Radiology, San Diego Veterans Administration Medical Center, La Jolla, California 92037*

Tessa Shercliff, BA *Research Assistant, Department of Engineering Science, University of Oxford, Oxford OX1 3PJ, England*

Stephen C. Shoemaker, MD *San Dieguito Orthopedic Medical Group, 9900 Genesee Avenue, La Jolla, California 92037*

Harry B. Skinner, MD, PhD *Professor, Department of Orthopaedic Surgery, University of California, San Francisco, School of Medicine, San Francisco, California 94143*

Hans-Ulrich Stäubli, MD *Professor, Department of Orthopedic Surgery, University of Bern, Inselspital, CH-3010 Bern, Switzerland, and Chief of Orthopaedics and Traumatology, Tiefenauspital der stadt und der Region Bern, Tiefenaustr. 112, CH-3004 Bern, Switzerland*

Mary Lou Stone, RPT *Registered Physical Therapist, Department of Orthopedics, Kaiser Permanente Medical Center, San Diego, California 92120*

H. von Schroeder, MD *Orthopedic Surgery Resident, Department of Surgery, Division of Orthopedics and Rehabilitation, University of California, San Diego, School of Medicine, La Jolla, California 92093*

Caroline W. Wang *Graduate Student, Orthopedic Bioengineering Laboratory, University of California, San Diego, School of Medicine, La Jolla, California 92093, and San Diego Veterans Administration Medical Center, La Jolla, California 92161*

Savio L-Y. Woo, PhD *Professor of Surgery and Bioengineering, Orthopaedic Bioengineering Laboratory, Division of Orthopaedic Surgery, University of California, San Diego, School of Medicine, La Jolla, California 92093, and San Diego Veterans Administration Medical Center, La Jolla, California 92161, and Executive Director, M. and D. Coutts Institute for Joint Reconstruction and Research, San Diego, California 92123*

Edmond P. Young, MD *Orthopedic Resident, Orthopedic Bioengineering Laboratory, Division of Orthopedic Surgery, University of California, San Diego, School of Medicine, La Jolla, California 92093*

Stephen Young, FRCS *Consultant Orthopaedic Surgeon, Department of Orthopaedic Surgery, South Warwickshire Hospital, Warwick CV34 5BW, England*

PART I

Patient Care

CHAPTER 1

Diagnosis of a Ligament Injury

Dale M. Daniel

Our study of knee ligaments begins with the patient. We identify problems. We go to the laboratory seeking solutions. We return to the patient. Thus in this book we shall begin with the patient. I shall present my approach to the evaluation and treatment of patients with knee ligament injuries. Case studies from my practice will be presented to share how one surgeon in the 1980s managed knee ligament injuries. The case presentations will raise questions that are being studied in the laboratory and will point the reader to chapters that discuss those questions.

Evaluation of the injured patient begins with the history of the injury event. There are certain scenarios that greatly increase the probability of a knee ligament injury. With a history like the following, the probability of an anterior cruciate ligament (ACL) disruption is greater than 70%: "I was playing basketball. Coming down from a rebound my knee popped and gave way. I could hear the pop. I tried to continue playing, but my knee felt too unstable and I had to quit. Within a couple of hours my knee was swollen." The history is helpful, it guides the work-up, but the *sine qua non* of a ligament disruption is the demonstration of abnormal knee motion. Disruption of a ligament will alter the limits of joint motion (Chapter 9).

The careful manual examination of joint motion will reveal most ligament disruptions. Patient relaxation is

important. The patient should lie supine on a firm but comfortable examining table with the limb supported. The motion resulting from a clinical test depends on the position of the limb at the initiation of the test, the force applied, point of application of the force, and point of detection of the displacement. Joint motion varies considerably within the normal population, but there is little right–left variation in a normal subject. Therefore in a patient with a unilateral knee injury, the motion of the injured knee should be compared to that of the normal knee. To compare the two limbs the examination conditions must be constant: starting position, applied force, and site of motion measurement. If the results of different examiners or serial examinations are to be compared, these elements must be constant.

Numerous tests have been described to detect pathologic knee motion. The pathologic motion resulting from certain tests are associated with a specific ligament or ligament complexes (Table 1-1). Primary tests render pathologic motion only if the specific ligament in question is injured. The injury of other ligaments may increase the pathologic motion being tested, provided that the primary ligament is disrupted (Chapter 9). On all displacement measurements the femur is held constant and tibial translation or joint space opening is measured. The starting position is the neutral resting position with the joint surfaces in contact. The applied force and site of motion measurement for each of the primary motion tests are presented in Table 1-2. The following tests are used as primary tests of ligament disruption.

D. M. Daniel: Department of Orthopedic Surgery, University of California, San Diego, School of Medicine, La Jolla, California 92037; and Kaiser Permanente Medical Center, San Diego, California 92120.

TABLE 1-1. *Primary clinical limits of motion tests*

Test	Ligament/ligament complex isolated injury[a]				
	ACL	PCL	MCC	LCC	PLC
Lachman	√				
Pivot shift	√				
Tibia posterior subluxation		√			
Abduction (25°)			√		
Adduction (25°)				√	
Reverse pivot shift					√

[a] ACL, anterior cruciate ligament; PCL, posterior cruciate ligament; MCC, medial collateral complex; LCC, lateral collateral complex; PLC, posterior lateral complex.

POSTERIOR CRUCIATE LIGAMENT

Both the anterior cruciate ligament (ACL) and the posterior cruciate ligament (PCL) limit the total anterior–posterior displacement of the tibia. The examination of the cruciate ligaments begins with the evaluation of the PCL. A PCL disruption results in greater posterior displacement of the tibia from the anatomic resting position, and an ACL disruption allows greater anterior displacement of the tibia from the anatomic resting position. To determine which structure(s) are disrupted, the clinician must be able to determine the neutral position. The neutral position is the resting position of the tibia supported by the intact PCL. The neutral po-

TABLE 1-2. *Tests of motion limits[a]*

Force[b]				Moment[b]				Measurement site[c]	Displacement measured[d]	Test identified by letter	
										Knee flexion position	
Ant	Post	Med	Lat	IR	ER	Valgus	Varus			25°	90°
+ +								TT (1)	Anterior	a	b
+ +					+			MC (2)	Anterior	c	d
+ +				+				LC (3)	Anterior	e	f
	+ +							TT (1)	Posterior	g	h
	+ +			+				MC (2)	Posterior	i	j
	+ +				+			LC (3)	Posterior	k	l
		+ +						MC (4)	Medial	m	
			+ +					LC (5)	Lateral	n	
										0°	25°
				−	−	+ +		MC (4)	Medial JSO[e]	o	p
				−	−		+ +	LC (5)	Lateral JSO[e]	q	r

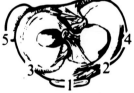

[a] Applied displacement forces and moments are noted for each test. The site of displacement measured, the translation for tests a through n, and the joint space opening for tests o through r are indicated by numbers that correspond to the numbers on the tibia diagram. Placed in boxes are the letters of the primary motion tests: a, h, p, and r. The other tests are performed in an attempt to characterize more completely the joint motion limits. Tests c, d, e, f, i, j, k, and l are performed to estimate compartment motions. Tests m and n are tests of medial and lateral tibial translation.

[b] Ant, anterior; Post, posterior; Med, medial; Lat, lateral; TT, tibial tubercle; MC, medial collateral; LC, lateral collateral; JSO, joint space opening; IR, internal rotation; ER, external rotation. + +, Primary force/moment; +, secondary moment to maximize displacement; −, motion constrained. Absence of a symbol indicates "motion unconstrained".

[c] Numbers in parentheses represent measurement sites located in the knee diagram in this table.

[d] Millimeters of displacement (measured or estimated) from the anatomic supine resting position.

[e] Referenced from joint surface contact position.

This table was developed in consultation with the International Knee Documentation Committee, chairpersons John Feagin (USA) and Werner Muller (Switzerland).

sition can be determined when the patient is lying supine with the knee at 90° of flexion (3). The resting position of the injured knee should be compared with the contralateral normal knee. If the PCL is disrupted, the tibia will sag posteriorly. The sag may be seen by looking at the knee profile, palpated by feeling the femoral condyle–tibia step-off, and confirmed by the quadriceps active test wherein contraction of the quadriceps pulls the tibia anteriorly (Fig. 1-1). To measure posterior displacement the tibia is first placed in the reduced position. If the tibia does not sag posteriorly and cannot be displaced posteriorly more than the contralateral knee with an intact PCL, the PCL is intact and the resting position is the anterior–posterior (A–P) neutral position.

ANTERIOR CRUCIATE LIGAMENT

Lachman Test

The *Lachman test* is an excellent test of the anterior tibia displacement limit (9,15). Prior to performing the Lachman test, the integrity of the PCL should be established with the quadriceps active test at 90° of flex-

ion (Fig. 1-1). To perform the Lachman test, the knee is placed in a position of 20–30° of flexion. The patient lies supine with a support under the thigh (Fig. 1-2). The clinician stabilizes the femur against the thigh support and applies an anterior displacement force to the proximal calf without enhancing or restraining axial rotation. The examiner senses the tibial displacement and the firmness of the displacement limit (end point). If both are normal, the Lachman test is negative. If either is pathologic, the Lachman test is positive. The displacement limit or "end point" may be graded and the side-to-side displacement difference estimated. End point is graded as firm (normal), marginal, or soft. Displacement is estimated in millimeters. An estimated right–left difference of 3 mm or greater is classified as pathologic (Chapter 24). If the PCL is intact, abnormal A–P displacement on the Lachman test indicates an ACL disruption. Examiners appear to be better able to detect end-point differences than displacement differences. An experienced examiner usually correctly diagnoses an ACL disruption, even when there is only a 4-mm right–left displacement difference, because of the alteration in end-point stiffness. However, following ACL surgery, the clinician will frequently state that a knee has a negative Lachman test when there is a

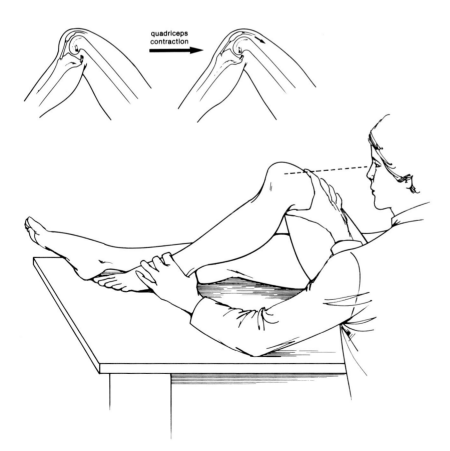

FIG. 1-1. The 90° quadriceps active test. Keeping the eyes at the level of the subject's flexed knee, the examiner rests the elbow on the table and uses the ipsilateral hand to support the subject's thigh and to confirm that the thigh muscles are relaxed. The foot is stabilized by the examiner's other hand, and the subject is asked to slide the foot gently down the table. Tibial displacement resulting from the quadriceps contraction is noted. (From ref. 3.)

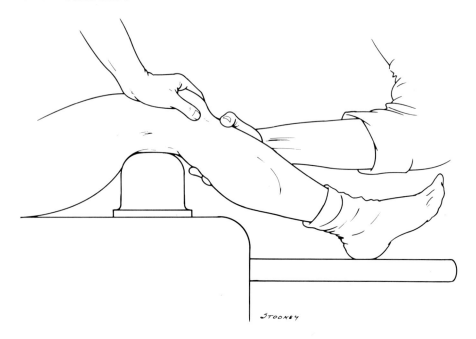

FIG. 1-2. The Lachman test. To facilitate patient relaxation, stabilize the femur, and control the joint flexion angle, the patient lies supine with the thigh supported in 20–30° of flexion. In this diagram the thigh is supported by the MEDmetric Knee Ligament Test Platform (MEDmetric Corporation, San Diego).

normal "end point" and a 4-mm right–left displacement difference documented by instrumented measurement.

Pivot Shift

Pivot shift tests are complex tests of the limits of knee motion. The pivot shift tests have been described by a number of authors as pivot shift test (5,6), Losee test (10), side lying test (14), and flexion–rotation drawer test (12). The test produces anterior subluxation and internal axial rotation in early flexion as a sequela of an ACL disruption. The posterior pull of the iliotibial tract reduces the tibia at 20–40° of flexion. The tests are performed by lifting the tibia and allowing the femur to fall posteriorly. As the knee is flexed and the iliotibial tract is tightened and moves from a position anterior to the axis of knee flexion to a position posterior to the axis of knee flexion, the anteriorly displaced and internally rotated tibia reduces. It is the relocation event that the clinician usually grades. The pivot shift is graded as 0 (absent), 1 + (slight slip), 2 + (moderate slip), or 3 + (momentary locking). Normal subjects are graded 0, and occasionally patients with greater normal anterior tibial motion are graded 1. The effect of tibial rotation on the pivot shift test (2,8) and the effect of hip abduction (1) have been reported. Internal rotation of the tibia and adduction of the hip both tighten the iliotibial tract; therefore the tibia reduces sooner, and the pivot shift grade is reduced. Disruption of the medial collateral ligament (MCL) allows the limb

to go into a valgus alignment and relax the iliotibial band. This reduction in the iliotibial band tone will result in a decrease in the pivot shift reduction event. Likewise, surgery altering the iliotibial band may alter the pivot shift reduction event, even when joint subluxation is not altered. This is important to consider when evaluating ACL reconstruction patients who have had an iliotibial band procedure. The pivot shift is consistently positive in the relaxed patient with a chronic ACL disruption and in the acutely injured anesthetized patient with an ACL disruption.

MEDIAL COLLATERAL LIGAMENT

The *valgus stress test* evaluates the MCL. The patient lies supine with the knees supported in 20–30° of flexion and neutral axial rotation (Fig. 1-3). The examination is performed as discussed in the legend of Fig. 1-3. The medial joint space opening, as well as stiffness of the motion limit, is estimated. The findings are compared to the patient's contralateral normal knee. In a first-degree injury, there is pain and tenderness at the site of the ligament injury; the end point is firm and the joint space opening is within 2 mm of the normal knee. In a second-degree injury, the end point is relatively firm and the joint space opening is increased 3–5 mm compared to that of the normal knee. In a third-degree injury, the end point is soft and the joint space opens more than 5 mm greater than that of the normal knee (4).

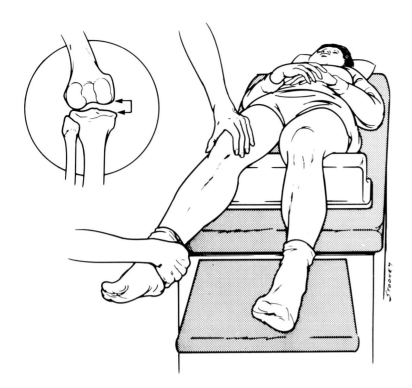

FIG. 1-3. Valgus stress test. To facilitate patient relaxation, stabilize the femur, and control the joint flexion angle, the patient lies supine with the thigh supported in 20–30° of flexion. With one hand, the examiner stabilizes the femur and palpates the medial joint line. With the other hand on the distal tibia, the examiner exerts an axial load to place the joint surfaces in contact; this is the test starting position. The leg is then abducted while constraining axial rotation. The medial joint space opening is estimated and the stiffness of the motion limit evaluated.

LATERAL COLLATERAL LIGAMENT

The *varus stress test* evaluates the lateral collateral ligament (LCL). The patient lies supine with the knees supported in 20–30° of flexion and neutral axial rotation. With one hand the examiner stabilizes the femur and palpates the lateral joint line. With the other hand on the distal tibia the examiner first exerts an axial load to place the joint surfaces in contact; this is the test starting position. The leg is then adducted while constraining axial rotation. The lateral joint space opening, as well as stiffness of the motion limit, is estimated. The grading system of injury is the same as for injuries to the MCL.

POSTERIOR LATERAL LIGAMENT COMPLEX

Axial Rotation

Most knee ligament injuries will affect axial rotation in addition to other motions (Chapter 9). When possible, primary clinical tests are selected which are diagnostic of a specific ligament injury, are easily performed, and can be confirmed by instrumented testing or stress radiographs. To evaluate the posterolateral ligamentous complex, the examiners must evaluate axial rotation and/or the posterior displacement of the lateral compartment. Compartment motion may be es-

timated by palpating the compartment while anteriorly and posteriorly displacing the compartment. This measurement may be made with stress radiographs (Chapter 25) but is very difficult to measure manually. The rotational position of the tibia can be determined by reference to the tibial tubercle, the malleolar axis, and the foot; however, the precise position of the femur cannot be determined. To evaluate the posterolateral ligament complex, the patient lies supine with the knee supported in 20–30° of flexion. Axial rotation is evaluated as described in Figs. 1-4 and 1-5. Axial rotation may also be evaluated similarly in 90° of flexion. Axial rotation near extension can be documented by stress radiograph compartment displacement measurements as discussed in Chapter 25.

Reverse Pivot Shift

The *reverse pivot shift test* is probably the most reliable clinical test of the posterior lateral ligament complex (7). The test is begun by supporting the limb with a hand under the heel, thereby placing the knee in full extension and neutral axial rotation. With the examiner's second hand on the lateral aspect of the calf, a mild valgus stress is applied and the knee is flexed. In a positive test, at about 20–30° of flexion the tibia will externally rotate; the lateral tibial plateau will displace posteriorly and will remain in this position during fur-

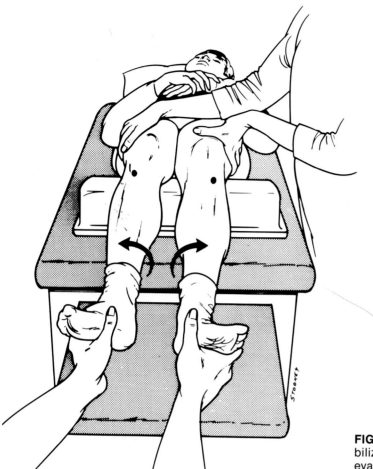

FIG. 1-4. Evaluation of axial rotation. An assistant stabilizes both femora. The examiner rotates the foot and evaluates tibial rotation by noting the external rotation of the tibial tubercle and the foot. The patient's left leg reveals greater external rotation.

ther flexion. When the knee is then extended, the tibia will reduce. In the standard pivot shift, the tibia is anteriorly displaced in early flexion and then reduces between 20° and 40° of flexion. In the reverse pivot shift, the tibia is initially reduced and then the lateral tibial plateau displaces posteriorly at 20°–30° of flexion. In a patient with a combined ACL and posterior lateral injury, one may observe the tibia go from an anterior position to a reduced position and then on to a posterior position. The reverse pivot shift is a useful test in the patient with a chronic injury. However, if the knee is acutely injured the patient is usually unable to relax enough to allow the test to be performed.

PRIMARY AND SECONDARY RESTRAINTS

The clinical examination is based on the correlation of the examination with surgical pathology and on laboratory ligament sectioning studies using nonconstrained testing devices (Chapter 9). A summary of the principal capsular and ligament structures around the knee are listed in Table 1-1 along with the tests that are most diagnostic of an isolated disruption. For a specific motion, the structure that provides the greatest limitation is considered the primary restraint. When a primary restraint is disrupted, motion in that plane is limited by the remaining structures. These are termed the *secondary restraints*. Disruption of a secondary restraint will not result in pathologic motion if the primary restraint is intact. However, sectioning a secondary restraint in the face of an absent primary restraint will enhance pathologic motion. One must also consider that a structure may function as a primary restraint to one motion and a secondary restraint to another. For example, the MCL is the primary restraint to valgus angulation and a secondary restraint to anterior translation. Sectioning the MCL does not affect anterior displacement, which is controlled by the ACL. However, if the ACL is disrupted, the MCL will now be one of the structures that limit anterior displacement. If the MCL is then disrupted, there is an increase in the anterior tibial displacement. It is important to note that the amount of increased motion

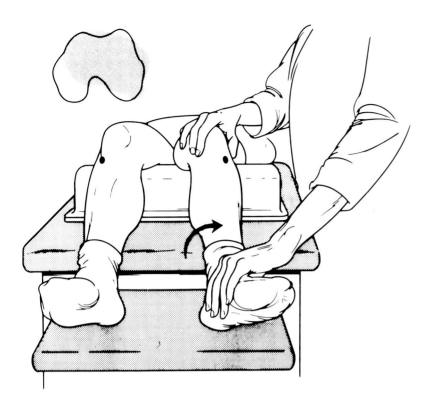

FIG. 1-5. Evaluation of compartment subluxation. If the axial rotation test illustrated in Fig. 1-4 reveals asymmetry of axial rotation, the examiner holds the thigh and palpates the tibial compartments while an external rotation torque is applied to the leg. This allows the examiner to discern if the rotation movement is due to posterior subluxation of the lateral tibial plateau or to anterior movement of the medial tibial plateau as is shown in the figure.

resulting from disruption of a single structure varies considerably from specimen to specimen and from patient to patient (Fig. 9-1).

OTHER DIAGNOSTIC TESTS

I routinely use instrumented measurement to evaluate patients with suspected cruciate ligament injuries. In addition to confirming the suspected diagnosis, the extent of pathologic motion can be documented (Chapter 24). Recently, magnetic resonance imaging (MRI) has been used to diagnose ligament disruptions (Chapter 26). In addition to disruption of the ligaments, the MRI may reveal meniscal injury. MRI studies are expensive, and at this time the role of MRI in patient management is controversial. Ligament disruptions may be diagnosed on manual examination by an experienced clinician with 90% accuracy. Diagnosis may be confirmed by instrumented measurement or stress x-rays. These examinations also provide the clinician with measurements of the pathologic motion, which help guide patient management decisions.

A more complete attempt at clinical documentation of knee motion was reported by Muller (11) and by Noyes (13). In addition to performing the examinations already described to document rotational pathology, the examiner estimates anterior and posterior displacement of the medial and lateral tibial plateaus individually as enumerated in Table 1-2. The relative motion of the two compartments is a measure of rotation. Compartment motion can be well documented on radiographs, as presented in Chapter 25. The accuracy of clinical assessment of compartment motion has not been established.

REFERENCES

1. Bach BR Jr, Warren RF, Wickiewicz TL. The pivot shift phenomenon: Results and description of a modified clinical test for anterior cruciate ligament insufficiency. *Am J Sports Med* 1988;16:571–576.
2. Clancy WG Jr, Ray JM. Anterior cruciate ligament autografts. In: Jackson DW, Drez D Jr, eds. *The anterior cruciate ligament deficient knee: new concepts in ligament repair.* St. Louis: CV Mosby, 1987;193–210.
3. Daniel DM, Stone ML, Barnett P, Sachs R. Use of the quadriceps active test to diagnose posterior cruciate-ligament disruption and measure posterior laxity of the knee. *J Bone Joint Surg* 1988;70A:386–391.
4. Ellison AE. Skiing injuries. *Clin Symp* 1977;29:2–40.
5. Fetto JF, Marshal JL. Injury to the anterior cruciate ligament producing the pivot-shift sign *J Bone Joint Surg* 1979;61A:710–714.
6. Galway HR, MacIntosh DL. The lateral pivot shift: a symptom and sign of anterior cruciate ligament insufficiency. *Clin Orthop* 1980;147:45–50.
7. Jakob RP. Observations on rotatory instability of the lateral compartment of the knee. *Acta Orthop Scand* 1981;52(Suppl 191):1–32.
8. Jakob RP, Stäubli HU, Deland JT. Grading the pivot shift: objective tests with implications for treatment. *J Bone Joint Surg* 1987;69B:294–299.

9. Jonsson T, Althoff B, Peterson L, Renstrom P. Clinical diagnosis of ruptures of the anterior cruciate ligament: a comparative study of the Lachman test and the anterior drawer sign. *Am J Sports Med* 1982;10:100–102.

10. Losee RE, Johnson TR, Southwick WO. Anterior subluxation of the lateral tibial plateau. A diagnostic test and operative repair. *J Bone Joint Surg* 1978;60A:1015–1030.

11. Müller W, Biedert R, Heft F, Jakob RP, Munzinger U, Stäubli HU. Oak knee evaluation: a new way to assess knee ligament injuries. *Clin Orthop* 1988;232:37–50.

12. Noyes FR, Bassett RW, Grood ES, Butler DL. Arthroscopy in acute traumatic hemarthroses of the knee. *J Bone Joint Surg* 1980;62A:687–695.

13. Noyes FR, Grood ES. Diagnosis of knee ligament injuries: clinical concepts. In: Feagin JA, eds. *The crucial ligaments*, vol. 1. New York: Churchill Livingstone, 1988;261–285.

14. Slocum DB, James SL, Larson RL, Singer KM. Clinical test for anterolateral rotatory instability of the knee. *Clin Orthop* 1976;118:63–69.

15. Torg JS, Conrad W, Kalen V. Clinical diagnosis of anterior cruciate ligament instability in the athlete. *Am J Sports Med* 1976;4:84–93.

CHAPTER 2

Principles of Knee Ligament Surgery

Dale M. Daniel

The goal of knee ligament surgery is to reestablish the normal knee motion limits. After each damaged structure is repaired or reconstructed, the knee should be ranged through an arc of 0–120° to confirm that joint flexion and extension have not been restricted. Disruption of repaired or reconstructed structures during this range of motion test reveals that they were incorrectly positioned or tensioned. Optimally, the strength of graft repairs and reconstructions will allow gentle testing of the knee motion limits at the conclusion of the surgical procedure.

The morbidity of ligament surgery is secondary to (a) surgical dissection to expose injured structures, (b) graft harvest, (c) graft implantation, and (d) restriction of limb function to protect the graft during the healing process. The surgical dissection should be minimized to expose only the ligamentous structures that will benefit significantly from surgical repair.

Midsubstance repairs of injured ligaments have not been demonstrated to be of benefit. Laboratory studies of medial collateral ligament (MCL) injury reveal better healing when the ligament is not sutured (Chapter 18). Clinical studies of isolated MCL injury reveal satisfactory results from nonsurgical treatment (Chapter 27). Laboratory studies of midsubstance anterior cruciate ligament (ACL) injury have revealed little potential for healing, and the clinical reports on the results

of midsubstance repairs are mixed (Chapter 19). When surgically treating a patient with a combined MCL–ACL injury, the ACL should be repaired or reconstructed. In the combined injury, a complete MCL tear should be repaired if it disrupted at or near its bone insertion. A midsubstance tear need not be surgically repaired or explored; the morbidity of the procedure probably outweighs the dubious benefit of a midsubstance repair. The site of the MCL injury can usually be determined by (a) localized tenderness or palpation of a defect, (b) bone avulsion seen on radiographs, (c) magnetic resonance imaging (MRI), or (d) a limited surgical exposure. The potential of a midsubstance posterior cruciate ligament (PCL) injury to heal is probably similar to that of the ACL. Healing of PCL and LCL ligaments have not been studied.

Ligament surgery, therefore, consists principally of fixing avulsed ligament structures and reconstructing midsubstance cruciate ligament disruptions. Technical aspects of surgery that will be discussed below are graft selection, placement, prefixation tensioning, and fixation.

GRAFT SELECTION

Ligaments have been reconstructed with biological tissues (autograft, xenograft, and allograft), synthetic material, and a combination of biological tissue and synthetic material (3,11). The structural properties of the human ACL and ligament graft tissues are the subject of Chapter 13. Experience with material other than

D. M. Daniel: Department of Orthopedic Surgery, University of California, San Diego, School of Medicine, La Jolla, California 92037; and Kaiser Permanente Medical Center, San Diego, California 92120.

autograft tissue is limited at this time and should be considered as experimental.

The most frequently used autograft tissues are the semitendinosus tendon, a portion of the patellar tendon and a portion of the distal iliotibial tract. Factors to consider in selecting an autograft are (a) the structural properties of the graft tissue (Chapter 13), (b) graft fixation, (c) fixation site healing, and (d) the graft site morbidity (Chapter 28). Following graft implantation, there is a considerable loss of graft strength (Chapter 21). Therefore, it is desirable to begin with a graft stronger than the tissue to be replaced. The patellar tendon graft is a strong structure with attached bone which allows optimum fixation. However, harvest of the middle third of the patellar tendon results in a higher incidence of anterior knee pain, flexion contracture, and extensor weakness than does harvest of a hamstring tendon (Table 28-3). I prefer to use the middle third of the patellar tendon when graft strength is the priority issue (Chapter 3, Case 1) and to use a hamstring tendon graft when there is greater concern about surgical morbidity (Chapter 3, Case 3).

Patellar Tendon Graft Harvest

An anterior medial incision is placed so that both the patellar and tibial bone blocks can be obtained and so that the tibial bone tunnel for graft passage can be drilled. The prepatellar retinaculum and epitenon are incised along the medial side of the patellar tendon and dissected across the front of the patella from medial to lateral (30). The patellar tendon width is measured. The middle one-third of the tendon or a 10-mm-wide strip, whichever is least, is harvested with attached patella and tibial bone (Fig. 2-1). The bone ends of the graft are then contoured so that the patellar end will pass snugly through a 9-mm tunnel and so that the tibial end will pass snugly through a 10-mm tunnel (Fig. 2-2). A No. 5 mersiline suture is passed through the bone tunnels (Fig. 2-3). The suture–graft complex is placed under tension for 10 min to set and stretch the sutures (Fig. 2-4). The graft is covered with a saline-soaked sponge to protect it from drying.

Hamstring Tendon Graft Harvest

A transverse incision is made in the crural fascia at the inferior border of the pes anserinus near the tibial insertion. The most inferior structure, the semitendinosus tendon, is identified and elevated sharply off the tibia. The fascial bands from the tendon which blend with the crural fascia are incised. The tibial end is then passed through a tendon stripper, and, while firmly pulling the tendon distally, the stripper is slid proximally to sever the tendon's connection to the muscle belly. A strip of tendon 22–30 cm in length is harvested. The tendon is cleaned of attached muscle fibers. A No. 2 mersiline suture is then placed in each end of the tendon using the technique described by Krackow (Fig. 2-19) (16,17).

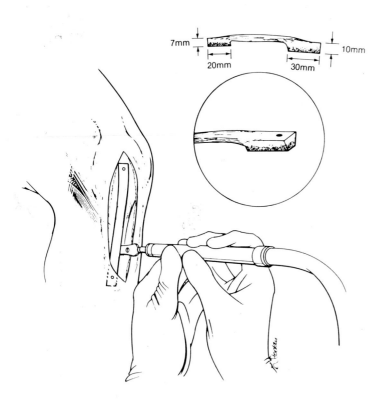

FIG. 2-1. Harvest of the middle one-third of the patellar tendon. The bone is harvested with a fine oscillating saw and delivered with a curved 6-mm osteotome. The Micro Aire 12-mm-wide short blade is used for the longitudinal bone cuts, and the 4-mm-wide blade is used for the horizontal cuts (Micro Aire, Valencia, California). The patellar bone harvested measures 20 × 9 × 7 mm, and the tibial bone measures 30 × 10 × 10 mm. Prior to removing the bone from its bed, 2-mm drill holes are placed in each bone plug. To facilitate passing the bone plug, the drill hole is placed 5 mm from the proximal end of the patellar block and 5–10 mm from the distal end of the tibial bone block.

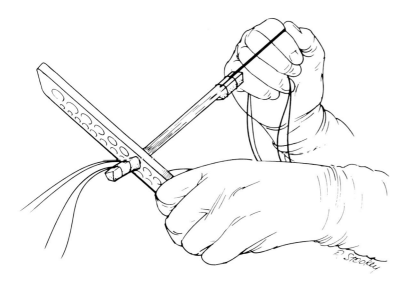

FIG. 2-2. Graft diameter is evaluated. In this figure, two sutures have been placed in each bone block in preparation to fix the graft with suture.

GRAFT PLACEMENT

ACL Graft Placement

Reconstruction of the cruciate ligaments consists of replacing a complex ligamentous structure with a cord of tissue or a prosthetic device. Within each of the

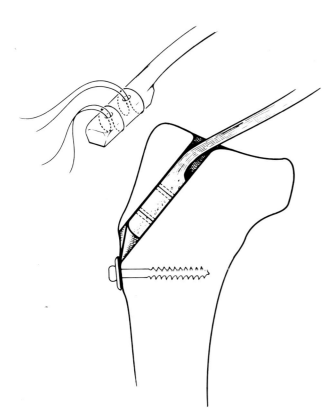

FIG. 2-3. Suture fixation of the graft with No. 5 mersiline suture (Ethicon, Summerville, New Jersey) using a grasping stitch placed through two bone holes and tied around a screw to fix the graft.

cruciate ligaments and within the MCL, there is a hypothetical neutral fiber that remains at constant length with passive knee motion (Chapter 10). The optimal graft placement is probably to center the graft at the attachment sites of this hypothetical fiber in order to minimize the length change of the fibers anterior and posterior to the neutral fiber (Fig. 2-5).

The surgical technique for achieving optimum graft placement is to select tibial and femoral attachment sites and then measure the length change between these attachment sites as the knee is passed through a range of motion. If flexion of the joint results in increasing length between attachment sites, then the course of the graft is anterior to the axis of joint rotation. If the distance between attachment sites decreases with joint flexion, then the course of the graft is posterior to the axis of rotation (Chapter 10). The proposed attachment sites should be adjusted until an acceptable site is identified. Movement of either tibial or femoral site will affect the distance measurements. Let us first consider the condition of moving the femoral site of attachment while maintaining the tibial site in the neutral position. The placement of the femoral tunnel is related to a coordinate system centered at the isometric point on the femur (Fig. 2-6). In this discussion, movement parallel to the roof of the intercondylar notch will be referred to as "anterior–posterior movement," and movement at a right angle to the roof will be called "superior–inferior movement." Moving the femoral attachment site posteriorly results in decreasing distance between attachment sites as the knee flexes. Placing the graft in the over-the-top position results in a decreasing distance between attachment sites in all studies reported (13,27,29). Moving the femoral attachment site anteriorly increases the distance between attachment sites as the knee is flexed (Table 2-1). Moving the femoral hole inferiorly, like moving

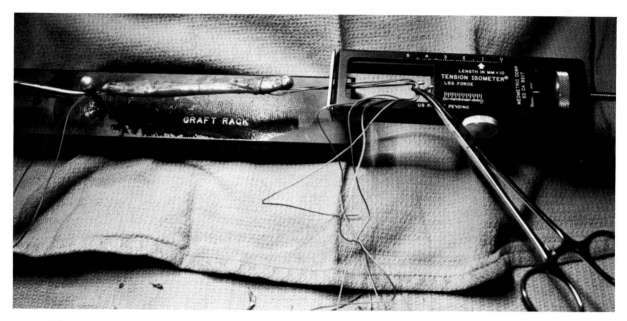

FIG. 2-4. Preloading the graft–suture complex (Graft Rack, MEDmetric Corporation, San Diego). The complex is loaded for 10 min. In practice, covering the graft with a saline-soaked sponge during the preloading period protects it from drying.

the femoral hole posteriorly, will result in shortening of the distance between attachment sites as the knee flexes. Exercises with a four-bar linkage model will assist the clinician in understanding the effect of tunnel placement on distance change between attachment sites with range of motion (Fig. 2-7). Figure 10-25 summarizes the effects of femoral hole placement on attachment site distance change with flexion. Movement of the tibial insertion site has less effect on distance change between attachment sites with range of motion

than does movement of the femoral attachment site because the tibial attachment site is farther from the joint axis of rotation.

In vitro studies by Penner (29) and Hoogland (13) revealed that when the femoral placement was in the over-the-top position, anterior movement of the tibial hole *decreased* the negative distance change with knee flexion, whereas posterior movement of the tibial hole *increased* the negative distance change. The surgeon must be aware, however, that anterior placement of

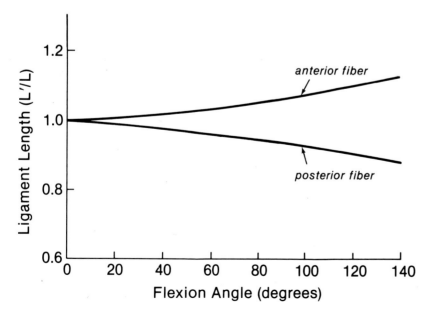

FIG. 2-5. Distance change between attachment sites of the anterior and posterior fibers of a graft 6 mm in diameter, the central fiber of which is at the isometric point. Calculated with a computer four-bar linkage model (Chapter 10).

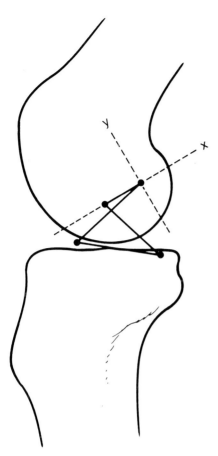

FIG. 2-6. The placement of the femoral hole is related to a coordinate system centered at the isometric point on the femur. The *x* axis passes through the isometric points of the posterior and anterior cruciate ligament insertions on the femur. The *y* axis passes through the ACL femoral isometric point at a right angle to the *x* axis. Bradley (4), studying four specimens, reported that the angle between the roof of the intercondylar notch and this line ranged from 5° to 10°. For practical purposes, the plane of the roof of the intercondylar notch can be considered to be parallel to the *x* axis and can be used to reference the movement of the femoral placement site. On lateral radiographs, the roof of the intercondylar notch is represented by Blumensaat's line. Anderson (1) reported that the mean angle between Blumensaat's line and the femoral shaft is 37°.

the tibial hole may result in graft impingement on the anterior portal of the intercondylar notch with knee extension. Penner (29) evaluated the surgical technique of modifying the over-the-top orientation by making an estimated 5-mm-deep posterior bone trough, thus bringing the femoral graft closer to the neutral site. The modified over-the-top position produced a mean 1.4-mm decrease in attachment site distance as the knee was flexed from 0° to 90° (seven specimens were studied).

Bone tunnels should be oriented and fashioned to minimize graft stress risers. Direction changes as a graft leaves a bone tunnel results in graft stress risers.

On the lateral aspect of the femur, the tunnel should be placed anterior to the intramuscular septum at the level of the lateral superior genicular artery to minimize direction change as the graft leaves the tunnel (Fig. 2-8). The tibial tunnel should begin 1–2 cm medial to the medial edge of the patellar tendon and at the superior edge of the pes anserinus insertion.

The ACL splays out as it inserts on the tibia (Fig. 4-22A). Therefore, anatomic reconstruction is not possible. To improve the mechanical advantage of the ACL graft to resist anterior tibial displacement, O'Brien (25) recommends placement of the guide pin for the anterior tibial tunnel 5 mm anterior to the anterior medial fibers of the ACL. A graft placed in this position will result in impingement of the graft as the knee goes into extension as demonstrated by O'Brien (25) in cadaveric studies. The authors, therefore, recommend that when the anterior placement site is used, the anterior portal of the intercondylar notch be enlarged, especially superiorly, to prevent impingement with terminal knee extension (Fig. 2-9). Yaru (33) studied the relationship between tibial graft placement and anterior portal impingement of a ligament graft as the knee goes into extension. The author demonstrated that anterior displacement of the tibia resulting from the anterior force of the patellar tendon pulling the knee into extension results in greater anterior graft impingement than does passive extension. Placement of a tibial pilot hole in the anterior medial fibers of the ACL (Fig. 2-10, site 4), about 6 mm anterior to the medial spine mated with a femoral pilot hole placement 3 mm anterior to the over-the-top position, results in 2–4 mm of decreasing length as the knee is flexed from 0° to 90°. When the pilot hole is enlarged to a 10-mm tunnel, this will result in near-isometric placement and little need for an anterior–superior notchplasty. My recommendations for two-tunnel ACL graft placement are listed below. These recommendations have evolved from those published in 1988 (7).

1. Place a pilot hole with a 2- to 4-mm pin or drill in the anterior medial fibers of the normal ACL (Fig. 2-10, site 4). If there is no anterior cruciate stump, the anterior insertion of the medial and lateral menisci and the medial intercondylar tubercle may serve to orient the guide pin placement.
2. Place a pilot hole at the junction of the roof and lateral wall of the intercondylar notch, 3 mm anterior to the over-the-top position.
3. Push a No. 5 braided suture down the femoral hole with a suture pusher (Synthes, Limited [USA], Wayne, Pennsylvania). A Hewson suture retriever (Richards Medical Company, Memphis, Tennessee) is passed through the tibial hole. The suture is passed through the femoral hole and grasped with an instrument that has been passed through

TABLE 2-1. *The change in length between the tibial and femoral anterior cruciate ligament graft sites with knee motion—in vitro studies*

Author	Range of motion	Orientation[a] Tibia	Orientation[a] Femur	Specimen number	Mean length change[b]
Odensten (27)[c]	0–135	N	N	10	0
Hoogland (13)[d]	0–130	N	N	4	−3 mm
Odensten	0–135	N	P	10	−10 mm
Hoogland	0–130	N	P	4	−8 mm
Penner (29)[e]	0–90	N	P	17	−4.5 mm
Odensten	0–135	N	A	10	+7 mm
Hoogland	0–130	N	A	4	+10 mm
Penner	0–90	N	A	8	+5.7 mm
Odensten	0–135	A	N	10	+5 mm
Hoogland	0–130	A	N	4	+3 mm
Odensten	0–135	P	N	10	−9 mm
Hoogland	0–130	P	N	4	−4 mm

[a] N denotes insertion neutral position (geographic center of the normal ligament attachment); P denotes posterior position, estimated to be 10–15 mm posterior to the neutral position; and A denotes anterior position, estimated to be 10–15 mm anterior to the neutral position. In Hoogland's study, the anterior data reported here was measured with the cable passed over the front of the tibia.
[b] A plus sign (+) denotes that the attachment-site distance increases with knee flexion, and a minus sign (−) denotes that the attachment-site distance decreases with knee flexion.
[c] Odensten did not apply a load to the measuring thread.
[d] Hoogland applied a 5-kg load to the measuring thread.
[e] Penner maintained constant tension on the tibial end of the polypropylene braid with a load cell.

the loop of the suture retriever. The suture is then pulled through the suture retriever and out through the tibial hole.

4. Clamp the suture with a hemostat as it exits the femoral hole. Attach the suture exiting the tibial hole to a measuring device. Measurement with the MEDmetric Tension/Isometer is illustrated in Fig. 2-11. The femoral holes should be adjusted until an acceptable position is obtained.

5. A guide pin is then placed in the femoral pilot hole, and a cannulated reamer is used to drill a tunnel 1 mm larger than the graft that will be passed into the femoral tunnel. A guide pin is placed in the tibial pilot hole, and a cannulated reamer is used to drill a tunnel that will allow passage of the fem-

oral end of the graft. The diameter of the reamer is the same as that of the tibial end of the graft.

6. A trial graft of dimensions similar to those of the biologic graft is passed, and isometry measurements are repeated (Fig. 2-12). If the distance between attachment sites decreases more than 3 mm as the knee is flexed from 0° to 90°, the intercondylar mouth of the femoral tunnel is enlarged anteriorly to allow the graft to move anteriorly. The isometry measurements are then repeated. If the distance between attachment sites increases more than 3 mm as the knee is flexed from 0° to 140° the femoral attachment site must be changed. The surgeon's choices are to go to an over-the-top graft orientation or to enlarge the femoral tunnel pos-

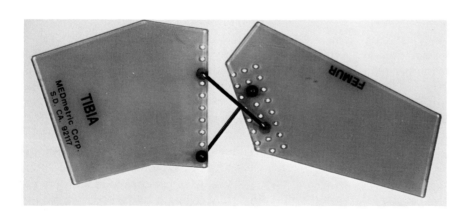

FIG. 2-7. Four-bar linkage model (MEDmetric Corporation, San Diego, California).

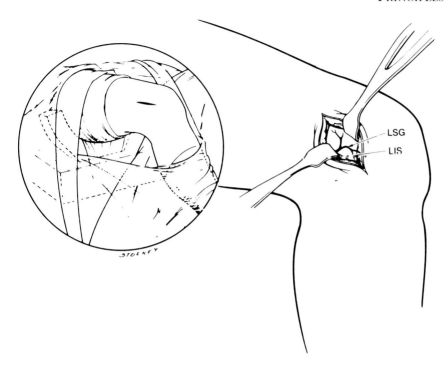

FIG. 2-8. The femoral drill hole begins on the lateral cortex anterior to the intramuscular septum (LIS) at the level of the lateral superior genicular (LSG) artery. Surgery is done with the surgeon sitting and the leg bent over the end of the table. The thigh is supported with a Surgi-assist limb support (MEDmetric Corporation, San Diego, California).

teriorly and place a bone graft taken from the lateral aspect of the femur on the anterior wall of the femoral tunnel.

7. A looped suture is passed through the femoral tunnel and out through the tibial tunnel. The graft is pulled up through the tibial tunnel and into the femoral tunnel.

Arthroscopically assisted cruciate graft implantation may decrease the surgical morbidity. For example, when using a semitendinosus graft to reconstruct the

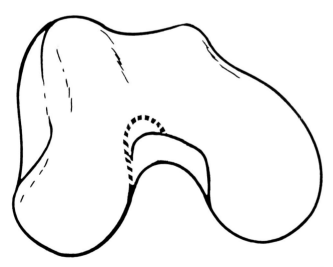

FIG. 2-9. Five to 10 mm of bone may need to be removed superolaterally to prevent graft impingement with knee extension if the graft is passed through an anterior tibial tunnel (Fig. 2-10, sites 1, 2, 3, and 5).

ACL, the joint trauma is reduced if the bone tunnels and graft passage are performed under arthroscopic observation as opposed to performing an arthrotomy. In contrast, when using a middle-third patellar tendon graft, there is little difference in joint morbidity between arthroscopically assisted graft placement and operating through the patellar tendon defect with the aid of a head lamp for intercondylar notch illumination (Fig. 2-13).

When performing a patellar tendon ACL reconstruction, I prefer to make the bone tunnels and pass the graft under arthroscopic control. Arthroscopic visualization of the femoral tunnel site is superior to visualization via an arthrotomy. To obtain adequate visualization of the intercondylar notch, soft tissue from the lateral side of the notch must be removed. Arthroscopically, this is achieved with a 5.5-mm motorized full-radius resector. Widening of the intercondylar notch 2–4 mm to obtain adequate exposure of the femoral tunnel site is frequently necessary. Arthroscopically, this is done by cutting through the hyaline cartilage and scoring the lateral femoral condyle with the use of a 6-mm osteotome. A grasper is used to remove bone fragments. The task is completed with the use of a motorized burr. After the graft is passed, the anterior fat pad is incised and the joint is directly visualized through the patellar tendon defect to evaluate graft impingement. Impingement on the roof of the anterior portal of the intercondylar notch is evaluated with the knee in full extension. A superior notchplasty is frequently necessary to relieve terminal extension impingement (Fig. 2-9).

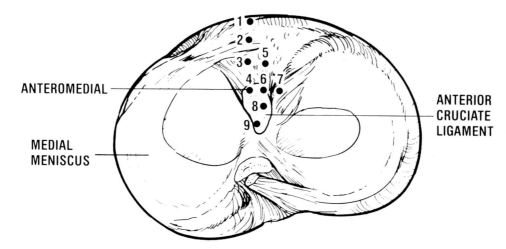

FIG. 2-10. Grafts placed through a tunnel at sites 1, 2, 3, 5, 6, and 7 resulted in graft impingement when the knee was extended. Sites 8 and 9 resulted in an increase in the distance between attachments sites as the knee was extended. Position 4 minimized the distance change between attachment sites with range of motion and did not result in graft impingement (32).

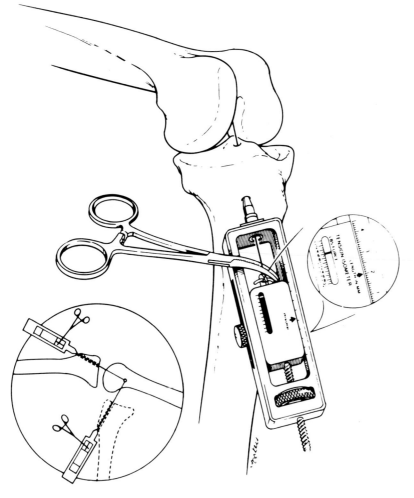

FIG. 2-11. The distance change between bone pilot holes with range of motion measured with the Tension/Isometer (MEDmetric Corporation, San Diego, California). A 4-lb force is applied, and the knee is ranged five times. With the knee in 90° of flexion, the force is again adjusted to 4 lb and the length scale is read. The knee is extended, the force scale is adjusted to 4 lb, and the length scale is read. The length change is calculated. Decisions are based on length changes with the knee flexion from 0° to 90°. The desired change is a decreased distance between the pilot holes of 2–3 mm as the knee is ranged from 0° to 90°. An increase in length should not be accepted.

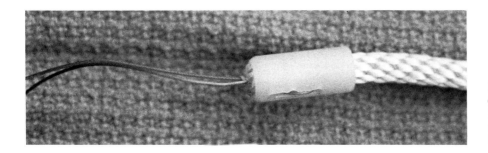

FIG. 2-12. Trial graft. A plastic tip on the tibial end minimizes friction in the tibia tunnel. (Courtesy of the MEDmetric Corporation, San Diego, California.)

PCL Graft Placement

After harvesting the middle one-third of the patellar tendon, the anterior aspect of the joint is visualized through the patellar tendon defect (Fig. 2-13). The posterior aspect of the joint is visualized through a 6-cm posterior medial incision entering the joint along the posterior edge of the posterior oblique ligament. Partial elevation of the capsule off the femur improves the posterior exposure. Through this exposure, the PCL stump can be visualized and the insertion site of the posterior cruciate ligament on the tibia can be palpated. A broad elevator may be placed to protect the posterior structures. A 2- to 4-mm pilot hole is placed from the anteromedial tibial surface along the superior edge of the pes anserinus insertion to the normal PCL

insertion site on the posterior surface of the tibia. This hole is then enlarged with a cannulated drill to accommodate the graft. A 10-cm incision is then made along the medial and inferior insertion of the vastus medialis. The vastus medialis is elevated to expose the medial side of the femur just superior to the synovial capsule. A 2- to 4-mm pilot hole is made through the medial side of the femur to enter the intercondylar notch just anterior and superior to the normal center of the PCL insertion. A No. 5 braided suture is then passed through the pilot holes. It is clamped on the front of the tibia, and the tension isometer is placed in the femoral hole. While supporting the tibia forward against the intact ACL, the knee is passed through a range of motion. Increasing distance between the tunnels with knee flexion indicates that the pilot hole is placed too

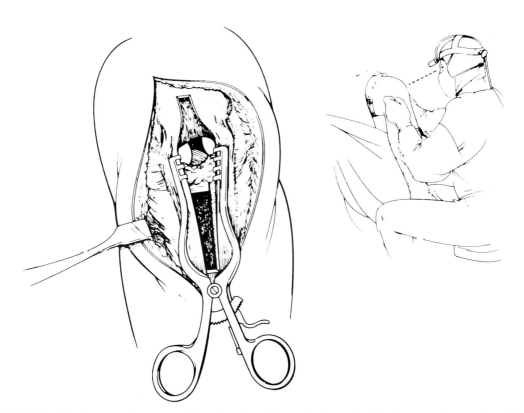

FIG. 2-13. The intercondylar notch is visualized through the defect in the patellar tendon. The patient's thigh is supported in a leg holder, and the knee is bent over the end of the table. The surgeon sits. The wound is illuminated with the use of a head lamp.

far anteriorly. If the distance between the tunnels decreases with knee flexion, this indicates that the femoral pilot hole is too far posterior. The femoral hole is adjusted until there is 1–3 mm of lengthening as the knee is flexed past 90°. The tunnels are then enlarged with a cannulated drill to accommodate the graft. The graft is pulled through the tibial tunnel and then into the femoral tunnel with the aid of a ligament graft passer (DePuy, Warsaw, Indiana).

GRAFT TENSIONING

Many authors have alluded to the need to apply some tension on the graft at the time of the graft fixation (10,14,15,24). Tension may be applied to precondition (a) the tissue (Chapter 13), (b) the prosthetic device (22), (c) the graft–suture interface (6), or (d) tissues of the knee that interface with the graft (22). The relationship between the tension applied and the joint stability will be dependent on the length of the graft and the graft stiffness. Burks (5) studied the relationship between prefixation graft load and anterior–posterior (A–P) tibial motion. In each of 10 human cadaveric specimens, he performed an ACL reconstruction with a patellar tendon bone–tendon–bone graft 10 mm in width, a double semitendinosus graft, and a 3-cm-wide band of the iliotibial tract. The graft was passed through tibial and femoral tunnels and fixed on the lateral aspect of the femur. A tensioning device was mounted on the tibia to ensure that the tibia was stabilized against the posterior restraining structures at the time of graft tensioning. The graft was loaded at the time of fixation to restore the specimen's normal A–P displacement. To restore the knee's cruciate intact A–P displacement, the mean graft load was: patellar tendon 16 N (3.6 lb), semitendinosus 38 N (8.5 lb) and iliotibial band 61 N (13.6 lb). Data from a single knee are presented in Fig. 2-14. The optimum prefixation graft tension has not been studied in the clinical setting. The graft tension decreases within minutes by stress relaxation (Chapter 13). Yoshiya (34) reported decreased vascularization of the graft when higher graft loads were applied at time of tensioning, 39 N versus 1 N in a dog model.

The MEDmetric Tension/Isometer (TI) may be used to tension the graft at time of fixation. The force is applied either through the TI mounted on the tibia (as illustrated in Fig. 2-15) or by pulling manually through the TI. The knee is placed at the flexion angle where there is the greatest distance between graft attachment sites. I have used a 22.5-N force for the patellar tendon graft and a 45-N force for the hamstring graft. After the wound is closed, a sterile adhesive drape is placed over the wound and then KT-1000 arthrometer measurements are performed (Fig. 2-16). The 89-N anterior

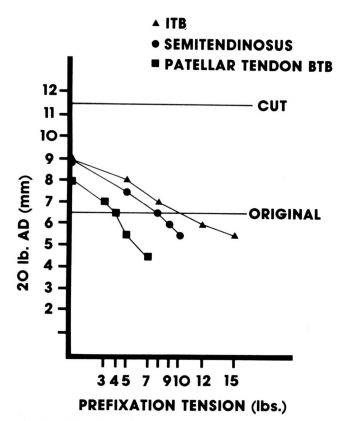

FIG. 2-14. Graft tension at the time of fixation versus the KT-1000 20-lb anterior displacement measurement in a single cadaveric knee (5).

displacement (injured knee minus normal knee) should be less than 3 mm. If this has not been accomplished, the limb is prepped, the graft exposed, the fixation evaluated, and the graft retensioned and fixed. At the San Diego Kaiser Hospital, retensioning has been required in five cases during the last 100 ACL reconstructions.

GRAFT FIXATION

Soft Tissue Fixation

Most graft failures occur during the first 6 months after surgery, many within 3 months of surgery (Chapter 29). The weak link in the repaired or reconstructed knee in the early postoperative period is the point of ligament or graft fixation. It behooves the surgeon to strive for maximum fixation strength, especially if the rehabilitation program includes an early motion program. Autograft strengths are in the order of 1000–2000 N (Chapter 13), whereas time-zero strength of fixation is 50–500 N. In a study of graft failure in a goat model, Holden (12) fixed fascia lata grafts with a staple or a reinforced bushing. Load-to-failure tests of the femur–graft–tibia unit at time zero revealed that 11 of 12 spec-

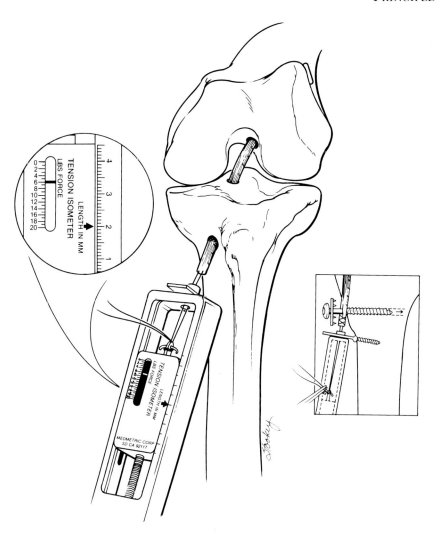

FIG. 2-15. Graft tensioning with the MEDmetric Tension/Isometer.

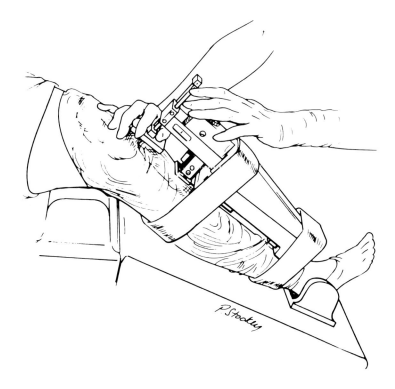

FIG. 2-16. After wound closure an adhesive drape is placed on the leg; displacement measurements are then performed with the KT-1000 arthrometer.

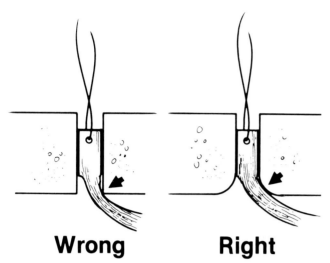

FIG. 2-17. The entrance into bone tunnels should be rounded to reduce graft impingement.

imens failed at the fixation site. Fixation site failure 2 weeks after surgery was 7 of 11, 4 weeks after surgery it was 4 of 13, and 8 weeks after surgery it was 0 of 13. Seventeen of the 26 nonfixation site failures occurred at the graft intraarticular exit of the tibial hole. This emphasizes the importance of tunnel orientation and of chamfering the tunnel entrance into the joint (Fig. 2-17). The angle change between the tunnel and intraarticular graft orientation with range of motion can be seen in Fig. 10-6.

Numerous studies on the soft-tissue-to-soft-tissue suturing technique are reported in the hand literature (20,21,28,32). Techniques studied that are applicable to ligament repair are shown in Figs. 2-18 and 2-19. Using a flexor tendon model in dogs, Urbaniak (32) found that the Bunnel and the Kessler suture techniques had similar initial strengths (39 N). The authors

performed an *in vivo* study of the Kessler and Bunnel suture techniques to compare the strengths during healing. The "grasping" suture of Kessler provided the strongest repair. At 5 days post-repair, the Kessler-repaired tendon strength was 18 N whereas the Bunnel-technique tendon strength was 6 N. The strength of all repairs reached a minimum between 3 and 12 days after surgery. Krackow (16,17) described a locking stitch using a single loop of No. 5 Ethibond (Fig. 2-19). He reported that the strength was 223 N. The author evaluated fixation techniques using glutaraldehyde-treated bovine knee collateral ligament specimens. The specimen preparations were cyclically loaded three times, to an upper limit of 50 N. This sequence was repeated, increasing the upper limit in 50-N increments, until failure. A summary of his work is presented in Fig. 2-20. The fixation of soft tissue with suture results in the graft pulling away from the fixation site when cyclical loading is applied. The suture elongates and then sinks into the soft tissue, and the suture knots tighten. Figure 2-21 demonstrates the elongation resulting from a biologic graft sutured to a synthetic graft when the biologic graft is fixed at one end and the synthetic graft is sutured to its other end.

Robertson (31) performed a series of studies using cadaveric tissue to compare the holding power of soft tissue by sutures, staples, and a screw with a plastic spiked washer or a screw with a metallic soft tissue plate (Table 2-2). The screw with spiked soft tissue washer or soft tissue fixation plate had the greatest holding power (Fig. 2-22). In describing the advantages of the toothed washer for soft tissue fixation, Müller (23) stated that the peripheral arrangement of the teeth firmly grasp the ligament over a broad area, and because of the design of the teeth and spacing of the teeth, the microcirculation to the tissue was not greatly altered. *In vivo* studies of ligament fixation to compare

A. Bunnell

C. Double Weave

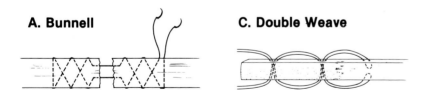

B. Kessler

D. Double Loop

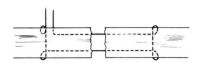

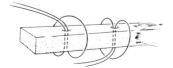

FIG. 2-18. A,B: Suture techniques in tendon tissue. **C,D:** Suture techniques in the bone attached to a patellar tendon graft (From ref. 31.)

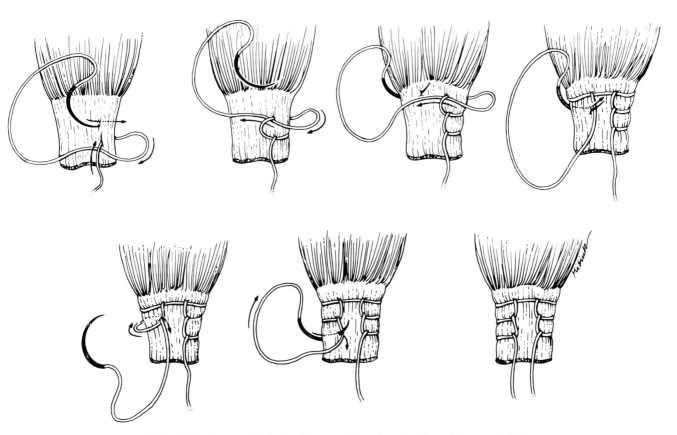

FIG. 2-19. A new stitch for ligament–tendon fixation. (From ref. 16.)

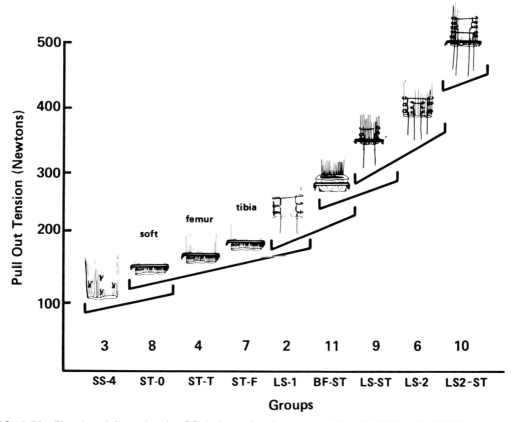

FIG. 2-20. Fixation failure loads. SS-4, four simple sutures (No. 5 Ethibond); ST-O, staple osteoporotic bone; ST-T, staple fixation tibia; ST-F, staple fixation femur; LS-1, single locking stitch; BF-ST, staple fixation over a cortical flap; LS-ST, single locking ligament suture plus staple; LS-2, two locking ligament sutures; LS2-ST, two locking ligament sutures plus staple. (From ref. 16.)

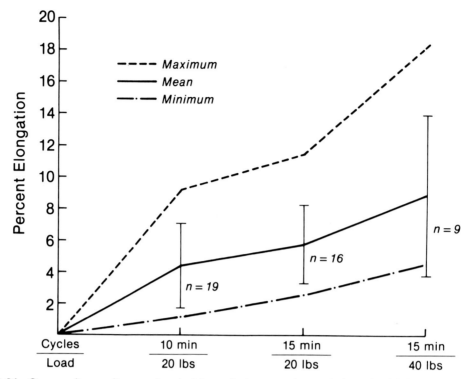

FIG. 2-21. Composite grafts constructed by suturing a polyprophylene braid (LAD, 3M Corporation, St. Paul, Minnesota) to one of five biological grafts (patellar tendon–bone, prepatellar retinaculum, semitendinosus tendon, gracilis tendon, and iliotibial band). The biologic tissue was anatomically attached or fixed distally with an AO screw and washer. The augmentation device was then sutured to the graft tissue and secured proximally to a hook attached to the load frame. The tests studied the device–suture–graft interface. Testing conditions consisted of preconditioning the grafts to 45 N (10 lb), 89 N, and then 45 N (each a single cycle) and then cycling the composite at 8 cycles/min. The elongations were measured at peak loads, and the failure cycle number and failure site were recorded. Preconditioning the composite grafts produced a 0–4% residual elongation. Forty cycles of loading to 89 N produced another 1–6% increase in elongation. Loading to higher peak forces produced further increases in elongation. (Investigation performed in UCSD laboratories by D. Penner, D. Flood, C. L. Van Kampen, S. May, and D. M. Daniel with funding from the 3M Corporation.)

TABLE 2-2. In vitro testing of soft tissue fixation[a]

	Mean failure load (newtons) Tissue type[b]		
	A	B	C
Screw			
Washer	211	180	225
Plate	266	238	202
Staple			
Stone	121	22	40
Barbed	76	13	81
Suture	99	72	202[c]

[a] From ref. 8.

[b] Type A tissue: Broad and thin. Medial and lateral capsule, medial ligament, and iliotibial track. Type B tissue: Narrow and cord. Lateral collateral ligament and hamstring tendons. Type C tissue: Thick. Quadriceps tendon and patellar tendon structures.

[c] Sutures passed through attached bone.

the use of barbed staples to the spiked washer and spiked fixation plate was reported in 1987 (8). The animals were sacrificed 6 weeks after surgery. Tissue under the staples appeared necrotic, whereas tissue under the spiked washers and plates appeared viable. Ligaments fixed with staples failed at a lower load than did those fixed with the soft tissue plate or the plastic washer (Table 2-3).

My choice for fixation of a semitendinosus graft ACL reconstruction is to use a screw with spiked soft tissue washer on both ends as demonstrated in Fig. 2-23. The graft must usually be greater than 25 cm in length to allow doubling of the graft and obtain screw fixation in strong tissue at both ends. If the graft is shorter, fixation with suture is used at one end.

In multiple-ligament injuries, I repair collateral ligaments or capsular structures back to their anatomic insertion with screws and soft tissue washers. After each structure is repaired, the knee is ranged from 0°

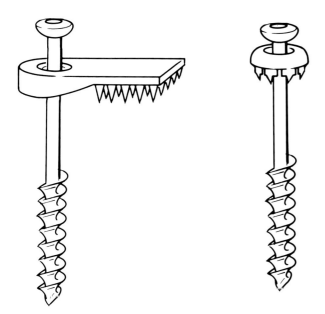

FIG. 2-22. Spiked washer and soft tissue fixation plate (Synthes, Limited [USA], Wayne, Pennsylvania).

to 120° of flexion to confirm proper tensioning and positioning of the repaired structure. If the tissue pulls out, it was inappropriately placed, tensioned, or fixed. Midsubstance tears are not repaired to bone. Shortening of ligament structures will result in a limitation of joint motion.

Patellar Tendon Graft Fixation

Patellar tendon with attached tibial tubercle and patellar bone are often used as an ACL graft. Robertson (31) evaluated securing patellar tendon with attached bone to a fixation post with suture. Techniques shown in Fig. 2-18C and D were utilized. The mean load to failure in 16 tests was 202 N (Table 2-2). In each preparation, care was taken to tie the knots down firmly with several square knots; nevertheless, the knots tightened down further and the sutures pressed into the tissue when cyclic loading was applied. The graft then pulled 2–4 mm away from the fixation site. Prefixation con-

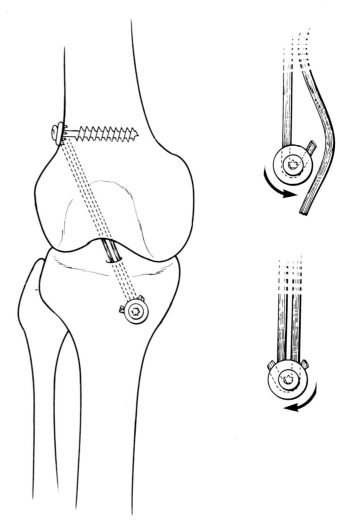

FIG. 2-23. ACL reconstructed with double semitendinosus graft fixed with screw and spiked washer at both ends.

ditioning of the graft with the graft rack can decrease the graft complex elongation after fixation (Fig. 2-4). In practice, the orientation of the fixation post screw is also a consideration (Fig. 2-24).

Lambert (19) reported use of an interference fit screw technique whereby the bone attached to patellar tendon graft source is pulled into the bone tunnel and secured with a 6.5-mm cancellous screw. The screw engages both the wall of the tunnel and the bone plug of the graft (Fig. 2-25). Kurosaka (18) evaluated the pull-out strength of the interface friction technique as well as other techniques. The grafts were fixed, the femur and tibia were secured at an angle of 45° of knee flexion, and the tensile test was performed with the tibia pulled parallel to the long axis of the femur. Tensile tests were performed at a speed of 30 mm/sec. The harvested bone was 25 mm in length, 10 mm in width, and 4 mm in depth. After careful bone trimming, the grafts were passed through 9.5-mm bone tunnels and

TABLE 2-3. *Canine MCL study[a]*

Fixation device	N	Failure load (newtons)[b]
Normal knee	2	694 ± 18
Ligament cut		
No fixation	6	283 ± 6
Washer	6	327 ± 32
Plate	5	292 ± 50
Staple	5	176 ± 23

[a] Animals were sacrificed 6 weeks after surgery. From ref. 8.
[b] Mean ± standard error.

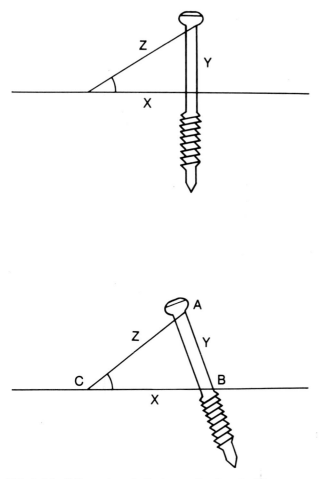

FIG. 2-24. If the suture is tied near the head of the screw, the fixation tension of the suture may be altered as the screw is inserted. It is best to tie the suture around the base of the screw (9).

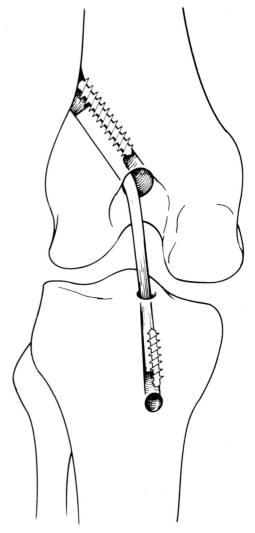

FIG. 2-25. Interference screw fixation technique using the Kurosaka screw design (DePuy, Warsaw, Indiana).

secured with a 6.5-mm AO screw. Placing a bone block with a cross-sectional area of 4 × 9.5 mm bone would leave a gap of 2–5 mm between the bone plug and the bone tunnel wall. Studies with tissue from seven human cadavers, mean age of 58.6 years, revealed significantly lower pull-out strength than did studies from three human cadaver knees with a mean age of 20.3. The pull-out strength was also increased when a larger screw size was used to better fill the gap between the bone tunnel and bone plug. Mean load-to-failure data from studies by Robertson (31) and Kurosaka (17) are presented in Fig. 2-26.

The strength of the interference screw technique is dependent on the bone quality, the compression of the bone plug in the tunnel, the length of screw-thread–bone contact, and the direction of the ligament forces. As demonstrated by Kurosaka (18), the better the bone quality and the greater the bone compression, the stronger the fixation. To provide the optimum fixation with an interface friction screw, the gap between the wall and the tunnel must be mated with the screw size.

Studies in our laboratory with pig bone reveal patellar tendon graft fixation strengths of 300–600 N. These are achieved with the interface friction technique when the screw is placed on the cortical side of the bone plug and when the outer diameter of the screw is 4 mm greater than the gap between the bone plug and the tunnel. In surgery, I use a gap gauge to measure the bone-plug–tunnel gap (Fig. 2-27), and then the fixation is selected so that the screw diameter minus the gap distance is 4–6 mm (Fig. 2-28). When inserting the screw, care is taken not to deflect the screw away from the bone plug into the metaphyseal bone (2). The screw should extend beyond all drill holes made in the bone but not beyond the end of the bone block, where it might abrade or incise the graft.

CONCLUSION

Ligament repair, graft harvest, placement, tensioning, and fixation are the tasks of ligament surgery; these

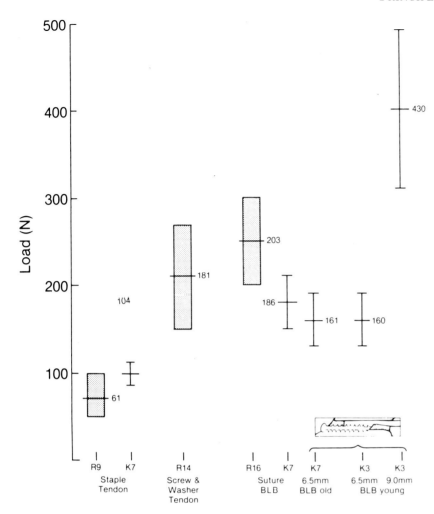

FIG. 2-26. *In vitro* studies of failure loads of graft fixation. R denotes Robertson study (31); K denotes Kurosaka study (17); BLB denotes bone–ligament–bone. Number after the author letter indicates the number of specimens studied (e.g., R9 indicates nine specimens studied).

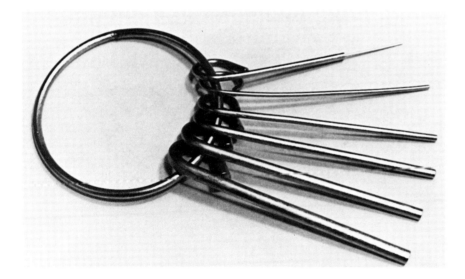

FIG. 2-27. Gap gauges (MEDmetric Corporation, San Diego, California).

BONE PLUG FIT

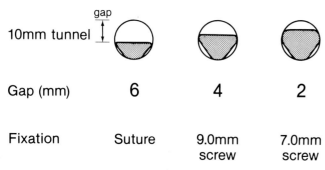

	gap		
10mm tunnel			
Gap (mm)	6	4	2
Fixation	Suture	9.0mm screw	7.0mm screw

FIG. 2-28. Fixation of a patellar tendon bone–tendon–bone ACL graft.

are the elements of the patient's care that the surgeon can best control. We can learn a great deal about the healing of biologic tissues from animal models. However, in the final analysis, the results of surgical procedures must be demonstrated on patients. Advancement of the field is dependent on careful documentation of the surgical procedure and the preoperative and postoperative knee evaluation.

The techniques and approaches presented in this chapter are based on *in vivo* and *in vitro* studies as well as clinical practice. My philosophical approach has changed little over the past decade, but with the use of newer instrumentation, the precision of graft harvest, placement, and fixation has improved. The surgical results presented in Chapters 3, 24, and 29 do not represent the outcome of surgical procedures performed precisely as described in this chapter. The procedures were performed between 1983 and 1988, a period in which these techniques were in evolution.

ACKNOWLEDGMENTS

Support from the following sources is gratefully acknowledged: 3M, St. Paul, Minnesota 55133; Depuy Orthopedics, Warsaw, Indiana 46580; Synthes, Limited [USA], Wayne, Pennsylvania 19087; and MEDmetric Corporation, San Diego, California 92121.

REFERENCES

1. Anderson AF, Lipscomb AB, Liudahl KJ, Addlestone RB. Analysis of the intercondylar notch by computed tomography. *Am J Sports Med* 1987;15:547–552.
2. Bach BR Jr. Potential pitfalls of Kurosaka screw interference fixation for ACL surgery. *Am J Knee Surg* 1989;2:76–82.
3. Balduni FC, Clemow AJT, Lehman RC. *Synthetic ligaments: scaffolds, stents, and prostheses.* Thorofare, NJ: Slack Inc., 1986.
4. Bradley J, FitzPatrick D, Daniel D, Shercliff T, O'Connor J. Orientation of the cruciate ligament in the sagittal plane. *J Bone Joint Surg* 1988;70B:94–99.
5. Burks RT, Leland R. Determination of graft tension before fixation in anterior cruciate ligament reconstruction. *Arthroscopy* 1988;4:260–266.
6. Butler DL. Evaluation of fixation methods in cruciate ligament replacement. *Instr Course Lect* 1987;36:173–178.
7. Daniel DM, Penner DA, Burks RT. Anterior cruciate ligament graft isometry and tensioning. In: Friedman MJ, Ferkel RD, eds. *Prosthetic ligament reconstruction of the knee*, vol. 1. Philadelphia: WB Saunders, 1988;17–21.
8. Daniel DM, Robertson DB, Flood DL, Biden EN. Fixation of soft tissue. In: Jackson DW, Drez D, eds. *The anterior cruciate deficient knee: new concepts in ligament repair.* St. Louis: CV Mosby, 1987;114–126.
9. Drez D. Personal communication.
10. Eriksson E. Reconstruction of the anterior cruciate ligament. *Orthop Clin North Am* 1976;7:167–179.
11. Friedman MJ, Ferkel RD, eds. *Prosthetic ligament reconstruction of the knee*, 1st ed. Philadelphia: WB Saunders, 1988.
12. Holden JP, Grood ES, Butler DL, et al. Biomechanics of fascia lata ligament replacements: early postoperative changes in the goat. *J Orthop Res* 1988;6:639–647.
13. Hoogland T, Hillen B. Intra-articular reconstruction of the anterior cruciate ligament. An experimental study of length changes in different ligament reconstructions. *Clin Orthop* 1984;185:197–202.
14. Insall J, Joseph DM, Aglietti P, Campbell RD Jr. Bone-block iliotibial-band transfer for anterior cruciate insufficiency. *J Bone Joint Surg* 1981;63A:560–569.
15. Jones KG. Reconstruction of the anterior cruciate ligament: a technique using the central one-third of the patellar ligament. *J Bone Joint Surg* 1963;45A:925–932.
16. Krackow KA, Thomas SC, Jones LC. A new stitch for ligament–tendon fixation. *J Bone Joint Surg* 1986;68A:764–766.
17. Krackow KA, Thomas SC, Jones LC. Ligament–tendon fixation: analysis of a new stitch and comparison with standard techniques. *Orthopedics* 1988;11:909–917.
18. Kurosaka M, Yoshiya S, Andrish JT. A biomechanical comparison of different surgical techniques of graft fixation in anterior cruciate ligament reconstruction. *Am J Sports Med* 1987;15:225–229.
19. Lambert KL. Vascularized patella tendon graft with rigid internal fixation for anterior cruciate ligament insufficiency. *Clin Orthop* 1983;172:85–89.
20. Mason ML, Shearon CG. Process of tendon repair: experimental study of tendon suture and tendon graft. *Arch Surg* 1932;25:615–692.
21. Mason ML. Primary and secondary tendon suture: a discussion of the significance of the technique in tendon surgery. *Surg Gynecol Obstet* 1940;70:392–402.
22. More RC, Markolf KL. Measurement of stability of the knee and ligament force after implantation of a synthetic anterior cruciate ligament. *J Bone Joint Surg* 1988;70A:1020–1031.
23. Müller W. *The knee: form, function, and ligament reconstruction*, 1st ed. New York: Springer-Verlag, 1983.
24. Noyes FR, Butler DL, Grood ES, et al. Biomechanical analysis of human ligament grafts used in knee ligament repairs and reconstructions. *J Bone Joint Surg* 1984;66A:344–352.
25. O'Brien WR, Henning CE. Anterior cruciate ligament substitute load versus tibial positioning: an *in vitro* study. Presented at the interim meeting of the AOSSM, San Francisco, California, January 1987.
26. O'Brien WR, Henning CE, Eriksson E. Femoral intercondylar notch impingement on anterior cruciate ligament substitutes. Presented at the 13th Annual Meeting of the AOSSM, Orlando, Florida, June 1987.
27. Odensten M, Gillquist J. Functional anatomy of the anterior cruciate ligament and a rationale for reconstruction. *J Bone Joint Surg* 1985;67A:257–262.
28. Peacock EE Jr. Some technical aspects and results of flexor tendon repair. *Surgery* 1965;58:330–342.
29. Penner DA, Daniel DM, Wood P, Mishra D. An *in vitro* study

of anterior cruciate ligament graft placement and isometry. *Am J Sports Med* 1988;16:238–243.

30. Roberts TS, Drez D Jr, Parker W. Prevention of late patellar fracture in ACL deficient knees reconstructed with bone–patellar tendon–bone autografts: a new technique. *Am J Knee Surg* 1989;2:83–86.

31. Robertson DB, Daniel DM, Biden E. Soft tissue fixation to bone. *Am J Sports Med* 1986;14:398–403.

32. Urbaniak JR, Cahill JD Jr, Mortenson RA. Tendon suturing methods: analysis of tensile strengths. Presented at the Symposium on Tendon Surgery in the Hand, Philadelphia, Pennsylvania, March 1974.

33. Yaru N. Personal communication.

34. Yoshiya S, Andrish JT, Manley MT, Bauer TW. Graft tension in anterior cruciate ligament reconstruction: an *in vivo* study in dogs. *Am J Sports Med* 1987;15:464–470.

CHAPTER 3

Case Studies

Dale M. Daniel and Mary Lou Stone

This chapter presents eight case studies of patients with ligament injuries. The indications for surgical care, rehabilitation regimens and the results of treatment will be discussed. A few notes about data presentation follow.

Knee flexion: Knee flexion is recorded using a convention commonly used in Europe. The flexion range is described with three numbers that denote (a) the beginning flexion, (b) the zero or neutral point, and (c) the maximum flexion. For example, 5/0/145 describes a knee that goes from 5° of hyperextension to 145° of flexion. A knee that lacks 15° of full extension and has 145° of flexion would be described by 0/15/145 (12).

Heel height difference: Injured knee extension relative to normal knee extension can be documented by measuring the heel height difference while the patient lies prone on the examining table with the lower limbs supported by the thighs (Fig. 3-1). One centimeter of heel height difference approximates one degree (Table 3-1).

Displacement measurements: Most displacement measurements are recorded as the injured knee minus normal knee difference ($I - N$). Normal knee data are presented to indicate the normal knee laxity as well as to give the reader an appreciation of the variation between measurements done on serial examinations. The patient's activity prior to examination, the level of relaxation during the examination, the precise placement of the testing instrument, and the direction of applied forces will alter the normal knee measured displacement. On all examinations the normal and injured knee are examined and decisions are made based on the normal knee minus injured knee difference ($N - I$). All follow-up measurements were made by one of the authors (MLS). Acute injury measurements and intraoperative measurements were made by various clinicians.

Thigh circumference: Thigh circumference measurements are made 10 cm proximal to the patella.

Pain and swelling: Pain and swelling are recorded for the activity performed at least 50 hours a year that causes the greatest symptoms. The symptoms are rated as 0 (absent), 1 (mild), 2 (moderate), and 3 (severe).

Giving way: Giving way is recorded as episodes per year. Full giving way is defined as an episode of giving way resulting in the patient falling or developing postevent swelling. Partial giving way is defined as a sensation of the knee giving way or a slight episode of giving way without the patient falling or experiencing postevent swelling.

Patient self-assessment: The patients record their

D. M. Daniel: Department of Orthopedic Surgery, University of California, San Diego, School of Medicine, La Jolla, California 92037; and Kaiser Permanente Medical Center, San Diego, California 92120.

M. L. Stone: Department of Orthopedics, Kaiser Hospital of San Diego, San Diego, California 92120.

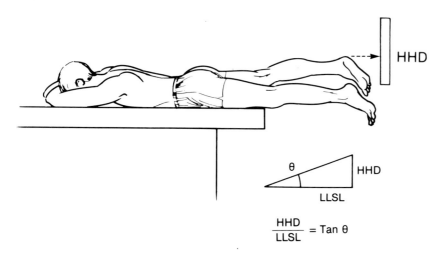

$$\frac{HHD}{LLSL} = Tan\ \theta$$

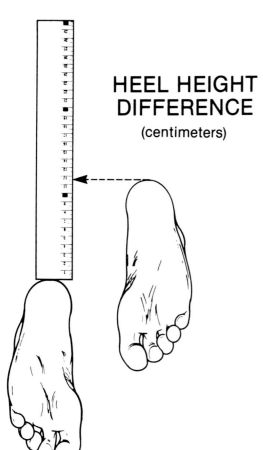

HEEL HEIGHT DIFFERENCE
(centimeters)

FIG. 3-1. Heel height difference. The patient lies prone on the examining table with the lower limbs supported by the thighs. The difference in heel height is measured. The conversion of heel height difference to degrees of extension loss is dependent on the leg length. The tangent of angle θ is the heel height difference (HHD) divided by the lower-leg segment length (LLSL). The lower-limb segment length is proportional to patient height (10). Table 3-1 presents the relationship between heel height difference (in centimeters) and angle θ, the degrees of extension deficit.

knee function for sports and occupational activities performed for 50 or more hours a year. Function is recorded as 0 (complete impairment) to 10 (preinjury function).

One-leg hop: The one-leg hop for distance is expressed as a percent of the patient's normal leg-hop distance (*I/N* × 100) (Chapter 29).

Strength testing: Knee extension and flexion strength is measured isokinetically with a Cybex dynamometer at 60°/sec. Data are given as a percentage of peak torque generated in relation to the patient's contralateral normal leg.

Shuttle run: The 40-yard shuttle run time is recorded (10).

TABLE 3-1. *Extension deficit (degrees)*

Patient height		Heel height difference (cm)					
cm	inches	2.5	5	7.5	10	12.5	15
157	62	3.3	6.6	9.8	13	16.1	19.1
168	66	3.1	6.2	9.2	12.2	15.1	18.0
178	70	2.9	5.8	8.7	11.5	14.3	17.0
188	74	2.8	5.5	8.2	10.9	13.6	16.1
198	78	2.6	5.2	7.8	10.4	12.9	15.4

CASE 1: ATHLETIC TEENAGER WITH ACL DISRUPTION

Acute Injury

History and Evaluation

A 15-year-old female soccer player twisted her left knee in a soccer game and had to discontinue play. An evaluation by an emergency room physician 2 days after injury revealed a "swollen stable knee with a limited range of motion." The following day the patient was evaluated in the orthopedic clinic (Table 3-2).

Arthroscopy revealed an anterior cruciate ligament (ACL) disruption near the femoral attachment. There was mild instability of the posterior horn of the medial meniscus. Visualization of the medial meniscus through the posterior medial portal revealed a peripheral tear of the medial meniscus 6 mm in length. A surgical reconstruction of the ACL was recommended. The patient obtained a second opinion, and she and her family elected not to have surgery.

Comment. For the following reasons a surgical repair was recommended: age less than 20, participates in a high-risk sport, meniscus tear, and moderate pathologic motion. The incidence of secondary knee

TABLE 3-2. *Case 1: examination after index injury without anesthesia*

Effusion (0–3)	2
Flexion	0/20/70
Posterior sag (70°)	0
Lachman	Positive
Valgus stress (25° I − N)	0
Varus stress (25° I − N)	0
KT-1000 30° anterior (mm)	
Normal 20 lb	8
Injured minus normal difference	4
20 lb	4
Manual maximum	8.5
Quadriceps active	3.5
Pivot shift	No test
Radiographs	No fractures Growth plates closed

injuries is higher in teenagers than in patients 20 years and older (Table 27-14). Jumping sports, as well as sports that involve shoe wear that restricts foot motion, place the ACL-disrupted patient at risk of injury. The risk of injury appears to correlate with the degree of pathologic motion (15). Most patients who cope with an ACL disruption (i.e., do not have secondary injuries or great disabilities) have a KT-1000 manual maximum difference of less than 8 mm (Fig. 24-15B).

Treatment

The knee was immobilized in 20° of flexion for 3 weeks. For 10 weeks the patient participated in a lower-limb strengthening program and refrained from running. Three months after injury, there was no effusion and symmetrical quadriceps and hamstring strength to manual testing. The examination of motion limits revealed the following: knee flexion 0/0/140, pivot shift 1+, and KT-1000 30° anterior manual maximum $I - N$ difference of 5 mm. A brace for running sports was recommended, and the patient selected a Don-Joy 4-Point Brace. An agility training program was initiated.

Second Injury

History and Evaluation

Five months after the index injury, she twisted her left knee while kicking a ball with her right foot in a soccer game. She was wearing her brace. Evaluation revealed a 2+ effusion, flexion 0/7/110, and medial joint line tenderness. Because of persistent symptoms and disability, 2 months later the patient had a surgical procedure to repair a medial meniscus tear 6 cm in length and to reconstruct the ACL.

Operative Procedure

For adequate visualization of the medial meniscus tear, the medial collateral ligament (MCL) femoral insertion was detached with a 15- × 15- × 10-mm bone block.

The synovial/capsular attachment to the meniscal rim was rasped to facilitate a healing response, and the meniscus was repaired with 10 vertically placed sutures. The MCL was then repaired with a 4-mm cancellous screw. The ACL was reconstructed with the middle one-third of the patellar tendon and the attached tibial bone and patellar bone. Evaluation of the graft placement revealed a 1-mm increase in distance between attachment sites as the knee was extended from 90° to 0° of flexion. A 6-lb load was placed on the graft at the time of fixation. After wound closure, KT-1000 measurements revealed the following: 30°/20-lb $I - N = -1.5$; manual maximum $= +0.5$. The patient was placed in a cylinder cast in 0° of flexion.

Rehabilitation Program After a Meniscus Repair and ACL Reconstruction with a Strong Graft

The rehabilitation program is designed to protect repaired structures and restore normal joint motion and limb strength. An outline of our rehabilitation program after an ACL reconstruction with a strong biologic graft is presented in Fig. 3-2. In a randomized study of 50 ligament surgeries limited to ACL reconstructions, we have not observed an advantage to passive motion 1 hour a day for the first 2 weeks after surgery in comparison to cast immobilization for the first 2 weeks after surgery. However, we have noted a higher joint stiffness rate in the patients with multiple-ligament surgery as compared to that in patients who had single ACL reconstructions (Chapter 28). Repair of the femoral origin of the MCL increases the risk of joint stiffness. Therefore, during weeks 1 and 2 after surgery, we did the following: Instead of being placed in a cylinder cast in extension, the patient was placed in a bivalve cast in extension which was removed for 1 hour each day for passive motion on a continuous passive motion (CPM) machine. To protect the meniscus repair, the rehabilitation program was modified to delay full weight-bearing until the seventh postoperative week. Squat exercises for quadriceps strengthening were also delayed until the seventh postoperative week. The patient's motion measurements after surgery are presented in Table 3-3.

Comment. The cylinder cast in extension for 2 weeks after surgery is used to prevent a flexion contracture. Prior to 1986, ACL surgery patients were placed in a cylinder cast in 30° of flexion for 3 weeks after surgery and then progressed to a 30° extension stop brace for 3–5 weeks. With this protocol, 30 of 105 patients (29%) with a single ACL reconstruction had a residual extension deficit of more than 5° one year after surgery. These patients had an increased incidence of anterior knee pain and a decrease in their knee extension strength (Chapter 28). In 1986 we changed to the protocol presented in Fig. 3-2. The incidence of an extension deficit more than 5° has decreased to 8% (Table 28-2). After the cylinder cast is removed, a range-of-motion brace is used during the day and an extension splint is used during hours of sleep, in order to maintain full extension. The brace is set with a 50° extension stop and no flexion stop. A hamstring and quadriceps strengthening program is initiated. In early flexion the patella tendon pulls the tibia forward and loads the ACL (Chapters 10 and 11). To reduce the quadriceps pull on the ACL graft, a 50° extension block brace limits motion. We advise quadriceps exercises where the patient pushes through the bottom of the foot; for example, squatting, cycling, and rowing machine. Patients are not to push through the front of the leg on an exercise machine. Machines that have the patient push through the front of the leg require active extension against a constant or increasing flexion moment. As the knee extends, the ACL/quadriceps tension ratio increases, placing the ACL graft at risk of disruptive loads (Chapter 11). The weak segment of the graft during the first 4–6 weeks is probably dependent on the fixation site (Chapters 2 and 21). The protection program during the first 6 weeks is to protect disruption of the graft fixation site. The protection program for the period of 6–52 weeks is to protect the remodeling graft (Chapters 20 and 21).

Follow-Up 1 Year After Injury

One year after surgery the patient returned to play on the high-school soccer team. The results of her 1-year postsurgery evaluation are presented in Table 3-4.

Comment. One year after surgery the patient had persistent mild pathologic laxity which is consistent with full knee function. She had knee extension weakness and thigh atrophy; surprisingly, however, her one-leg hop for distance was normal. Exercises to obtain an extension strength of 80% or more of the normal side is recommended prior to the patient's return to competitive soccer. We recommended she continue her quadriceps exercise program with a goal of 90–100% of the normal side strength.

CASE 2: RECREATIONAL ATHLETE WITH ISOLATED ACL DISRUPTION

Acute Injury

History and Evaluation

A 25-year-old male engineer twisted his right knee while dribbling down the court in a basketball game.

	WEEK								MONTH						
	1	2	3	4	5	6	7	8	3	4	5	6	7/8	9/12	13/24

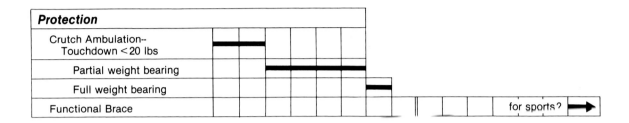

Immobilization

| | | | | | | | | |
Cast in extension — 10-14 days
Hours of sleep only
Brace—Motion 50°—120°

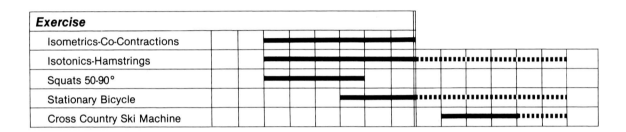

Protection

Crutch Ambulation-- Touchdown <20 lbs
Partial weight bearing
Full weight bearing
Functional Brace — for sports? ➤

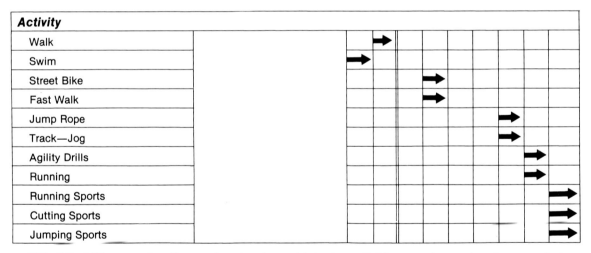

Exercise

Isometrics-Co-Contractions
Isotonics-Hamstrings
Squats 50-90°
Stationary Bicycle
Cross Country Ski Machine

Activity

Walk
Swim
Street Bike
Fast Walk
Jump Rope
Track—Jog
Agility Drills
Running
Running Sports
Cutting Sports
Jumping Sports

FIG. 3-2. ACL reconstruction protocol—strong biologic graft. The exercise protocols presented in Figs. 3-2 and 3-3 are specific to the knee musculature. In practice, we instruct and encourage the patient to also follow a program of general total-body stretching, cervical through heel-cord. Additionally, we recommend a trunk and lower-extremity strengthening program for all patients recovering from knee ligament injury or surgery. These programs are generally initiated at week 4, when swelling and pain resolve.

TABLE 3-3. *Case 1: postoperative motion limits*

Week:	2	3	4	5	6	8	12	16	20	24
Heel height difference (cm):	0	0	0	6	4	6	0	0	0	0
Knee flexion:	40	55	65	80	90	110	130	135	140	140
KT-1000 30° anterior (mm) Injured minus normal difference										
20 lb						−3		0		2
Manual maximum						−3		0		2

The patient felt his knee go out of place and then relocate. As he described the injury he moved his hands in a way that demonstrated anterior tibial translation and relocation. He tried to continue playing, but the knee went out on two more occasions and he discontinued play. He had no prior knee problems, and, for the year prior to injury, his sports activities were football or basketball once a week and racquetball three times a week (150 hours per year). He was examined in the orthopedic clinic 2 days after injury (Table 3-5). Examination under anesthesia revealed a 1+ pivot shift, and arthroscopy revealed a midsubstance ACL disruption and no meniscal or joint surface injuries.

Comment. The incidence of a meniscus tear in an acute ACL disruption is greater than 50% in most studies (Tables 27-5 and 27-13). In our experience, 31% of the patients arthroscoped acutely had meniscus surgery. Many of those patients had a small posterior horn lateral meniscus fragment that was removed. However, meniscus tears in this vascular region may not require surgery. We presently leave many of these lesions alone. Only 6% of acutely injured patients, in our experience, require a meniscus repair (Table 27-13), though others have reported a higher incidence (Table 27-9). We have used four methods to evaluate the meniscal condition in an ACL injured patient: (i) repeated clinical examination over an 8- to 12-week period, (ii) arthrogram, (iii) magnetic resonance imaging (MRI) and (iv) arthroscopy. Selection of the evaluation plan is largely a socioeconomic decision. In our experience, arthroscopy is the most accurate method of diagnosing a surgical meniscus tear followed by arthrogram, MRI, and clinical examination, in that order. We cannot diagnose accurately on the clinical examination which patients with an acute ACL disruption have a meniscus tear. Posterior medial joint line tenderness increases the possibility of a peripheral medial meniscus tear. However, there are more lateral meniscus tears associated with an acute ACL disruption than with medial tears (Tables 27-5 and 27-13), and many do not have joint line tenderness. The use of MRI is discussed in Chapter 26. It is important to grade the MRI meniscus image (17). Grade I and II meniscal signals do not indicate a surgical meniscus injury. Only the Grade III signal is a probable surgical meniscus injury. With greater experience, the accuracy of identifying surgical meniscal tears with MRI will undoubtedly improve. In

TABLE 3-4. *Case 1: evaluation 1 year after surgery*

Symptoms	
Pain and swelling	0
Giving way, partial or full	0
Ability to walk, squat, run, jump, cut	Full
Examination	
Effusion	0
Tenderness, crepitus, irritability	0
Thigh circumference (*I − N*)	2.5 cm
Knee flexion	0/0/140
Valgus stress (25° *I − N*)	0
KT-1000 30° anterior (mm)	
Normal 20 lb	7
Injured minus normal difference	
20 lb	2.5
30 lb	2.5
Manual maximum	4
Quadriceps active	3
Function	
40-yard shuttle run	10.4 sec
One-leg hop for distance (*I/N* × 100)	102%
Cybex at 60°/sec	
Knee extension	76%
Knee flexion	104%

TABLE 3-5. *Case 2: examination without anesthesia 2 days after injury*

Effusion	1+
Flexion	0/0/130
Posterior sag (70°)	0
Lachman	Positive
Valgus stress (25° *I − N*)	0
Varus stress (25° *I − N*)	0
KT-1000 30° anterior (mm)	
Normal 20 lb	9
Injured minus normal difference	
20 lb	3
Manual maximum	6
Quadriceps active	4
Pivot Shift	1
Radiographs	No fractures

this case, the treating surgeon elected to perform arthroscopy.

Treatment

This patient is a 25-year-old male with moderate involvement in high-risk sports activities There is no meniscus pathology. The pathologic joint motion is mild. It was elected not to reconstruct the ACL.

Rehabilitation

A 3-month activity restriction and limb-strengthening program was followed (Fig. 3-3). To allow healing of unrecognized capsular, ligamentous, and meniscal lesions as well as to allow time for adaptation of muscle firing patterns that may minimize pathologic joint motion (Chapter 14), no running or jumping is permitted for 3 months.

Follow-Up

The patient now plays racquetball and states that his knee function in that activity is 90% of the preinjury level. He occasionally plays touch football and states that his knee function in football is 75% of the preinjury level. He is unable to play basketball. A functional knee brace is used when participating in sports. Three years after the index knee injury, the patient was evaluated in the orthopedic clinic because he had knee swelling following a twisting event while playing racquetball. No surgical procedure was performed. The patient has been evaluated frequently as part of an NIH-funded ACL natural history study (NIH Grant No. 01-990-6813). Study radiographs taken 5 years after injury are normal, and a technetium bone scan performed 5 years after injury revealed no increase in medial or lateral compartment uptake and a mild increase in patella uptake bilaterally. Data from the clinical evaluations are presented in Table 3-6.

Comment. The patient is marginally coping with his ACL-disrupted knee. He has moderate pathologic motion and good knee function. He continues to play a sport that involves lateral movement; while wearing his brace, he has a couple partial giving-way episodes a year. If the patient continues playing racquetball and experiencing giving-way episodes, it is likely that he will tear a meniscus. To date he has not torn a meniscus and his bone scan does not reveal post traumatic arthritis.

CASE 3: CHRONIC ACL TEAR AND PERIPHERAL MENISCUS TEAR

Acute Injury

History and Evaluation

A 43-year-old female recreational soccer player injured her left knee in a soccer game while cutting to the right. She tried to continue playing but had to stop. The patient was seen in the emergency room 2 days after injury. It was noted she had a swollen stable knee with "no ACL laxity." She was referred to the orthopedic clinic. The results of examination 6 days after injury are presented in Table 3-7.

Treatment

The patient was placed on the activity–exercise program presented in Fig. 3-3. Because of persistent swelling 3 months after injury, an arthrogram was performed which did not reveal meniscus injury. Twelve months after injury the patient requested a functional knee brace and stated that she planned to play recreational soccer.

Second Injury

History and Evaluation

Thirteen months after her index injury, the patient's left knee gave way while she was walking downstairs. Physical examination revealed a small flexion contracture and anterior medial joint line tenderness. Because the patient was leaving for Europe, she delayed any further evaluation or treatment for 6 weeks. A diagnostic arthroscopy 15 months after the index injury and 6 weeks after the second injury revealed a large displaced medial meniscus tear with some fissuring of the meniscus fragment. The displaced tear was reduced, and it was noted that the tear was 3 cm in length and 3 mm from the periphery. Surgical care of the knee was postponed to allow the patient to review the surgical options in relation to the meniscus lesion (repair or excise) and a possible ACL reconstruction.

Treatment

The patient elected to have a meniscus repair and ACL reconstruction with a low-risk graft source (ipsilateral semitendinosus tendon). One week after the diagnostic arthroscopy, the meniscus was repaired and the ACL

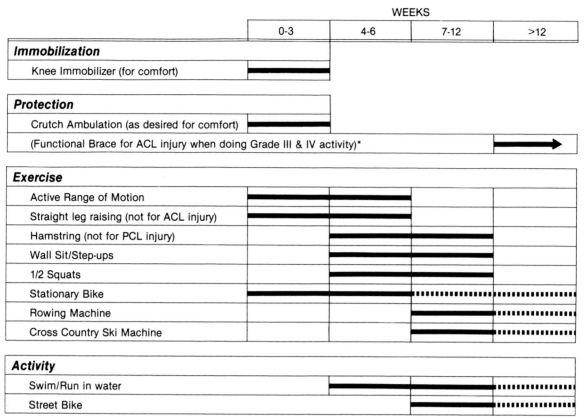

	WEEKS			
	0-3	4-6	7-12	>12
Immobilization				
Knee Immobilizer (for comfort)	▬▬			
Protection				
Crutch Ambulation (as desired for comfort)	▬▬			
(Functional Brace for ACL injury when doing Grade III & IV activity)*				▬▬➤
Exercise				
Active Range of Motion	▬▬	▬▬		
Straight leg raising (not for ACL injury)	▬▬	▬▬		
Hamstring (not for PCL injury)		▬▬	▬▬	
Wall Sit/Step-ups		▬▬	▬▬	
1/2 Squats		▬▬	▬▬	
Stationary Bike	▬▬	▬▬	▬▬ ····	····
Rowing Machine			▬▬	····
Cross Country Ski Machine			▬▬	····
Activity				
Swim/Run in water		▬▬	▬▬	····
Street Bike			▬▬	····

At 12 wks if there is no pain or swelling, full range of motion, and satisfactory strength, activities may progress in this order:

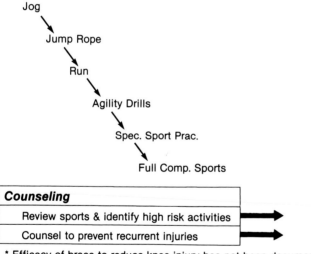

Jog
→ Jump Rope
→ Run
→ Agility Drills
→ Spec. Sport Prac.
→ Full Comp. Sports

Counseling	
Review sports & identify high risk activities	▬▬➤
Counsel to prevent recurrent injuries	▬▬➤

* Efficacy of brace to reduce knee injury has not been documented.

FIG. 3-3. Nonoperative rehabilitation protocol—single-ligament injury. See legend to Fig. 3-2 for further details.

reconstructed with a double semitendinosus passed through bone tunnels under arthroscopic control. The distance between graft attachment sites at full extension was 1 mm greater than the distance at 90° of flexion. A 4-lb fixation load was applied to the graft with a tibial-mounted MEDmetric Tension/Isometer at the time of graft fixation (Fig. 2-13). Because the graft was not of sufficient length to be well fixed with a screw on the anterior aspect of the tibia, the screw fixation was augmented with sutures through the graft which were tied to the screw. The patient's rehabilitation program was similar to the program described for Case 1.

TABLE 3-6. *Case 2: periodic evaluations*

	Time since injury				
	6 months	1 year	2 years	4 years	5 years
Racquetball (hr/year)	156	80	24	100	24
Symptoms (0–3)					
Pain	1	2	1	1	1
Swelling	1	1	2	1	1
Giving-way episodes (no./year)					
Partial	0	1	2	0	3
Complete	0	0	0	0	0
Impairment (0–3)					
Walking	0	0	0	0	1
Squatting	1	1	1	1	1
Running	0	1	1	1	1
Jumping	1	1	1	1	1
Cutting	1	1	1	1	1
One-leg hop for distance ($I/N \times 100$)	101%	99%	96%	96%	97%
Patient assessment of knee function (0–10)	9	9	9	9	9
Heel height difference	0	0	0	0	0
Flexion (F = full)	F	F	F	F	F
KT-1000 30° anterior (mm)					
Normal 20 lb	10	9	9	7	6
Injured minus normal difference					
20 lb	6	3	4	4	2
30 lb	—	—	—	—	3
Manual maximum	5	5	4	6	9
Quadriceps active	2	4	3.5	5	3
Pivot shift	2	2	1	2	2

Follow-Up

Twenty-four months after surgery the patient states that she has no functional impairment. Radiographs of her reconstructed knee showing the course of the graft tunnels and the screws used for graft fixation are shown in Fig. 3-4. By history and examination it ap-

TABLE 3-7. *Case 3: examination without anesthesia 3 days after injury*

Effusion	1+
Flexion	0/0/130
Posterior sag (70°)	0
Lachman	Positive
Valgus stress (25° $I - N$)	0
Varus stress (25° $I - N$)	0
KT-1000 30° anterior (mm)	
Normal 20 lb	6
Injured minus normal difference	
20 lb	4
Manual maximum	8
Quadriceps active	3.5
Pivot shift	No test
Radiographs	No fractures

pears that the patient has a stable meniscus. The patient did not return to play soccer. She bicycles regularly. Follow-up data are presented in Table 3-8.

Comment. We have routinely managed acute ACL ligament injuries in patients over 30 years old without ligament reconstruction unless there is a reparable meniscus. In the case of a reparable meniscus, the meniscus is repaired and the ACL is reconstructed. It is unlikely that a 44-year-old patient will successfully return to a Level 4 sport (Chapter 29) with or without a ligament reconstruction. Prior to this patient returning to soccer, she tore her medial meniscus walking down stairs. A previous arthrogram had not demonstrated a meniscus tear. At surgery the displaced meniscus fragment was seen to be damaged. Because of the appearance of the meniscus, the length of time the meniscus had been displaced, the age of the patient, and the mechanism of second injury, we believed the meniscus fragment was degenerative and damaged. The likely possibility that the repaired meniscus would not heal satisfactorily was discussed with the patient, who chose to have a meniscus repair. We consider meniscus repair to be a relative indication for ACL reconstruction. The reconstruction is performed to decrease

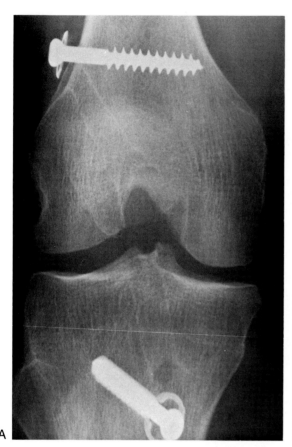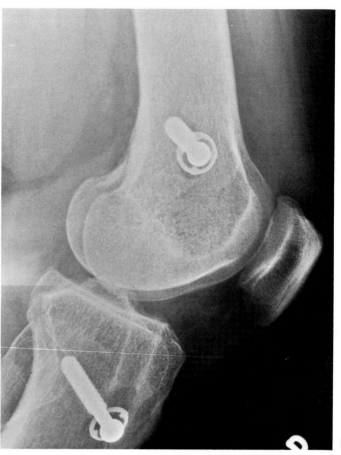

A

B

FIG. 3-4. Case 3. Radiograph taken 2 years after ligament surgery. The semitendinosus graft was fixed on the femur and the tibia with a 6.5-mm screw and a spiked soft tissue washer as illustrated in Fig. 2-22. The position of the bone tunnels may be seen. **A:** The anterior–posterior (A–P) radiograph shows that the tunnel enters the lateral aspect of the femur at the level of the lateral superior genicular artery (Fig. 2-7). **B:** The lateral radiograph shows that the posterior edge of the tibia tunnel is at the anterior edge of the intercondylar tubercles.

the meniscus trauma secondary to joint subluxation. In older patients we recommend semitendonsus as the graft source as opposed to the stronger patellar tendon. The incidence of joint stiffness and quadriceps weakness is less after using a hamstring graft than after using the patellar tendon (Table 28-2). The opportunity for fixation in this patient's graft was believed to be inadequate to tolerate a fixation load of greater than 4 lb. Hamstring grafts require approximately an 8-lb load to reduce the anterior tibial displacement to between 5 and 7 mm (Table 2-12). The restraint obtained with the hamstring tendon was accepted. Because of the poor graft fixation and the repair of a degenerative meniscus, consideration was given to an immobilization period of 4 weeks. However, because of the patient's age of 44, there was a desire to minimize knee immobilization. The compromise was to begin motion in the third postoperative week.

CASE 4: CHRONIC ACL DISRUPTION WITH DEGENERATIVE TEAR OF MEDIAL MENISCUS

Acute Injury

History and Evaluation

A 27-year-old male desk clerk injured his right knee while playing football at age 17. After the injury he had partial giving-way episodes three to four times per year. Because of a fear of injuring his knee after the index injury, he didn't play football or basketball. He did play racquetball two to three times per month. For the past 3 months he experienced medial knee pain and an occasional locking sensation. The results of his knee examination are presented in Table 3-9.

TABLE 3-8. *Case 3: Evaluation preoperatively (PO), under anesthesia prerepair (PR) and after reconstruction (REC) and 6, 12, and 24 months after reconstruction*

	Anesthesia					
	PO	PR	Rec	6 months	12 months	24 months
Symptoms (0–3)						
Pain	1				1	1
Swelling	3				1	0
Giving-way episodes (no./year)						
Partial						
Complete	1				0	0
Impairment (0–3)						
Walking	1				0	0
Squatting	1				0	0
Running	3				0	0
Jumping	3				0	0
Cutting	3					
One-leg hop for distance	0				56%	101%
Patient assessment of knee function (0–10)	?					
Heel height difference	5	0	0	0	0	0
Flexion	100			135	135	135
KT-1000 30° anterior (mm)						
Normal 20 lb	6	3	3	7	4	6
Injured minus normal difference						
20 lb	2	6	5	1	3	2
30 lb	—	7.5	—	1	4	2
Manual maximum	4	9	5	2	5	4
Quadriceps active	1	—	—	4	3	4
Pivot shift (0–3)		1		0	0	0

Treatment

Arthroscopy revealed a degenerative tear of the medial meniscus. The lateral meniscus was normal. The joint surfaces were normal. There was an attenuated ACL ligament. The degenerative portion of the medial meniscus was removed, leaving a stable medial meniscus rim.

Follow-Up Evaluation

At our request, the patient returned for a follow-up evaluation 2 years after surgery. He reported that he

TABLE 3-9. *Case 4: examination 10 years after index injury*

Effusion	0
Tenderness	Medial joint line
Flexion	0/0/130
Posterior sag (70°)	0
Lachman	Positive
Valgus stress (25° I − N)	0
Varus stress (25° I − N)	0
KT-1000 30° anterior (mm)	
20-lb injured minus normal difference	6

was playing racquetball 3 days a week. The results of the evaluation are presented in Table 3-10.

Comment. The patient probably disrupted his ACL at age 17. He modified his life style by not participating in football or basketball (high-risk sports) but was able to participate in a moderate-risk sport, racquetball. Ten years after the ACL injury, he presents with symptoms of a medial meniscus tear. In this situation, our approach is to care for the meniscus lesion and to allow the patient to demonstrate if there still is a significant impairment. Two years after surgery the patient was pleased with his knee function. Measurements of joint subluxation and of pivot shift, as well as KT-1000 measurements, did not reveal an increase in joint instability.

CASE 5: ACUTE MCL INJURY

Acute Injury

History and Evaluation

A 21-year-old female waitress slipped while dancing. She felt her knee "pop" and fell to the floor. Examination in the emergency room revealed a stable knee with limited range of motion. She was evaluated in the

TABLE 3-10. *Case 4: Evaluation 2 years after meniscus surgery, 12 years after index injury*

Symptoms (0–3)	
Pain	0
Swelling	0
Giving-way episodes (no./year)	
Partial	0
Complete	0
Impairment (0–3)	
Walking	0
Squatting	0
Running	0
Jumping	0
Cutting	0
One-leg hop for distance	95%
Patient assessment of knee function (0–10)	10
KT-1000 30° anterior (mm)	
Normal 20 lb	7
Injured minus normal difference	
20 lb	5
Manual maximum	7
Quadriceps active	4
Pivot shift	2

orthopedic clinic 4 days after injury (Table 3-11). Arthroscopy revealed that the ACL was intact. Both menisci were intact. The medial meniscus could be raised off the tibial surface about 4 mm, indicating a tear of the meniscal tibial ligament. The joint surfaces were intact.

Treatment

The rehabilitation course followed the outline given in Fig. 3-3. The patient was given a knee immobilizer for

TABLE 3-11. *Case 5: examination of acute injury*

Examination without anesthesia	
Effusion	2+
Tenderness	Diffuse medial
Flexion	0/10/80
Posterior sag (70°)	0
Lachman	+/−
Valgus stress (25° I − N)	Pain, soft end point
Varus stress (25° I − N)	0
Radiographs	No fractures
Examination under general anesthesia	
Posterior sag (70°)	0
Valgus stress x-ray, 25°/6-lb-ft I − N	4
KT-1000 30° anterior (mm)	
Normal 20 lb	6
Injured minus normal difference	
20 lb	0.5
30 lb	0.5
Manual maximum	3.5

TABLE 3-12. *Case 5: Evaluation 6 months after injury*

Symptoms (0–3)	
Pain	0
Swelling	0
Giving-way episodes (no./year)	
Partial	0
Complete	0
Impairment (0–3)	
Walking	0
Squatting	1
Running	0
Jumping	0
Cutting	1
One-leg hop for distance (I/N × 100)	100%
Patient assessment of knee function (0–10)	9
Valgus stress x-ray, 25°/6-lb-ft I − N	3 mm
KT-1000 30° anterior	
Normal 20 lb	8
Injured minus normal difference	
20 lb	1
30 lb	1
Manual maximum	1
Quadriceps active	3

comfort and was allowed to ambulate without crutches. Two weeks after surgery she began riding a stationary exercise bicycle. Six weeks after surgery she had a full range of motion and no pain.

Follow-Up Evaluation

Six months after injury the patient returned for an evaluation at our request (Table 3-12). She had returned to her preinjury activities including dancing 8 hours a week.

Comment. The patient with an isolated MCL tear will frequently have greater pain and restriction of motion than will a patient with an isolated ACL disruption. The anterior displacement is within normal limits or very slightly increased, as was seen in this case (Table 9-2). It has been well documented in laboratory studies (Chapter 18) and clinical reviews (Chapter 27) that the isolated MCL heals satisfactorily without surgical intervention or cast immobilization. For 2–4 weeks after injury we recommend immobilization as needed for comfort, and for 12 weeks after injury we recommend no running, jumping, or activities that would place a valgus or twisting stress on the knee.

CASE 6: ACUTE ACL AND MCL DISRUPTION

Acute Injury

History and Evaluation

A 23-year-old female research biologist "twisted" her right knee when she quickly changed directions while

TABLE 3-13. Case 6: examination of acutely injured knee

Examination without anesthesia	
Effusion	2+
Tenderness	MCL tibia insertion
Flexion	0/5/90
Posterior sag (70°)	0
Lachman	Positive
Valgus stress (25° I − N)	Pain, soft end point
Varus stress (25° I − N)	0
KT-1000 30° anterior	
Normal 20 lb	8
Injured minus normal difference	
20 lb	3
Manual maximum	5
Quadriceps active	−4.5
Radiographs	No fractures
Examination under anesthesia	
Posterior sag (70°)	0
Lachman	Positive
Valgus stress x-ray (Fig. 3-5), 25°/6-lb-ft I − N (Fig. 3-6)	5 mm
Valgus stress 0° I − N)	0
KT-1000 30° anterior	
Normal 20 lb	5
Injured minus normal difference	
20 lb	6.5
Manual maximum	7

playing soccer. She heard a "ripping sound" in her knee, fell to the ground, and experienced intense pain. She stated that she was not a soccer player but that she was playing in an informal game with some friends. She was a recreational runner and ran 8 hours a week. The results of an examination 2 days after injury in the orthopedic clinic and 5 days after injury under anesthesia are presented in Table 3-13. Radiographs performed under anesthesia at 25° of flexion with a 6-lb-ft valgus stress (Fig. 3-5) revealed an injured minus normal medial joint line opening of 5 mm (Fig. 3-6).

Arthroscopy revealed a parrot-beak tear of the lateral meniscus which was excised. With the application of valgus stress, the medial meniscus pulled away from the medial tibial plateau but was attached to the meniscal tibial ligament, indicating a tear of the meniscal tibial ligament at its insertion site on the tibia. There was a tear of the ACL near its femoral attachment. Articular surfaces were normal.

Treatment

Through an anterior medial longitudinal incision the middle third of the patella tendon was harvested (Fig. 2-1). A transverse incision was made in the crural fascia along the inferior margin of the pes anserinus where

it crosses the MCL. Retraction of the pes tendons proximally revealed that the superficial MCL had avulsed from the tibia. The ACL was reconstructed with the patellar tendon graft, and the superficial MCL was attached to its anatomic tibial insertion site with a screw and spiked soft tissue washer. The deep MCL insertion and the posterior medial corner were not explored. Postrepair KT-1000 30°/20-lb I − N was 0. The patient was placed in a cylinder cast in 0° of flexion.

Rehabilitation and Follow-Up

Her rehabilitation program is outlined in Fig. 3-2. Distal fixation of the superficial MCL without performing a wide medial exposure adds little to the risk of postoperative joint stiffness. We therefore did not use an early passive motion program for this patient. A record of postoperative range of motion, thigh atrophy, and arthrometer measurements is presented in Table 3-14. Two years after surgery the patient jogs 4 hours per week at her preinjury level. She is currently a medical student in another state. Inventory of her symptoms and impairments is presented in Table 3-15.

Comment. We have managed patients who participate in sports activities with an ACL and MCL disruption by routinely repairing or reconstructing the ACL ligament. If a nondamaged ACL is avulsed from the bone, the ligament is reattached. In all intraligamentous injuries, irrespective of how close the injury is to the ligament insertion site, the ligament is reconstructed. In the athletic patient, the stronger patellar tendon graft source is used. To establish the point of MCL disruption, patient tenderness is carefully evaluated and the preoperative radiographs are reviewed for bone avulsion. Arthroscopy also aids in evaluating the site of collateral ligament origin. There will probably be a rent in the joint capsule, therefore an outflow drainage system should be maintained at all times during the arthroscopy. The surgeon should recognize the potential of arthroscopy irrigation fluid extravasating into the soft tissues and initiating a compartment syndrome (Chapter 28). Little additional dissection is needed to expose the tibial insertion of the MCL ligament through the incision used to harvest the patellar tendon graft. By incising the crural fascia along the inferior edge of the pes anserinus and then retracting the pes tendons proximally, the superficial MCL insertion may be exposed. Except in the medial injury with significant valgus instability in full extension, complete exposure of the medial side of the knee to repair an MCL disruption is of greater morbidity than benefit. Lifting the medial flap to expose the entire MCL and the posterior oblique ligament increases the risk of sensory nerve injury and postoperative joint stiffness.

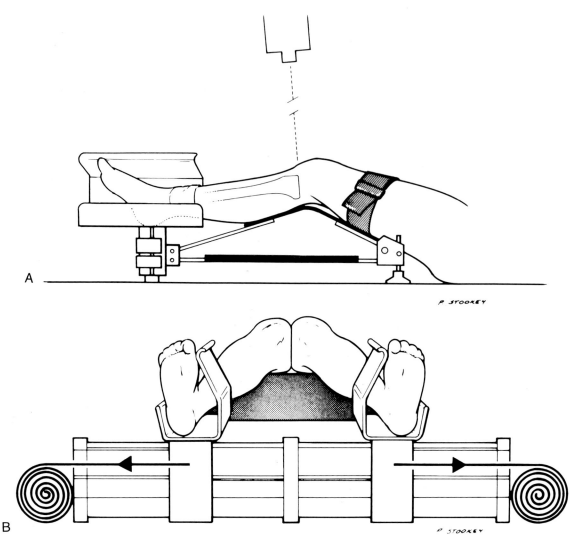

FIG. 3-5. Valgus stress radiographic technique. The abduction stress radiograph is performed with a stress radiograph device designed by the MEDmetric Corporation, San Diego, California. **A:** The knee is positioned in 20° of flexion. A restraining strap is used to hold the thighs together. **B:** The foot support cradles the foot to resist axial limb rotation. A 5-, 10-, or 15-lb force is applied to each leg, producing a 6-, 13-, or 19-lb-ft moment. The distance between the joint line and the point of force application is 15 inches. The tibia is supported parallel with the x-ray plate.

CASE 7: BILATERAL ISOLATED PCL DISRUPTION

Left Knee Injury

History and Evaluation

A 32-year-old male custodian injured his left knee when he caught his foot in a hole while running. The knee twisted and he fell to the ground onto his knee. Evaluation in the emergency room revealed a positive drawer test, and a diagnosis of a cruciate ligament injury was made ("anterior and/or posterior"). The results of the evaluation in the orthopedic clinic are listed in Table 3-16. Arthroscopy revealed both menisci, and all cartilage surfaces were intact. The ACL was intact. There was a midsubstance tear of the posterior cruciate ligament (PCL).

Treatment

The ligament was not repaired or reconstructed. The patient was placed on a 3-month bicycle program and then allowed to return to full activity. Examination 4 months after injury revealed no effusion, full flexion, and a 4-mm posterior tibial sag. The patient returned to full activity.

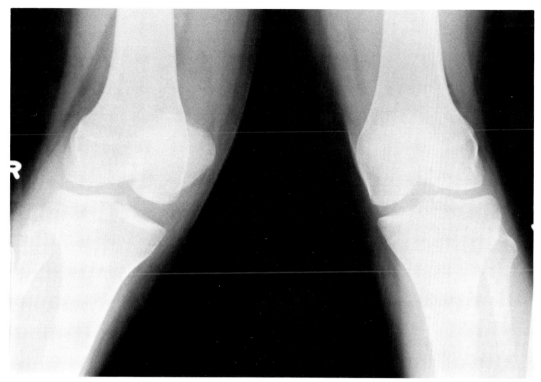

FIG. 3-6. Case 6. Valgus stress radiograph. Abduction stress radiograph taken under anesthesia 5 days after injury. A 6-lb-ft abduction stress was applied with the testing device illustrated in Fig. 3-5. The medial joint space opening on the right is 5 mm greater than that on the left. Note that there is greater limb rotation on the right.

Right Knee Injury

History and Evaluation

Six months after his left knee injury he slid on his right knee to catch a ball in a baseball game. Shortly after that, while running to first base, his knee popped and gave way. He was seen 3 days after injury in the orthopedic clinic (Table 3-17). Arthroscopy of the right knee revealed that the menisci, the joint surfaces, and the ACL were normal. There was a midsubstance acute tear of the PCL.

Treatment and Follow-Up

Ligament repair or reconstruction surgery was not performed. The patient was placed on a bicycle program

TABLE 3-14. *Case 6: knee motion limits after surgery*

	Weeks				Months		
	4	6	8	12	4	6	12
Heel height difference (cm)	4	7	10	8	7	5	5
Flexion (degrees)	60	85	90	95	115	115	125
Thigh circulation difference (cm)				4	2	4	1
Valgus stress (25° $I - N$)						0	0
KT-1000 30° anterior							
Normal 20 lb			8			8	8
Index minus normal difference							
20 lb			−2			0.5	1
30 lb			—			1	1
Manual maximum			−2			1	1
Quadriceps active			−2			0	1
Pivot shift							0

TABLE 3-15. *Case 6: inventory of symptoms and impairments after surgery*

Years since surgery	1	2
Symptoms (0–3)		
Pain	1	1
Swelling	2	1
Giving-way episodes (no./year)		
Partial	0	0
Complete	0	0
Impairment (0–3)		
Walking	0	0
Squatting	1	1
Running	0	0
Jumping	—	0
Cutting	—	0
One leg hop for distance ($I/N \times 100$)	100%	
Patient assessment of knee function (0–10)	7	9

for 3 months and then he returned to full activity. Three years after the patient's initial injury he returned for an evaluation at our request (Table 3-18). He reported that he was not playing any sports because of lack of time.

Comment. PCL injuries are sustained in sports activities as well as in motor vehicle accidents. We have evaluated a number of patients who sustained an isolated PCL disruption while playing baseball (Table 27-2). PCL disruptions can be consistently diagnosed by carefully documenting a posterior tibial sag (5). PCL midsubstance repairs have not been successful, and reconstructions have been only marginally successful. We have routinely treated acute isolated PCL disruptions nonoperatively. There is a low incidence of associated meniscus tears in the PCL-injured patient with a single-ligament injury (Table 27-16). Arthroscopic examination, arthrogram, or MRI to document

TABLE 3-16. *Case 7: examination after left knee injury*

Examination without anesthesia	
Contusions/abrasions	None
Flexion	0/0/90
Effusion	2+
Tenderness	Posterior
Posterior sag (90°)	Positive
Lachman (anterior end point)	Firm
Valgus stress (25° $I - N$)	0 cm
Varus stress (25° $I - N$)	0
Examination under spinal anesthesia	
KT-1000 total A–P displacement (mm)	
30°/20 lb	
Normal right knee	8
$I - N$	3
70°/20 lb	
Normal right knee	6.5
$I - N$	9

TABLE 3-17. *Case 7: isolated bilateral PCL disruptions[a]*

Contusions/abrasions	None
Flexion	0/0/120
Effusion	2+
Tenderness	None
Posterior sag (90°) right and left	Positive
Lachman (anterior end point)	Firm
Valgus stress (25° $I - N$)	0 cm
Varus stress (25° $I - N$)	0
KT-1000 70° anterior quadriceps active displacement (mm)	
Left	4
Right	5

[a] Examination 3 days after right knee injury, 6 months after left knee injury.

joint surface or meniscal injury is optional. For a few years after injury, many patients with an isolated PCL disruption have good function (Table 27-20). Unfortunately, many patients with a PCL disruption develop degenerative arthritis (Table 27-18). It has not been established that the current level of success of PCL reconstructive surgery will increase the patient's function or decrease the incidence of degenerative arthritis.

CASE 8: ACL, PCL, AND MCL DISRUPTION

Acute Injury

History and Evaluation

A 35-year-old female emergency room physician sustained an injury to her left knee while skiing. She was

TABLE 3-18. *Case 7: three years after bilateral PCL injuries*

	Right	Left
Symptoms (0–3)		
Pain	0	0
Swelling	0	0
Giving way episodes (no./year)		
Partial	0	0
Complete	0	0
Impairment (0–3)		
Walking	0	0
Squatting	0	0
Running	0	0
Jumping	0	0
Cutting	0	0
One-leg hop for distance (inches)	72	77
Patient assessment of knee function (0–10)	10	10
KT-1000		
70° quadriceps active	4 mm	6 mm
30°/20-lb total A–P	15 mm	17 mm
70°/20-lb total A–P	14 mm	15 mm

TABLE 3-19. *Case 8: PCL, ACL, MCL disruption*

Examination without anesthesia	
Flexion	0/0/45
Effusion	1+
Posterior sag (45°)	Positive
Lachman (anterior end point)	Soft
Valgus stress (25° I − N)	10 cm
Varus stress (25° I − N)	0
Peripheral pulses	Right–left symmetry
Neurologic examination	intact
Radiographs	Fig. 3-7A
Examination with general anesthesia	
Valgus stress (0° I − N)	5 mm
Varus stress (25° I − N)	20 mm
KT-1000 (injured minus normal)	
30°/20-lb total A–P	10 mm
30°/manual maximum total A–P	21 mm
90°/20-lb posterior	10 mm

evaluated by a physician at the ski area and then transferred to our hospital. The results of her examination are presented in Table 3-19, and a lateral radiography of her knee is shown in Fig. 3-7A.

Treatment

The operative findings and treatment are presented in Table 3-20. At the conclusion of the procedure the patient's knee could be ranged from 0° to 100°. The KT-1000 30°/20-lb total A–P injured − normal knee difference was 1.5 mm. The patient was placed in a cast in full extension.

Comment. The patient had a three-ligament injury without a history of joint dislocation. She was 3 days post-injury, and there had been no signs or symptoms of neurologic or vascular injury; therefore an arteriogram was not performed (15). The bone fragment in the anterior aspect of the joint on the lateral radiograph (Fig. 3-7A) was the tibial bone attached to the avulsed PCL. Sutures were passed through the base of the ligament and passed through 2.5-mm drill holes in the tibia. Because the patellar tendon was injured, it was not used as a graft source. A consent had been obtained to use graft tissue from the normal right knee. However, in this 35-year-old M.D. the surgeons decided to use the graft source of lower morbidity, the ipsilateral hamstring tendon. After the cruciate mechanism had been restored, the medial structures were repaired. After each structure was repaired, the knee was ranged from 0° to 100° to verify that the repair had not limited the joint flexion.

The position selected for immobilization following surgery was full extension, for two reasons: First, to avoid a postoperative flexion contracture; second, there is less tendency for the tibia to sag posteriorly with the knee in full extension. The fixation of the PCL with suture to the tibia was believed to have a holding power of less than 30 lb, and the suture was believed to be at risk of abrasion on the tibial bone tunnels with joint motion. Therefore, despite the significant risk of joint stiffness secondary to the patellar ligament injury and medial capsular and collateral ligament repair, it was elected to wait 2 weeks before beginning a passive range-of-motion program.

Rehabilitation Program

Weeks 0–2: Cylinder cast in extension. Crutch ambulation.

Weeks 3–6: Bivalve cast in full extension. Crutch ambulation. Thigh muscle isometric co-contractions in the cast. Eight hours a day, the cast was removed and the knee was ranged on a continuous passive motion machine. She was instructed to manipulate the patella daily to improve patellar mobility.

Weeks 7–16: No immobilization. Gradual progression from crutch ambulation to ambulation without crutches. Daily range-of-motion program and pool exercises. Passive stretching by a physical therapist three times a week. She was unable to ride an exercise cycle because of limited motion.

Weeks 17–24: A modified exercise cycle was used to allow cycling with a limited range of motion. Adjustment of the seat height and pedal shank length accommodated the cycle to the patient's available range of motion (Fig. 3-8).

Weeks 24–52: Continued cycle exercise and swimming. Increased use of non-impact-loading gym exercise and equipment where force is applied through the sole of the foot.

The patient lived a 3-hr drive from our office and was seen less frequently than is customary. Recovery of flexion after surgery proceeded as follows: 6 weeks—55°; 8 weeks—70°; 16 weeks—70°; 24 weeks—95°; 52 weeks—120°. Her examination 1 year after surgery is presented in Table 3-21.

Comment. Three months after surgery a lateral radiograph revealed inferior position of the patella (Fig. 3-7B). The patient had a Stage II infrapatellar contracture syndrome (13), presumably secondary to patellar tendon trauma. This condition is discussed in Chapter 28. The patient reported that the modified exercise bike was very helpful in regaining motion and limb strength. It is our experience that when the patient is working diligently in a daily exercise and range-of-motion program, closed manipulation under anesthesia

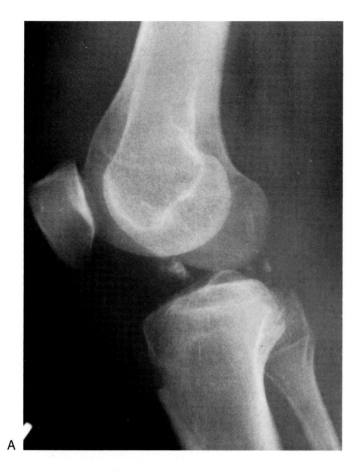

A

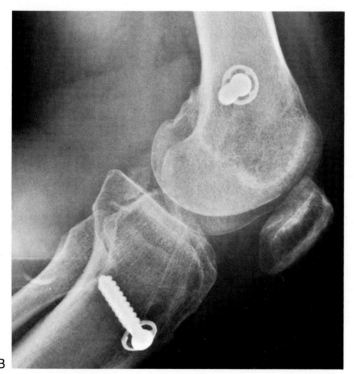

B

FIG. 3-7. Case 8. **A:** Lateral radiograph taken the day of injury. Note the fracture fragment off of the tibial tubercle. The large fracture fragment in the anterior aspect of the intercondylar notch was bone attached to the tibial end of the PCL. **B:** Radiograph 3 months after injury. The bone attached to the avulsed PCL ligament has not united to the tibia. On this slightly oblique radiograph, the femoral tunnel for the ACL graft appears to be in an anterior position. The patella is displaced distally. The preoperative radiograph patellar tendon/patella ratio is 1.4, and the 3 months postoperative radiograph patellar tendon/patella ratio is 1.1.

TABLE 3-20. *Case 8: operative findings and surgery performed*

Findings	Action
Complex lateral meniscus tear	Excised
Hyaline cartilage fracture, 8 × 8-mm lateral femoral condyle	Excised
Tear medial one-third of patellar tendon	No surgical treatment
Avulsion of PCL from tibia with bone fragment	Repaired with suture through tibia drill holes
Midsubstance tear ACL	Reconstructed with ipsilateral double semitendinosus
MCL tear	Suture repair
PCL tear	Suture repair

is of little benefit. The patient may lose motion secondary to the postmanipulation inflammation. If the patient is not working actively in a therapy program, manipulation under anesthesia may gain motion, but the manipulation must be followed with a disciplined daily range-of-motion program to maintain that motion, which usually requires 5–10 days of postmanipulation hospitalization. We have no personal experience with the operative care of the infrapatellar contracture syndrome as discussed by Paulos (13).

KNEE BRACES

Several types of knee braces are commercially available. The American Academy of Orthopedic Surgery's 1984 *Knee Brace Seminar Report* classified three brace types.

Prophylactic: Prophylactic braces have been designed to prevent injury. There is no knee brace designed to protect the normal knee against ACL injury. Several investigators have studied the use of a single-sided hinge brace to reduce the incidence of MCL injuries sustained in football (1,6,7,14,16). The routine use of prophylactic knee braces currently available has not been proven effective in reducing the number or severity of knee injuries. In some circumstances, such braces may even have the potential to be a contributing factor to injury (5).

Postoperative knee braces: For most knee ligament surgeries, postoperative protocols include a period of joint immobilization. There are four reasons why joint motion may be limited: (i) for patient comfort, (ii) to prevent deformity, (iii) to limit ligament injury secondary to passive joint motion, and (iv) to protect repaired ligaments from muscle forces. For the first 10–

14 days we place the patient in a cylinder cast with the knee in full extension to avoid the development of a joint flexion contracture. We then begin a program of extension bracing during hours of sleep to maintain full extension. During the day, a range-of-motion brace is used to allow joint motion and muscle strengthening activities. To minimize the ACL graft tension resulting from a quadriceps contraction, the range-of-motion brace is set to block the terminal 50° of extension. In addition to restricting the flexion arc, postoperative knee braces have been demonstrated to provide anterior, valgus, and axial rotational knee stability (8).

Functional knee braces: Functional knee braces are used by patients to minimize joint impairment and to lower the risk of injury. Functional braces have been recommended for patients with pathologic knee motion secondary to ligament disruptions or for patients following knee ligament surgery. The proposed mechanisms of action are a mechanical constraint of joint motion and improvement of joint position sense.

A number of investigators have demonstrated that functional knee braces decrease anterior joint subluxation in the ACL-disrupted knee at low loads, but do not eliminate joint subluxation (2,4,10,11). Mortensen (11) measured anterior displacement with the KT-2000 in 10 cadaveric knees with the ligaments intact and the ACL sectioned. He then repeated the measurements after applying a commercial knee brace (Fig. 3-9). Custom braces were made from plaster molds of the limbs. Eleven brace designs were tested on 10 knees. Six were custom braces (CTI, Indiana, Lenox Hill, MKS III, Omni TS-7, and Townsend) and five were "off-the-shelf" braces (Don-Joy 4-Point, Ecko, Lerman multiligament, Lorus, and Nuko). One brace design, the Generation II brace, was tested on five knees. Data

TABLE 3-21. *Case 8: one year after ligament surgery (8 months pregnant)*

Symptoms (0–3)	
Pain	0
Swelling	0
Giving way episodes (no./year)	
Partial	0
Complete	0
Impairment (0–3)	
Walking	0
Squatting	3
Heel height difference	5
Knee flexion	120
KT-1000 70° quadriceps active	+1
KT-1000 (injured minus normal)	
30°/20-lb total A–P	1
30°/manual maximum total A–P	4
70°/20-lb posterior	0

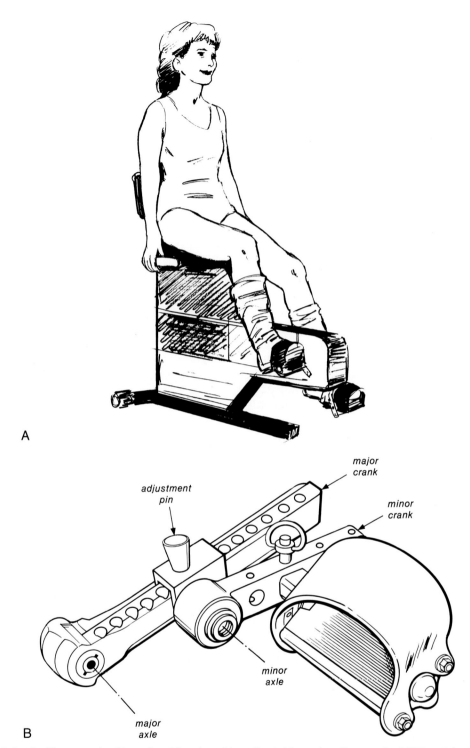

FIG. 3-8. A: Flexercycle (Exercise bicycle with adjustable epicyclic crank, MEDmetric Corporation, San Diego, California). **B:** Adjustable epicyclic crank. **C:** Pedal orbits. The outer perimeter of the dashed area marks the orbit of a pedal in the standard position on the major crank. Positioning the minor axle and placement of the pedal on the minor crank as shown allows an infinite number of pedal orbits within the dashed area. The pedal orbits may be round or oval. The epicycle crank allows the pedal orbit to accommodate the patient's knee flexion range.

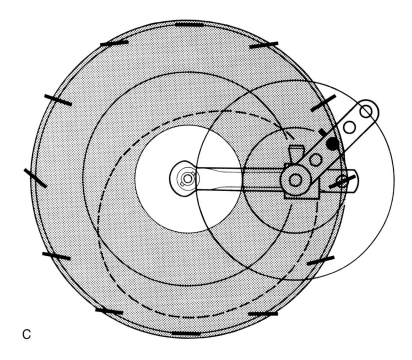

C

FIG. 3-8. (*continued*)

on 40-lb load anterior displacement are presented in Fig. 3-10. At a 20-lb load, the anterior displacement in the ACL-disrupted knee was reduced 3 mm or more in 10 of 12 braces; at the 40-lb load, a similar reduction occurred in 4 of 12 braces. The pathologic quadriceps displacement was reduced by 50% in 9 of 12 braces (Fig. 3-11). Mortensen (11) also tested the specimens on the Oxford testing rig (Chapter 12). Sectioning the ACL resulted in a small increase in internal tibial rotation in the quadriceps-stabilized knee. Functional

knee bracing did not constrain axial rotation. The author did not note a significant difference between custom braces and "off-the-shelf" braces. Mishra (10) evaluated 42 patients with an ACL-disrupted knee who used a functional knee brace. KT-1000 arthrometer testing was performed as part of the evaluation. When measuring the braced knee, the tibial tubercle sensor was replaced by a hook that fit under the brace to contact the tibial sensor with the skin over the tibial tubercle (Fig. 3-12). In the unbraced state, the 20-lb *I*

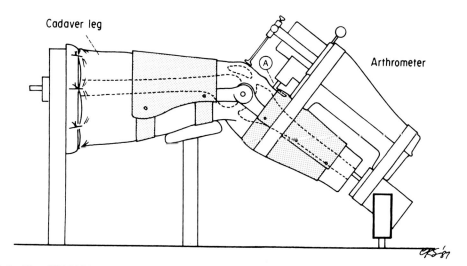

FIG. 3-9. The KT-2000 arthrometer (MEDmetric, San Diego, California) was used to test A–P displacement in a cadaver limb. The fresh-frozen limbs were 23 inches in length and were mounted with femoral and tibial intramedullary rods. The thigh soft tissues were sutured to a proximal plate, and a canvas strap was sutured to the patellar tendon to do the quadriceps displacement test. The tibial tubercle pad was replaced with a hook (A) to allow the sensor to be in direct contact with the skin.

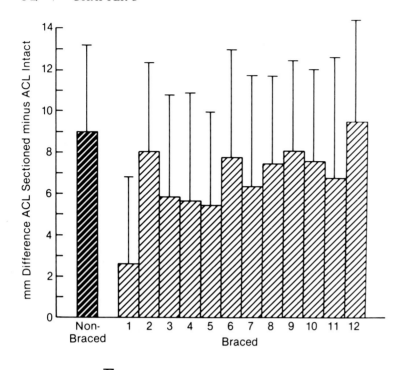

FIG. 3-10. Anterior displacement tests with the KT-2000 with a 40-lb displacement force. The injured minus intact displacement difference for the unbraced ACL-disrupted knee and the braced ACL-disrupted knees for each brace is given. The results of braces 2 through 12 are similar. The displacement for brace 1 is less than that of the other 11 braces. Brace 1 was a custom-made brace. The brace fit very tightly and caused significant soft tissue deformity that the investigators believed could not be tolerated by a patient.

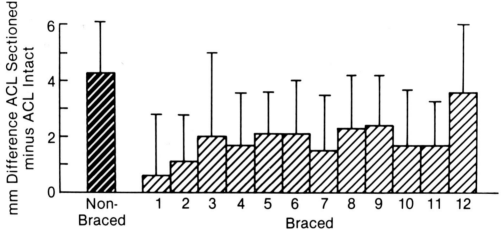

FIG. 3-11. Quadriceps active displacement was achieved by extending the leg by pulling a strap attached to the quadriceps tendon. The increased displacement after sectioning the ACL is shown for the unbraced and braced condition.

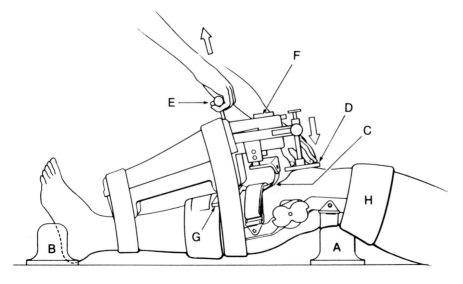

FIG. 3-12. KT-1000 arthrometer adapted for knee brace. A, thigh support; B, foot rest; C, hook adapter for tibial sensor; D, patella sensor; E, force handle; F, displacement dial; G, wooden block adapter for knee brace bulk; H, functional knee brace.

TABLE 3-22. *Comparison of mean side-to-side differences (mm)*

Group	N		Passive 20-lb anterior drawer at 30°	Passive anterior drawer maximum excursion at 30°	Quadriceps active anterior drawer at 30°
All braces	42	I − N[a]	5.00 ± 2.04	6.45 ± 2.36	4.06 ± 1.71
		B − N	1.41 ± 2.25	2.75 ± 2.32	1.70 ± 1.65
		p Value[b]	<.001	<.001	<.001
Don-Joy 4-Point	20	I − N[a]	5.16 ± 1.46	6.29 ± 2.32	4.05 ± 1.94
		B − N	0.47 ± 1.98	1.97 ± 1.70	1.37 ± 1.58
		p Value[b]	<.001	<.001	<.001
CT	6	I − N[a]	4.75 ± 4.31	7.42 ± 1.50	5.08 ± 2.06
		B − N	1.17 ± 2.04	2.58 ± 2.29	1.25 ± 1.97
		p Value[b]	<.05	<.006	<.003
Lenox Hill	7	I − N[a]	5.07 ± 1.43	6.79 ± 2.93	4.29 ± 0.95
		B − N	3.00 ± 2.06	4.07 ± 2.32	3.07 ± 1.30
		p Value[b]	<.006	<.001	<.043
RKS	9	I − N[a]	4.75 ± 1.56	5.81 ± 2.58	3.13 ± 0.88
		B − N	2.44 ± 2.29	3.56 ± 3.17	1.63 ± 1.53
		p Value[b]	<.001	<.009	<.003

[a] I − N, injured minus normal; B − N, braced injured knee minus normal.
[b] Matched t tests (injured no brace minus normal) versus (injured with brace minus normal).

− N displacement difference was 5 mm. Bracing reduced the displacement but did not return it to normal (Table 3-22). There are no published data on braces reducing posterior subluxation in the PCL-injured knee.

Branch (3) investigated the concept that braces may function to enhance joint proprioception. An electromyogram (EMG) study was performed on ACL-injured patients in and out of brace to determine if the use of a brace altered the EMG muscle firing pattern. There was no significant difference between the braced and unbraced condition. Investigators have also evaluated brace use by performing functional tests in brace users in and out of their brace. Houston (9) performed

Cybex strength testing on seven male athletes. Their peak torque was greater at all speeds without the brace. A 15-min endurance test showed 41% higher blood lactate with brace use. Houston concluded that functional knee braces impair muscle performance. Zetterlund (18) studied energy expenditure resulting from running on a treadmill. A small, but significant, increase in oxygen consumption and heart rate were noted with brace use. Mishra (10) had brace users perform the 40-yard shuttle run and one-leg hop for distance in and out of the brace. Statistical analysis of the results of the 42 patients tested showed no significant difference with brace use. Some of the more impaired patients did increase their one-leg hop for distance per-

TABLE 3-23. *Summary of specific task performance, knee pain with sports, knee swelling with sports*

	Specific task performance ratings[a]				
	Good	Fair	Poor	Unknown	Total number of patients
Without brace	10	25	7	0	42
Braced	22	16	1	3	42
	Knee pain with sports				
	No pain	Mild	Moderate	Severe	Unknown
Without brace	26	11	1	2	2
Braced	35	4	2	0	1
	Knee swelling with sports				
	No swelling	With strenuous activity	Moderate	Severe	Unknown
Without brace	26	11	2	1	2
Braced	34	6	1	0	1

[a] The specific task performance rating is discussed in Chapter 29.

TABLE 3.24. *Sport I performance[a] levels: all braces[b]*

	Unable to compete	100%	90%	75%	50%	25%	Severe	Unknown
No brace	8	4	1	10	4	3	5	7
Wearing brace	4	1	11	10	7	0	2	7

Sport I class: Strenuous = 24 Moderate = 18
Preinjury hours/year: $\bar{x}$ = 210 Range 100–1600
Postinjury hours/year: − $\bar{x}$ = 112 Range 0–1600

[a] Preinjury performance established as 100%.
[b] Sport I was the subject's sport of greatest participation prior to injury. A strenuous sport was defined as a sport involving jumping or cutting. A moderate sport was defined as a sport involving running or lateral motion, but not involving jumping or cutting (Chapter 29).

TABLE 3-25. *Giving-way episodes post-injury[a]*

Giving way	N	Gives way	Does not give way	Unknown
No brace (pooled)	42	24	15	3
All braces (pooled)		6	34	2
Without Don-Joy 4-Point	20	10	7	3
With Don-Joy 4-Point		1	17	2
Without CT	9	4	5	0
With CT		0	9	0
Without Lenox Hill	6	5	1	0
With Lenox Hill		2	4	0
Without RKS	7	5	2	0
With RKS		3	4	0

[a] Giving-way episodes equals total giving-way episodes plus partial giving-way episodes.

formance with brace use. In contrast to the lack of objective documentation that braces are very useful, many patients believe they have better function in a brace and thus participate more vigorously in sports activity as reported by Mishra (Tables 3-23 and 3-24) (10).

The following question remains to be answered: Does the use of a functional brace prevent injury? Functional braces are used in the unstable knee to prevent further injury and in the reconstructed knee to prevent graft failure. Mishra (10) reported that patients state that they have fewer giving-way episodes in the brace (Table 3-25). However, there are no published data to support the thesis that braces prevent injury or graft failure.

It is the authors' custom to recommend brace use for patients with ACL disruptions when they participate in Class III or IV sports (Chapter 29). If knee ligament surgery restores the normal knee motion limits, we do not advise brace use after reconstruction. If the surgery is marginally successful or unsuccessful, we do advise that a brace be used for Class III or IV sports.

ACKNOWLEDGMENTS

Support from the following sources is gratefully acknowledged: DonJoy, Inc., Carlsbad, California 92008; Innovation Sports, Irvine, California 92718; Sutter Biomedical, San Diego, California 92123; MEDmetric, San Diego, California 92121; and Lennox Hill, Long Island City, New York 11101.

REFERENCES

1. Anderson G, Zeman SC, Rosenfeld RT. The Anderson knee stabler. *Physician Sportsmed* 1979;7:125–127.
2. Beck C, Drez D Jr, Young J, Cannon WD Jr, Stone ML. Instrumented testing of functional knee braces. *Am J Sports Med* 1986;14:253–256.
3. Branch TP, Hunter R, Donath M. Dynamic EMG analysis of anterior cruciate deficient legs with and without bracing during cutting. *Am J Sports Med* 1989;17:35–41.
4. Branch T, Hunter R, Reynolds P. Controlling anterior tibial displacement under static load: a comparison of two braces. *Orthopedics* 1986;9:1249–1252.
5. Garrick JG, Requa RK. Prophylactic knee bracing. *Am J Sports Med* 1987;15:471–476.
6. Hansen BL, Ward JC, Diehl RC. The preventive use of the Anderson knee stabler in football. *Physician Sportsmed* 1985;13:75–81.
7. Hewson GF Jr, Mendini RA, Wang JB. Prophylactic knee bracing in college football. *Am J Sports Med* 1986;14:262–266.
8. Hofmann AA, Wyatt RW, Bourne MH, Daniels AU. Knee stability in orthotic knee braces. *Am J Sports Med* 1984;12:371–374.
9. Houston ME, Goemans PH. Leg muscle performance of athletes with and without knee support braces. *Arch Phys Med Rehabil* 1982;63:431–432.
10. Mishra DK, Daniel DM, Stone ML. The use of functional knee braces in the control of pathologic anterior knee laxity. *Clin Orthop* 1989;241:213–220.
11. Mortensen W, Foreman K, Focht L, Daniel D, Biden E. An *in*

vitro study of functional orthoses in the ACL disrupted knee. *Trans Orthop Res Soc* 1988;13:520.

12. Noyes FR, Grood ES, Torzilli PA. Current concepts review: the definitions of terms for motion and position of the knee and injuries of the ligaments. *J Bone Joint Surg* 1989;71A:465–472.

13. Paulos LE, Rosenberg TD, Drawbert J, Manning J, Abbott P. Infrapatellar contracture syndrome. An unrecognized cause of knee stiffness with patella entrapment and patella infera. *Am J Sports Med* 1987;15:331–341.

14. Rovere GD, Haupt HA, Yates CS. Prophylactic knee bracing in college football. *Am J Sports Med* 1987;15:111–116.

15. Sisto DJ, Warren RF. Complete knee dislocation. A follow-up study of operative treatment. *Clin Orthop* 1985;198:94–101.

16. Teitz CC, Hermanson BK, Kronmal RA, et al. Evaluation of the use of braces to prevent injury to the knee in collegiate football players. *J Bone Joint Surg* 1987;69A:2–9.

17. U.S. Department of Commerce. Statistical Abstract of the United States 1988, p. 100.

18. Zetterlund AE, Serfass RC, Hunter RE. The effect of wearing the complete Lenox Hill Derotation Brace on energy expenditure during horizontal treadmill running at 161 meters per minute. *Am J Sports Med* 1986;14:73–76.

PART II

Structure

Knee Ligaments: Structure, Function, Injury, and Repair, edited by D. Daniel, et al.

CHAPTER 4

Gross Anatomy

Robert T. Burks

MEDIAL KNEE ANATOMY

It is helpful to describe the supportive structures on the medial side of the knee as constituting three layers (Fig. 4-1) (49). The most superficial is layer I, which is the extension of the deep fascia covering the quadriceps and continues on as the deep fascia of the leg (Fig. 4-2). It invests the sartorius and serves as that muscle's insertion, unlike the discrete tendons of insertion of the underlying gracilis and semitendinosus (Figs. 4-1 and 4-2). Layer II is the superficial medial collateral ligament (MCL). Layers I and II blend together approximately 1–2 cm anterior to the leading edge of the superficial MCL, these fibers join with fibers from the vastus medialis to form the medial patellar retinaculum (Fig. 4-1). Layer I completely covers the medial aspect of the knee and is infrequently torn with injury. Therefore this layer usually needs to be incised to find the underlying pathology. Incising layer I on the more posterior aspect of the knee allows it to be separated from the superficial MCL (Fig. 4-3) (49). The only area on the medial aspect of the knee where all three layers can be found together is directly over the superficial MCL.

The gracilis and semitendinosus run between layers I and II, and they insert distal to the tibial tuberosity. They overlie the tibial attachment of the superficial MCL (Figs. 4-3 and 4-4). Although these tendons have discrete insertions on the tibia, they also have attach-ments to the deep fascia. These fibers need to be cut in order to harvest the tendons for use in knee reconstructive procedures.

Layer II is the superficial MCL, which originates at the medial femoral epicondyle. It runs approximately 10–11 cm to its tibial insertion, where it is covered by the gracilis and semitendinosus (Fig. 4-4) (10,11,50). This has been called either the medial collateral ligament, the tibial collateral ligament, or the superficial medial ligament (29,49). Posterior to the long vertical fibers of the superficial MCL, layers II and III merge together. Along with the semimembranosus tendon and sheath, they form the posteromedial corner of the knee (Fig. 4-1). Warren (50) demonstrated different strain patterns within the fibers of the superficial MCL when the knee was placed through a range of motion. He felt that the ligament should not be viewed as a single homogeneous unit, since its anterior fibers behaved differently from the more posterior fibers. Others have confirmed this and have shown that the anterior fibers tighten and show increased strain during the first 70–105° of flexion, and the more posterior fibers relax and have decreased strain (3,9).

As the knee flexes, the femur moves posteriorly on the tibia, and the superficial MCL slides posteriorly over the proximal tibia, helping to maintain a more uniform tension in the fibers (Figs. 4-4 and 4-5) (10,11). The posterior sliding is accentuated by external rotation of the tibia in relation to the femur. Because of this, there can be no meniscal attachment to the superficial MCL, since this would preclude its change in position (35).

The posteromedial corner of the knee is an area of

R. T. Burks: Department of Orthopedic Surgery, Division of Sports Medicine, University of Utah Medical Center, Salt Lake City, Utah 84132.

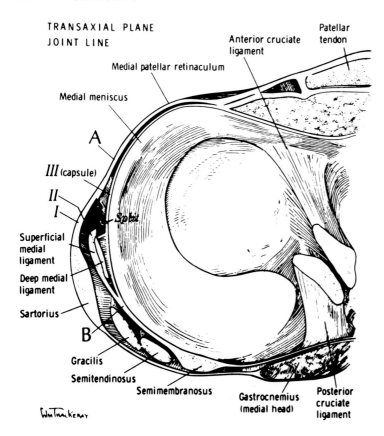

TRANSAXIAL PLANE
JOINT LINE

Anterior cruciate ligament

Patellar tendon

Medial patellar retinaculum

Medial meniscus

A

III (capsule)

II

I

Sartorius

Superficial medial ligament

Deep medial ligament

B

Gracilis

Semitendinosus

Semimembranosus

Gastrocnemius (medial head)

Posterior cruciate ligament

FIG. 4-1. A transverse section at the joint line of a right knee illustrating the medial layers. Point A is the junction of layers I and II anteriorly, and point B is the merging of layers II and III posteriorly. (From ref. 49.)

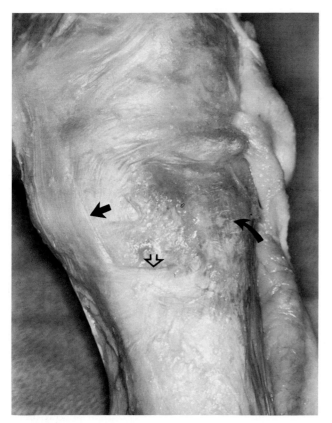

FIG. 4-2. Skin reflected from a left knee to expose layer I. The closed arrow indicates the leading edge of the superficial MCL. The open arrow indicates the top edge of the sartorius fibers in layer I. The curved arrow is on the tibial tubercle.

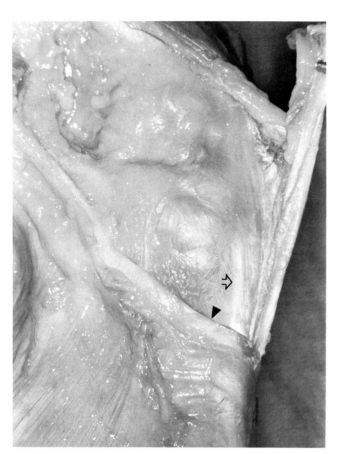

FIG. 4-3. A left knee with layer I and the sartorius reflected anteriorly. The arrowhead indicates the gracilis tendon, and the open arrow indicates the posterior edge of the superficial MCL.

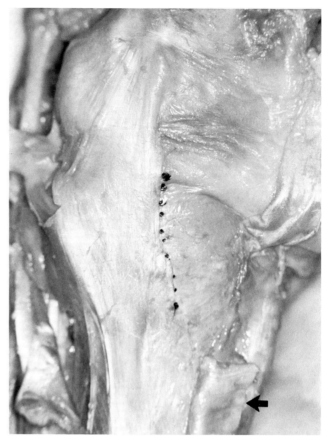

FIG. 4-4. A left knee in full extension, with ink outlining the anterior edge of the superficial MCL. The closed arrow indicates the cut edge of the pes tendons that have been folded back anteriorly to show the proximal aspect of their tibial attachments.

blending of layers II and III. This area is confluent with the posterior edge of the superficial MCL, and it runs obliquely to the tibia (Fig. 4-6). This area has been termed the "posterior oblique ligament" by Hughston (23). It has also been referred to as the oblique portion of the tibial collateral ligament or, simply, the posteromedial corner (10,11,31,50). Hughston (23) reported that the origin of this ligament is from the adductor tubercle, slightly posterior and proximal to the femoral epicondyle, and propose it as a distinctly separable ligament. Warren (49) was unable to identify a discrete separable ligament, and since the fibers are in the same layer as the superficial MCL, he preferred to call it the oblique fibers of the superficial medial ligament. This chapter will describe the structure as the "oblique fibers of the superficial medial collateral ligament." The attachment sites of the fibers in this area move toward each other with increasing flexion and therefore relax. Hughston (23) measured this distance change to be 8–18 mm with a progressively decreasing distance with knee flexion. The more posterior proximal fibers also move underneath, or they move deep to the more anterior fibers with knee flexion

(Fig. 4-5) (9). All authors (10,11,23,27,49) call attention to the fact that the oblique fibers are reinforced by the semimembranosus and its tendon sheath.

Layer III is the capsule of the knee joint and attaches primarily to the articular margins (49). It is thin anteriorly and provides little stability to the knee. The part of the capsule that holds the meniscal rim to the tibia is called the coronary ligament. It is short and holds the meniscus tighter in relationship to the tibia than to the femur. Beneath the superficial MCL, this layer is thickened and called the deep MCL. It has also been named the deep medial ligament, deep collateral, or middle capsular ligament (Fig. 4-7) (29,45,50). The deep MCL may be divided into the meniscofemoral and meniscotibial ligaments, which run from the meniscus to the femur and from the meniscus to the tibia, respectively. Layers II and III are readily separable at their midportion. However, approximately 1–2 cm behind the anterior edge of the superficial MCL, layers II and III blend into the posteromedial corner of the knee. The peripheral fiber system of the medial meniscus is intimately blended with this area, but many

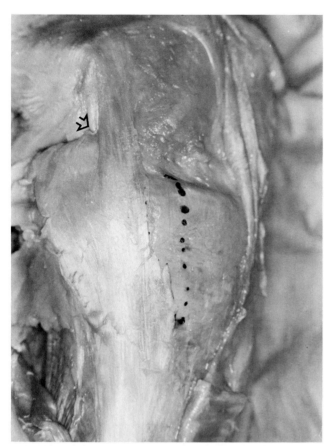

FIG. 4-5. A left knee in 90° of flexion and some external tibial rotation, demonstrating the posterior displacement of the superficial MCL as shown by the distance of the ligament from the original ink line. The open arrow indicates the posterior oblique fibers folding deep to the superficial MCL.

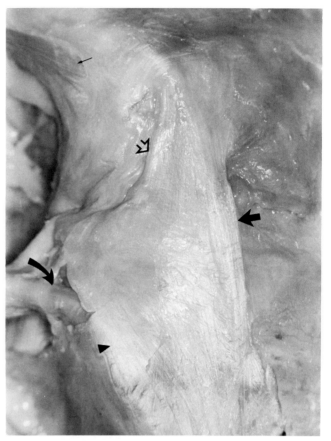

FIG. 4-6. A left knee showing a close-up of the medial side. The open arrow indicates the oblique fibers of the superficial MCL. The closed arrow indicates the leading edge of the superficial MCL. The arrowhead points to the obliquely oriented fibers of the distal aspect of the superficial MCL and the area of contribution from the semi-membranosus tendon sheath. The curved arrow is on the semimembranosus tendon (the sheath has been opened). The small arrow shows the adductor magnus tendon.

of the capsular fibers run uninterrupted from the femur to the tibia (10,11,35). The capsule posterior to the oblique fibers of the superficial MCL is redundant with knee flexion. An arthrotomy to gain access to the posterior aspect of the knee should be made in this redundant capsule, avoiding the oblique fibers of the superficial MCL.

The semimembranosus and its tendon sheath are important contributors to the posteromedial corner anatomy (27,45,49). The tendon is described as having five arms of insertions (Fig. 4-7). The first is a direct attachment to the posteromedial tibia just below the joint line. The second direct attachment proceeds anteriorly just beneath the superficial MCL. A third arm, more from the tendon sheath, runs to blend with the posteromedial capsule. A fourth contributes substantially to the oblique popliteal ligament which runs over the posterior surface of the joint capsule. The fifth arm blends with the superficial MCL distally.

LATERAL KNEE ANATOMY

Seebacher (44) divided the lateral side of the knee into three layers, as Warren did on the medial side (Fig. 4-8) (49). Hughston (21) prefers to divide it into three areas from anterior to posterior. Both systems may be useful in organizing the anatomical areas of importance, but the emphasis here will be on the layer approach. The superficial layer is the deep fascia of the thigh and calf, with the laterally condensed fibers that make up the iliotibial tract. This layer is continuous from the prepatellar bursa to the fascia over the popliteal fossa. The iliotibial tract is connected with the intermuscular septum down to the supracondylar tubercle of the femur. It then continues free of connection until it inserts on Gerdy's tubercle (25). There are capsulo-osseous attachments of the iliotibial tract that Terry (46) reports are important for lateral knee sta-

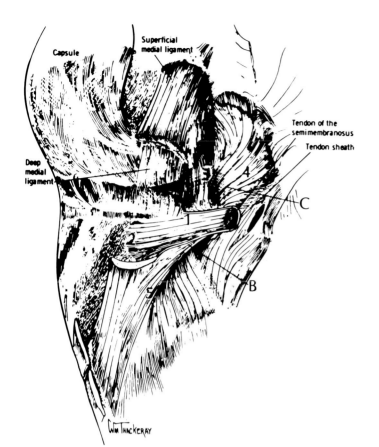

FIG. 4-7. A right knee demonstrating the five arms of the semimembranosus and its sheath. Points 1 and 2 are direct insertions of the tendon, Point 3 is the contribution of the sheath to the posterior oblique fibers. Points 4 and C are the oblique popliteal ligament. Point 5 and B are the fiber contribution to the distal superficial MCL. Point C is the oblique popliteal ligament. (From ref. 49.)

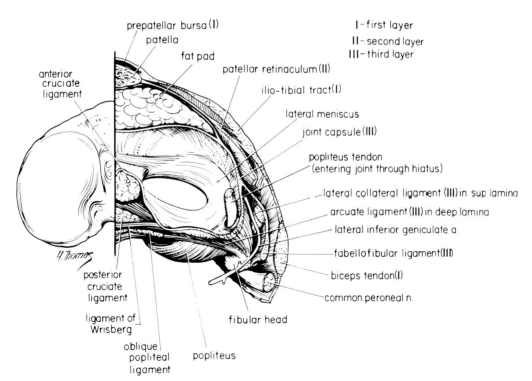

FIG. 4-8. A view of a right knee after removal of the femur. Note the division of the fabellofibular ligament and lateral collateral ligament from the arcuate ligament by the lateral inferior geniculate artery. (From ref. 44.)

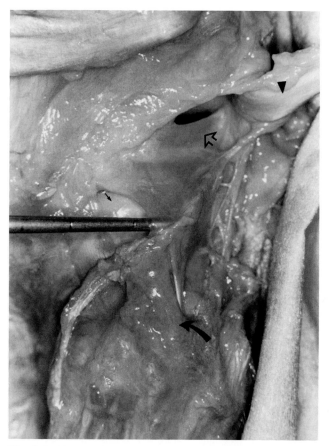

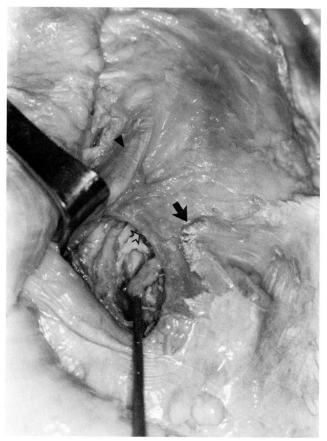

Fig. 4-9. Posterolateral aspect of a right knee. The closed arrow is the reflected popliteus tendon. The open arrow indicates the "bare" area of the lateral meniscus. The small arrow shows the tibial articular cartilage. The probe is deep to the coronary ligament, with some of the distal fibers running to the fibular head being shown by the curved arrow.

FIG. 4-10. A right knee showing the superficial lamina of layer III. The closed arrow indicates the cut edge of the iliotibial band. The open arrow shows the posterior edge of the fabellofibular ligament. The probe is holding up the lateral inferior geniculate artery. The arrowhead is on the lateral head of the gastrocnemius.

bility, and he has termed them an "anterolateral ligament of the knee." Some fibers sweep anteriorly to the lateral border of the patella, and they join with fibers of the vastus lateralis to form the lateral retinaculum (25,40). Confluent with this layer is the biceps tendon, which lies posteriorly and is considered in the superficial layer much as the sartorius is on the medial side. The biceps tendon has a complex lateral insertion, and Marshall (34) found three layers. There are important attachments to Gerdy's tubercle, fibers that blend with the crural fascia of the leg, fibers that loop around the lateral collateral ligament (LCL), and fibers that insert on the styloid process and head of the fibula.

Deep to the superficial fascia is the retinaculum of the quadriceps and the patellofemoral ligaments (44). The patellofemoral ligaments run from the patella to (a) the terminal fibers of the intermuscular septum, (b) the lateral epicondyle, and (c) the fabella or posterolateral capsule. Reider (40) found that the more a patella tended toward a Wiberg III, the larger the lateral

patellofemoral ligament would be. It was felt that this helped explain the greater tendency toward subluxation with the Wiberg III patella. The patellomeniscal ligament runs roughly parallel to the patellar tendon and attaches to the margin of the lateral meniscus and terminates at Gerdy's tubercle (44).

The third or deepest layer comprises the lateral capsule as well as the LCL. This arrangement, therefore, differs from that on the medial side. The capsule attaches primarily to the articular margin region. The lateral meniscus is held to the tibia by the coronary ligament which is longer than that for the medial meniscus. This allows greater excursion for the lateral meniscus. The coronary ligament at the posterolateral corner may attach to the head of the fibula (Fig. 4-9). The lateral meniscus has a bare area, or hiatus, of no capsular attachment; this hiatus is approximately at the midportion of the lateral meniscus and averages 1.3 cm in length (12).

Just posterior to the midportion of the joint, the capsule divides into two laminae (44). The superficial lam-

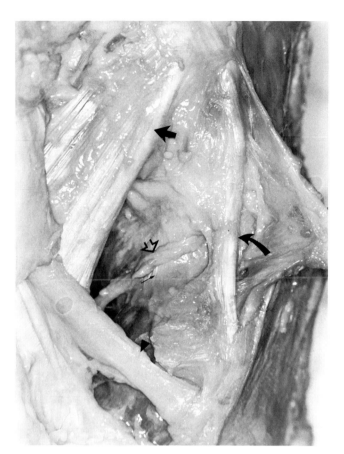

FIG. 4-11. The superficial lamina of layer III in a right knee has been reflected to show the LCL (*curved arrow*). Note its attachment on the lateral aspect of the fibular head. The open arrow points to the lateral inferior geniculate artery. This is running superficial to the underlying arcuate ligament (*small arrow*). The arrowhead shows the peroneal nerve, and the closed arrow is on the lateral border of the lateral head of the gastrocnemius.

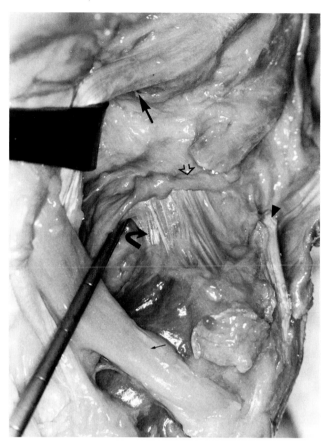

FIG. 4-12. A right knee where the LCL has been excised (*arrowhead*). The curved arrow indicates the arcuate ligament. The open arrow is on the lateral inferior geniculate artery. The closed arrow shows the lateral head of the gastroc. The small arrow is on the peroneal nerve.

ina encompasses the LCL, and it ends posteriorly in a variably sized fabellofibular ligament (Figs. 4-8 and 4-10). It is because of this investment that Seebacher (44) considers the LCL as part of the deepest or capsular layer. The LCL runs from the lateral epicondyle of the femur to the proximal lateral aspect of the fibular head (Fig. 4-11). Because of its location behind the axis of rotation, the LCL is tightest in extension but relaxes in flexion, especially at angles greater than 30° (10,27,37,48). In the past, the LCL has been given a minor role in varus stability; however, it is now believed to be the primary restraint to varus stress (18,37).

The deeper lamina runs along the posterolateral meniscus and comprises the coronary ligament (20). This layer then ends in the arcuate ligament. The arcuate ligament spans from the styloid process of the fibular head, and it interdigitates with and crosses over the popliteus muscle–tendon junction. It inserts in the pos-

terior capsule near the termination of the oblique popliteal ligament (Figs. 4-11 and 4-12). This deeper lamina is always separated from the LCL by the inferior lateral geniculate artery, which also separates the fabellofibular ligament from the arcuate ligament (Figs. 4-11 and 4-12) (26,44).

The term "short lateral ligament" appears in descriptive anatomy articles (26,31). It is unclear whether this structure is the arcuate ligament, the fabellofibular ligament, or a different ligamentous structure from these two. Kaplan (26) called the fabellofibular ligament the true short lateral ligament. However, when the fabellofibular ligament is not present (due to absence of the fabella), he described the lateral fibers of the arcuate as constituting the short lateral ligament. It is confusing to label ligaments by giving them different names depending on how large they are or depending on what other ligaments are present. Since the inferior lateral geniculate artery runs between the arcuate and fabellofibular ligaments and clearly separates them, it seems reasonable to simply use the term "arcuate ligament" for that which runs deep to the

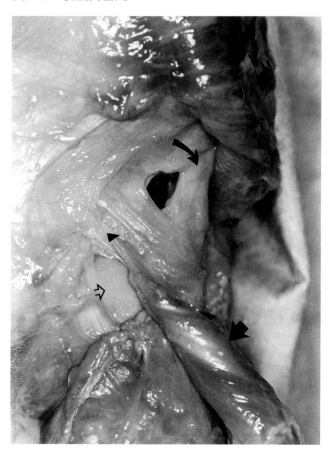

FIG. 4-13. In a right knee, the popliteus has been detached from the tibia and rolled laterally (*closed arrow*). The arrowhead is on the interdigitation of fibers from the popliteus and arcuate ligament with the posterior aspect of the lateral meniscus. The curved arrow is on the popliteus tendon as it runs toward its femoral attachment. The open arrow is on the tibial articular cartilage.

artery and crosses over the popliteus. Likewise, it seems reasonable to call the structure from the lateral head of the gastrocnemius to the fibular styloid which is superficial to the inferior lateral geniculate artery the "fabellofibular ligament" (44). The term "short lateral ligament" would then be deleted. Seebacher (26) and Kaplan (44) have pointed out that the fabellofibular ligament is usually attenuated when the fabella is not present, conversely, this ligament is very robust when a large fabella is present.

Most current articles on surgical repair of this area do not delineate the anatomy in such a detailed fashion. In fact, De Lee (15) said it was of no particular significance. He and others refer to this area simply as the "arcuate complex," which is made up of the arcuate ligament, the LCL, the popliteus, and the lateral head of the gastrocnemius (8,21,22,24).

The popliteus originates obliquely over the posterior proximal tibia and is covered by its own fascial investment. It has a firm connection to the posterior horn of the lateral meniscus and to the arcuate ligament as well (Fig. 4-13) (32). It then runs extrasynovially within the joint and terminates on the lateral femoral condyle, just distal and slightly posterior to the femoral attachment of the LCL (12). It is important to understand the complex attachment of the popliteus to the lateral

meniscus, arcuate ligament, posterior capsule, and lateral femoral condyle in order to appreciate the role it can play in static stability. It is not simply a muscle–tendon unit with simple origin and insertion from tibia to femur.

The posterior capsule is attached to the popliteal surface of the femur, proximal to the femoral condyles and inferiorly to the upper surface of the tibia (20). The capsule is thin over the posterior aspect of the femoral condyles, where it is supported by the two heads of the gastrocnemius. The medial head of the gastrocnemius originates slightly more proximally than the lateral head. The capsule is reinforced by the oblique popliteal ligament, which runs diagonally from the semimembranosus tendon sheath toward the lateral head of the gastrocnemius. The capsule is also reinforced by the arcuate ligament laterally as has been described (Fig. 4-14).

CRUCIATE LIGAMENT ANATOMY

Histologic Anatomy

The anterior and posterior cruciate ligaments (ACL and PCL, respectively) are intracapsular but extra-

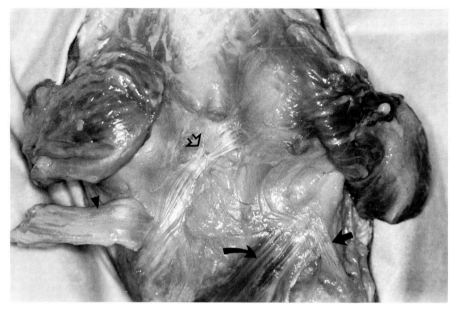

FIG. 4-14. The posterior capsule of a right knee. The two heads of the gastrocnemius have been transected and displaced medially and laterally. The open arrow indicates the oblique popliteal ligament. The arrowhead is on the semimembranosus tendon, the curved arrow is on the popliteus, and the closed arrow is on the arcuate ligament.

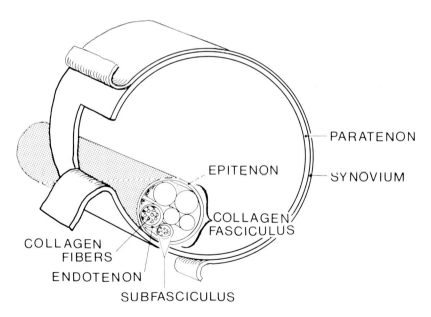

FIG. 4-15. A diagrammatic view of a cruciate ligament down to the collagen fiber level.

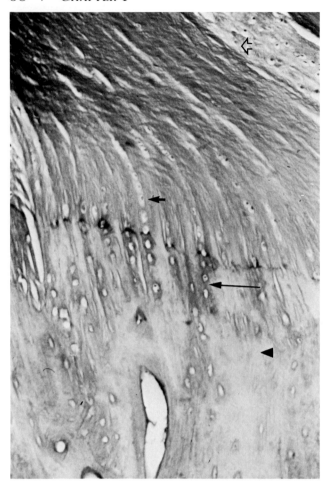

FIG. 4-16. Photomicrograph of the anterior cruciate insertion. The open arrow is on the ligament (zone I). The small closed arrow is on zone II. The long arrow is on zone III, while the arrowhead is on zone IV. (Photomicrograph courtesy of Dr. Steven Arnoczky.)

synovial ligaments. These ligaments appear crossed (hence "cruciate") on viewing the knee anteriorly or laterally (39). Most of the microscopic anatomy has been done on the ACL by Danylchuk (14). The ligament is composed of collagen fibrils, 150–250 μm in diameter, which appear parallel at high magnification. These fibrils form fibers 1–20 μm in diameter, and the majority of these fibers run parallel to the long axis of the ligament. A large number of collagen fibers merge together to make the subfascicular unit, which varies from 100 to 250 μm. A thin band of loose connective tissue called the *endotenon* surrounds the subfasciculus. In humans the amount of endotenon is great, which makes the ligament appear to be made of bundles and less uniform. Three to 20 subfasciculi are bound together to form the collagen fasciculus, which ranges from 250 μm to several millimeters in diameter. The epitenon then surrounds the fasciculus and is more dense than the endotenon. Surrounding the entire ligament is the paratenon, which blends with the epitenon. The synovium then covers the ligament, thus making it extrasynovial (Fig. 4-15).

An important aspect of cruciate anatomy is the change from flexible ligamentous tissue to rigid bone, mediated by a transitional zone of fibrocartilage and mineralized cartilage (Fig. 4-16) (4). This helps prevent stress concentration at the attachment site by allowing a gradual change in stiffness (4). Cooper (13) characterized four discrete regions in this transition. Zone I is composed of wavy collagen fibers. Zone II is the fibrocartilage zone with chondrocytes being the predominant cell. In zone III the ground substance becomes mineralized. In zone IV the bone matrix collagen fibers blend with the mineralized fibrocartilage. A dark stained line is seen between zones II and III (Fig. 4-16).

Vascular Anatomy

The cruciate ligaments are covered by a synovial fold that originates at the posterior inlet of the intercondylar notch and extends to the anterior tibial insertion of the ACL (4,7,33,41). Here it joins with the synovium from the joint capsule distal to the fat pad. The predominant source of blood supply is the middle geniculate artery, which leaves the popliteal artery and directly pierces the posterior capsule (2,4,5,7,33,41). Figure 4-17 shows the vascularity of both the ACL and the PCL. The cruciates have an arborization of the

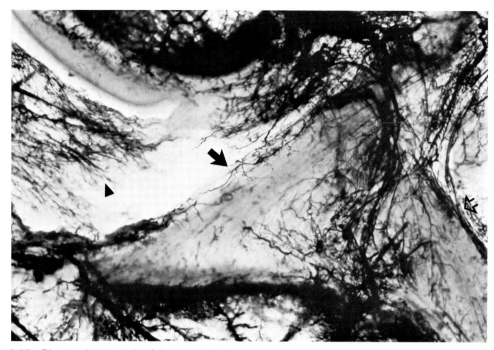

FIG. 4-17. Photomicrograph of the vascularity to the cruciate ligaments. The arrowhead indicates the fat pad. The closed arrow is on the anterior edge of the ACL. The open arrow is on the posterior edge of the PCL. (From ref. 4.)

vessels which penetrate the ligament transversely. These vessels anastomose with endoligamentous vessels that lie parallel to the collagen bundles in the ligaments (4,33). The osseous attachments of the cruciates contribute little to their vascularity (7,33). There is a significant blood supply from the fat pad via the inferior medial and lateral geniculate arteries, which may play a more important role when the ligament is injured (6,7).

Neurologic Anatomy

Nerve fibers, of the size most consistent with transmitting pain, are readily visualized in the intrafascicular spaces occupied by the vessels (28,43). These are presumably terminal branches from the tibial nerve in the popliteal fossa (30). In 1984, Schultz (42) investigated mechanoreceptors in cruciate ligaments and

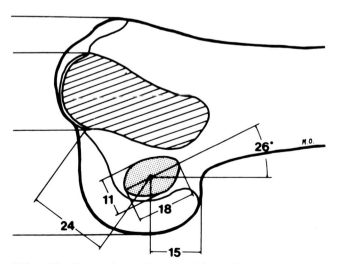

FIG. 4-18. Femoral attachment of the ACL as determined by Odensten. The measurements are in millimeters. (From ref. 38.)

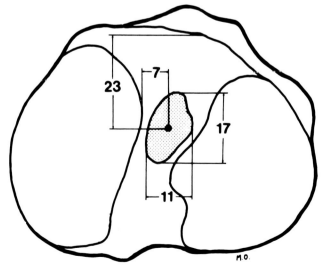

FIG. 4-19. Tibial attachment of ACL with measurements in millimeters as determined by Odensten. (From ref. 38.)

found a few thin axons in the substance of the ligaments, as well as bundles of axons running on the surface of the ligament. "Mechanoreceptors" were identified in the ligament and were felt to be similar to golgi tendon organs. They were mostly on the surface of the ligament, well beneath the synovial lining and primarily at the insertion sites. They were postulated to respond as proprioceptors and to signal potentially injurious deformation of the ligaments and joint. Schutte (43) studied the neuroanatomy of the human ACL and found three morphological types of mechanoreceptors as well as free nerve endings. The three mechanoreceptors were as follows: Ruffini endings, which are slow-adapting and respond to slight changes in ligament tension; a second type of Ruffini mechanoreceptor, which is also slow-adapting, resembling a golgi tendon organ; and a pacinian corpuscle, which is a rapidly adapting mechanoreceptor. Free nerve endings for transmitting pain were also identified but were far more scarce than the mechanoreceptors.

Insertion Site Anatomy

The bony attachments of the cruciates have been investigated by several authors. In 1975, Girgis (17) presented the ACL and PCL attachments in detail. More recently, Odensten (38) published his examinations of the ACL. In our laboratory, dissections were performed on ACLs and PCLs, measuring orientation and anatomy of the cruciate insertions for comparison with the prior two studies; for the most part, our findings concur with those of Odensten. Compared to Girgis, the ACL femoral attachment of Odensten is oval and therefore wider (Fig. 4-18) (38). The overall location, however, is fairly similar to that of Girgis (17). Tibial ACL attachments are shown for the Odensten study in Fig. 4-19. All authors agree that the femoral attachment is oriented primarily in the longitudinal axis of the femur, and the tibial attachment is longitudinal in the anteroposterior axis of the tibia. This arrangement leads to the well-known twist of the ACL fibers when

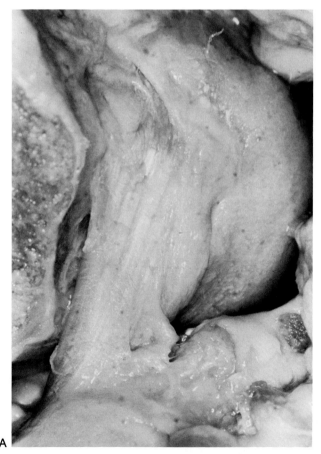
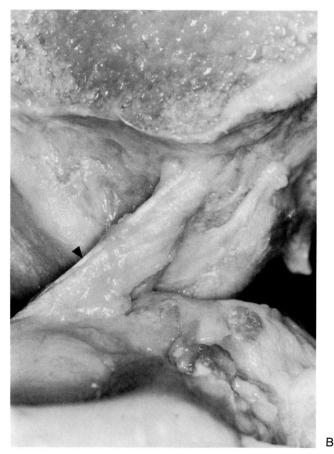

A

B

FIG. 4-20. A: A right knee in full extension with the medial femoral condyle removed. B: The same knee in 90° of flexion showing the twist of the ACL fibers. The arrowhead indicates the anteromedial fibers which are taut.

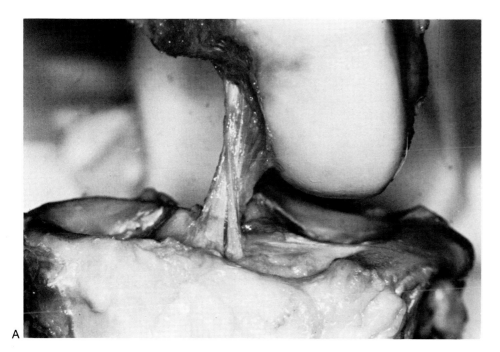

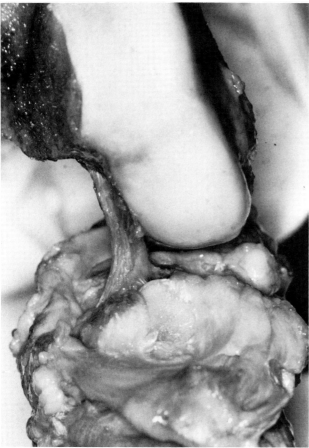

FIG. 4-21. **A:** An anterior view of a left knee. The medial femoral condyle and all ligaments except the ACL have been removed. The tibia is being held in its normal position. **B:** The same knee with the tibia being allowed to rotate freely. Note the 90° internal rotation of the tibia in relation to the femur.

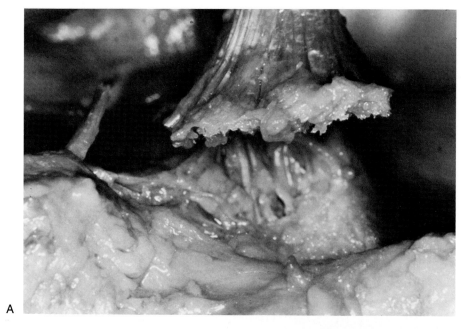

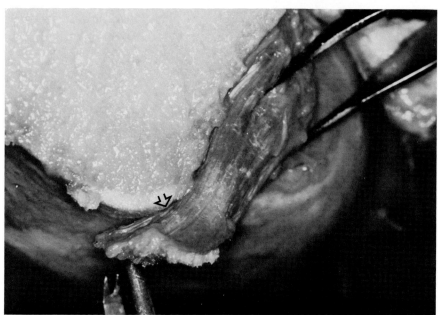

FIG. 4-22. A: An anterior view of a right knee with tibial attachment of the ACL avulsed from the tibia, demonstrating the "foot" region. **B:** A lateral view of the same knee with the ACL held in the normal position for full knee extension. The open arrow is on the area of potential impingement.

the knee moves from extension to flexion (Fig. 4-20A and B) (17). There is also a twist of the ACL fibers in the coronal plane with external rotation of the fibers by approximately 90° as they approach the tibial surface (38). In 1986, van Rens (47) reported that in dogs, cutting of all ligaments except the ACL and letting the tibia hang free resulted in a 180° derotation in a normal ACL. The same relationship in a human knee, which agrees with the 90° twist of the fibers described by

Odensten, is shown in Fig. 4-21A and B. In the saggital plane, the average angle between the long axis of the femur and the ACL with the knee flexed 90° is 28° ± 4° (38).

The ACL tibial attachment fans out and forms a "foot" region. This allows the ACL to tuck under the roof of the intercondylar notch (Fig. 4-22A and B). This unique attachment of the ACL causes concern for a certain ACL reconstruction technique. If an anteriorly

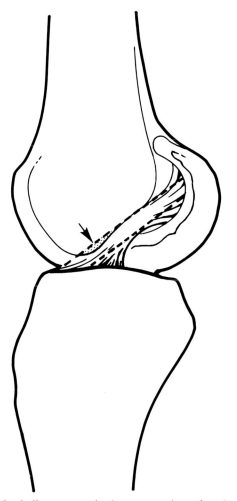

FIG. 4-23. A diagrammatic demonstration of replacing an ACL with a "foot" region by a straight graft. If the anterior fibers of the ACL are used as a guide for the drill hole, the dashed line representing the anterior edge of the new graft is seen to intersect with the notch when the knee is in full extension. This dotted area (*arrow*) is the location of possible impingement.

placed drill hole is used with a graft whose fibers do not possess a "foot"-type region, the graft might be predisposed to impingement on the roof of the inter-condylar notch. As one can see in Fig. 4-23, a dashed line representing the borders of a straight graft material is shown to impinge on the notch with the knee in full extension. However, with the same starting point, the fibers of a normal ACL can slip under this point as a result of their sweeping nature.

The PCL femoral attachment as determined by Gir-gis (17) is half-moon-shaped as shown in Fig. 4-24. Our mapping of the femoral attachment of the PCL in 15 specimens showed it to be 21 mm × 10 mm with the longitudinal axis in the anteroposterior plane of the femur. However, the attachment is positioned more at the apex of the intercondylar notch, and less so on the inner wall (Fig. 4-26A and Fig. 4-27A and B). As one

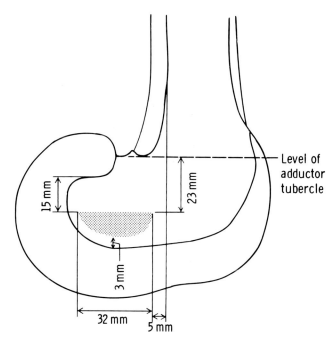

FIG. 4-24. Diagrammatic representation of the femoral attachment of the PCL. (From ref. 17.)

can see in Fig. 4-26A, if the meniscofemoral ligaments are included, the femoral attachment appears larger, closer to the articular cartilage, and more on the inner wall. The tibial attachment of the PCL is below the level of the joint (in the middle of the posterior tibia) and is rectangular in shape. The mapping of this area by Girgis is shown in Fig. 4-25. It is important to note that although the tibial attachment of the PCL is significantly below the joint surface, it is intraarticular to the posterior capsular attachment (22).

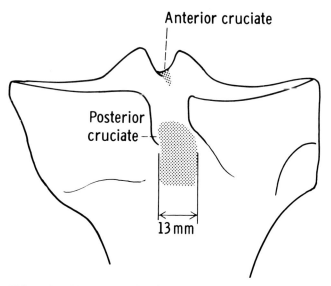

FIG. 4-25. Diagrammatic tibial attachment of the PCL. (From ref. 17.)

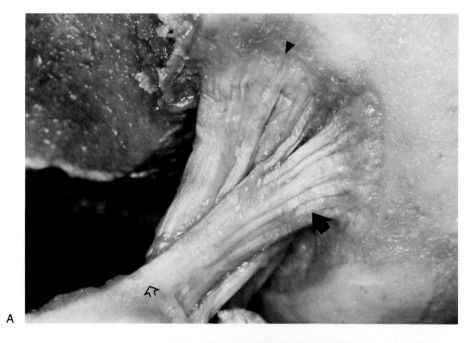

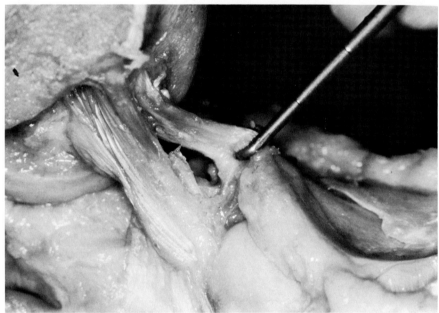

FIG. 4-26. A: A right knee with the lateral femoral condyle and ACL removed. The closed arrow is on the ligament of Humphrey. The open arrow indicates the same fibers as they join the posterior horn of the lateral meniscus. The arrowhead shows where the PCL attaches more on the roof of the intercondylar notch and not soley on the inner wall of the medial femoral condyle. **B:** A posterior view of the same knee with a probe on the ligament of Humphrey.

The ligaments of Humphrey and of Wrisberg are intimate with the PCL femoral attachment and are meniscofemoral ligaments that run from the posterior horn of the lateral meniscus to blend with the PCL (19). In Fig. 4-26A and B, a ligament of Humphrey is shown as it runs to insert anterior to the PCL. The ligament of Wrisberg attaches on the posterior aspect of the femoral insertion of the PCL.

Fiber Orientation

Many authors have described anatomically separate bands in the ACL and the PCL (1,16,17). For the ACL, the bands are called *anteromedial* and *posterolateral*, with some including an intermediate band (36). The appearance of anatomically different bands may be due to the increased amount of loose connective tissue (en-

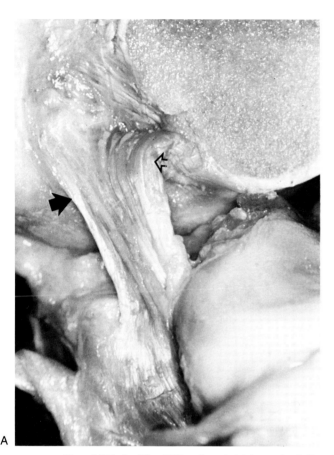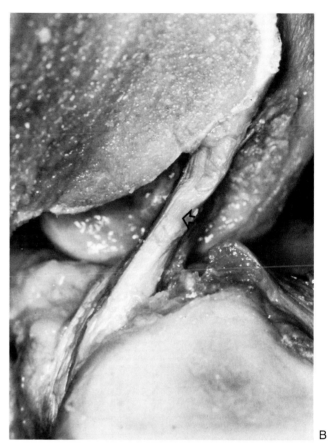

A

B

Fig. 4-27. A: The PCL of a right knee in full extension viewed posteriorly. The closed arrow is on the tight posterior fibers (posteromedial band) of the PCL, and the open arrow is on the more lax anterior fibers. **B:** The same knee in 90° of knee flexion. The more anterior fibers (anterolateral band) are now tight (*open arrow*).

dotenon) that is seen in human cruciate ligaments (14,28). Although there is disagreement on the actual anatomic division of the ligament, it seems agreed that ACLs have "functional bands" so that tension is varied among the fibers in the ligament with range of motion (4).

For the ACL, the anteromedial part is tighter in flexion and the posterolateral part is tighter in extension (Fig. 4-20A and B) (16,17). Hughston (22) refers to the PCL as having an anterolateral band and a posteromedial band. In extension, the posterior fibers are taut, whereas the bulk of the ligament is relaxed (Fig. 4-27A) (17,22). Conversely, the more posterior fibers become lax in flexion, whereas the remainder (anterolateral) become taut (Fig. 4-27B).

REFERENCES

1. Abbott LS, Saunders JB, De CM, Bost FC, Anderson CE. Injuries to the ligaments of the knee joint. *J Bone Joint Surg* 1944;26:503–521.
2. Alm A, Stromberg G. Vascular anatomy of the patellar and cruciate ligaments: a microangiographic and histologic investigation in the dog. *Acta Chir Scand [Suppl]* 1974;44:25–35.
3. Arms S, Boyle J, Johnson R, Pope M. Strain measurement in the medial collateral ligament of the human knee: an autopsy study. *J Biomech* 1983;16(7):491–496.
4. Arnoczky SP. Anatomy of the anterior cruciate ligament. *Clin Orthop* 1983;172:19–25.
5. Arnoczky SP. Blood supply to the anterior cruciate ligament and supporting structures. *Orthop Clin North Am* 1985;16(1):15–28.
6. Arnockzky SP. The vascularity of the anterior cruciate ligament and associated structures. In: Jackson DW, Drez D Jr, eds. *The anterior cruciate deficient knee*. St. Louis: CV Mosby, 1987;27–54.
7. Arnoczky SP, Rubin RM, Marshall JL. Microvasculature of the cruciate ligaments and its response to injury. *J Bone Joint Surg* 1979;61A:1221–1229.
8. Baker CL, Norwood LA Jr, Hughston JC. Acute posterolateral rotary instability of the knee. *J Bone Joint Surg* 1983;65A:614–618.
9. Bartel DL, Marshall JL, Schieck, RA, Wang JB. Surgical repositioning of the medial collateral ligament. *J Bone Joint Surg* 1977;59A:107–116.
10. Brantigan OC, Voshell AF. The mechanics of the ligaments and menisci of the knee joint. *J Bone Joint Surg* 1941;23:44–66.
11. Brantigan OC, Voshell AF. The tibial collateral ligament: its function, its bursae, and its relation to the medial meniscus. *J Bone Joint Surg* 1943;25:121–131.

12. Cohn AK, Mains DB. Popliteal hiatus of the lateral meniscus. *Am J Sports Med* 1979;7(4):221–226.
13. Cooper RR, Misol S. Tendon and ligament insertion: a light and electron microscopic study. *J Bone Joint Surg* 1970;52A:1–20.
14. Danylchuk KD, Finlay JB, Kreck JP. Microstructural organization of human and bovine cruciate ligaments. *Clin Orthop* 1978;131:294–298.
15. De Lee JC, Riley MB, Rockwood CA Jr. Acute posterolateral rotary instability of the knee. *Am J Sports Med* 1983;11(4):199–206.
16. Furman W, Marshall JL, Girgis FG. The anterior cruciate ligament: a functional analysis based on postmortem studies. *J Bone Joint Surg* 1976;58A:179–185.
17. Girgis FG, Marshall JL, Al Monajem ARS. The cruciate ligaments of the knee joint: anatomical, functional and experimental analysis. *Clin Orthop* 1975;106:216–231.
18. Grood ES, Noyes FR, Butler DL, Suntay WJ. Ligamentous and capsular restraints preventing medial and lateral laxity in intact human cadaver knees. *J Bone Joint Surg* 1981;63A:1257–1269.
19. Heller L, Langman J. The menisco-femoral ligaments of the human knee. *J Bone Joint Surg* 1964;46B:307–313.
20. Hollinshead WJ. *Anatomy for surgeons, vol III: the back and limbs.* New York: Harper & Row, 1969.
21. Hughston JC, Andrews JR, Cross MJ, Moschi A. Classification of knee ligament instabilities part II: the lateral compartment. *J Bone Joint Surg* 1976;58A:173–179.
22. Hughston JC, Bowden JA, Andrews JR, Norwood LA. Acute tears of the posterior cruciate ligament. *J Bone Joint Surg* 1980;62A:438–450.
23. Hughston JC, Eilers AF. The role of the posterior oblique ligament in repairs of acute medial (collateral) ligament tears of the knee. *J Bone Joint Surg* 1973;55A:923–940.
24. Hughston JC, Norwood LA Jr. The posterolateral drawer test and external rotational recurvatum test for posterolateral rotary instability of the knee. *Clin Orthop* 1980;147:82–87.
25. Kaplan EP. The iliotibial tract. *J Bone Joint Surg* 1958;40A:817–832.
26. Kaplan EB. The fabellofibular and short lateral ligaments of the knee joint. *J Bone Joint Surg* 1961;43A:169–179.
27. Kaplan EB. Some aspects of functional anatomy of the human knee joints. *Clin Orthop* 1962;23:18–29.
28. Kennedy JC, Alexander IJ, Hayes KC. Nerve supply of the human knee and its functional importance. *Am J Sports Med* 1982;10(6):329–335.
29. Kennedy JC, Fowler PJ. Medial and anterior instability of the knee. *J Bone Joint Surg* 1971;53A:1257–1270.
30. Kennedy JC, Weinberg HW, Wilson AS. The anatomy and functions of the anterior cruciate ligament. *J Bone Joint Surg* 1974;56A:223–235.
31. Last RJ. Some anatomical details of the knee joint. *J Bone Joint Surg* 1948;30B:683–688.
32. Last RJ. The popliteus muscle and the lateral meniscus. *J Bone Joint Surg* 1950;32B:93–99.
33. Marshall JL, Arnoczky SP, Rubin RM, Wickiewicz TL. Micro-vasculature of the cruciate ligaments. *Physician Sports Med* 1979;7(3):87–91.
34. Marshall JL, Girgis FG, Zelko RR. The biceps femoris tendon and its functional significance. *J Bone Joint Surg* 1972;54A:1444–1450.
35. Müller W. *The knee form, function, and ligament reconstruction.* Berlin: Springer-Verlag, 1983.
36. Norwood LA, Cross MJ. Anterior cruciate ligament: functional anatomy of its bundles in rotary instabilities. *Am J Sports Med* 1979;7(1):23–26.
37. Noyes FR, Grood ES, Butler DL, Paulos LE. Clinical biomechanics of the knee: ligamentous restraints and functional stability. In: Funk FJ, Jr, ed. *American Academy of Orthopedic Surgeons' Symposium on the Athlete's Knee.* St. Louis: CV Mosby, 1980; 1–35.
38. Odensten M, Gillquist J. Functional anatomy of the anterior cruciate ligament and a rationale for reconstruction. *J Bone Joint Surg* 1985;67A:257–261.
39. Palmer I. On injuries to the ligaments of the knee joint: a clinical study. *Acta Chir Scand [Suppl]* 1938;53.
40. Reider B, Marshall JL, Koslin RT, Elmsford BR, Girgis FG. The anterior aspect of the knee joint. *J Bone Joint Surg* 1981;63A:351–356.
41. Scapinelli R. Studies on the vasculature of the human knee joint. *Acta Anat* 1968;70(3):305–331.
42. Schultz RA, Miller DC, Kerr CS, Micheli L. Mechanoreceptors in human cruciate ligaments. *J Bone Joint Surg* 1984;66A:1072–1076.
43. Schutte MJ, Dabezies EJ, Zimny Ml, Happel LT. Neural anatomy of the human anterior cruciate ligament. *J Bone Joint Surg* 1987;69A:243–247.
44. Seebacher JR, Inglis AE, Marshall JL, Warren RF. The structure of the posterolateral aspect of the knee. *J Bone Joint Surg* 1982;64A:536–541.
45. Slocum DB, Larson RL, James SI. Late reconstruction of ligamentous injuries of the medial compartment of the knee. *Clin Orthop* 1974;100:23–55.
46. Terry GC, Hughston JD, Norwood LA. The anatomy of the iliopatellar band and iliotibial tract. *Am J Sports Med* 1986;14:39–45.
47. van Rens TJG, van den Berg AF, Huiskes R, Kuypers W. Substitution of the anterior cruciate ligament: a long-term histologic and biomechanical study with autogenous pedicled grafts of the iliotibial band in dogs. *Arthroscopy* 1986;2(3):139–154.
48. Wang CJ, Walker PS, Wolf B. The effects of flexion and rotation on the length patterns of the ligaments of the knee. *J Biomech* 1973;6:587–596.
49. Warren LF, Marshall JL. The supporting structures and layers on the medial side of the knee. *J Bone Joint Surg* 1979;61A:56–62.
50. Warren LF, Marshall JL, Girgis F. The prime static stabilizer of the medial side of the knee. *J Bone Joint Surg* 1974;56A:665–674.

Knee Ligaments: Structure, Function, Injury, and Repair, edited by D. Daniel, et al.
© 1990 by Raven Press, Ltd. All rights reserved.

CHAPTER 5

Ligament Structure, Chemistry, and Physiology

David Amiel, E. Billings, Jr., and Wayne H. Akeson

For many years, tendons and ligaments have been classified together as dense, regularly arranged connective tissue (14,18,32). It became common to think of these tissues as "similar" to the point that the terms "tendon" and "ligament" were sometimes used interchangeably in the literature (1,5,53).

Although both are organized, regular connective tissue, they are entirely different functionally. Tendons are a conduit connecting muscle to bone, thereby allowing movement of a joint complex through muscle contraction or relaxation. Ligaments, on the other hand, are short bands of fibrous tissue which bind bone to bone and provide support for internal organs. Ligaments are relatively inelastic. In concert with the bony geometry and the dynamic effects of muscle and tendon (51,55), they limit and guide joint motion. The functional differences between ligaments and tendons prompted a more thorough evaluation with regard to their histological and biochemical properties. Substantial differences were noted in this assessment (6).

This chapter describes ligamentous tissue through its recognized constitutional differences with tendon, and it also attempts to ascribe these differences to function.

STRUCTURE

The histology of periarticular tendons and ligaments is a much neglected area of investigation. As mentioned

above, most histology texts combine these tissues with the reticuloendothelial system and describe them as "dense, regular connective tissue" (4,12,35,65). This description is accurate but incomplete. Certain types of ligaments and tendons are sufficiently characteristic to be distinguishable from each other based upon their histological appearance (Fig. 5-1). This distinction is analogous to the microscopic dissimilarity between cardiac and skeletal muscle tissues.

The following histological analysis describes some of the basic differences among a variety of tendons and ligaments. The variables considered are collagen bundle width, cell morphology and size, as well as "crimp." Crimp is a feature of both tendons and ligaments, and it represents a regular sinusoidal pattern in the matrix. The periodicity and amplitude of crimp appear to be structure-specific features, and they are best evaluated under polarized light. The simple functional explanation for this accordion-like pattern in the matrix is that it provides a "buffer" in which slight longitudinal elongation may occur without fibrous damage. It also provides a mechanism for control of tension and acts as a "shock absorber" along the length of the tissue. When physiologic mechanical limits of this crimp are exceeded, however, irreversible damage occurs and the physical properties of the tissue are changed (70).

Although both ligaments and tendons have crimping within their fascicles, there appear to be differences in the crimp pattern between these two structures (72). In the canine anterior cruciate ligament (ACL) and patellar tendon, two patterns of crimping are noted. The centrally located fascicles in the ACL are either

D. Amiel, E. Billings, Jr., and W. H. Akeson: Department of Surgery, Division of Orthopaedics and Rehabilitation, University of California, San Diego, School of Medicine, La Jolla, California 92093.

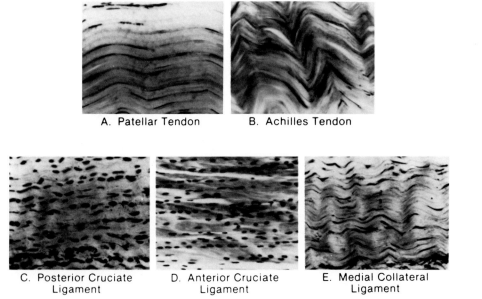

A. Patellar Tendon

B. Achilles Tendon

C. Posterior Cruciate
Ligament

D. Anterior Cruciate
Ligament

E. Medial Collateral
Ligament

FIG. 5-1. Midsubstance frozen sections of various tendons and ligaments [hematoxylin and eosin (H&E), original magnification ×250]. (From ref. 6.)

straight or undulated in a planar wave pattern (Fig. 5-2), whereas those located at the periphery are arranged in a helical wave pattern (Fig. 5-3). In the patellar tendon, all the fascicles are found to undulate in the helical wave pattern.

The following histological description refers to rabbit tendons and ligaments unless otherwise specified.

Microscopic examination of patellar tendon sections that have been stained with hematoxylin and eosin, or evaluated directly under polarized light, reveals the presence of longitudinally oriented bundles of collagenous tissue. These bundles are approximately 20 μm in width and have the characteristic crimp pattern of regular connective tissue. In patellar tendon, the crimp

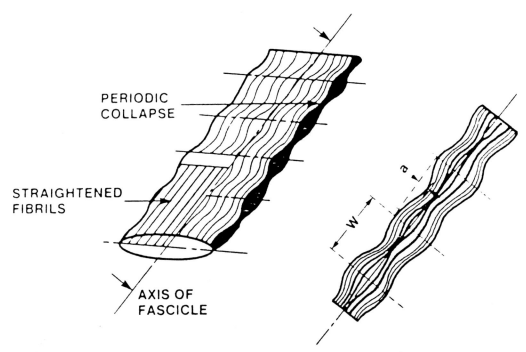

PERIODIC COLLAPSE

STRAIGHTENED FIBRILS

AXIS OF FASCICLE

FIG. 5-2. Schematic diagram of the collagenous fascicle showing the planar waveform model. (From ref. 72.)

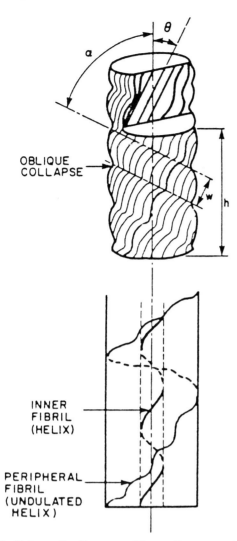

OBLIQUE
COLLAPSE

INNER
FIBRIL
(HELIX)

PERIPHERAL
FIBRIL
(UNDULATED
HELIX)

FIG. 5-3. Schematic diagram of the collagenous fascicle showing the helical wave form model. θ, helix angle; α, inclination angle; w, wavelength; h, apparent half-pitch. (From ref. 72.)

period is approximately 120 μm in length, with a corresponding amplitude of about 15 μm. On either side of the bundles or fascicles, spindle-shaped fibroblasts approximately 25 μm in length are observed. These are aligned longitudinally. Cytoplasm is indistinct, and only nuclei can be seen. More cellular areas within areolar connective tissue are observed. These sites, which are actually investing layers of tissue, are called "peritendineum" (Fig. 5-4) and have been previously described as a site of reserve cells (36). They also mark the site of nerve and blood supply to the tendon.

Rabbit Achilles tendon demonstrates cell morphology, cell size, bundle width, and crimp period that are similar to those of patellar tendon. A difference between the crimp amplitude of these tissues is present, with Achilles tendon having almost three times (40 μm) the wave height relative to patellar tendon. This may

relate to an increased margin of shock absorbance for this tendon.

Histological assessment of the ACL demonstrates longitudinally oriented bundles of collagen with a width of about 20 μm as seen in the patellar tendon. The crimp period in the cruciate ACL, however, is considerably shorter (45–60 μm), and the amplitude is less than 5 μm. Fibroblasts are located on either side of the collagenous bundles, but the ligament is considerably more cellular than the tendon (Fig. 5-5). ACL fibroblasts are round to ovoid and are substantially different in appearance from the fibroblasts in the patellar tendon. They measure about 5–8 μm in diameter and 12–15 μm in length. Cells are arranged longitudinally along the borders of the fascicles. Like the patellar tendon, groups of cells which concentrate in areolar connective tissue are observed (Fig. 5-5). These have not been previously described and may be the ligamentous correlate to the peritendineum areas.

The medial collateral ligament (MCL) of the knee is notable for rod-shaped and spindle-shaped cells of length intermediate to patellar tendon and ACL cells. The MCL is observed to have cells measuring 15 μm in length and 3–5 μm in width. Crimp period measures approximately 45 μm with a 10-μm amplitude, and collagen bundle width is approximately 20 μm as seen in the other structures discussed. Measurements of cell size, shape, crimp specifics, and bundle width of the tendons and ligaments are provided in Table 5-1.

Assessment of the ACL and the MCL by transmission electron microscopy (TEM) characterizes the ultrastructural differences and illustrates the heterogeneity of these two periarticular ligaments (41). The fibrils of the ACL exhibit a wide range of diameters. The fibroblasts are ovoid and lie in columns between layers of compact parallel bundles of collagen fibrils (Fig. 5-6A and B). These fibroblasts have abundant cellular organelles, indicating a high level of cellular activity. These cells have multiple small cellular processes, or microvilli, which project into a surrounding area of amorphous ground substance with reticular fibers but not into the compact parallel collagen fibrils.

The MCL has predominantly large-diameter collagen fibrils. The MCL fibroblasts are spindle-shaped and lie in the midst of compact parallel collagen fibrils with little or no surrounding amorphous ground substance (Fig. 6C and D). These fibroblasts have an abundance of cellular organelles, indicating a high level of cellular activity. They also have long thin cellular processes extending from the main body of the cell out into the areas of densely packed collagen fibrils.

These substantial differences in morphology and ultrastructure may reflect both the functional and environmental differences between these two periarticular ligaments, the ACL and MCL. The cellular morphological characteristics of the MCL are those of

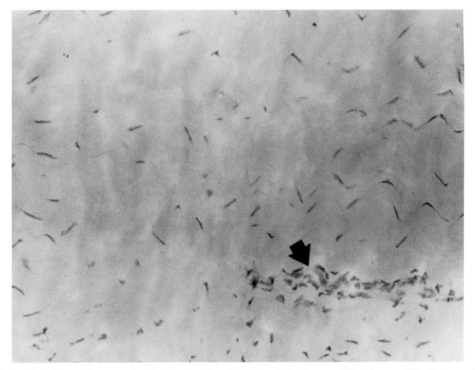

FIG. 5-4. Histology of normal patellar tendon (H&E, original magnification ×50). Note spindle-shaped fibroblasts, coarse fibrillar crimp, and peritendineum (*arrow*).

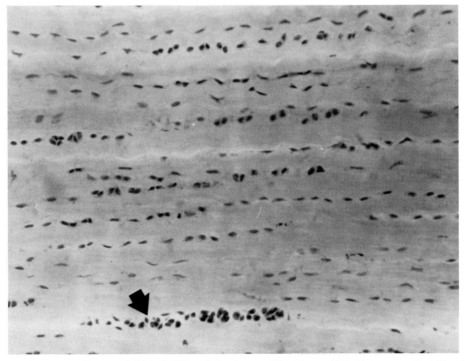

FIG. 5-5. Histology of normal ACL (H&E, original magnification ×50). Note rounded fibroblasts, fine fibrillar crimp and cluster of potential reserve cells (*arrow*).

TABLE 5-1. *Summary of histological observations of rabbit periarticular connective tissue[a]*

Tissue	Collagen bundle width (μm)	Crimp period (μm)	Crimp amplitude (μm)	Cell shape	Cell size (μm × μm)
Patellar tendon	20	120	15	Spindle	3–5 × 15
Achilles tendon	20	120	40	Spindle	3–5 × 15
Anterior cruciate ligament	20	45–60	<5	Round to ovoid	5–8 × 12–15
Medial collateral ligament	20	45	10	Rod to spindle	3–5 × 15

[a] From ref. 7.

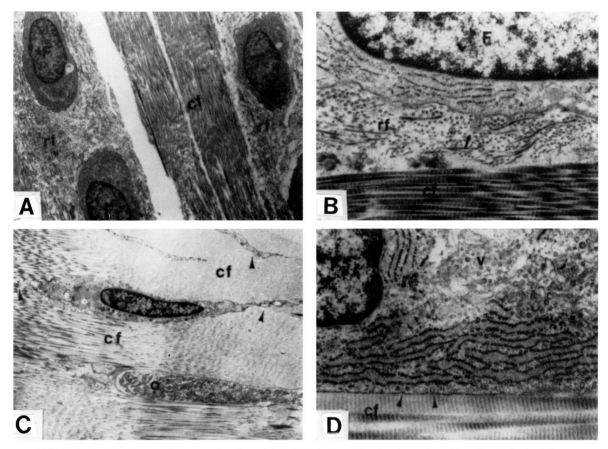

FIG. 5-6. A: Electron micrograph of a rabbit ACL in longitudinal section. The fibroblasts (F) are ovoid and arranged into rows between compact parallel collagen fibril bundles (cf). These fibroblasts have many microvilli that extend into the surrounding area of amorphous ground substance and reticular fibers (rf). **B:** Electron micrograph showing a rabbit ACL in longitudinal section. The fibroblast (F) has an abundance of organelles and microvilli (*arrow*) extending out into an area of reticular fibers (rf) which surrounds the cell. The well-organized, compact parallel collagen fibrils (cf) are separated from the cell membrane by this area of amorphous ground substance. **C:** Electron micrograph of a rabbit MCL in longitudinal section, demonstrating fibroblasts (F) with abundant organelles (o) lying in the midst of compact parallel collagen fibrils (cf). These cells have long cellular processes extending out between compact fibrils (*arrowheads*). **D:** Electron micrograph showing a high-power view of an MCL fibroblast (F) that has its cell membrane immediately adjacent to the compact parallel collagen fibrils (cf). The cytoplasm has an abundance of cellular organelles and vesicles (v). Note the vesicles along the cell membrane which are presumably emptying their contents into the extracellular space (*arrowheads*).

all fibroblasts, whereas the ACL cellular characteristics are similar to fibrocartilage cells. These observations lead to a series of profound and important questions concerning the differences in function, homeostasis, and repair between the ACL and MCL.

BIOCHEMISTRY

The biochemical parameters used to assess the constitutional properties of collagenous tissue include collagen typing, collagen reducible and nonreducible crosslink analysis, and ground substance content. The value of each of these variables relates to its importance in the study of both (a) soft tissue injury and healing and (b) the response to exercise and the deleterious effects of immobilization. It is obvious that a more complete understanding of these problems could improve various treatment modalities and place them on firm scientific ground. This is particularly the case when one considers that most investigations of tissue injury and healing involve skin and not tendons and ligaments (17,19,30).

Collagen is the key protein for the stabilization of the musculoskeletal system. It provides the mechanical properties that impart the "connect" function to connective tissue. It constitutes 65–80% of the mass by dry weight of specialized connective tissues such as tendon, ligament, skin, joint capsule, and cartilage.

Tropocollagen

The collagen molecule is one of the largest in the body, appearing rod-like with dimensions of 300 nm in length and 1.5 nm in diameter. These rods are termed "tropocollagen." They are assembled in a three-dimensional array in the extracellular environment, being influenced by environmental stresses and additional biologic factors. The sum of these extracellular influences affects the orientation and size of fibrils that are assembled from the tropocollagen units. The assembly is typically patterned in a quarter stagger (Fig. 5-7), which is seen as 64-nm subbonding on transmission electron micrographs. A small gap exists between the head-to-tail linear assembly of the tropocollagen units and may be of functional importance in bone as a nucleation site of apatite crystals in the process of matrix mineralization of osteoid (23).

The individual tropocollagen units are made up of three chains that are independently synthesized in the manner of other proteins. The length of the messenger RNA molecule required for the synthesis is extraordinary, since each chain contains about 1000 amino acids. Most of the chains (called α chains) are precisely ordered with a general sequence of glycine-proline-hydroxyproline, glycine-proline-x-, or glycine-x-proline,

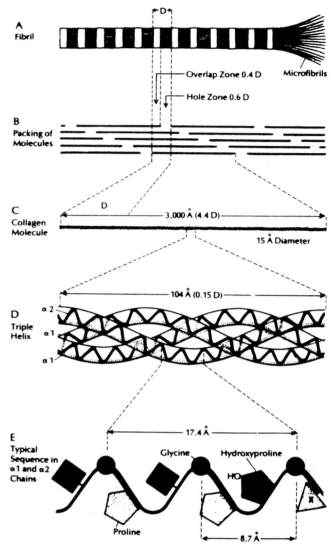

FIG. 5-7. Diagram showing the relationship between the single-strand protein of the α chain to the triple helix, the collagen molecule, and the fully developed fibril. The characteristic feature of the collagen molecule is its rigid, very long, narrow, rod-like structure, which is created by the tight winding of three α chains into a triple helix termed "tropocollagen." (From ref. 64.)

where x is another amino acid (31). The amino acids glycine, proline, and hydroxyproline make up the bulk of the primary structure and are unique to collagen (Fig. 5-7). Glycine is the smallest amino acid and permits the close packing necessary for the assembly of the three α chains into tropocollagen. Proline and hydroxyproline are cyclic imino acids whose structure presumably imparts rigidity to the final triple-helix configuration. Further details of the collagen molecular arrangements are presented in recent reviews (34,42,46,49,63). Collagen undergoes numerous modifications following ribosomal assembly, which are initiated by intracellular or extracellular enzymes. Examples of these processes include (a) hydroxylation of proline or lysine and (b) glycosylation of hydroxyly-sine. These modifications are termed "secondary features," as distinguished from the direct-coded structure (Fig. 5-8). The functional importance of these secondary features is uncertain, but various effects have been postulated such as aiding stability, regulating synthesis, controlling fiber diameter, and influencing collagen–proteoglycan interaction.

The structure of ligaments can be described from microscopic to macroscopic (29) (Fig. 5-9). The linear polypeptide chains folded into the α-helix chain, and three of these chains associate to form the triple helix or tropocollagen molecule. These units are packed together in the quarter-stagger arrangement to form microfibrils that aggregate to comprise the ligament.

The assembly of the three α chains into tropocollagen is facilitated by a group of amino acids at the end of each α chain that are called "registration pep-tides." The triple helix plus its registration peptide is larger than the tropocollagen molecule and is called "procollagen." Once the assembly of the triple helix is completed, the registration peptides are no longer needed and are cleaved by an enzyme, procollagen peptidase, as the procollagen passes through the cellular membrane into the extracellular space.

The α chains are not identical among species or within a single species. Early data on mammalian skin collagen showed two types of α chain, α_1 and α_2, present in a ratio of 2 to 1. Three types of α chains were identified in codfish skin collagen: α_1, α_2, and α_3 (59). Since these initial studies, a variety of collagen types have been described. A summary of the makeup and distribution of the major collagen types accepted at present is given in Table 5-2. The precise functional importance of these different types of collagen is presently unresolved (50). It is clear that the type of col

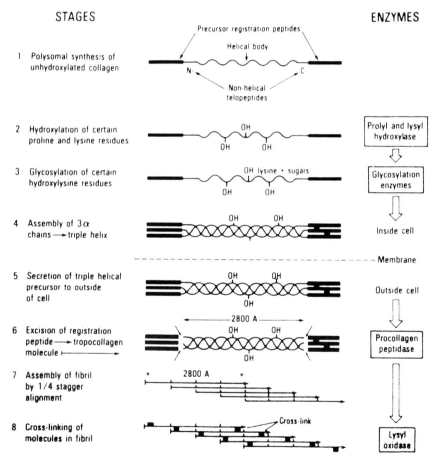

FIG. 5-8. The enzymatic stages in maturation of collagen. Several enzymatic steps are necessary for creation of the final collagen molecule and its maturation into a collagen fibril. These enzymatic steps take place partly within the cell and partly outside the cell. Even those steps that occur inside the cell are posttranslational; that is, they are not directly under genetic control. However, they are very essential for the proper development of the final structure. Defects in many of the steps have been identified in a variety of heritable disorders of connective tissues. The final aggregation of collagen into a structure that becomes crosslinked is essential in order to produce the requisite tensile stress-resistant properties characteristic of mature connective tissue. (From ref. 38.)

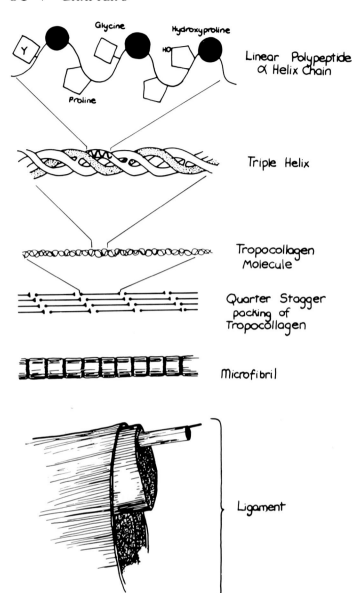

Glycine Hydroxyproline

Proline

Linear Polypeptide α Helix Chain

Triple Helix

Tropocollagen Molecule

Quarter Stagger packing of Tropocollagen

Microfibril

Ligament

FIG. 5-9. The structure of ligaments, from microscopic to macroscopic. A linear polypeptide chain is folded into the α helix, and three chains associate to form the triple helix or tropocollagen molecule. These are packed in quarter-stagger arrangement to form microfibrils that aggregate to comprise the ligament. (From ref. 28.)

lagen influences the type of aggregates that interact to form the complex structure, and the different properties of tendon, ligament, bone, or integument result.

It is apparent that a composite combination of the appropriate collagens are seen in normal connective tissues. Excessive amounts or lack of the appropriate collagen type is associated with pathology. For example, atherosclerotic plaques contain a high proportion of Type I collagen (43), and the lack of Type III collagen in the skin of Ehlers–Danlos IV patients has been associated with their extensible, fragile skin (62).

The dry weight collagen content has been found to be higher in the tendinous tissues studied (Achilles and patellar tendon) than in the ligamentous tissues (ACL and MCL) (Table 5-3) (6). Collagen typing analysis reveals that the tendons contain no detectable Type III collagen and that this form makes up 9–12% of the collagen in periarticular ligaments (Table 5-3). Type

III collagen is also observed in healing (17,30) and embryonic tissue (20). The fact that a less "mature" form of collagen is present may reflect the tissue response to a broad range of stresses, with the percentage of Type III collagen changing relatively rapidly as a function of applied forces. Alternatively, the Type I/III ratio endows the tissue with specific structural properties, allowing it to cope with the wide varieties of force and force vectors that ligaments are subjected to.

Collagen Crosslinks

Structural collagen obtains its stability from its unique molecular coil configuration, the quarter-staggered packing of tropocollagen units (58), and its ability to form covalent intramolecular and intermolecular

TABLE 5-2. *Types and characteristics of known collagens*[a]

Type	Chains	Characteristics	Aggregate form	Localization
I	$\alpha_1(I)$, $\alpha_2(I)$	(Hybrid composed of two kinds of chains) Most abundant; low in hydroxylysine and glycolysate hydroxylysine	Small 67-nm banded fibril	Bone, tendon, skin, dentin, ligament, fascia, uterus, and artery
Type I trimer	$\alpha_1(I)$	Increased content of 3- and 4-hydroxyproline and hydroxylysine as compared to the heteropolymer		Fetal tissues, inflammatory and neoplastic states
II	$\alpha_1(II)$	Abundant; relatively high in hydroxylysine and glycosylated hydroxylysine	Small 67-nm banded fibril	Hyaline cartilage, vitreous humor
III	$\alpha_1(III)$	High in hydroxylysine containing interchain disulfide bonds	Small 67-nm banded fibril	Skin, artery, and uterus
IV	$\alpha_1(IV)$, $\alpha_2(IV)$	High in hydroxylysine and glycosylated hydroxylysine; may contain large globular regions	Nonfibrillar network	Basement membranes
V	$\alpha_1(V)$, $\alpha_2(V)$, $\alpha_3(V)$	Similar to Type IV	Small fibers	Most interstitial tissues
VI	$\alpha_1(VI)$, $\alpha_2(VI)$, $\alpha_3(VI)$	Microfibrils	100-nm banded fibrils	Most interstitial tissues
VII	?	Long chain	FLS-like dimer[b]	Anchoring fibrils
VIII	$\alpha_1(VIII)$	Small helice linked in tandem	?	Some endothelial cells
IX	$\alpha_1(IX)$, $\alpha_2(IX)$, $\alpha_3(IX)$	Minor cartilage protein; contains attached glycosaminoglycan	?	Cartilage
X	$\alpha_1(X)$	Short chain	?	Hypertrophic mineralizing cartilage

[a] From ref. 7.
[b] The term "FLS" refers to collagen molecules arranged in an antiparallel, partially and overlapping array.

crosslinks (9,11,27,45,57,66,69). The former occur between α chains of the same tropocollagen molecule, and the latter occur between adjacent tropocollagen molecules. Crosslinks are key to both tensile strength characteristics and resistance to chemical or enzymatic breakdown. Their absence causes the collagen fibers to be extremely weak and friable. The classic manifestation of this problem is lathyrism, which is induced in animals ingesting the common sweet pea.

Curvature of the spine, rupture of the aorta, and fragile skin are common consequences. The biochemical problem is due to the presence of β-cyanoalanine and its decarboxylated product β-aminoproprionitrile in the seeds of the sweet pea (15). These compounds are potent inhibitors of lysyl oxidase, an enzyme of vital importance in the creation of crosslinks (48).

The crosslinks result from enzyme-mediated reactions involving mainly lysine and hydroxylysine. The

TABLE 5-3. *Biochemical properties of tendons and ligaments*[a]

Tissue	Total collagen (mg/g dry tissue)	Type of collagen			Glycosaminoglycan content (mg hexosamine/g dry tissue)
		I	II	III	
Patellar tendon	867.2 ± 8.9	>95	—	<5	3.92 ± 0.16
Achilles tendon	868.2 ± 10.2	>95	—	<5	2.75 ± 0.20
Anterior cruciate ligament	802.6 ± 9.8	88 ± 2	—	12 ± 2	9.89 ± 0.56
Medial collateral ligament	797.1 ± 11.1	91 ± 2	—	9 ± 2	4.56 ± 0.26

[a] From ref. 6.

lysine and hydroxylysine molecules have secondary amine groups on terminal projections extending laterally from the α chain, which are available for cross-linking reaction. The initial reaction in this process is the oxidative deamination of the terminal amine to an aldehyde by the enzyme lysyl oxidase (Fig. 5-10). These reactions have general similarity to the reactions that stabilize elastin. The resulting allysyl residues condense with one another to form an aldol condensation product (60) characteristic of intramolecular crosslinks (Fig. 5-11A) (24,42). Intermolecular crosslinks characteristically form in the reaction of allysine with lysine or hydroxylysine to form a Schiff base (δ-semialdehyde) (Fig. 5-11B). These aldol condensation and Schiff-base reaction products possess double bonds that apparently are reduced to more stable forms *in vivo* with the passage of time. Intramolecular crosslinks of the aldol type seem to be restricted to the N-terminal region of the collagen molecules in which they occur. The reactions leading to the formation of the intramolecular (aldol) and intermolecular (Schiff base) crosslinks are shown in Fig. 5-11A and B). In addition to lysinonorleucine (a compound first identified in elastin), other bimolecular Schiff bases of importance in ligaments are hydroxylysinonorleucine (HLNL) and dihydroxylysinonorleucine (DHLNL) Fig. 5-12A). Although these hydroxylysine-containing crosslinks are the most prevalent intermolecular crosslinks in native insoluble collagen, other more complex combinations also exist, including histidinohydroxymerodesmosine (HHMD), a tetramolecular crosslink (Fig. 12B). Most studies on crosslinking of collagen in the past decade have utilized the presence of the double bond of the unsaturated compound to label the "reducible" crosslinks with tritium. Typically, this has been done by reducing the aldol condensation product (namely, δ-semialdehyde) with tritium-labeled sodium borohydride. The reduced product is thereby labeled with tritium, and it can be detected following acid hydrolysis and column chromatography utilizing separation systems similar to those used in amino acid analysis.

The type of intermolecular collagen reducible crosslinks present in patellar and Achilles tendon differs considerably from those in the MCL and ACL (6). The tendinous tissue has a considerably different collagen reducible cross link elution profile than that of ligamentous tissue. The reducible crosslinks studied include DHLNL, HLNL, and HHMD. The relative concentrations of the crosslinks can be expressed as ratios for the tendinous and ligamentous tissues (Table 5-4). The ligaments are seen to have 12 to 17 times the DHLNL/HLNL ratio as the tendons, and three to four times the [DHLNL + HLNL]/HHMD ratio. The ACLs were observed to have the highest ratios of these crosslinks.

In addition to the reducible collagen crosslinks, isolation of a naturally fluorescing nonreducible crosslinking amino acid has been accomplished and was subsequently identified as pyridinoline (Fig. 5-12C) (22,25,26). It has been observed in tendon, ligament, and hyaline cartilage in order of increasing concentration. A three- to fivefold difference in its concentration is seen between rabbit ACL and patellar tendon, with MCL being intermediate in concentration.

Pyridinoline's proposed pathway of formation involves a spontaneous interaction of the two hydroxylysine-containing dysfunctional reducible crosslinks, resulting in a rearrangement to hydroxypyridinium (21). This pathway suggests an age-related transformation of the reducible crosslink, DHLNL, to a more stable nonreducible crosslink, pyridinoline. This may explain why the concentration of reducible, keto-imine crosslinks decreases with age in connective tissues (67).

The functional importance of the different crosslink species present in tendon and ligament is unknown. It is worth recalling, however, that DHLNL is the major collagen reducible crosslink in embryonic and healing tissue (10,23). In healing tissue, HLNL gradually replaces it (10). This suggests that a less "mature" or more mutable crosslink is present in ligament, perhaps again to allow reaction to a wide range and variety of forces.

Ground Substance

"Ground substance" is the term used to refer to the portion of connective tissue consisting of proteogly-

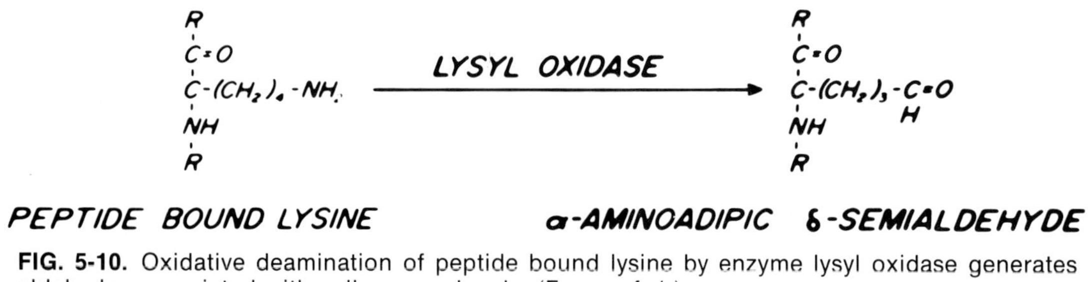

FIG. 5-10. Oxidative deamination of peptide bound lysine by enzyme lysyl oxidase generates aldehydes associated with collagen molecule. (From ref. 1.)

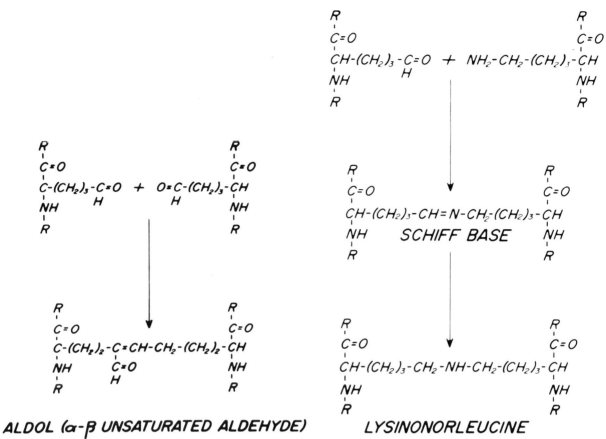

FIG. 5-11. A: Aldol condensation reaction involving lysine-derived aldehydes located near the N terminal of the molecule. This aldol condensation is responsible for formation of intramolecular crosslink. (From ref. 1.) **B:** Schiff-base reaction occurring between a lysine-derived aldehyde and an unmodified ε-amino group. This interaction is primarily responsible for the formation of intermolecular crosslinks and can involve either of the lysines of hydroxylysine. It is acid-labile and seems to require further stabilization to render the collagen fiber heat- and acid-stable. The reduced forms (lysinonorleucine or its hydroxylated derivatives) can be isolated after reduction. (From ref. 1.)

cans and glycosaminoglycans (GAGs). On a dry weight basis, the ground substance constituents of tendon comprise less than 1% of the total tissue and slightly more in ligament. Water, however, comprises 60–80% of the total wet weight, and a significant part of that water is associated with the ground substance. This material and water provide lubrication and spacing that are crucial to the gliding function at intercept points where fibers cross in the tissue matrices (54). Gliding is an essential physical property of tendons and ligaments. The water and ground substance also confer viscoelastic properties to these tissues. The movement of water in the system is inhibited by its entrapment between the large, highly charged molecules of proteoglycans.

Proteoglycans are relatively uniform chemically in the different periarticular connective tissues. The proteoglycan subunit consists of a core protein with protein-linked GAG side chains. Hyaluronic acid, chondroitin 4-sulfate, chondroitin 6-sulfate, and dermatan

sulfate represent the majority of the GAG present. Except for hyaluronic acid, the GAGs are covalently linked to proteins to create aggregate molecules of massive molecular weight. They are highly negatively charged and possess a large number of hydroxyl groups. These hydroxyl groups attract water through hydrogen binding, contributing important features to the collagen-fiber–ground-substance interaction, and may relate to some of the differences in mechanical properties between tendon and ligament.

The concentration of GAGs present in the rabbit ligamentous tissue studied differs significantly from that present in tendinous tissue. The ACLs have the highest proportion of GAGs, two to four times the amount observed in the tendons studied. MCL also demonstrates a higher GAG concentration than the tendons (Table 5-3)(6).

The functional importance of these differences is unknown; however, the higher the GAG content, the more water is associated with the complex. This nat-

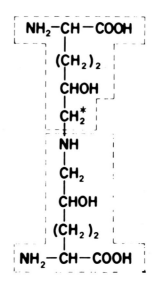

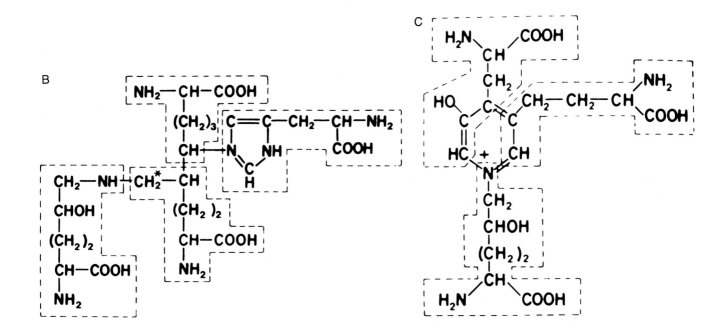

FIG. 5-12. A: Bimolecular reducible crosslinks. Structures of most abundant crosslinks in ligament after reduction with NaBH₄. Asterisks indicate sites of tritium labeling with radioactive isotope reduction. Basic amino acid skeletons contributing to crosslinks are enclosed by dashed lines. (From ref. 1.) **B:** Tetramolecular reducible crosslinks. Structures of most abundant crosslinks in ligament after reduction with NaBH₄. Asterisks indicate sites of tritium labeling with radioactive isotope reduction. Basic amino acid skeletons contributing to crosslinks are enclosed by dashed lines. (From ref. 1.) **C:** This trifunctional crosslink, which joins three adjacent collagen molecules, can be generated by one hydroxylysine residue and two hydroxylysine-derived aldehydes or by spontaneous interaction of two hydroxylysine-5-ketonorleucine residues formed from a hydroxylysine and a hydroxylysine aldehyde. (From ref. 1.)

TABLE 5-4. Reducible crosslink distribution[a]

Tissue	DHLNL/HLNL[b]	[DHLNL + HLNL]/HHMD[b]
Patellar tendon	0.16 ± 0.06	1.47 ± 0.23
Achilles tendon	0.15 ± 0.04	1.32 ± 0.06
Anterior cruciate ligament	2.77 ± 0.73	4.64 ± 0.73
Medial collateral ligament	1.86 ± 0.17	3.17 ± 0.37

[a] From ref. 7.
[b] DHLNL, dihydroxylysinonorleucine; HLNL, hydroxylysinonorleucine; HHMD, histidinohydroxymerodesmosine.

urally alters the viscoelastic properties of these tissues and may represent an additional "shock-absorbing" feature in ligament (optimized in the cruciate ligaments) which is unnecessary in tendon.

Glycoproteins

The important role of glycoproteins such as fibronectin (61) and actin in tendons and ligament in the complex interaction of cells of these tissues and their environment during growth, healing, and remodeling are poorly understood. Fibronectins are important in an array of cellular function, particularly those involving a cell's interaction with its surrounding extracellular matrix. They are high-molecular-weight extracellular glycoproteins whose functions include intra- and extracellular matrix morphology, cellular adhesion (both cell-to-cell and cell-to-substratum), cell adhesion, and cell migration. Fibronectins have adhesive domain specific to fibrin, actin, hyaluronic acid, cell surface factors and collagen. They function to attract and couple key elements in normal, healing, and growing tissues. They are of particular importance in soft connective tissues, where the major components are cells, collagen, and ground substance (61).

A heterogeneity of the morphological and biochemical properties of the various periarticular tissues such as the ACL, posterior cruciate ligament (PCL), MCL, and patellar tendon have been previously noted. Fibronectin has also been shown in both ligament and tendon tissues (13,55,68,71). In the periarticular tissues and plasma of the rabbit, fibronectin levels have been quantified in our laboratory (Table 5-5). Although fibronectin quantities of the ACL and PCL are similar,

they differ significantly from those of the MCL and patellar tendon. This represents two to three times more fibronectin in the intraarticular ACL and PCL (which are surrounded by a synovial sheath) than in the extraarticular MCL and patellar tendon (which have no synovial covering).

These results confirm the heterogeneity among ligaments and tendons. The periarticular tissues have been studied in order to describe ligaments that are more metabolically active than tendons (6). This was indicated by a higher level of cellularity, proteoglycan content, and Type III collagen, each of which may act as an adherent factor for fibronectin. Increased cellularity and Type III collagen are also seen in healing tissues, where fibronectin levels have been observed to increase (33,37,71). In fact, fibronectin has been shown to facilitate wound healing (47) and to be required for normal collagen organization and deposition by fibroblasts *in vitro* (44). Clearly, the role of fibronectin is important for the morphological and biochemical characteristics among ligaments and tendons following injury and during development.

NUTRITION OF PERIARTICULAR TENDONS AND LIGAMENTS

Nutritional contribution to tendons and ligaments of the knee and flexor tendons of the hand have been investigated in an attempt to understand and improve the healing limitations of the affected tissue. The vascular anatomy of the canine and human patellar tendon has been described using microangiographic and tissue clearing techniques (3,56). These studies demonstrate that the blood supply to the tendon anteriorly is based upon the retinacular vessels originating from the recurrent tibial, inferior lateral geniculate, superior lateral geniculate, and inferior medial geniculate arteries. The latter vessel also supplies the anterior fat pad, which, in turn, provides branches to the posterior portion of the patellar tendon. In the dog, the anterior fat pad contribution to the patellar tendon is more significant than in humans. Branches of these arteries within the tendon substance anastomose and branch off into slender, longitudinally oriented vessels that form cap-

TABLE 5-5. Amount of fibronectin

Tissue	Mean ± standard deviation (μg/mg dry tissue)
Anterior cruciate ligament	2.02 ± 0.27
Posterior cruciate ligament	1.90 ± 0.38
Medial collateral ligament	0.80 ± 0.22
Patellar tendon	0.70 ± 0.16

illary channels about the collagenous bundles. Intraarticular injection of tritiated proline demonstrates that the patellar tendon derives its nutritional source from blood, and it also demonstrates that synovial fluid makes no detectable contribution to tendon nutrition (5).

Anatomic and physiological studies of digital flexor tendons have been performed demonstrating the contribution of both blood supply and synovial fluid to tendon nutrition (39,40,52). Blood supply to the tendon is generated through the vincular system via branches from the digital artery, distally at the insertion to bone, proximally at the origin of the synovial sheath, and through muscular attachment. Synovial fluid bathes the tendon within the sheath and is presumed to be especially important at the avascular and hypovascular areas of the tendon. These areas include the space between the vincular systems and the bifurcation of the superficialis tendon, respectively.

The MCL derives a blood supply from the inferior medial geniculate artery and from its osseous attachments. In addition to this, synovial fluid is observed to make a nutritional contribution in a rabbit model (5). The ACL is known to have a limited healing capacity (16). Studies have shown that the blood supply to the ligament is poor, and authors have suggested that this may explain the poor repair potential of this structure (3,8). It has been recently demonstrated that the ACL is capable of deriving nutrition from synovial fluid, and this source may be the primary nutritional source for the tissue (5). As a result, nutrition per se may not explain the limited repair potential observed in this ligament.

ACKNOWLEDGMENTS

Support from the following sources is gratefully acknowledged: NIH Grants AR34264, AR14918, and AR38159; the San Diego Veterans Administration Medical Center; the Easter Seals Research Foundation; and the Malcolm and Dorothy Coutts Institute for Joint Reconstruction and Research. We would also like to thank Mrs. Fran Shepherd for her word-processing assistance.

REFERENCES

1. Akeson WA. In: Hunter LY, Funk FJ, eds. *Rehabilitation of the injured knee*, vol 3. St. Louis: CV Mosby, 1984.
2. Alm A, Ekstrom H, Stromberg B. The anterior cruciate ligament: a clinical and experimental study on tensile strength, morphology and replacement by patellar ligament. *Acta Chir Scand [Suppl]* 1974;445:15.
3. Alm A, Stromberg B. Vascular anatomy of the patellar and cruciate ligaments. *Acta Chir Scand [Suppl]* 1974;445:25.
4. Amenta P. *Histology*, 3rd ed. New Hyde Park, NY: New York Medical Examination Publishing Company, 1983;70.
5. Amiel D, Abel MF, Kleiner JB, Akeson WH. Synovial fluid nutrient delivery in the diarthrial joint: an analysis of rabbit knee ligaments. *J Orthop Res* 1986;4:90–95.
6. Amiel D, Frank CB, Harwood FL, Fronek J, Akeson WH. Tendons and ligaments: a morphological and biochemical comparison. *J Orthop Res* 1984;1(3):257.
7. Amiel D, Kleiner JB. In: Nimni ME, Olsen B. Biochemistry of tendon and ligament. *Collagen. Biotechnology, vol III*. Cleveland: CRC Press, 1988;223–251.
8. Arnoczky SP, Rubin RM, Marshall JL. Microvasculature of the cruciate ligaments and its response to injury. An experimental study in the dog. *J Bone Joint Surg* 1979;61A:1221.
9. Bailey AJ. The nature of collagen. In: Florkin M, Stotz E, eds. *Comprehensive biochemistry*, vol 26B. Amsterdam: Elsevier, 1968;297.
10. Bailey AJ, Robins SP. Embryonic skin collagen replacement of the type of aldimine cross-links during the early growth period. *FEBS Lett* 1972;21:330.
11. Bailey AJ, Robins SP, Balian G. Biological significance of the intermolecular cross-links of collagen. *Nature* 1974;251:105.
12. Bailey FR. *Bailey's textbook of microscopic anatomy*, 18th ed. Kelly DE, Wood RL, Enders AC, eds., Baltimore: Williams and Wilkins, 1984;172.
13. Banes AJ, Link GW, Bevin AG, et al. Tendon synovial cells secrete fibronectin *in vivo* and *in vitro*. *J Orthop Res* 1988;6(1):73.
14. Bloom W, Fawcett DW. *A textbook of histology*, 8th ed. Philadelphia: WB Saunders, 1962;105.
15. Bornstein P. The biosynthesis of collagen. *Annu Rev Biochem* 1974;43:567.
16. Clayton ML, Miles JS, Abdulla M. Experimental investigations of ligamentous healing. *Clin Orthop* 1968;61:146.
17. Clore JN, Cohen K, Diegelmann RF. Quantitation of collagen types I and III during wound healing in rat skin. *Proc Soc Exp Biol Med* 1979;161:337.
18. Copenhaver WM, Bunge RP, Bune, MB. *Bailey's textbook of histology*, 16th ed. Baltimore: Williams and Wilkins, 1971;125.
19. Dunphy JE. *Wound healing*. New York: Medcom Press, 1974;22.
20. Epstein EH, Munderloh NH. Isolation and characterization of CNBr peptides of human $\{\alpha1(III)\}_3$ collagen and tissue distribution of $\{\alpha1(I)\}_2$ $\alpha2$ and $\{\alpha1(III)\}_3$ collagens. *J Biol Chem* 1975;250:9304.
21. Eyre DR, Oguchi H. Collagens: their measurement, properties and a proposed pathway of formation. *Biochem Biophys Res Commun* 1980;92(2):403.
22. Eyre DR, Koob TJ, Van Ness KP. Quantitation of hydroxypyridinium crosslinks in collagen by high-performance liquid chromatography. *Ann Biochem* 1984;137:380.
23. Forrest L, Shuttleworth A, Jackson D, Mechanic GL. A comparison between the reducible intermolecular cross-links of the collagens from mature dermis and young dermal scar tissue of the guinea pig. *Biochem Biophys Res Commun* 1972;46:1776.
24. Franzblau C. Elastin. In: Florkin M, Stotz E, eds. *Comprehensive biochemistry*, vol 3. Amsterdam: Elsevier, 1971;659.
25. Fujimoto D. Isolation and characterization of a fluorescent material in bovine Achilles tendon collagen. *Biochem Biophys Res Commun* 1977;76(4):1124.
26. Fujimoto D, Moriguchi T. Pyridinoline, a non-reducible cross-link of collagen. *J Biochem* 1978;83:863.
27. Gallop PM, Blumenfeld OO, Henson E, Scheider AL. Isolation and identification of α-amino aldehydes in collagen. *Biochemistry* 1968;7:2409.
28. Gamble JG, Edwards CC, Max SR. Enzymatic adaptation in ligament during immobilization. *Am J. Sports Med* 1984;12(3):224.
29. Gamble JG, Edwards CC, Max SR. Enzymatic adaptation in ligament during immobilization. *Am J Sports Med* 1984;12(3):221–228.
30. Gay S, Viljanto J, Rackallio J, Penttinen R. Collagen types in early phases of wound healing in children. *Acta Chir Scand* 1978;144:205.
31. Glimcher MJ, Krane SM. The organization and structure of bone, and the mechanism of calcification. In: Gould BS, ed.

Treatise on collagen, vol 2: biology of collagen. New York: Academic Press, 1968;67.

32. Ham AW. *Histology,* 6th ed. Philadelphia: JB Lippincott, 1974;374.

33. Kurkinen M, Alitalo K, Vaheri A, Stenman S, Saxen L. Fibronectin in the development of embryonic chick eye. *Dev Biol* 1979;69:589–600.

34. Lane JM, Weiss C. Review of articular cartilage collagen research. *Arthritis Rheum* 1975;18:553.

35. Leeson CR. In: Leeson CR, Leeson TS, eds. *Textbook of histology,* 5th ed. Philadelphia: WB Saunders, 1985;97.

36. Leeson TS, Leeson CR. *A brief atlas of histology.* Philadelphia: WB Saunders, 1979;47.

37. Lehto M, Duance VC, Restall D. Collagen and fibronectin in a healing skeletal muscle injury. *J Bone Joint Surg* 1985;67B(5):820–828.

38. Levene CI. Diseases of the collagen molecule. *J Clin Pathol* 1978;12:82.

39. Lundborg GN, Myrhage R, Rydevik B. The vascularization of human flexor tendons within the digital synovial sheath region—structural and functional aspects. *J Hand Surg* 1977;2(6):417.

40. Lundborg GN, Rank F. Experimental studies on cellular mechanisms involved in healing of animal and human flexor tendon in synovial environment. *Hand* 1980;12(1):3.

41. Lyon RM, Billings E Jr, Woo SL-Y, Ishizue KK, Kitabayashi L, Amiel D, Akeson WH. The ACL: a fibrocartilaginous structure. Presented at Transactions of the 35th Meeting of the Orthopedic Research Society, Las Vegas, February 6–9, 1989.

42. Mathews MB, Collagen. In: *Connective tissue: macromolecular structure and evolution.* New York: Springer-Verlag 1975;15.

43. McCullagh KA, Balian G. Collagen characterization and cell transformation in human atherosclerosis. *Nature* 1975;258:73.

44. McDonald JA, Kelly DG, Broekelmann TJ. Role of fibronectin in collagen deposition: Fab' to the gelatin-binding domain of fibronectin inhibits both fibronectin and collagen organization in fibroblast extracellular matrix. *J Cell Biol* 1982;92:485–492.

45. Mechanic GL. An automated scintillation counting system for continuous analysis: cross-links of (^{3}H)NaBH$_4$ reduced collagen. *Anal Biochem* 1974;62:349.

46. Miller EJ. The collagen of the extracellular matrix. In: Lash JW, Burger MM, eds. *Cell and tissue interactions.* New York: Raven Press, 1977;71.

47. Nagelschmidt M, Becker D, Bonninghoff N, Engelhardt GH. Effect of fibronectin therapy and fibronectin deficiency on wound healing: a study in rats. *J Trauma* 1987;27(11):1267–1271.

48. Narayanan AS, Siegal RC, Martin GR. On the inhibition of lysyl oxidase by β aminoproprionitride. *Biochem Biophys Res Commun* 1972;46:745.

49. Nimni ME. Molecular structure and function of collagen in normal and diseased tissue. In: Burleigh PMC, Poole AR, eds. *Dynamics of connective tissue macromolecules.* New York: American Elsevier, 1975.

50. Nimni ME. Collagen: structure, function and metabolism in normal and fibrotic tissues. *Semin Arthritis Rheum* 1983;13:1.

51. Noyes FR, Grood ES, Butler DL, Paulos LE. Clinical biomechanics of the knee: ligament restraints and functional stability. In: *Surgical repair reconstruction.* American Academy of Orthopedic Surgeons' Symposium on Athlete's Knee. St Louis: CV Mosby, 1980;1.

52. Ochiai MN, Matsui T, Miyaji N, Merklin RJ, Hunter JM. Vascular anatomy of flexor tendons. I. Vincular system and blood supply of the profundus tendon in the digital sheath. *J Hand Surg* 1979;4(4):321.

53. O'Donoghue DH, Rockwood CA, Zaricznyj B, Kenyon, R. Repair of knee ligaments in dogs. I. The lateral collateral ligament, *J Bone Joint Surg* 1961;43A:1167.

54. Ogston AG. The biological functions of the glycosaminoglycans. In: Balasz EA, ed. *Chemistry and molecular biology of the intercellular matrix,* vol 3. London: Academic Press, 1970:1231.

55. Palmer I. On injuries to the ligaments of the knee joint. *Acta Chir Scand [Suppl]* 1938;53:1.

56. Paulos LE, Butler DL, Noyes FR, Grood ES. Intra-articular cruciate reconstruction. *Clin Orthop* 1983;172:78.

57. Paz MA, Henson EH, Rombauer R, Abrash L, Glumenfeld OO, Gallop PM. Alpha-amino alcohols as products of a reductive side reaction of denatured collagen with sodium borohydride. *Biochemistry* 1970;9:2123.

58. Petruska JA, Hodge AJ. A subunit model for the tropocollagen macromolecule, *Proc Natl Acad Sci USA* 1964;51:871.

59. Piez KA. Characterization of a collagen from codfish skin containing three chromatographically different alpha chains. *Biochemistry* 1965;4:2590.

60. Piez KA. Cross-linking of collagen and elastin. *Annu Rev Biochem* 1968;37:547.

61. Pitaru S, Aubin JE, Bhargava U, Melcher AH. Immunoelectron microscopic studies on the distributions of fibronectin and actin in a cellular dense connective tissue: the periodontal ligament of the rat. *J Periodont Res* 1987;22:64–74.

62. Pope FM, Martin GR, Lichtenstein JR. Patients with Ehlers-Danlos syndrome type IV lack type III collagen. *Proc Natl Acad Sci USA* 1975;72:1314.

63. Serafini-Fracassini A, Smith JW, Collagen. In: *The structure and biochemistry of cartilage,* Edinburgh: Churchill Livingstone, 1974;29.

64. Prockop DJ. The biosynthesis of collagen and its disorders. *N Engl J Med* 1979;301:13.

65. Snell RS. *Clinical and functional histology for medical students,* 1st ed. Boston: Little, Brown, 1984;107.

66. Tanzer ML. Crosslinking of collagen. *Science* 1973;180:561.

67. Tanzer ML. Cross-linking. In: Ramuchandran GN, Reddi AH, eds. *Biochemistry of collagen.* New York; Plenum, 1976;137.

68. Taylor CM, Oelbaum RS, Grant ME. The biosynthesis of glycoproteins by cultured bovine tendon fibroblasts. *Connect Tissue Res* 1982;10:319–331.

69. Traub W, Piez KA. The chemistry and structure of collagen. *Adv Protein Chem* 1971;25:243.

70. Viidik A. Simultaneous mechanical and light microscopic studies of collagen fibers. *Z Anat Entwicklungsgesch* 1972;136:204.

71. Williams IF, McCullagh KG, Silver IA. The distribution of types I and III collagen and fibronectin in the healing equine tendon. *Connect Tissue Res* 1984;12:211–227.

72. Yahia LH, Drouin G. Microscopical investigation of canine anterior cruciate ligament and patellar tendon: collagen fascicle morphology and architecture. *J Orthop Res* 1989;7:243–251.

PART III

Function

Knee Ligaments: Structure, Function, Injury, and Repair, edited by D. Daniel, et al.

CHAPTER 6

The Sensory Function of Knee Ligaments

Robert L. Barrack and Harry B. Skinner

Ligaments have two major roles in maintaining normal knee joint kinematics. They act as a dynamic guide to knee motion and also act as a passive mechanical restraint that prevents abnormal translations from occurring when stressful loads are applied. Ligament tears disrupt these functions and often lead to symptomatic instability. The biomechanical abnormalities of joint motion which result have been outlined in the instant-center-of-rotation analysis of Frankel (26) as well as in the four-bar linkage model that has been described by Müller (60) and O'Connor (Chapter 10). The clinical consequences of knee instability include giving way with stressful activities, reinjuries, and early degenerative arthritis (49,55,56). Kennedy (54) has noted that the early clinical result will often be satisfactory initially, particularly in the case of anterior cruciate ligament (ACL) tears. He observed, however, that the instability will often be progressive in nature, leading to a dramatic increase in disability over a period of time. In later years, observations by Kennedy (54) led him to the conclusion that the clinical decline

commonly observed following knee ligament injuries was not only the result of the loss of a passive restraint but also the result of neurologic feedback. He hypothesized that knee injury led to ligamentous laxity which resulted in failure of mechanoreceptor feedback and loss of reflex muscular contractions. This, he felt, contributed to the repetitive injuries and clinical decline (Fig. 6-1).

In reviewing the literature, we found that this was not a new concept in orthopedics. In 1944, Dr. LeRoy Abbott (1) published a treatise on injuries of ligaments of the knee joint in which he concluded that ligaments have a rich sensory innervation that allows them to act as the first link in the "kinetic chain." He stated that impulses arising in the ligaments are transmitted through the central nervous system back to the effector muscles, allowing for maintenance of normal, smooth, coordinated motion of the joint. He went on to state that abnormally strong impulses, such as initiated when a ligament is overstretched, results in contraction of allied muscle groups, thereby protecting the ligaments and preventing further injury and subluxation of the knee.

In the next decade, another astute observer of knee ligament injury, Ivar Palmer (66), expressed interest in proprioceptive input from knee ligaments. He demonstrated reflex contraction of the medial hamstring and vastus medialis in response to stimulation of the

R. L. Barrack: Department of Orthopaedic Surgery, U. S. Naval Hospital, Oakland, California 94627, and Department of Orthopaedic Surgery, University of California, San Francisco, School of Medicine, San Francisco, California 94143.

H. B. Skinner: Department of Orthopaedic Surgery, University of California, San Francisco, School of Medicine, San Francisco, California 94143.

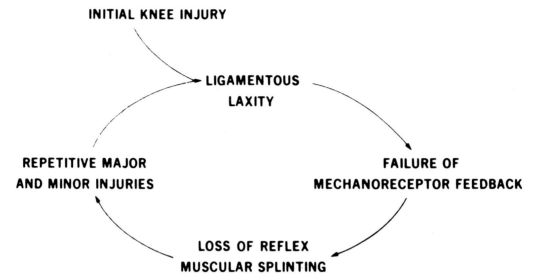

FIG. 6-1. Hypothesized neurogenic contribution to progressive knee instability. (From ref. 54.)

deep capsular portion of the medial collateral ligament (MCL) and further showed that the reflex is weakened in the traumatized joint and loses its selectivity.

Sensation originating in joints has long been recognized by physiologists as the source of proprioceptive and kinesthetic ability (2,81,89). The French neurologist, Duchenne, was among the first to emphasize the clinical importance of articular sensations in his nineteenth-century writings (68). The recent demonstration of mechanoreceptors in human knee ligaments, as well as the realization of the long-term effects of ligament injuries, has renewed interest and research into the neurologic function of knee ligaments (73,74). The purpose of this chapter, therefore, is to review previous knowledge of joint sensation, including basic anatomy and physiology, and to review current research in this area, including its application to knee injuries, rehabilitation, and reconstruction.

PHYSIOLOGY OF JOINT SENSATION

Terminology and Basic Principles

Awareness of the body and its relationship with the surrounding environment is mediated through the phenomenon of sensation. The senses are broadly divided into special (sight, hearing, taste, smell) and somatic or somesthetic (pain, temperature, touch). Each specific type of sensation is called a *modality*. Every sensory modality has a specific end-organ that responds to a stimulus in a characteristic way. The stimulus is converted to an electrical potential and is conducted along nerve fibers specific to each sensory modality. The impulses are carried along established neural path-

ways to either elicit an appropriate reflex response or reach the cortical level (and thus conscious awareness) of a stimulus.

Sensations originating about joints are specialized variations of the sense of touch referred to as *proprioception* and *kinesthesia*. Proprioception refers to the conscious awareness of the limb position in space. Kinesthesia implies awareness of joint motion (59,91). These sensory modalities originate by stimulation of specialized nerve endings referred to as *mechanoreceptors* (Fig. 6-2). These specialized end-organs (mechanoreceptors) function as transducers, converting the mechanical energy of physical deformation into the electrical energy of a nerve action potential (Fig. 6-3).

An important characteristic of mechanoreceptor response is that of adaptation. All receptors are maximally stimulated (i.e., they generate the maximal number of electrical impulses) immediately after a new stimulus is detected. If a stimulus is continually applied, receptors differ as to how they continue to respond. Some receptors rapidly decrease the number of impulses generated per second to extinction within milliseconds of the stimulus onset, even though the stimulus persists. These are rapidly adapting (i.e., phasic) receptors. Other receptors decline to a constant steady state of a fairly high level of impulses per second in the presence of continued stimulation. These are slowly adapting (i.e., tonic) receptors. The different receptor types serve different functions. Rapidly adapting receptors such as pacinian corpuscles and hair receptors respond to small changes in pressure with a sudden burst of high-frequency impulses followed by rapid deterioration even though the stimulus (pressure) is maintained. They are, therefore, very sensitive to the onset of sudden changes in pressure or

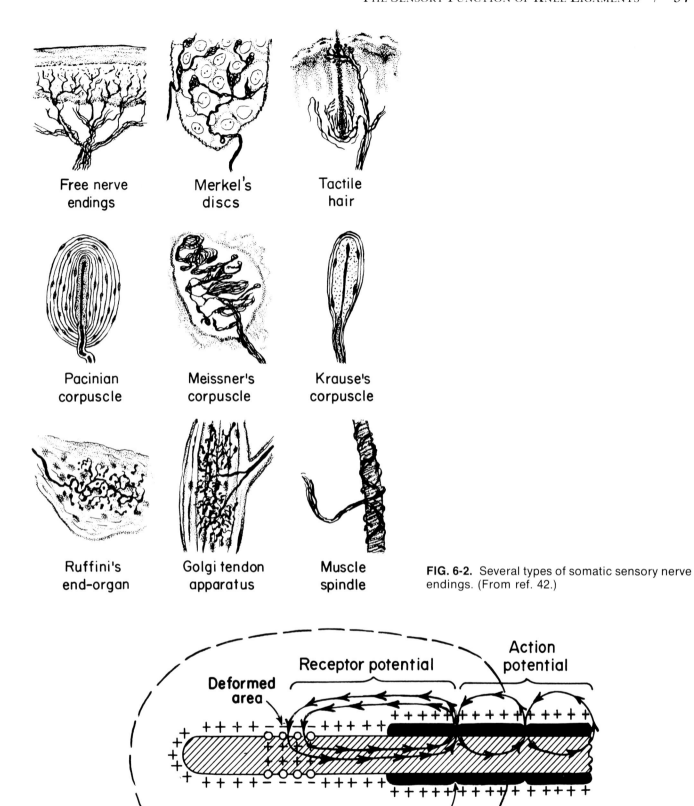

Free nerve endings

Merkel's discs

Tactile hair

Pacinian corpuscle

Meissner's corpuscle

Krause's corpuscle

Ruffini's end-organ

Golgi tendon apparatus

Muscle spindle

FIG. 6-2. Several types of somatic sensory nerve endings. (From ref. 42.)

Action potential

Receptor potential

Deformed area

Node of Ranvier

FIG. 6-3. Excitation of a sensory nerve fiber by a receptor potential produced in a pacinian corpuscle. (From ref. 42.)

movement but not to slow or constant pressures. Slowly adapting receptors such as joint receptors and muscle spindles are always generating impulses depending on the relative position of muscles and joints. Thus, they are always sensitive to the position of body parts and changes in position, since these changes are reflected by differing rates of impulse generation throughout the range of motion of joints (Fig. 6-4). Rapidly adapting receptors are therefore stimulated by initiation or termination of motion or rapid change in velocity or direction of movement. They would be more likely to be stimulated by rapid loading or change in tension of the joint capsule or ligaments. Slowly adapting receptors, on the other hand, give steady-state information on joint position as well as sensing motion and angle of rotation.

Impulses are transmitted from receptors to the central nervous system via nerve fibers that are specific for each sensory modality (Table 6-1). Joint sensation is carried along large myelinated fibers with high conduction velocities which allow for rapid response to change in tension in ligaments. Pain fibers, in contrast, have slow conduction velocities.

Sensory information is transmitted from the joints via articular nerves through posterior roots to the spinal cord. Impulses are then transmitted through the dorsal-column–lemniscal (posterior column) system to the cerebral cortex, where there is a high degree of spatial orientation (Figs. 6-5 and 6-6). Müller (60) has noted that there is a disproportionately high cortical representation for the lower limb, which he takes as evidence of the importance of proprioceptive input from the lower extremity.

Joint Innervation

Over 100 years ago, Hilton (43) described the nerve supply to joints. He stated that joints are innervated by articular branches of the nerves supplying the muscles that cross that joint, a principle that has come to be known as *Hilton's law*. Physiological studies examining proprioceptive or kinesthetic responses of the knee joint have most often been recorded from the posterior articular nerve in feline specimens (12,14,16,31,39). However, medial and lateral articular branches have also been described as providing significant afferent input (15,81). The most extensive studies of the innervation of the human knee joint were performed by Jeletsky in 1931 (50) and Gardner in 1948 (33). Both showed variability in distribution and consistency of some articular branches, but they were able to establish a predominant pattern of human knee joint innervation.

More recently, a review of histological studies and dissections by Kennedy (54) best summarized the current understanding of the specific pattern of innervation of the human knee. This investigator described two distinct groups of articular nerves. The posterior group consisted of (a) the prominent posterior articular

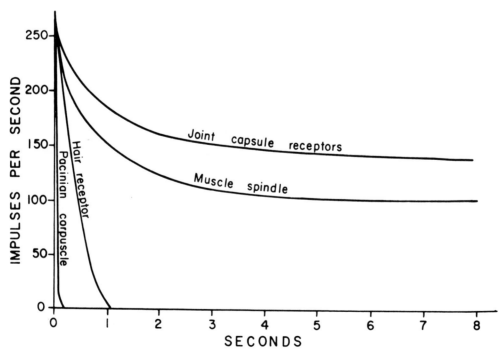

FIG. 6-4. Adaptation of different types of receptors, showing rapid adaptation of some receptors and slow adaptation of others. (From ref. 42.)

TABLE 6-1. *Conduction velocities of various types of nerve fiber*

Type of fiber	Diameter (μm)	Approximate conduction velocity (m/sec)	Function
A (α)	15–70	100	Motor muscle proprioception
A (β)	10–15	30–70	Touch, kinesthesia
A (γ)	4–8	30	Touch, muscle spindle
A (δ)	1–4	10	Pain, heat, cold
B	1–3	5	Preganglionic autonomic
C	0.2–1.0	1	Postganglionic autonomic

nerve, arising as a branch of the tibial nerve, and (b) a terminal branch of the obturator nerve. The anterior group consisted of articular branches of the femoral, common peroneal, and saphenous nerves. Consistent with numerous physiology studies over preceding decades, Kennedy (54) found the largest and most prom-

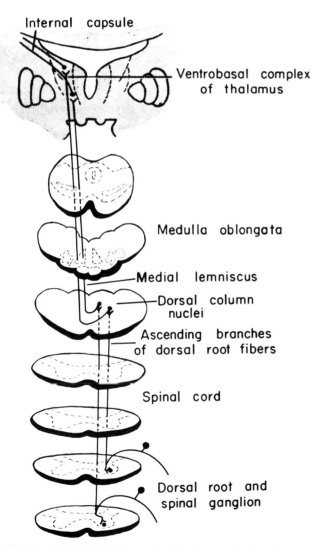

FIG. 6-5. The dorsal column and spinocervical pathways for transmitting critical types of tactile signals. (From ref. 42.)

inent articular nerve to be the posterior articular nerve. This has also been described by other authors as the predominant nerve supply of the posterior capsule and cruciate ligaments (39,81). This nerve branches from the posterior tibial nerve above the knee in the popliteal fossa (Fig. 6-7). It then wraps around the popliteal artery and vein before forming the popliteal plexus, which penetrates the posterior capsule (Fig. 6-8). Branches of this plexus are described to course through the synovial lining of the cruciate ligaments and extend as far anteriorly as the infrapatellar fat pad.

Anteriorly, the capsule is innervated by terminal branches of the femoral, common peroneal, and saphenous nerves. Femoral nerve branches to the vastus lateralis, intermedius, and medialis contribute articular branches to the lateral, central, and medial portions of the capsule, respectively (Fig. 6-9A and B). The common peroneal nerve contributes two branches anteriorly which innervate capsular structures. The lateral articular nerve innervates the posterolateral corner of the knee (Fig. 6-10), whereas the recurrent peroneal gives off a branch to the anterolateral capsule (Fig. 6-11). The final anterior articular afferent nerve is the infrapatellar branch of the saphenous nerve, which innervates the anteromedial capsule. This branch has particular clinical significance because it also provides sensory branches to the patellar tendon. Freeman (29) has demonstrated mechanoreceptors within the patellar tendon, at least in animal specimens, and patellar tendon is frequently utilized as a graft tissue in cruciate ligament reconstructions.

Mechanoreceptor Function

The specific receptors responsible for joint position sense are Ruffini end-organs, pacinian corpuscles, and Golgi tendon organs (Fig. 6-2). Ruffini and Golgi receptors are slowly adapting and have previously been described as the dominant receptor type in joint capsules (2,64,81,90). They respond to active or passive motion throughout the range of knee motion (41). Maximal response has been demonstrated at the extremes of knee motion (36,38,40). External rotation also ac-

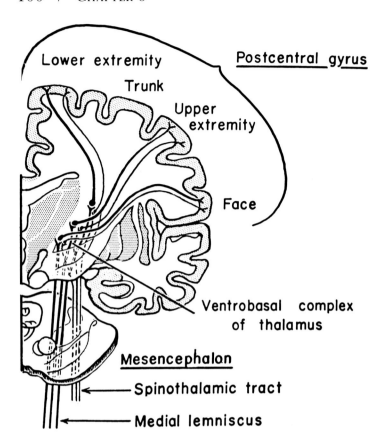

Lower extremity
Trunk
Upper extremity
Face
Postcentral gyrus

Ventrobasal complex of thalamus

Mesencephalon

Spinothalamic tract

Medial lemniscus

FIG. 6-6. Projection of the dorsal-column–lemniscal system from the thalamus to the somatic sensory cortex. (From ref. 42.)

centuates discharge of these receptors (14,15,36,81). Since both of these positions are suggestive of possible injury situations for the knee, it seems likely that these receptors may play a role in signaling impending injury. Response from these receptors has been obtained by passive motion of the knee performed while directly monitoring the articular nerves (15,16). Clinically,

slow passive motion has been utilized to measure the threshold to detection of change in position of the knee (6–9,44,53,77–80). These slowly adapting receptors were, therefore, thought to play a dominant role in signaling joint position. Stimulation of these same receptors, however, has repeatedly demonstrated the generation of reflex muscular contraction about the af-

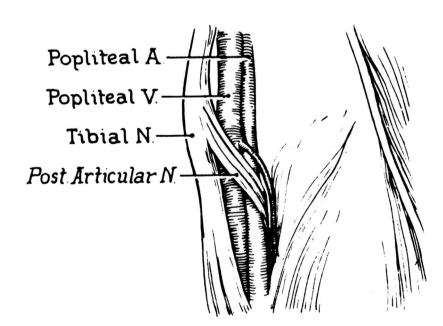

Popliteal A.
Popliteal V.
Tibial N.
Post. Articular N.

FIG. 6-7. Origin of the posterior articular nerve from the posterior tibial nerve in the popliteal fossa. (From ref. 54.)

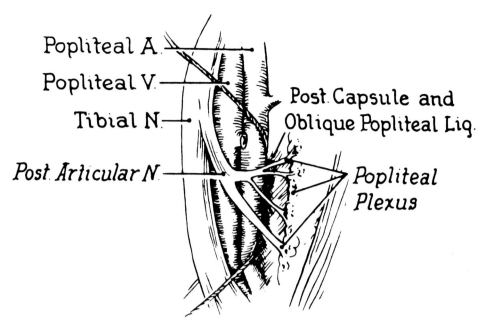

FIG. 6-8. Popliteal plexus deep in the popliteal fossa. (From ref. 54.)

fected joint (20,28). Freeman (27) demonstrated reflex contraction of the gastrocnemius muscle resulting from ankle joint movement that persisted in spite of division of tendons and removal of skin and any other source of reflex initiation other than the joint capsule. Dee (18) similarly demonstrated reflex activity of muscles around the hip, which was only abolished by local anesthetic instillation into the joint. He believed that protective reflexes were mediated through the ligamentum teres. Intraarticular anesthetic was also found to cause a disturbance of posture and gait in experimental animals (25). This was not, however, demonstrated in humans, at least in gait analysis during normal walking with intraarticular anesthesia (7). Rapidly adapting pacinian corpuscles have been described more often at ligament insertions rather than at joint capsules. Since they respond to sudden acceleration, they too are in a position to initiate protective reflexes.

These mechanoreceptors have been consistently demonstrated in various dissections of animal knees. In addition to the feline ACL (12,29,32), receptors have been demonstrated in the MCL (3,62) and in the menisci (54), particularly in the posterior horns (63). Receptors in these structures were also demonstrated to initiate reflex muscular contraction that was thought to be protective (5,65). The reflex most often elicited was that of inhibition of extension and facilitation of flexor muscle groups (81).

The role of receptors in muscles, such as muscle spindles, is a subject of debate. While some investigators feel that muscle receptors contribute to position sense (35,72), the majority believe that they only mediate muscle tension via subcortical reflexes and that

none of the sensory input reaches conscious awareness (41,51). Muscular activity, however, can have a prominent effect on position sense indirectly. Grigg (36) has suggested that muscles which cross a joint can activate joint afferent receptors when they contract. Anatomically, the close integration of muscle and tendinous insertions with the joint capsule has been demonstrated on the medial side of the knee (45,46,86,89) as well as on the lateral side (75). Hughston (45,46) described (a) the capsular arms of the semimembranosus and (b) the effect of muscle contraction in tightening the capsule. He emphasizes the importance of restoring this relationship in repair or reconstruction of the medial side of the knee.

The specific response characteristics of mechanoreceptors were recently described by Grigg (39) in a feline model. The "mechanically sensitive" neurons located in the posterior capsule were calibrated prior to testing. They were then loaded, and recordings were obtained during knee rotation. The mechanoreceptors were found to function as load cells from which it was possible to estimate loading of the posterior capsule. Additionally, the fraction of an applied moment that the posterior capsule sustained during knee extension could be estimated (Fig. 6-12).

Conclusions from animal studies cannot automatically be extrapolated to humans, however, since differences are known to exist in morphology and population density of mechanoreceptors among various species (67). In addition, the nature of mechanoreceptors of human knee ligaments has just recently been described. Neuroanatomical studies by Kennedy (54,55) revealed variability in the innervation of the

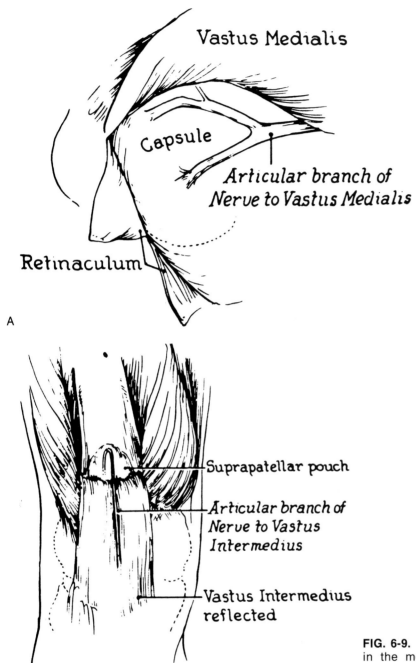

FIG. 6-9. **A**: Nerve to the vastus medialis terminating in the medial capsule. (From ref. 54.) **B**: Articular branch of the nerve to the vastus intermedius arising from the suprapatellar pouch. (From ref. 54.)

human knee. He found mechanoreceptors within multiple clefts in the tibial origin of the ACL and within the vascular synovial covering. None, however, were found within the ligament. These were usually associated with vasculature, and it was concluded that they must serve a vasomotor function. In reviewing the studies by Kennedy and Freeman, however, Müller (60) concluded that tension perception took precedence over pain sensation or vasoregulation in the sensory function of the cruciate or collateral ligaments.

In 1984, Schultz (73) reported the presence of mech-

anoreceptors in human cruciate ligaments. Fusiform corpuscles were found only at the surface of the ligaments. The receptors were 200 μm long by 75 μm wide, were oriented parallel to the fibers of the ligament, and had the morphological appearance of a Golgi tendon organ (Fig. 6-13A and B). There was only one receptor found in each ligament, and they were present in both the anterior and the posterior cruciate ligaments. No receptors were found within the menisci themselves. This finding is consistent with the work of Kennedy (54), who described abundant neural ele-

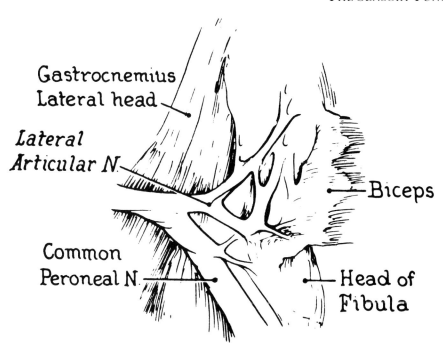

FIG. 6-10. Origin of the lateral articular nerve from the common peroneal nerve. (From ref. 54.)

ments in the perimeniscal capsular tissues but not within the meniscus itself. These findings differ markedly from those of Wilson (92), who reported penetration of the nerve supply to the peripheral one-half of the meniscus. Schultz (73) also described an absence of mechanoreceptors in the capsular ligaments with only free nerve endings present. Receptors were frequently deformed or absent in end-stage arthritic knees, implying that mechanoreceptor function might play a role in the disease process. The possibility of a proprioceptive role for the cruciate ligaments was suggested.

More recently, Schutte (74) performed an in-depth analysis of the neural anatomy of the human ACL. In addition to standard histologic staining techniques, computerized image analysis was performed to determine the population density of any receptors encountered. The ACL was found to have a high density of various neural elements within the collagenous structure of the ligament. In contrast, Kennedy (55) found receptors only at the tibial origin and in the vascular synovial covering, and Schultz (73) described a small population of Golgi-type receptors on the surface of the ligament. Schutte (74) demonstrated mechanore-

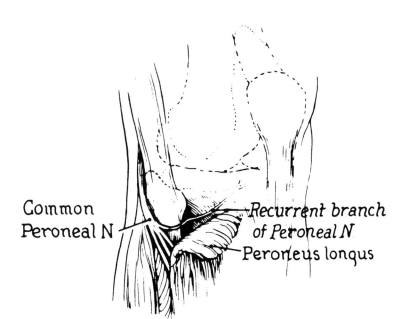

FIG. 6-11. Recurrent peroneal nerve ascending the anterolateral tibia to enter the knee joint. (From ref. 54.)

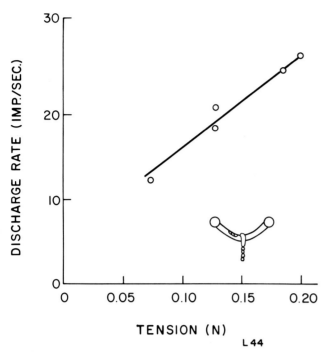

FIG. 6-12. The response of joint capsule receptors as a function of load. (Courtesy of Peter Grigg, Ph.D.)

ceptors that morphologically resembled Ruffini end-organs, Golgi tendon organs, and pacinian corpuscles (Fig. 6-14A through C). There were few free nerve endings demonstrated, suggesting that the ligament itself is relatively insensitive to pain. The few nerve endings present were observed primarily within 5 mm of the femoral origin. The characteristic twist in the ligament was relatively free of neural elements. Most mechanoreceptors were demonstrated from the point distal to the twist in the ligament (approximately 12 mm from the femoral origin) to the tibial insertion. These findings of a preponderance of receptors at the tibial insertion coincide with those of Kennedy and other previous investigators. The neural elements constituted 1% of the total ligament area. The pacinian corpuscle was the most common receptor type observed. The high density of specialized mechanoreceptors led the authors to conclude that the ligament must have an important sensory function.

CLINICAL STUDIES

The histologic confirmation of the presence of mechanoreceptors in the human ACL led recent investigators to suggest that knee ligaments must have a significant sensory function (5,73,74). This echoes the previously stated hypothesis of Kennedy (54) that the failure of mechanoreceptor feedback is a contributing factor to the clinical decline following knee ligament injuries (Fig. 6-1). This also supports the clinical impression of Abbott (1). In recent years, loss of proprioceptive feedback has been suggested as a significant factor in a number of other clinical conditions affecting the knee.

Gait Analysis

In an early study involving biomechanical gait analysis of patients with rheumatoid and osteoarthritis of the knees, Stauffer (83) described a number of gait abnormalities. Numerous gait parameters were found to differ significantly from age-matched controls. These included an increase in medial–lateral shear forces underfoot, indicating exaggerated medial–lateral displacement of the body center. This resulted in a "waddling"-type gait. The author suggested that the loss of proprioceptive feedback from diseased knee joints might require a wider-based gait for better balance. Overall, it was concluded that the gait mechanics of patients with diseased knee joints were a compromise between attempts to decrease pain and increase proprioceptive feedback from the diseased knee. The author felt that increased proprioceptive feedback would result, thereby, in an increase in dynamic muscle control and stability. Therefore, it was again hypothesized that knee capsular and ligament receptors have a clinically important role in providing afferent sensory input and generating stabilizing reflexes.

Prodromos (70) utilized gait analysis to study patients who had undergone proximal tibial osteotomy for medial gonarthrosis. He found that patients who walked with a high adduction moment about the knee preoperatively tended to maintain this gait pattern postoperatively. These patients had a poor clinical result. A proprioceptive neural mechanism was again suggested as a means by which some patients utilized a compensatory gait pattern in the face of a pathologic knee condition.

Andriacchi (4) examined patients following total knee arthroplasty with various prosthetic designs. He discovered that even patients who were completely asymptomatic following surgery had significant gait abnormalities. Patients with implants that retained the cruciate ligaments performed better than those with cruciate-sacrificing prostheses. It was not clear whether this was due to (a) better maintenance of mechanical restraint, (b) better joint kinematics, or (c) afferent sensory input from the cruciates. It was suggested by the author, however, that loss of proprioceptive control might be a factor in the clinical result. He further speculated that different prosthetic designs impose different strains on the capsular tissues where mechanoreceptors are located, and might therefore alter feedback on joint position.

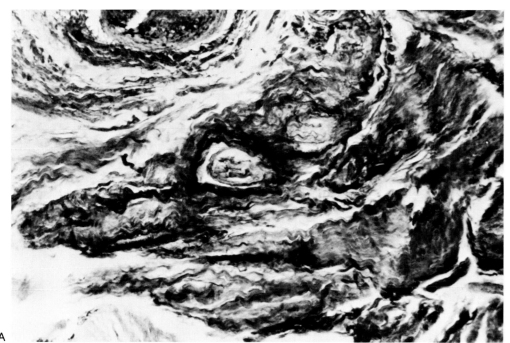

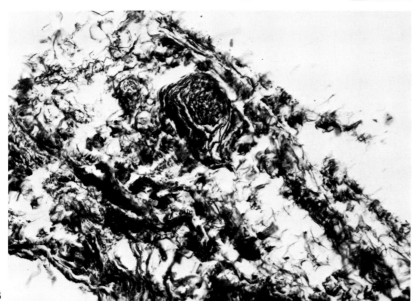

FIG. 6-13. A: A mechanoreceptor just beneath the surface of the cruciate ligament (parallel collagen bundles). This is near the ligament's femoral attachment (Ranvier gold chloride, ×235). (From ref. 73.) **B**: Cross section of a mechanoreceptor just beneath the surface of a human cruciate ligament. Note the similarity to the Golgi tendon organ (Bodian, ×160). (From ref. 73.)

Proprioception Measurements on Normal Subjects

In spite of the hypothesized role of sensory input from knee ligaments in a number of traumatic and degenerative conditions of the knee, clinical measurement of knee joint proprioception or position sense has infrequently been described. Grigg (37) measured position sense of the hip following total hip replacement. Horch (44) applied a similar measurement technique to the knee. The threshold to detection of slow passive change in position of the knee was reported as 2–4° in normal subjects when angular velocities in the range of 0.5°/sec were used. Under these conditions, the slowly adapting Ruffini- or Golgi-type mechanoreceptors are thought to be selectively stimulated. The ability to re-position the knee to an angle at which it was previously placed passively has also been utilized as a test of position sense or proprioception.

Effect of Age and Arthrosis

Applying these methods to normal control group, Skinner (77) reproduced the findings of Horch (44) for normal young adults but further discovered that proprioceptive ability as measured by these tests declined as

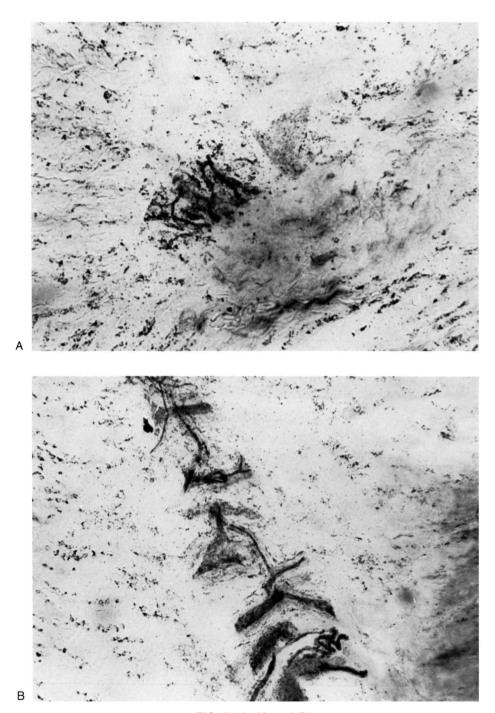

FIG. 6-14. (A and B)

part of normal aging (Fig. 6-15). Other investigators have verified the decline in proprioception with age (53). It has been hypothesized that loss of proprioceptive input might play a factor in geriatric orthopedic problems such as hip fractures that result from an increased incidence of falls along with a lack of reflex muscular splinting (52,53). At least two groups of investigators studied (a) subjects with degenerative arthritis of the knee and (b) those with total knee re-placement. Decline in proprioceptive function was found to occur secondary to the arthritic process, which was not any better or worse following joint replacement (9,23). This is interesting in light of the histologic findings of Schultz (73), who noted the relative absence of mechanoreceptors in ligament tissue removed from arthritic knees during total knee replacement compared to histologic findings in amputation specimens of disease-free knees. It is also consistent

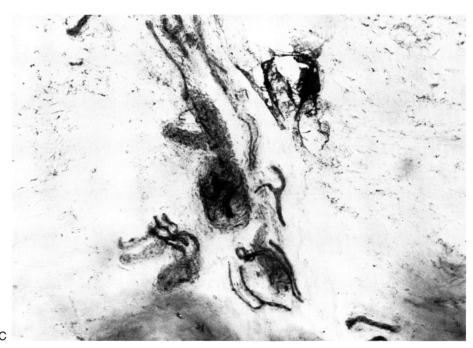

FIG. 6-14. Light micrograph of the ACL showing (**A**) a Ruffini end-organ (×175), (**B**) a mechanoreceptor resembling a Golgi tendon organ (×150), and (**C**) a pacinian corpuscle (×215). (From ref. 74.)

with the findings of Andriacchi (4) and others who have found that gait parameters remain abnormal following total knee replacement in spite of complete alleviation of pain and correction of deformity. In a study that examined gait and proprioception parameters following total knee replacement, proprioceptive loss was found to correlate with gait abnormalities at least as well as any clinical rating parameters (78).

Effect of Athletic Training

Studies on athletic populations indicated that extensive training might improve proprioceptive ability (6). Conversely, the effect of muscle fatigue was found to cause a temporary diminution in joint position sense (80). The mechanism by which this occurs is not clear, however. Since fatigue would apparently seem to affect muscle tissue the most dramatically, diminished position sense with fatigue might be thought to be secondary to loss of input from muscle receptors. Two groups of investigators, however, have demonstrated that fatigue is associated with a temporary increase in laxity of the knee joint (79,84). Fatigue might therefore be equally likely to produce an altered response from ligament receptors. Strain within the knee ligaments, particularly the ACL, has been shown to be closely linked to activity within the hamstrings and quadriceps (71). Loss of tone in the hamstrings would therefore be expected to increase strain in the ACL.

Effect of Injury

Attempts have been made to neutralize ligament receptors with intraarticular anesthesia and to measure the effect on position sense. At least one study was unable to demonstrate any effect on proprioception or gait parameters during normal walking (7). Although capsular receptors would be expected to be anesthetized by intraarticular anesthesia, recently described receptors within the cruciate ligaments might be unaffected. The cruciate ligaments are intraarticular but are extrasynovial, and mechanoreceptors were recently shown by Schutte (74) to be within the substance of the ligaments. Both factors might prevent local anesthesia from affecting these receptors. Tibone (87) examined gait parameters in patients without an ACL and found no abnormalities in basic gait parameters in straight-ahead walking. Dynamic electromyogram (EMG) during running, however, showed longer duration of activity in the medial hamstrings. Force-plate analysis also demonstrated diminished lateral shear forces for the affected limb during cross-cutting maneuvers. Attainment of normal strength in the hamstring muscle group was not adequate to prevent occurrence of the observed abnormalities. It was not clear whether these were the result of (a) loss of proprioceptive feedback from the torn ligaments, (b) simple loss of mechanical restraint, or (c) both in combination.

A recent gait study utilizing dynamic EMG during

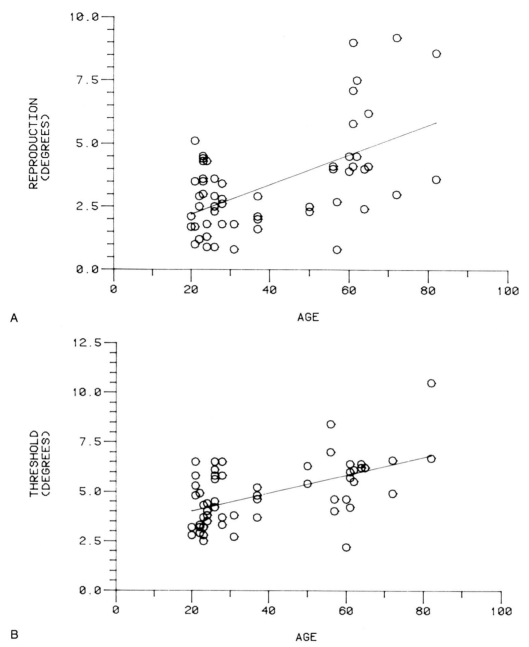

FIG. 6-15. The relationship of kinesthesia and reproduction with age. **A**: Reproduction. **B**: Kinesthesia. (From ref. 77.)

walking did, however, show numerous differences in muscle synergy patterns in patients with ACL deficiency (57). Among the observed differences were increased activity in the hamstrings and diminished activity in the quadriceps and gastrocnemius during joint loading in the swing-to-stance transition. Since the ACL was absent, this response was likely to be the result of stimulation of capsular or tendinous mechanoreceptors. These receptors are stimulated by the slightly abnormal strain they might experience in the absence of a functioning cruciate ligament. It is also possible that this represents a simple muscle-spindle

stretch reflex, but this seems unlikely in normal straight-ahead walking.

A recent report by Barrack (8) quantified proprioception in the ACL-deficient knee. The threshold to the detection in change of position of the knee was measured. Patients with arthroscopically documented absence of the ACL were tested. Threshold values were compared between injured and normal uninjured knees in the test group of young adults. An age-matched control group was also tested. Normal controls were found to have virtually identical threshold values between their right and left knees, with a variation of less than 2%. The test group, however, had a significantly higher threshold value for the injured knee compared to the normal knee, with a variation of over 25% overall. Patients with both acute and chronic ACL instability were tested. No difference was seen between the two groups, implying that the deficit occurred primarily, at the time of injury, rather than secondarily, as a result of progressive laxity over time. Quadriceps atrophy is known to accompany ACL insufficiency in many patients (10). Therefore, thigh circumference and isokinetic testing was also performed to determine if any correlation existed between loss of muscle tone or function and proprioceptive measurements. Since no relationship was observed, proprioceptive loss was, therefore, attributed to absence of the ACL rather than to muscle atrophy. This study by Barrack (8) examined conscious awareness of joint position, which is one major function of mechanoreceptors. The other major sensory afferent role of joint receptors is that of reflex generation. This aspect of knee joint proprioception has also been investigated.

Kennedy (54) examined the effect of knee joint effusions on reflex inhibition of quadriceps muscle contraction. He injected 10-ml increments of fluid into the knee while EMG response amplitude was recorded from the vastus medialis, vastus lateralis, and quadriceps femoris. A 30–50% inhibition of reflex-evoked quadriceps contraction was found to result from 60-ml infusion of normal saline. Inhibition of the vastus medialis was most marked, and maintenance of the effusion for a period of time showed no diminution in the degree of inhibition. This is typical of the response pattern of slowly adapting mechanoreceptors. Injection of local anesthetic prior to infusion of fluid into the joint effectively blocked the inhibition that had previously been demonstrated. Capsular receptors were therefore believed to be responsible for generating this reflex quadriceps inhibition. A subsequent study quantified the loss of muscle strength associated with joint effusion and also concluded that joint afferents played a role in generating this reflex (22). A similar mechanism has been suggested for reflex inhibition of quadriceps activity following meniscectomy and arthrotomy (76,85).

Neural Response Times

Based on his histologic findings and studies on reflex inhibition, Kennedy (54) suggested that loss of mechanoreceptor feedback could lead to reinjury and progressive laxity. A prior study by Pope (69) examined the possible role of reflex muscle contraction in preventing an acute injury. He first showed that contraction of the medial hamstring muscles and the quadriceps substantially increased the valgus stiffness of the

medial ligaments by 104% and 164%, respectively, thus providing substantial potential protection from injury. It was shown, however, that with tactile or visual stimulus to prophylactic muscle contraction, there was insufficient time for the contraction to be of value in sports situations (Fig. 6-16). Pope (69) assumed, however, that the stimulus for muscle contraction was the appreciation of pain or that of a visual stimulus. Impulses from free nerve endings, which are responsible for pain when the knee is stressed, are conducted much more slowly than proprioceptive impulses originating in mechanoreceptors (Table 6-1). Pain is not produced even when mechanoreceptors are maximally stimulated, and these receptors were found more frequently than free nerve endings in knee ligaments (74). Reflex muscle contraction originates via change in tension of knee ligaments. This physically deforms Golgi, Ruffini, or pacinian end-organs, thereby initiating reflex muscle contraction that would occur an order of magnitude faster than if elicited by appreciation of pain or a visual stimulus. Response time would therefore be expected to be significantly faster than estimated in Pope's study (69). Pope states, however, that the magnitude of many sports injuries, such as a linebacker striking the lateral side of a running back's knee at high speed, far exceeds the force necessary to disrupt the knee ligaments even with the benefit of maximal muscle contraction. Guyton (41) emphasizes the speed with which mechanoreceptive sensations are conducted, particularly from rapidly adapting pacinian corpuscles. The potential of these corpuscles to modulate muscle tension during sports activities (such as running) in an almost predictive manner is also emphasized (41). It is likely, therefore, that proprioceptive input does occur through a mechanism which is adequate to serve a protective and/or stabilizing function during normal daily function and even during the moderate stress of most sporting activities. The high energies involved in catastrophic injuries of many contact sports, however, exceed the ability of muscular contraction to prevent ligament rupture.

The synergy between ligaments and muscles in stabilizing the knee was recently examined by Solomonow (82). The knees of experimental animals and of human subjects were loaded with and without an ACL in a manner known to stress the ACL while simultaneously recording electromyographic response in the hamstrings and quadriceps. The test demonstrated a primary rapid reflex arc from mechanoreceptors in the ACL to the hamstring muscle group. There was also a moderate inhibitory effect on the quadriceps. A secondary reflex arc originating in either capsular or muscle tendon receptors was demonstrated in the absence of an ACL, which initiated hamstring contraction in response to knee joint instability. This reflex was found to have a longer response time and to also involve si-

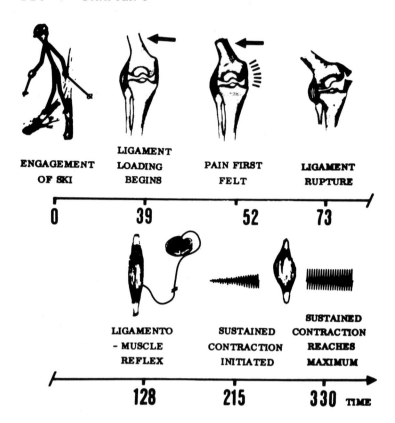

ENGAGEMENT OF SKI — 0

LIGAMENT LOADING BEGINS — 39

PAIN FIRST FELT — 52

LIGAMENT RUPTURE — 73

LIGAMENTO - MUSCLE REFLEX — 128

SUSTAINED CONTRACTION INITIATED — 215

SUSTAINED CONTRACTION REACHES MAXIMUM — 330 TIME

FIG. 6-16. The inadequate response time of a reflex arc initiated by pain. (From ref. 69.)

multaneous quadriceps inhibition. Based on this finding, a potential beneficial effect of hamstring strengthening was suggested by the author.

CLINICAL IMPLICATIONS

Joint position sense or knee joint proprioception has been a topic of extensive research by physiologists since Sir Charles Bell and G. B. Duchenne debated the relative contributions of muscle versus joint receptors over 100 years ago (68). Only in recent years, however, have these findings been applied to topics of concern to the orthopedic surgeon. While our present understanding of the role of mechanoreceptor feedback in the function of the normal and injured knee is certainly incomplete, certain principles do have clinical relevance to the treatment of knee ligament injuries.

Knee Effusions

Perhaps the most basic reflex is the mechanoreceptive reflex, which has now been well documented to inhibit quadriceps contraction when a knee effusion is present (22,54). This inhibition is mediated by slowly adapting receptors and can therefore be maintained indefinitely in the presence of a persistent stimulus. This would lead to rapid muscle atrophy and obviously would have a deleterious effect on rehabilitation. Relief of effusion

either post-injury or post-surgery is, therefore, advantageous on a neuromuscular basis. This could be done through joint aspiration, through application of compression, or through joint motion, either by active muscle contraction or by continuous passive motion. The beneficial effects of immediate motion following knee reconstruction have been outlined by Noyes (62). Although a certain amount of knee effusion is unavoidable postoperatively, the negative effect on quadriceps tone may be partially overcome by bypassing the mechanoreceptors reflex and resorting to direct electrical stimulation of the affected muscle group. Erikkson (21) and subsequently Morrissey (58) have reported beneficial effects of direct electrical stimulation of muscle in diminishing the amount of muscle atrophy that invariably follows knee ligament surgery.

Orthoses

Although there is little doubt that orthoses should be utilized until healing is complete, the role they serve beyond that point is uncertain. They are probably not physically strong enough to prevent sudden overload in the case of a traumatic episode. It has been suggested that such devices may be beneficial because, among other things, they provide proprioceptive input. This hypothesis was tested recently by Branch (13). Dynamic electromyography was performed on patients with ACL tears during cutting maneuvers with and without a knee brace. No difference in the reflex contraction time of the hamstrings could be demonstrated with the addition of bracing. Thus, the ability of knee braces to provide proprioceptive input to the postinjury or postsurgical knee remains unproven.

Palmer (66) believed that knee injuries intensified afferent protective reflexes leading to hamstring spasm, quadriceps inhibition, and the typical semi-flexed posture of the injured knee. He believed that this could lead to irreversible contracture and atrophy if steps were not taken to reverse this process. Palmer also stressed that the injured knee was more susceptible to reinjury or to further, more serious injury, due to alteration or loss of protective proprioceptive reflexes. This sentiment has recently been echoed by Müller (60), who emphasizes the need for protected weight-bearing following knee surgery until proprioceptive control mechanisms return. Protective bracing following knee ligament injuries treated nonoperatively or through primary repair and/or reconstruction, therefore, probably has a neuromuscular basis. Overload of the healing ligament or ligament repair should theoretically be prevented by bracing and protected weight-bearing until proprioceptive reflexes are reestablished.

Proprioceptive Training

Following knee ligament injury and resultant instability, it now seems likely that some patients suffer a proprioceptive deficit, both in position sense (8) and in slowing or diminution of protective reflexes (82). This has relevance in the patient's subsequent rehabilitation, particularly following nonoperative treatment. Proprioceptive training has been suggested as a beneficial aspect of rehabilitation following knee injury or reconstruction (11). Agility training has also been advocated following ligament reconstruction (17). The neuromuscular basis for this concept arises from a study on the ankle by Freeman in 1967 (30). The author described a proprioceptive deficit following ankle ligament injuries. He believed that injury or degenerative diseases affecting the joint capsule led to loss of mechanoreceptor input with resultant impairment of postural and kinesthetic sensation (30). Proprioceptive training through "stabilometry" or training on an unstable board was shown to significantly reduce episodes of giving way. This concept has been applied to knee ligament injuries. Giove (34) reported a high clinical success rate with ability to return to competitive sports simply by achieving adequate hamstring rehabilitation. Walla (88) went one step further and found that active hamstring control reducing the pivot shift was present in 95% of patients who had successfully

avoided surgery following an ACL injury. Further, he found that the ability to achieve "reflex level" hamstring control was most closely correlated with a successful clinical outcome. More recently, Ihara (47) described the beneficial effect of "dynamic joint control." Patients underwent a course of training using unstable boards and were taught to react to suddenly applied forces. A significant improvement in hamstring reaction time (peak torque time) was achieved. The strength of contraction was also significantly improved as reflected by an increase in peak torque value. There was no correlation, however, between isometric muscle strength and reaction times, implying that simple muscle strengthening does not have the beneficial effect found with dynamic training. It appears that neuromuscular training can, to some degree, substitute for the lost sensory input following knee ligament injuries.

Ligament Reconstruction

The final topic of relevance of sensation originating in the knee is in the area of knee ligament repair or reconstruction. Loss of sensory input has concerned knee surgeons for many years. Du Toit (19) postulated that Hey Groves' free fascial substitutions failed, in part, because of loss of proprioceptive feedback and designed the gracilis transfer with the expectation of maintaining this function. Insall (48) believed that his iliotibial bone block transfer maintained proprioceptive ability. Finally, Noyes (61) described the potential benefit of maintaining a vascular supply to a patellar tendon graft as not only preventing complete necrosis but as also maintaining neural connections. Whether proprioceptive ability can be maintained through acute ligament repair or restored through ligament reconstruction is an important question that remains unanswered. In the case of acute injuries, it is probably a mistake to focus on a single anatomic structure such as the ACL. When anterolateral, anteromedial, or combined instability results from an injury, numerous structures are injured, including the capsular ligaments as well as the ACL. Other anatomic relationships are also disrupted, including injuries to the meniscocapsular junction and the musculotendinous unit complex (86). Hughston (46) emphasized the close relationship of the semimembranosus to the MCL and capsular ligament as well as to the medial meniscus. All of these structures have been demonstrated to provide mechanoreceptor input. Repair of these disrupted structures may minimize the disability resulting from loss of input from the ACL. By restoring the normal relationship of the medial ligaments and semimembranosus and repairing the medial meniscus to the capsule, Hughston (45) was able to achieve clinical success with a large group of patients, even when the torn ACL itself was ignored.

Restoration of appropriate length and tension in capsular ligaments would appear to give the best chance of maintaining proprioceptive input from ligament mechanoreceptors. While this is a logical conclusion of all that is presently known about knee joint sensation, it has admittedly not been proven clinically or in experimental models. Müller (60), however, emphasizes the importance of the deep capsular ligaments in providing proprioceptive stability control and stresses the importance of restoring normal length to the capsular ligaments for this reason.

Whether an acutely repaired ACL retains any sensory function is uncertain. Kennedy (55) believed that the ACL had an adequate blood supply for primary healing to potentially take place. Repair of the ligament alone, however, has generally resulted in persistent instability, implying that neither mechanical nor sensory function is successfully restored (24).

Whether proprioceptive input through reconstruction of a chronically unstable knee is restored is unknown. Certainly, a prosthetic ligament has no potential for sensory input. Free grafts may or may not restore sensory afferent function. While the graft material, such as patellar tendon, may originally contain mechanoreceptors, neural connections are severed and the graft tissue undergoes necrosis. It is unknown whether any mechanoreceptor function returns with graft revascularization. Reconstructions that restore a normal amount of tension to lax capsular structures do have the potential of improving sensory input as do transfers that remain viable. Whether this, in fact, is achieved is a topic for future research.

From a neuromuscular viewpoint, choice of graft material for the ACL reconstruction is somewhat narrow. A report by Limbird (57) demonstrated the importance of the hamstrings in dynamic compensation for ACL deficiency, suggesting that sacrifice of these tendons for reconstruction may hinder the final result. Several other reports (34,87,88) note the importance of the hamstring musculature in achieving a successful clinical outcome. Studies showing protective reflex hamstring activity in ACL-deficient knees (82) provide further evidence that hamstring sacrifice for ligament reconstruction should be considered a last resort in order to maintain rehabilitation potential from a dynamic and proprioceptive viewpoint.

CONCLUSION

In addition to providing passive restraint to abnormal motion, knee ligaments provide sensory input that is responsible for conscious appreciation of joint position as well as for initiation of stabilizing and protective reflexes. This function diminishes by a certain degree as part of normal aging. More marked diminution is associated with degenerative joint disease. This may explain the abnormal gait pattern observed in patients with degenerative arthritis of the knee. It may also explain why normal gait is not restored following total knee arthroplasty, and in some cases following proximal tibial osteotomy in spite of absence of pain or deformity. Knee ligament disruption and resultant instability also seem to result in some loss of sensory feedback. Diminution in appreciation of joint position as well as in protective reflexes has recently been demonstrated following ACL tears. Neuromuscular training seems to be beneficial by substituting mechanoreceptor feedback from capsular and tendinous receptors for that of the lost cruciate ligament. There is no current evidence that bracing restores any proprioceptive feedback. Acute repair of disrupted capsular and collateral ligaments, as well as restoration of the normal relationship between the menisci and tendinous expansions inserting on the capsule, have the potential of maintaining the mechanoreceptor function known to be present in all of these tissues. The question remains, however, whether the proprioceptive function of the cruciate ligaments can be maintained by acute repair or restored by chronic reconstruction.

The opinions or assertions expressed herein are those of the authors and are not to be construed as official or as necessarily reflecting the views of the Department of the Navy or of the naval service at large.

REFERENCES

1. Abbott LC, Saunders JB, Dec M, et al. Injuries to the ligaments of the knee joint. *J Bone Joint Surg* 1944;26:503–521.
2. Adams JA. Feedback theory of how joint receptors regulate the timing and positioning of a limb. *Psychol Rev* 1977;84:504–523.
3. Andrew BL. The sensory innervation of the medial ligament of the knee joint. *J Physiol (Lond)* 1954;123:241–250.
4. Andriacchi TP, Galante JO, Fermier RW. The influence of total knee-replacement design on walking and stair-climbing. *J Bone Joint Surg* 1982;64A:1328–1335.
5. Arnoczky SP. Anatomy of the anterior cruciate ligament. *Clin Orthop* 1983;172:19–25.
6. Barrack RL, Skinner HB, Brunet ME, Cook SD. Joint kinesthesia in the highly trained knee. *J Sport Med Phys Fitness* 1983;24:18–20.
7. Barrack RL, Skinner HB, Brunet ME, Haddad RJ Jr. Functional performance of the knee after intraarticular anesthesia. *Am J Sports Med* 1983;11(4):258–261.
8. Barrack RL, Skinner HB, Buckley SL. Proprioception in the anterior cruciate deficient knee. *Am J Sports Med* 1989;17:1–6.
9. Barrack RL, Skinner HB, Cook SD, Haddad RJ Jr. Effect of articular disease and total knee arthroplasty on knee joint-position sense. *J Neurophysiol* 1983;50(3):684–687.
10. Baugher WH, Warren RF, Marshall JL, Joseph A. Quadriceps atrophy in the anterior cruciate insufficient knee. *Am J Sports Med* 1984;12(3):192–195.
11. Blackburn TA Jr. Rehabilitation of anterior cruciate ligament injuries. *Orthop Clin North Am* 1985;16(2):241–269.

12. Boyd IA. The histological structure of the receptors in the knee-joint of the cat correlated with their physiological response. *J Physiol* 1954;124:476–488.

13. Branch TP, Hunter R, Donath M. Dynamic EMG analysis of anterior cruciate deficient legs with and without bracing during cutting. *Am J Sports Med* 1989;17:35–41.

14. Burgess PR, Clark FJ. Characteristics of knee joint receptors in the cat. *J Physiol* (Lond) 1969;203:317–335.

15. Clark FJ. Information signaled by sensory fibers in medial articular nerve. *J Neurophysiol* 1975;38:1464–1472.

16. Clark FJ, Burgess PR. Slowly adapting receptors in cat knee joint: can they signal joint angle? *J Neurophysiol* 1975;38:1448–1463.

17. Curl WW, Markey KL, Mitchell WA. Agility training following anterior cruciate ligament reconstruction. *Clin Orthop* 1983;172:133–136.

18. Dee R. Structure and function of hip joint innervation. *Ann R Coll Surg Engl* 1969;45:357–374.

19. Du Toit GT. Knee joint cruciate ligament substitution. The Lindemann (Heidelberg) operation. *S Afr J Surg* 1967;5:25–30.

20. Ekholm J, Eklund G, Skoglund S. On the reflex effects from the knee joint of the cat. *Acta Physiol Scand* 1960;50:167–174.

21. Eriksson E, Häggmark T. Comparison of isometric muscle training and electrical stimulation supplementing isometric muscle training in the recovery after major knee ligament surgery. *Am J Sports Med* 1979;7:169–171.

22. Fahrer H, Rentsch HU, Gerber NJ, Beyeler C, Hess CW, Grünig B. Knee effusion and reflex inhibition of the quadriceps. A bar to effective retraining. *J Bone Joint Surg* 1988;70B:635–638.

23. Faris PM, Jiang CC, Otis JC, Manouel M. Proprioceptive input of the posterior cruciate ligament in knee prostheses. *Trans Orthop Res Soc* 1988;13:358.

24. Feagin JA Jr. The syndrome of the torn anterior cruciate ligament. *Orthop Clin North Am* 1979;10:81–90.

25. Ferrell WR, Baxendale RH, Carnachan C, Hart IK. The influence of joint afferent discharge on locomotion, proprioception and activity in conscious cats. *Brain Res* 1985;347:41–48.

26. Frankel VH, Burstein AH, Brooks DB. Biomechanics of internal derangement of the knee. Pathomechanics as determined by analysis of the instant centers of motions. *J Bone Joint Surg* 1971;53A:945–962.

27. Freeman MAR, Dean MRE, Hanham IWF. The etiology and prevention of functional instability of the foot. *J Bone Joint Surg* 1985;47B:678–685.

28. Freeman MAR, Wyke B. Articular contributions to limb muscle reflexes. An electromyographic study of the influence of ankle-joint mechanoreceptors upon reflex activity in the gastrocnemius muscle of the cat. *J Physiol* 1964;171:20P–21P.

29. Freeman MAR, Wyke BD. The innervation of the knee joint. An anatomical and histological study in the cat. *J Anat* 1964;101:505–532.

30. Freeman MAR, Wyke B. Articular reflexes of the ankle joint. An electromyographic study of normal and abnormal influences of ankle-joint mechanoreceptors upon reflex activity in leg muscles. *Br J Surg* 1967;54:990–1001.

31. Gardner E. Reflex muscular responses to stimulation of articular nerves in the cat. *Am J Physiol* 1950;161:133–141.

32. Gardner ED. The distribution and termination of nerves in the knee-joint of the cat. *J Comp Neurol* 1944;80:11–32.

33. Gardner E. The innervation of the knee joint. *Anat Rec* 1948;101:109–130.

34. Giove TP, Miller SJ 3rd, Kent BE, Sanford TL, Garrick JG. Non-operative treatment of the torn anterior cruciate ligament. *J Bone Joint Surg* 1983;65A:184–192.

35. Goodwin GM, McCloskey DI, Matthews PB. The persistence of appreciable kinesthesia after paralysing joint afferents but preserving muscle afferents. *Brain Res* 1972;37:326–329.

36. Grigg P. Mechanical factors influencing response of joint afferent neurons from cat knee. *J Neurophysiol* 1975;38:1473–1484.

37. Grigg P, Finerman GA, Riley LH. Joint position sense after total hip replacement. *J Bone Joint Surg* 1973;55A:1016–1025.

38. Grigg P, Hoffman AH. Properties of Ruffini afferents revealed by stress analysis of isolated sections of cat knee capsule. *J Neurophysiol* 1982;47:41–54.

39. Grigg P, Hoffman AH. Neuronal mechanoreceptors as a probe for tissue mechanics. Presented at the Annual Meeting of the American Academy of Orthopaedic Surgeons, Atlanta, Georgia, February 1988.

40. Grigg A, Hoffman AH, Fogarty KE. Properties of Golgi–Mazzoni afferents in cat knee joint capsule as revealed by mechanical studies of isolated joint capsule. *J Neurophysiol* 1982;47:31–40.

41. Guyton AC. *Textbook of medical physiology*, 6th ed. Philadelphia: WB Saunders, 1980.

42. Guyton AC. *Textbook of medical physiology*, 7th ed. Philadelphia: WB Saunders, 1986.

43. Hilton J. *On the influence of mechanical and physiological rest in the treatment of accidents and surgical diseases, and the diagnostic value of pain*. A course of lectures. London: Bell and Daldy, 1863.

44. Horch KW, Clark FJ, Burgess PR. Awareness of knee joint angle under static conditions. *J Neurophysiol* 1975;388:1436–1447.

45. Hughston JC, Barrett GR. Acute anteromedial rotatory instability. Long-term results of surgical repair. *J Bone Joint Surg* 1983;65A:145–153.

46. Hughston JC, Eilers AF. The role of the posterior oblique ligament in repairs of acute medial (collateral) ligament tears of the knee. *J Bone Joint Surg* 1973;55A:923–940.

47. Ihara H, Nakayama A. Dynamic joint control training for knee ligament injuries. *Am J Sports Med* 1986;14:309–315.

48. Insall J, Joseph DM, Aglietti P, Campbell RD Jr. Bone-block iliotibial-band transfer for anterior cruciate insufficiency. *J Bone Joint Surg* 1981;63A:560–564.

49. Jacobsen K. Osteoarthrosis following insufficiency of the cruciate ligaments in man: a clinical study. *Acta Orthop Scand* 1977;48:520–526.

50. Jeletsky AG. On the innervation of the capsule and epiphysis of the knee. *Vestn Khir* 1931;22:74–112.

51. Jewett DL, Rayner MD. *Basic concepts of neuron function*. Boston: Little, Brown, 1984.

52. Johnson JT. Neuropathic fractures and joint injuries: pathogenesis and rationale for prevention and treatment. *J Bone Joint Surg* 1967;49A:1–30.

53. Kaplan FS, Nixon JE, Reitz M, Rindfleisch L, Tucker J. Age-related changes in joint proprioception and sensation of joint position. *Acta Orthop Scand* 1985;56:72–74.

54. Kennedy JC, Alexander IJ, Hayes KC. Nerve supply of the human knee and its functional importance. *Am J Sports Med* 1982;10:329–335.

55. Kennedy JC, Weinberg HW, Wilson AS. The anatomy and function of the anterior cruciate ligament, as determined by clinical and morphological studies. *J Bone Joint Surg* 1974;56A:223–235.

56. Lane JM, Chisena E, Black J. Experimental knee instability: early mechanical property changes in articular cartilage in a rabbit model. *Clin Orthop* 1979;140:262–265.

57. Limbird TJ, Shiavi R, Frazer M, Borra H. EMG profiles of knee joint musculature during walking: changes induced by anterior cruciate ligament deficiency. *J Orthop Res* 1988;6:630–638.

58. Morrissey MC, Brewster CE, Shields CL Jr, Brown M. The effects of electrical stimulation on the quadriceps during postoperative knee immobilization. *Am J Sports Med* 1985;13:40–45.

59. Mountcastle VS. *Medical physiology*. 14th ed. St. Louis: CV Mosby, 1980.

60. Müller W. *The knee: form, function and ligament reconstruction*. Berlin: Springer-Verlag, 1982.

61. Noyes FR, Butler DL, Paulos LE, Grood ES. Intra-articular cruciate reconstruction, part I: perspectives on graft strength, vascularization and immediate motion after replacement. *Clin Orthop* 1983;172:71–77.

62. Noyes FR, Mangine RE: Early knee motion after open and arthroscopic anterior cruciate ligament reconstruction. *Am J Sports Med* 1987;15:149–160.

63. O'Connor BL. The mechanoreceptor innervation of the posterior attachments of the lateral meniscus of the dog knee joint. *J Anat* 1984;138:15–26.

64. O'Connor BL, Gonzales J. Mechanoreceptors of the medial collateral ligament of the cat knee joint. *J Anat* 1979;129:719–729.

65. O'Connor BL, McConnaughey JS. The structure and innervation of cat knee menisci and their relation to a 'sensory hypothesis' of meniscal function. *Am J Anat* 1978;153:431–442.

66. Palmer I. Pathophysiology of the medial ligament of the knee joint. *Acta Chir Scand* 1958;115:312–318.

67. Polocek P. Differences in the structure and variability of encapsulated nerve endings in joints of some species of mammals. *Acta Anat* 1961;47:112–124.

68. Poore GV. Paralysis of the muscular and articular sensibility. In: *Selections from the clinical works of Dr. Duchenne*. London: New Sydenham Society, 1883;378–398.

69. Pope MH, Johnson RJ, Brown DW, Tighe C. The role of the musculature in injuries to the medial collateral ligament. *J Bone Joint Surg* 1979;61A:398–402.

70. Prodromos CC, Andriacchi TP, Galante JO. A relationship between gait and clinical changes following high tibial osteotomy. *J Bone Joint Surg* 1985;67A:1188–1194.

71. Renstrom P, Arms SW, Stanwyck TS, Johnson RJ. Strain within the anterior cruciate ligament during hamstring and quadriceps activity. *Am J Sports Med* 1988;14:83–87.

72. Roland PE. Do muscular receptors in man evoke sensations of tension and kinaesthesia? *Strain Technol* 1975;50:162–165.

73. Schultz RA, Miller DC, Kerr CS, Micheli L. Mechanoreceptors in human cruciate ligaments. A histologic study. *J Bone Joint Surg* 1984;66A:1072–1076.

74. Schutte MJ, Dabezies EJ, Zimny ML, Happel LT. Neural anatomy of the human anterior cruciate ligament. *J Bone Joint Surg* 1987;69A:243–247.

75. Seebacher JR, Inglis AE, Marshall JL, Warren RF. The structure of the posterolateral aspect of the knee. *J Bone Joint Surg* 1982;64A:536–541.

76. Shakespeare DT, Stokes M, Sherman KP, Young A. Reflex inhibition of the quadriceps after meniscectomy: lack of association with pain. *Clin Phys* 1985;5:137–144.

77. Skinner HB, Barrack RL, Cook SD. Age-related decline in proprioception. *Clin Orthop* 1984;184:208–211.

78. Skinner HB, Barrack RL, Cook SD, Haddad RJ Jr. Joint position sense in total knee arthroplasty. *J Orthop Res* 1984;1:276–283.

79. Skinner HB, Wyatt MP, Hodgdon JA, Conard DW, Barrack RL. Effect of fatigue on joint position sense of the knee. *J Orthop Res* 1986;4:112–118.

80. Skinner HB, Wyatt MP, Stone ML, Hodgdon JA, Barrack RL. Exercise-related knee joint laxity. *Am J Sports Med* 1986;14:30–34.

81. Skoglund ST. Joint receptors and kinesthesis. In: *Handbook of sensory physiology*. Vol. 2 Springer-Verlag, 1973;111–136.

82. Solomonow M, Baratta R, Zhou BH, Shoji H, Bose W, Beck C, D'Ambrosia R. The synergistic action of the anterior cruciate ligament and thigh muscles in maintaining joint stability. *Am J Sports Med* 1987;15:207–213.

83. Stauffer RN, Chao EY, Györy AN. Biomechanical gait analysis of the diseased knee joint. *Clin Orthop* 1977;126:246–255.

84. Steiner ME, Grana WA, Chillag K, Schelberg-Karnes E. The effect of exercise on anterior–posterior knee laxity. *Am J Sports Med* 1986;14:24–29.

85. Stokes M, Young A. The contribution of reflex inhibition to arthrogenous muscle weakness. *Clin Sci* 1984;67:7–14.

86. Terry GC, Hughston JC. Associated joint pathology in the anterior cruciate ligament-deficient knee with emphasis on a classification system and injuries to the meniscocapsular ligament-musculotendinous unit complex. *Orthop Clin North Am* 1985;16:29–39.

87. Tibone JE, Antich TJ, Fanton GS, Moynes DR, Perry J. Functional analysis of anterior cruciate ligament instability. *Am J Sports Med* 1986;14:276–284.

88. Walla DJ, Albright JP, McAuley E, Martin RK, Eldridge V, El-Khoury G. Hamstring control and the unstable anterior cruciate ligament-deficient knee. *Am J Sports Med* 1985;13:34–39.

89. Warren LF, Marshall JL. The supporting structures and layers on the medial side of the knee: an anatomical analysis. *J Bone Joint Surg* 1979;61A:56–62.

90. Williams WJ. A systems-oriented evaluation of the role of joint receptors and other afferent in position and motion sense. *Crit Rev Bio Med Eng* 1981;7:23.

91. Willis WP, Grossman RG. *Medical neurobiology*, 3rd ed. St. Louis: CV Mosby, 1981.

92. Wilson AS, Legg PG, McNeur JC. Studies on the innervation of the medial meniscus in the human knee joint. *Anat Rec* 1969;165:485–491.

Knee Ligaments: Structure, Function, Injury, and Repair, edited by D. Daniel, et al.
© 1990 by Raven Press, Ltd. All rights reserved.

CHAPTER 7

Fundamental Studies in Knee Ligament Mechanics

Savio L-Y. Woo, Edmond P. Young, and Michael K. Kwan

The ligaments of the knee are well designed for their role in the maintenance of normal joint kinematics, with each ligament oriented in the direction needed to provide joint stability. Ligaments are unique connective tissues. Their densely packed collagen fiber bundles are arrayed in parallel along the length of the tissue substance to allow for the most efficient resistance of tensile loads. Like other soft connective tissues, ligaments are characterized by a nonlinear mechanical behavior. Their nonlinear properties have been modeled by Viidik (50) as a parallel array of individual linearly elastic components that represent the fibrillar components of the tissue, primarily collagen (Fig. 7-1). Because of varying amounts of folding or "crimp" present in the collagen fibrils, "recruitment" of additional fibrils occurs with increasing tensile deformation. As increasing numbers of these fibrils become load-bearing, an increase in tissue stiffness is seen and a nonlinear load–deformation curve results. During normal motion, this nonlinear behavior allows the ligaments to provide gentle guidance to maintain normal joint kinematics without sustaining substantial loads or deformations. Yet, when the knee is subjected to ab-

normally large forces, the nonlinear properties help the ligaments to rapidly provide additional protection to the joint. Excessive joint motion is limited by the increasing stiffness of the ligament in response to potentially deforming loads.

Ligament insertions to bone are also well adapted to their intended function. Force dissipation is achieved through a gradual transition from ligament to fibrocartilage to bone. Disruption is less likely to occur in this transition region than in the bone or peri-insertional tissue substance (37–39). As with all physiological systems, there are functional adaptations of the ligament and its insertion sites to age, temperature, sex, levels of stress and motion, and any number of other unknown parameters. The mechanism of adaptation may well involve changes in the biochemical content and organization of the ligament substance.

Much research has been performed to date in an effort to elucidate the specifics of ligament mechanics. The acquisition of quantitative information regarding ligament function has important applications to both our fundamental understanding of normal knee mechanics and our management of knee ligament injury. These studies also provide baseline data for the analysis of knee motion as well as reference criteria for the design of ligament replacements. In discussing the tensile properties of ligaments, it is important to distinguish between the structural properties of the bone–

S. L-Y. Woo, E. P. Young, and M. K-W. Kwan: Orthopaedic Bioengineering Laboratory, University of California, San Diego, La Jolla, California, and San Diego Veterans Administration Medical Center, La Jolla, California 92093.

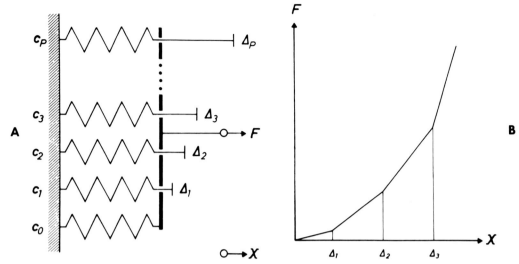

FIG. 7-1. A: Model of nonlinear elasticity based upon progressive recruitment of individual linearly elastic components. **B:** The resultant nonlinear load–deformation curve. (From ref. 15.)

ligament–bone complex and the mechanical properties of the ligament itself. The structural properties (e.g., ultimate load, ultimate deformation, linear stiffness, and energy absorbed at failure) describe the tensile behavior of the bone–ligament–bone complex as a functional composite and can be obtained from the load–deformation curve. The mechanical properties (e.g., tangent modulus, tensile strength, and ultimate strain) are measurements of the material characteristics of the ligament substance itself and can be obtained from the stress–strain curve. These structural and mechanical parameters will be discussed further in later sections.

EXPERIMENTAL TECHNIQUES

The experimental determination of the mechanical properties of ligaments poses a number of technical hurdles, including the accurate measurement of specimen dimensions and the isolation of the properties of the tissue substance from those of its connecting structures. The simplest case, testing of an isolated segment of ligament, is complicated by difficulties in effectively securing the cut ends of the specimen. Ligaments are typically insufficient in length to allow convenient clamping of the isolated substance for tensile testing. Furthermore, clamping of the free ends generally results in damage and weakening of the underlying tissue, eventually contributing to premature failure. The use of a bone–ligament–bone preparation provides more secure clamping and may provide a better approximation of *in situ* loading conditions; however, it becomes difficult to isolate the tensile properties of the ligament substance from those of the insertion sites

(58). We shall review the current progress in this area of study and specifically discuss the newly developed techniques used in our laboratory to overcome some of these difficulties.

Determination of Cross-Sectional Area

Because stress is defined as the load per unit area, the accurate measurement of ligament cross-sectional area is essential for the determination of this mechanical property. Conventional mechanical measurement methods, such as vernier calipers, have been used to measure the width and thickness of ligaments, with the area calculated by assuming a rectangular cross section. The cross-sectional shapes of many ligaments are irregular and geometrically complex, however, and large errors in measurements can result. Early attempts to determine cross-sectional areas of soft tissues include those by Gratz (18), Cronkite (8), Nunley (40), and Rigby (42). In the 1960s, the gravimetric method, which calculated the cross-sectional area through division of the specimen's volume (calculated from its weight) by the length, was used by Abrahams (1), Elden (11), Matthews (30), and VanBrocklin (48). In recent years, a number of other methods have been used. Haut (21) assumed the cross-sectional shape of canine anterior cruciate ligament (ACL) to be elliptical and calculated the cross-sectional area by measuring the major and minor axes with a micrometer. The area micrometer system determines cross-sectional areas by compressing the specimen in a rectangular slot of known width and then measuring the specimen height with a micrometer. This method was described by Ellis (13) for the measurement of cross-sectional areas of tendons. Walker (51) also used an area micrometer to measure tendon cross-sectional areas, whereas Butler (7) used a modification of this method to determine the cross-sectional area of the ACL and of other soft tissues. However, measurements made using the area micrometer method have been shown to be dependent upon the pressure applied to the specimen, as demonstrated by Allard (3). Woo (55,58) used a micrometer system that applied a minimal compressive force to the specimen during thickness measurements of canine and swine medial collateral ligament (MCL). The widths of these specimens were measured with a cathetometer, and the areas were calculated by assuming the cross-sectional shape to be rectangular. Shrive (43) designed a thickness caliper to measure the area of the rabbit MCL by determining the thickness profile along the width of the tissue.

A number of noncontact image reconstruction techniques have been described (12,19,24,36). Ellis (12) used a "shadow amplitude method" to determine the radius of specimen profiles in order to reconstruct the specimen cross section. Gupta (19) used a rotating microscope to determine the profile of the canine ACL, from which the cross-sectional area was calculated. Njus (36) used a video dimension analyzer system to measure profile widths.

The laser micrometer method is a new, noncontact,

automated system developed in our laboratory to determine cross-sectional area and shape of ligaments using a collimated laser beam and digital image reconstruction (27). The specimen is placed perpendicular to the path of the laser beam and is then rotated through 180° by a computer-controlled drive system. The profile width for each increment of rotation is recorded simultaneously via a microprocessor. The center of rotation and upper and lower boundaries of the object are then determined for each incremental rotation, and an iterative procedure is used to digitally reconstruct the cross-sectional shape. The cross-sectional area can then be calculated by computer. For determination of both cross-sectional shape and area of the ACL, the laser micrometer method proved to be both highly accurate and reproducible in its reconstruction of the complex ligament geometry, as verified by histological sections (Fig. 7-2). In addition, this technique has been used to measure the variation in shape and cross-sectional area along the length of a ligament. It is unlikely that conventional methods could have reproduced these complex cross sections.

Recently, a study was performed to compare three methods for cross-sectional area measurements of the rabbit MCL: (i) the laser micrometer method, (ii) the vernier caliper method, and (iii) the area micrometer method. Each of the three methods was used to mea-

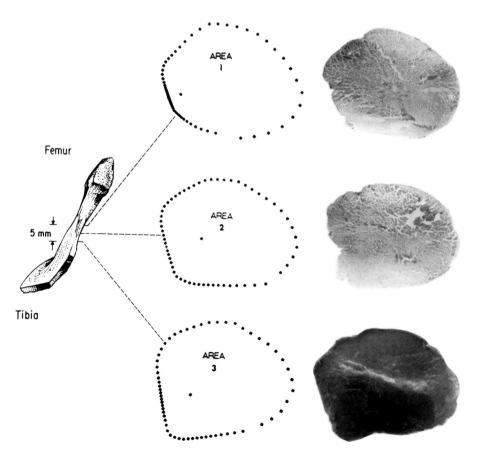

FIG. 7-2. Laser micrometer reconstructions of the cross section of the ACL at three locations, demonstrating good agreement with the corresponding histological sections. (From ref. 27.)

sure the cross-sectional area at identical locations along the midsubstance of the rabbit MCL. The areas obtained using the area micrometer method were, on average, 21.9% lower than the areas obtained using the laser micrometer method. This is consistent with the difference obtained previously by Lee for the ACL (27). Because of the external pressure applied by the area micrometer to the ligament, we believe the specimen was forced to conform to an area other than its natural shape, thus leading to a lower value of cross-sectional area measurements. The vernier calipers, on the other hand, slightly underestimated the cross-sectional area by an average of 2.3%. This suggests that the assumption of a rectangular cross section is reasonable for the rabbit MCL. Recently, Shrive (43) also showed a near-rectangular cross section for the MCL and presented a new device, consisting of a thickness caliper and a displacement transducer, for measurement of cross-sectional area. However, the area measurements given by this device were reported to be 43% less than those obtained by using the vernier calipers. This large discrepancy may have been due to distortion of the ligament cross section as the thickness caliper was dragged across the width of tissue.

Determination of Strain

Historically, changes in ligament length have been reported as testing-machine cross-head or clamp-to-clamp displacement. When testing a bone–ligament–bone complex, however, these values reflect only the structural properties of the complex as a whole, and they fail to isolate the mechanical properties of the ligament substance from those of the insertion sites and other interposed soft tissues. In contrast, ligament strain is a material property of the isolated ligament substance and is expressed as the deformation of the ligament substance normalized to a defined initial (reference) length. Ligament strain has been estimated by a wide variety of methods (5,7,10,28,31,32,47,53). Kennedy (25) performed one of the first important studies of knee ligament strain using a liquid-mercury strain gauge sutured to the ligament. Others have also used liquid-metal strain gauges to measure strains in the tissue substance (22,31,32). Dorlot (10) measured the change in insertion site separation during knee flexion as an estimation of ligament strain. A Hall effect strain transducer has been developed by Arms (5) which uses changes in an electromagnetic field to determine length changes in the ligament (Fig. 8-17). Buckle transducers have been used by others to measure the forces in the ligament substance (Fig. 8-16) (2,28). These systems rely on direct contact with the test specimen, however, and may impose artifact upon the measured quantities.

The video dimension analyzer (VDA), developed more than a decade ago by our laboratory, provides an excellent tool for the measurement of tissue strain which requires no direct contact with the specimen. This method relies instead on a recorded video image of the test specimen (Fig. 7-3). Prior to testing, two or more reference lines (markers for gauge length) are drawn on the tendon or ligament perpendicular to the loading axis with a Verhoff's elastin stain (62). Tensile testing is then performed, and the data are recorded by a video camera and a videocassette recorder. The taped image is then played back through the VDA system, which superimposes two electronic "windows" over the reference lines. These windows automatically track the movement of the reference lines throughout the test and convert the horizontal scan time between lines into an output voltage. The voltage change, expressed as a function of the initial voltage, can then be calibrated to correspond to percent strain of the tissue. The frequency response of the VDA system is as high as 120 Hz, and errors in linearity and accuracy are less than 0.5% (57).

There are a number of advantages in using noncontact methods such as the VDA system to measure strains of ligaments as compared to other methods involving mechanical or electronic gauges: (a) There is no physical contact with the specimen during testing; (b) strains can be measured in the midsubstance independent of the insertion sites; (c) strain values can be obtained from different regions of the same specimen simply by selective placement of the reference lines (gauge lengths); (d) video recording of testing permits the data to be conveniently analyzed after the test and provides a permanent record; and (e) the advent of high-speed video recorders allows high-strain-rate testing to be videotaped with strain analysis done at slower playback speeds (41).

RECENT FINDINGS ON BIOMECHANICAL PROPERTIES

Equipped with recent technological developments, such as those just described, several new fundamental investigations into the tensile properties of ligaments are possible. Again, it is important to distinguish between the structural properties of the bone–ligament–bone complex and the mechanical properties of the ligament itself. Direct experimental measurement of load (using a load cell) and deformation (based on test-machine cross-head or clamp-to-clamp displacement) are reasonably straightforward. The structural properties, represented by the load–deformation curve, are measurements of the tensile behavior of the bone–ligament–bone complex as a functional composite (Fig. 7-4A). Other parameters, such as linear stiffness, en-

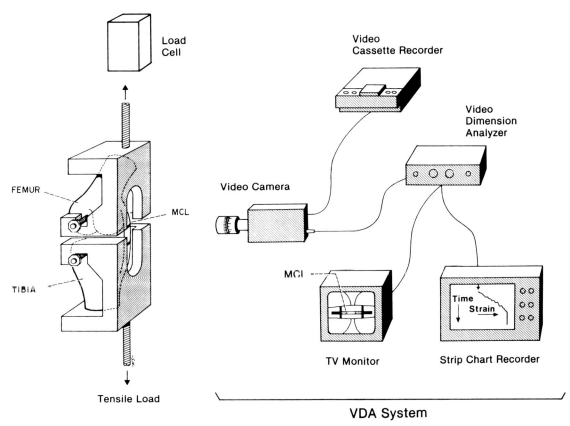

FIG. 7-3. The VDA system as configured to measure the tensile strain in the MCL. The system records the strain history from the two ligament stain lines (gauge lengths) by means of the video camera, videocassette recorder, dimension analyzer, and strip chart recorder. (From ref. 62.)

ergy absorbed at failure, ultimate load, and ultimate deformation, can be determined from the load–deformation curve. However, these structural properties represent the behavior of the complex as a whole and are dependent upon a number of other parameters, including (a) the mechanical properties of the tissue substance, (b) the geometry of the tissue (cross-sectional area, length, and shape), and (c) the properties of the bone–ligament junction. On the other hand, the mechanical (material) properties, represented by the stress–strain curve, are measurements of the material characteristics of the ligament substance itself, reflecting the organization and/or orientation of its collagen fibers as well as the interactions of the various other constituents (Fig. 7-4B). Other parameters, such as the tangent modulus, tensile strength, and ultimate strain, can be determined from the stress–strain curve. These parameters will remain constant for a given tissue regardless of its size or shape.

The experimental determination of the structural and mechanical properties of knee ligaments involves a number of variables in the testing environment, including the method of storage, temperature of the test environment, specimen age, skeletal maturity, and applied strain rate. Our laboratory has evaluated the ef-

fects of these different factors on the properties of ligaments.

Temperature-Dependent Properties

An important consideration when testing ligaments is the influence of the environmental temperature on their biomechanical behavior. Most tests have been performed with the specimens in air at room temperature. Others have immersed the specimen in a bath, such as an isotonic solution, where pH and temperature can be closely controlled. Rigby (42) suggested that no changes occur in the mechanical properties of ligaments between 0°C and 37°C. Apter (4), however, reported that the elastic modulus of collagen varies inversely with temperature from 0°C to 70°C. Hunter (23) found an inverse relationship between joint stiffness and temperature. A similar temperature dependence has been documented by our laboratory for articular cartilage (26).

The effect of temperature on ligament properties was studied using the adult canine femur–MCL–tibia complex (FMTC) (61). The specimen was mounted in clamps and submerged in a physiologic saline bath with a heating and cooling system monitored and controlled

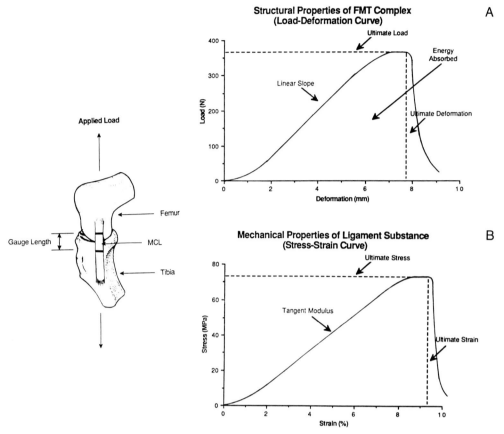

FIG. 7-4. Typical results of tensile testing to failure. The structural properties are obtained from the load–deformation curve (**A**), whereas the mechanical properties are obtained from the stress–strain curve (**B**).

by a thermostat (accuracy within 0.5°C). Cyclic testing was performed at temperatures ranging from 2°C to 37°C at a pH of 7.4. Hysteresis curves were measured for cycling between 0 and 2 mm extension (i.e., ligament strains of approximately 0% and 3.5%). Additional cycles were performed between 1 and 2 mm extension to determine the temperature-dependent viscoelastic properties.

The peak loads during cyclic testing were seen to equilibrate at progressively lower levels as the testing temperature was increased. When the peak load for the first cycle is normalized to the first cycle load at 22°C, the decrease in peak load with temperature can be expressed by a simple linear relationship (Fig. 7-5). By the 10th cycle, the peak load for the FMTC was reduced to 92 ± 1%, 90 ± 1%, and 88 ± 1% of the first cycle load for 2°C, 22°C, and 37°C, respectively. The area of hysteresis reflected a similar inverse relationship with temperature, characterized by a decrease in the area of the first cycle with increasing temperature. It is particularly important to note that because of time- and history-dependent viscoelastic properties, the ligament requires 1–2½ hours between temperature changes to regain its untested, resting

characteristics. These viscoelastic properties have not been addressed in previous studies and may explain why our findings differ from those obtained by others. It also demonstrates that experimental protocols for future studies should include standardization of test temperature, since variations in temperature can have profound effects on ligament behavior.

Effects of Storage by Freezing

Biomechanical testing of ligaments has evolved into very complex procedures that occasionally require testing to be extended over several days. Thus, storage by freezing of the specimens before as well as between testing sessions becomes a necessity. Additionally, there is an increasing clinical interest in the use of ligament allografts, and some preservation protocols require that the allograft be frozen. Consequently, the effects of frozen storage on the mechanical properties of these tissues must be addressed.

The effects of postmortem storage on the properties of soft tissues were studied as early as 1847 by Wertheim (54), who found no difference in the modulus of

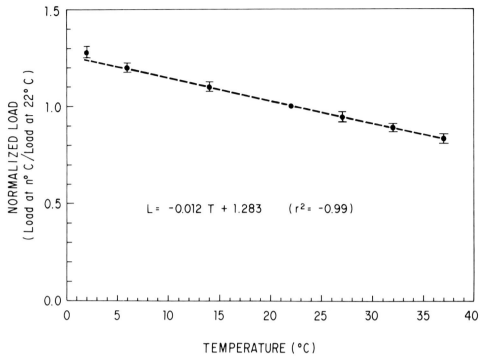

$$L = -0.012 \ T + 1.283 \qquad (r^2 = -0.99)$$

FIG. 7-5. Normalized peak load for the first cycle with respect to the first cycle load at 22°C, as a function of temperature. The decrease in peak load with temperature can be expressed by a simple linear relationship. (From ref. 61.)

elasticity between canine tendons tested fresh and those tested 5 days later. Smith (44) reported that the rabbit ACL became less extensible within 1 hour after death, whereas Viidik (49) found no consistent changes in the properties of the femur–ACL–tibia complex after up to 96 hours post-mortem. In a subsequent study, Viidik (50) tested the rabbit femur–ACL–tibia complex following storage at −20°C for 1 week and found no consistent changes in the load–deformation properties. Matthews (30) compared the cyclic behavior between fresh and frozen cat extensor tendons and found that the overall stiffness did not change significantly in the first 3 hours after death. More recently, Noyes (38) examined the effect of 4 weeks of frozen storage at −15°C on the monkey ACL and found no changes in the structural properties of bone–ligament–bone specimens. Barad (6) also studied the monkey ACL and found a slight (but not significant) decrease in the structural and mechanical characteristics of the ligament after deep freezing at −80°C for 3–5 weeks. Others have reported a slight increase in linear stiffness (10).

In all, the literature to date has been conflicting and inconclusive, due in part, perhaps, to differences in measurement techniques. A study was performed in our laboratory to examine possible changes in the structural properties of the FMTC, as well as the mechanical properties of the rabbit MCL substance, following 45 days of limb storage at −20°C (59). Fresh

contralateral limbs were dissected immediately at sacrifice and were tested as controls. Experimental ligaments were stored with muscle and other tissues left in place rather than in the completely dissected state. Each specimen was then double-wrapped in saline-soaked gauze and sealed in an airtight plastic bag. Specimens were thawed at refrigerator temperatures (4°C) overnight prior to the day of testing. After allowing temperature equilibration to 37°C, specimens were subjected to cyclic testing in order to characterize the hysteresis curves. The FMTC was then tensile tested to failure to obtain load–deformation curves for the FMTC (structural properties) and stress–strain curves for the MCL substance (mechanical properties).

In general, no significant differences in the measured parameters were noted between fresh and frozen samples (Table 7-1). The one exception was the area of hysteresis. Frozen samples demonstrated significant decreases in the area of hysteresis during the first few cycles of loading and unloading when compared to fresh, contralateral controls. These differences diminished and became insignificant with further cycling. It is conjectured that these changes may result from some insult to cellular integrity or associated ground substance (49) or from changes in ligament fluid dynamics (45).

Thus, storage by freezing does not appear to significantly affect the properties of ligaments, except the

TABLE 7-1. *Areas of hysteresis and structural properties of the rabbit FMTC (skeletally mature animals) comparing fresh and frozen bone–ligament–bone preparations*

	Fresh (n = 5)	Stored 45 days (n = 5)
Area of hysteresis		
1st cycle (N-mm)	5.86 ± 1.60	2.20 ± 0.54[a]
10th cycle (N-mm)	1.36 ± 0.50	0.58 ± 0.30
Structural properties (at failure)		
L_{max} (N)	368.4 ± 15.0	316.2 ± 22.3
d_{max} (mm)	6.6 ± 0.5	6.6 ± 0.5
A_{max} (N-mm)	1330.0 ± 200.0	1170.0 ± 200.0

[a] $p < 0.05$.
[b] L_{max} is the ultimate load in newtons; d_{max} is the deformation at failure; A_{max} is the energy absorbed.

area of hysteresis, which may be a more sensitive indicator with which to detect minor changes. Freezing did not appear to affect the ligament insertion sites, since the mode of failure was not altered between the experimental and control specimens. It is necessary, however, to reiterate that care must be taken in preparing the tissue sample prior to freezing in order to protect the sample from dehydration.

Effects of Skeletal Maturity

Several effects of skeletal maturity on the properties of ligaments and their insertions have been demonstrated. Several authors, using rat-tail tendons, have described age-dependent increases in collagen fibril size, ultimate load, and tensile strength from puberty to adulthood (20,33,34). Once skeletal maturity was achieved, no changes were observed until senescence, where decreases in these structural properties may result (38). Tipton (46) examined the junctional strength of the rat FMTC over the first 2 years of life and noted that junctional strength increased most rapidly between 15 and 90 days. Failure energy and linear stiffness were also shown to increase with age. Limited information exists, however, regarding age-related changes in the mechanical properties of the ligament substance.

The effects of skeletal maturity on ligament mechanics were studied in our laboratory using four age groups of male New Zealand white rabbits. Animals were aged 1½ months (open epiphysis by radiological examination), 4–5 months (open epiphysis), 6–7 months (closed epiphysis), 12–15 months (closed epiphysis), and 40 months (closed epiphysis). There was a striking similarity between the trends for cross-sectional area of the MCL and body weight of the animals as functions of age. Both the cross-sectional area and

body weight increased as the animals matured, ultimately reaching a plateau at about 6–7 months of age (Fig. 7-6). The structural properties of the FMTC underwent dramatic changes from 1 to 7 months of age, after which time the differences between groups diminished (Fig. 7-7). The mechanical properties of the ligament substance demonstrated relatively early maturation by 6–7 months of age, as the stress–strain curves within the functional range were similar to those of the adults (Fig. 7-7). During this early maturation process, the ligament showed drastic increases in tensile strength and ultimate strain; after the animals became mature, these increases were greatly diminished (Fig. 7-8). It was also demonstrated by histological examination that the tibial insertion site of the MCL is affected by its proximity to the growth plate, where rapid remodeling activity weakens the subperiosteal attachment for the younger animals. The failure modes reflect these findings (Fig. 7-9). All rabbits with open epiphyses failed by tibial avulsion, and all rabbits older than 1 year old failed by tearing in the ligament substance.

Effects of Aging

Several investigations have been performed to determine the changes in ligament mechanics that occur with senescence. Noyes (38) found that the structural properties were two to three times greater in young versus old groups of human cadaver femur–ACL–tibia preparations. Furthermore, the failure mode of young knees was more commonly by midsubstance failure, whereas older knees failed by bony avulsion. The effects of aging were studied in our laboratory using pairs of human cadaveric knees obtained from young donors (22–41 years, mean age = 35 years) and older donors (60–97 years, mean age = 76 years).

One knee of each pair was randomly assigned to be tensile tested to failure along the ACL axis, whereas the contralateral knee was tested along the tibial axis. The femur–ACL–tibia complexes were all tested at a knee flexion angle of 30°. The results demonstrated a significant effect of age on linear stiffness, defined as the slope of the linear portion of the load–deformation curve (Fig. 7-10). Both specimen age and loading axis had a significant effect on ultimate load at failure (Fig. 7-11). The mean ultimate load of the younger specimens was higher than that of the older specimens, and the mean ultimate load of the ACL-axis-tested specimens was higher than that of the tibial-axis-tested specimens. A decrease in ultimate load was seen with increasing age, regardless of loading axis; moreover, the difference in ultimate load between the ACL and tibial loading axis decreased with increasing age. Femur–ACL–tibia failure mode was affected by both

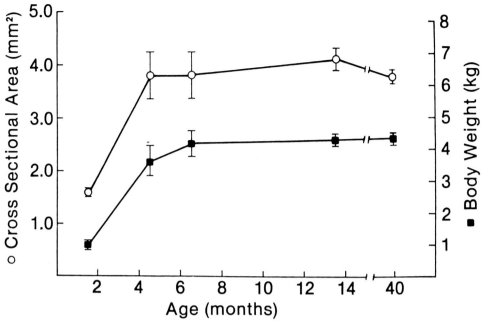

FIG. 7-6. The cross-sectional area of the MCL and body weight of the animal as functions of age.

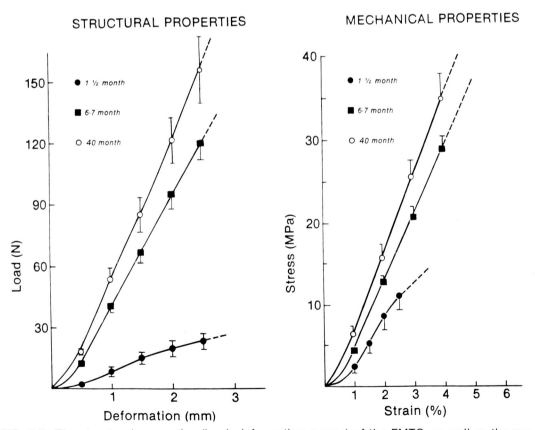

FIG. 7-7. The structural properties (load–deformation curves) of the FMTC, as well as the mechanical properties (stress–strain curves) of ligament substance, for three age groups: $1\frac{1}{2}$ months (open epiphysis), 6–7 months (closed epiphysis), and 40 months (closed epiphysis).

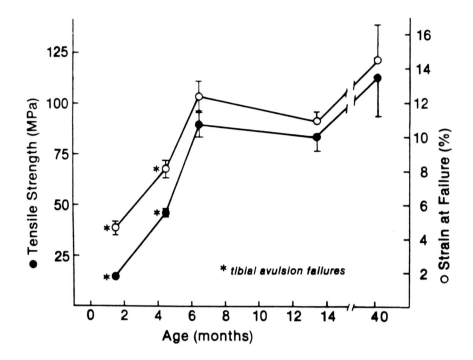

FIG. 7-8. The tensile strength and strain at failure of MCL as functions of age.

specimen age and loading axis. Older specimens had a higher incidence of midsubstance failure than did younger specimens, regardless of loading axis. Specimens tested along the ACL axis had a higher percentage of midsubstance failure than did those tested along the tibial axis, regardless of specimen age (57% of the younger age group and 86% of the older age group). The effects of aging on the structural properties of the femur–ACL–tibia have been clearly shown; therefore, specimen age must be considered in the de-

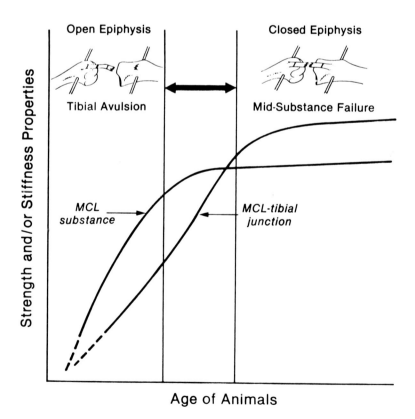

FIG. 7-9. A schematic diagram depicting the relationship between failure mode and age, hypothesizing the asynchronous rates of maturation of the bone–ligament–bone complex and the ligament substance. (From ref. 60.)

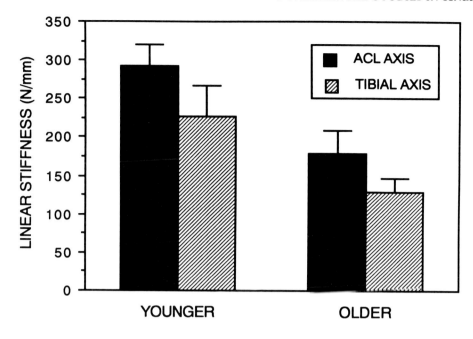

FIG. 7-10. The linear stiffness of human femur–ACL–tibia complex with respect to age and loading axis.

sign and interpretation of future biomechanical investigations.

Effects of Strain Rates

Considerable attention has been given to the effects of the rate of stretch on the failure mode of the bone–ligament–bone complex. Some investigators have felt that the generally poor success in producing ligament substance failure experimentally has been due primarily to the employment of lower strain rates (9,20,37). Others have shown that skeletal maturity can

have a significant effect on the failure mode (60). For example, when tested at a relatively low strain rate (0.3%/sec), the FMTC from rabbits with open epiphyses all failed by tibial avulsion, whereas those from older animals (12–15 months) with closed epiphyses failed by substance tear (60).

The effects of strain rate on the structural and mechanical properties of the MCL have recently been investigated using the FMTC of two groups of New Zealand white rabbits: (i) open epiphysis ($3\frac{1}{2}$ months old) and (ii) closed epiphysis ($8\frac{1}{2}$ months old). The specimens were subjected to uniaxial tensile tests at five different extension rates (0.008–113 mm/sec), corre-

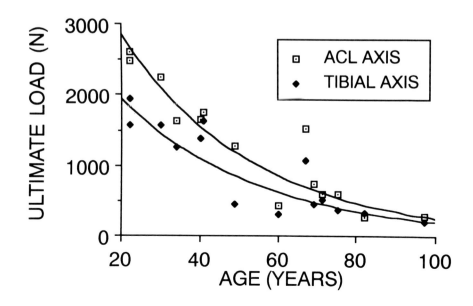

FIG. 7-11. A plot depicting the decreasing load at failure of the human femur–ACL–tibia complex with increasing age for two axes of loading.

sponding to ligament substance strain rates of 0.01%/sec to over 200%/sec. In the case of high strain rates, a high-speed video recording system was used to tape the test at 2000 frames/sec for data analysis to be performed at normal playback speed of 60 frames/sec (41).

For the open-epiphysis group, the structural properties (load–deformation curves) of the FMTC were found to be dependent on the extension rate (Fig. 7-12). The ultimate load and energy absorbed increased 2.5 and 3.0 times, respectively, between the lowest and highest strain rates. For the closed-epiphysis group, the ultimate load and energy absorbed also increased with increasing extension rates, but to a lesser degree. The mechanical properties (stress–strain curves) of the MCL substance in the prefailure range paralleled the results obtained for the structural properties (Fig. 7-13). The tensile strength of the MCL in the closed-epiphysis group increased significantly with strain rate, but only by 60% from the lowest to the highest strain rates.

Thus, differences in skeletal maturity, rather than strain rate, produced the greatest changes in the structural and mechanical properties. Failure modes were also significantly affected by skeletal maturity and were independent of strain rate. All failures in animals with open epiphyses occurred by tibial avulsion, whereas all failures in animals with closed epiphyses occurred by ligamentous disruption either at midsubstance or near the tibial insertion site (but with no bony avulsion). These results were confirmed by photomicrograph. We therefore believe that the age of the animals is a much more important factor in determining failure mode than is strain rate.

VISCOELASTIC PROPERTIES

Ligaments display time- and history-dependent viscoelastic behaviors that reflect the complex interactions of the collagen and the surrounding proteins and ground substance. Unlike purely elastic materials, the shape of the load–deformation curve for a ligament will vary depending upon the previous loading history. For instance, the loading and unloading curves of these tissues do not follow the same path as a result of internal energy losses, forming a hysteresis loop. In addition, ligaments demonstrate *creep*, an increase in deformation over time under a constant load (Fig. 7-14A), and *stress relaxation*, a decline in stress over time under a constant deformation (Fig. 7-14B).

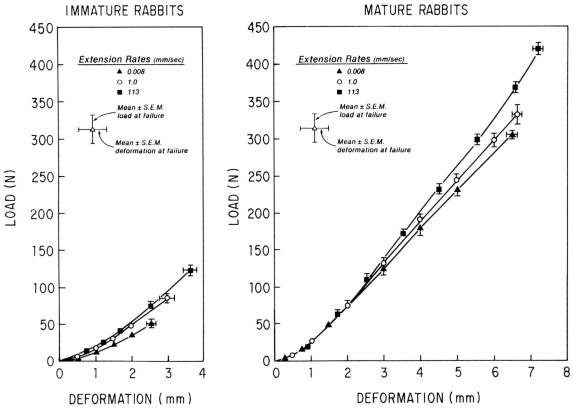

FIG. 7-12. The structural properties (load–deformation curves) of the FMTC in skeletally immature (**left**) and mature (**right**) rabbits as a function of extension rate.

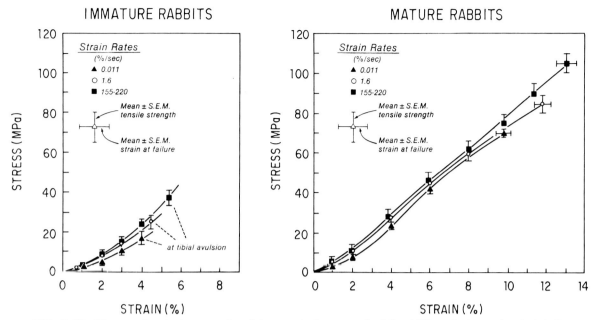

FIG. 7-13. The mechanical properties (stress–strain curves) of the MCL substance in skeletally immature (**left**) and mature (**right**) rabbits as a function of strain rate.

The viscoelastic behavior of ligaments has important clinical as well as physiological significance. The phenomenon of stress relaxation becomes important during walking or jogging, in which the applied strains are repetitive and nearly constant (56,57). Cyclic stress relaxation will effectively reduce the stress in the tissue substance, a phenomenon that may help to prevent fatigue failure of ligaments under prolonged cyclic loading. On the other hand, repetitious loading to a constant load results in a gradual increase in deformation, demonstrating creep behavior of the ligaments. These changes have been noted clinically with temporary softening and increases of test excursion (laxity) in exercised joints. After a short recovery period there is a return to normal joint stiffness, and the ligament returns to its original length.

The viscoelastic behavior of ligaments can be described mathematically by a theoretical relationship for soft tissues first proposed by Fung (16,17). This mathematical relationship, known as the quasi-linear viscoelastic (QLV) theory, assumes that the stress response $\sigma(t)$ of a tissue to an applied strain history $\epsilon(t)$ can be expressed as an integral sum of the individual responses to a series of infinitesimal step increases in strain, in terms of a *reduced relaxation function* $G(t)$ and the *elastic response* of the tissue, $\sigma^e(\epsilon)$:

$$\sigma(t) = \int_0^t G(t - \tau) \frac{\partial \sigma^e(\epsilon)}{\partial \epsilon} \frac{\partial \epsilon}{\partial \tau} \, d\tau \qquad [1]$$

The reduced relaxation function is defined as $G(t) =$

$\sigma(t)/\sigma(0)$ and has the property that $G(0) = 1$. The common expressions chosen for $G(t)$ and $\sigma^e(\epsilon)$ are

$$G(t) = \frac{1 + C\left[E_1\left(\dfrac{t}{\tau_2}\right) - E_1\left(\dfrac{t}{\tau_1}\right)\right]}{1 + C \ln\left(\dfrac{\tau_2}{\tau_1}\right)} \qquad [2]$$

$$\sigma^e(\epsilon) = A(e^{B\epsilon} - 1) \qquad [3]$$

These expressions contain the material constants C, τ_1, τ_2, A, and B which describe the viscoelastic properties of the tissue and can be determined experimentally. Recently, the QLV theory has been further refined to apply to a ramp loading condition, since a true step load (or infinite strain rate) is experimentally impossible to achieve (29). This refined theory has been successfully used to determine the viscoelastic constants for the anteromedial bundles of porcine ACL (29). The constants C, τ_1, τ_2, A, and B were determined from the results of an experimental stress relaxation test using a nonlinear least-square curve-fitting procedure. It can be seen that the QLV theory agreed sufficiently well with the experimental data (Fig. 7-15A). Using the constants determined, the reduced relaxation function and the elastic response (for porcine ACL anteromedial bundles) were found to be

$$G(t) = 0.858 - 0.049 \ln(t) \qquad [4]$$

$$\sigma^e(\epsilon) = 210(e^{0.63\epsilon} - 1) \qquad [5]$$

The expressions for $G(t)$ and $\sigma^e(\epsilon)$ shown in Eqs. [4]

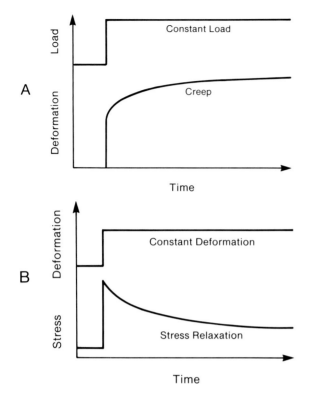

FIG. 7-14. Schematic representation of (**A**) creep behavior (increasing deformation over time under a constant load) and (**B**) stress relaxation (decreasing stress over time under a constant deformation).

and [5] were validated by a second experiment in which these equations were used to predict the behavior of the tissue under cyclic loading between 1% and 5% strain. As shown in Fig. 7-15B, the predicted peak and valley stresses matched well with the experimental data. Thus, the QLV theory is shown to provide an accurate mathematical description of the time- and history-dependent viscoelastic properties of the ACL.

DETERMINATION OF *IN SITU* STRESSES AND STRAINS

An understanding of the magnitudes of stresses and strains present in the knee ligaments during joint motion is an important prerequisite for the understanding of joint function. Because of a number of technical problems associated with the measurement of ligament stresses and strains *in situ*, little data are currently available in the literature. The majority of studies of ligament behavior during joint motion have focused on the changes in ligament strain. Warren (53) placed pins in the tibial and femoral insertion sites of the human MCL to measure changes in ligament strain as a function of knee flexion angle. France (14) monitored strains on the bone surface near the ligament insertion sites as a means of measuring tension. Arms (5) at-

tached Hall effect transducers to the ligament substance to measure strain. Liquid-mercury strain gauges of various sizes have also been used by a number of investigators (22,25,31,32). Still others have used spatial kinematic linkages to study the length changes of the knee ligaments during joint motion. Special devices such as the buckle transducer (28) have been used to measure the ligament forces *in situ*. Ahmed (2) further refined this technique to study ligament tensions *in situ* during tibial anterior translation and axial rotation. There is some disagreement among the results of these studies, which may be a result of artifact imposed upon the measured quantities due to direct contact by the various transducers.

Using the VDA system discussed previously, a new noncontact method was developed to determine the ligament strains, stresses, and forces *in situ* as a function of knee flexion angle, as well as skeletal maturity. The experimental method can be described in the following steps (Fig. 7-16):

Step 1. With the knee joint at 90° flexion, two parallel lines, 0.5 cm proximal and distal to the joint line, were stained across the width of the MCL using a Verhoeff's elastin stain. The distance between these markers was measured using the VDA system and represented the *in situ* length of the ligament. Then, the knee was flexed between 60° and 120° and the length changes in three regions of the MCL (anterior, middle, and posterior thirds) were recorded relative to the *in situ* length of the MCL at 90°.

Step 2. The knee was then refixed at 90° and dissected free of all soft tissues with the exception of the MCL, thus relieving all external load and allowing the FMTC to retract completely. The distance between the markers was measured and defined as the *stress-free, zero length*. The *in situ* strains for the three regions of the MCL were defined as $(l - l_0)/l_0$, that is, the length of the ligament in the intact knee (l) at 60°, 90°, and 120° of flexion with respect to the stress-free, zero length (l_0) at 90°.

Step 3. After the cross-sectional area of the MCL was obtained, the FMTC was mounted for tensile testing. To mimic the *in vivo* conditions, the specimen was first stretched to an average *in situ* strain level as determined from the *in situ* length obtained at 90°. The FMTC was then cycled between the maximum and minimum *in situ* strain values (obtained previously) until the loading and unloading curves became the same in order to minimze the viscoelastic effects. By assuming that the material properties of the MCL are similar in each of the three regions (anterior, middle, and posterior), the recorded loads could be divided equally among the three regions. By dividing the load for each region by one-third of the total cross-sectional area, the *in situ* stresses, as well as the stress–strain

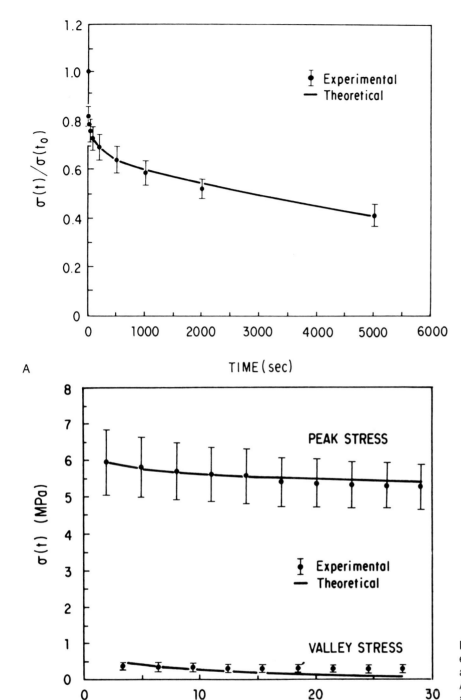

FIG. 7-15. Theoretical prediction versus experimental results for (**A**) stress relaxation of anteromedial bundle of porcine ACL following application of a ramp load and (**B**) peak and valley stress relaxation for the anteromedial bundle under cyclic loading. (From ref. 29.)

curves, were calculated for the individual regions. By summing the *in situ* stresses, the total load in the ligament *in situ* was also determined.

For rabbit knees, the total load *in situ* at 90° of knee flexion was determined to be 1.5 ± 0.2 N and 3.0 ± 0.4 N for skeletally immature and mature groups, respectively. Similarly, the individual stresses for all regions were significantly greater for those which were skeletally mature. There was a significant difference

in the stress and strain levels among the three regions at 60° and 120° flexion (Fig. 7-17): The anterior region demonstrated the greatest stress and strain levels at 120° flexion, whereas the posterior region showed the greatest levels at 60° flexion. There were no significant differences among the three regions at 90° flexion. Interestingly, the middle region did not show significant variation in stress or strain levels between any of the flexion angles examined. The maximum stress and

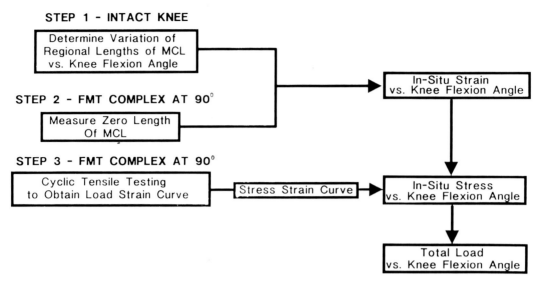

FIG. 7-16. A flow chart delineating the experimental procedure for determination of the *in situ* stresses and strains in MCL.

strain in the MCL for both the skeletally immature and mature groups occurred in the posterior region at 60° flexion, with average values of 2.4 ± 0.4 MPa and 4.0 ± 0.2% for the former and 4.0 ± 0.5 MPa and 5.4 ± 0.2% for the latter. In general, these data indicate an increase in ligament tension with skeletal maturity and also document a variation in stress and strain values across the ligament substance during passive knee flexion.

SUMMARY AND FUTURE DIRECTIONS

This chapter has reviewed some of the recent advances in the study of the biomechanics of ligaments. The development of normal- and high-speed video recorders, the video dimension analyzer system, the laser micrometer, and other new bioengineering tools has permitted the accurate determination of stress and strain in the ligament substance, providing new insights into biomechanical properties of the knee ligaments. Using these tools, a number of important principles have been demonstrated. The tensile behavior of ligaments (and probably most musculoskeletal soft tissue) is based upon an inverse relationship between ligament stiffness and temperature. This study reinforces the need for a standardized testing procedure, since any change in environmental temperature may influence the results. Given proper protection against dehydration, storage by freezing does not appear to significantly affect the mechanical properties of ligaments, allowing greater flexibility in ligament storage and testing protocols.

Another important concept presented in this chapter is the distinction between the properties of the ligament substance and those of the ligament–bone insertion sites under various conditions. Investigations concerning the strain rate sensitivity of ligaments have reinforced the concept that mechanical properties of the ligaments, like most other soft tissues, are relatively insensitive to rates of stretch. The properties of the insertion sites (and thus the structural properties) are, however, significantly dependent upon skeletal maturity. Despite variations in strain rate over four orders of magnitude, all FMTCs from animals with open epiphyses failed by tibial avulsion, whereas complexes that were skeletally mature failed within the MCL substance. The mechanical properties of the MCL substance were not nearly as affected by age as were the structural properties of the FMTC. Thus, the rates of maturation of the insertion sites and the MCL substance appear to be asynchronous. The effect of age on joint function is also demonstrated by the study of *in situ* strain levels and strain distributions in the MCL. The strain distribution in the ligament is non-homogeneous during various phases of joint motion, and strain levels suggest an increase in ligament tension with maturation.

The understanding of the biomechanics of normal ligaments is an important prerequisite for the study of both their normal function and the healing processes that occur in response to injury. Much of our current understanding of the biomechanical properties of ligaments has come from the development and application of new technologies that have afforded us the ability to examine old ideas more thoroughly and accurately. Even more importantly, these examinations have provided both the impetus and the means for the exploration of new areas.

IN-SITU LIGAMENT STRAIN vs. KNEE FLEXION ANGLE

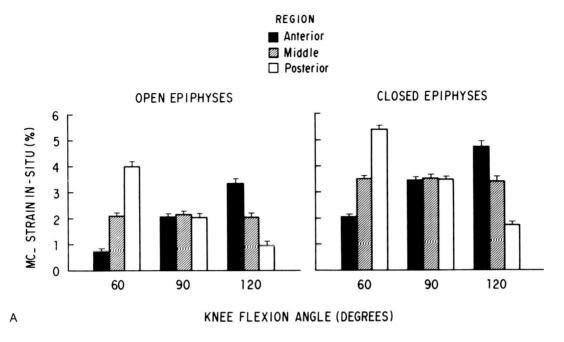

A

IN-SITU LIGAMENT STRESS vs. KNEE FLEXION ANGLE

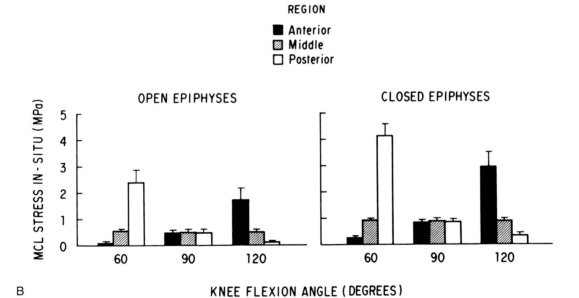

B

FIG. 7-17. Comparison of *in situ* strain (**A**) and *in situ* stress (**B**) in the MCL substance at three flexion angles for skeletally immature and mature specimens.

GLOSSARY

Biomechanics The study of the mechanics of biological materials.

Creep A viscoelastic behavior characterized by a change in strain or deformation of a specimen with time under a constant applied stress (Fig. 7-14A).

Deformation (*d*) The change in a dimension of a specimen under external loading. For example, the increase in length of a bone–ligament–bone complex under tensile loading.

Elastic response ($\sigma^e(\epsilon)$) A mathematical expression used in the QLV theory to describe the instantaneous stress–strain relationship of viscoelastic materials.

Energy absorbed at failure (A_{max}) The energy required to fail a specimen under tensile loading, represented by the area under the load–deformation curve up to the point of failure.

Failure mode The form of mechanical failure produced by tensile testing. In bone–ligament–bone specimens, failure may occur (a) in the ligament substance, (b) by avulsion at the insertion sites (with bony debris at rupture sites), or (c) by soft tissue pulling-out at or near the epiphysial region (with no bony involvement at the failure site).

Gauge length The initial (reference) length used for measurements of strain.

Hysteresis A path-dependent characteristic of viscoelastic materials, such that the load–deformation or stress–strain curve obtained during loading differs from that obtained during unloading due to internal energy losses. For a single loading–unloading cycle, these loading and unloading curves form a closed loop (hysteresis loop).

Linear stiffness For a load–deformation curve with a curvilinear shape, the slope of the curve over a range of deformation where the curve is most nearly linear.

Load (*L*) The external force applied to a specimen (ligament). Loads may be further characterized as tensile, compressive, shear, bending, or torsional.

Load–deformation curve The relationship between the applied load and the corresponding deformation of a specimen obtained during testing (e.g., tensile testing of a bone–ligament–bone complex, Fig. 7-12).

Mechanical (material) properties The tensile properties of the ligament substance as a material, represented by the stress–strain curve. Properties such as tangent modulus, tensile strength, and ultimate strain can be determined from the stress–strain curve (Fig. 7-13).

Mechanics The study of the force, motion, deformation, and strength of materials in response to externally applied loads.

Modulus The slope of the stress–strain curve in the linear region.

QLV theory Quasi-linear viscoelastic theory. A mathematical model to describe the nonlinear viscoelastic behavior of soft connective tissues, first developed by Fung (16).

Reduced relaxation function ($G(t)$) A mathematical expression used in the QLV theory to describe the stress relaxation characteristics of a tissue. It is defined as the time-dependent stress divided by the initial stress.

Stiffness The slope of the load–deformation curve for a specimen with a linear load–deformation relationship.

Strain (ϵ) The change in specimen dimension under external loading divided by the initial (reference) dimension of the specimen, expressed as a percentage. For example, the change in length with respect to initial length of a ligament during tensile testing.

Strain gauge An electronic device used for the measurement of small deformation (or strain).

Strain rate The rate at which a specimen is deformed, expressed in terms of strain per unit time.

Stress (σ) The load in a specimen divided by its cross-sectional area measured perpendicular to the axis of loading.

Stress relaxation A viscoelastic behavior characterized by a decrease in stress in a specimen with time under a constant applied strain or deformation (Fig. 7-14B).

Stress–strain curve The relationship between the applied stress and corresponding strain present in a specimen (e.g., the ligament substance) during testing (Fig. 7-13).

Structural properties The tensile properties of the bone–ligament–bone complex as a structural unit, represented by the load–deformation curve. Properties such as linear stiffness, ultimate load, ultimate deformation, and energy absorbed at failure can be obtained from the load–deformation curve (Fig. 7-12).

Tangent modulus The slope of a line tangent to a segment of the stress–strain curve within a specified range of strain.

Tensile properties The characteristics of a material that describe its behavior under a tensile load.

Tensile strength (σ_{max}) The maximum stress that can be sustained by a specimen prior to failure.

Ultimate load (L_{max}) The maximum load that can be sustained by specimen prior to failure.

Ultimate deformation (d_{max}) The maximum deformation that can be sustained by a specimen prior to failure.

Ultimate strain (ϵ_{max}) The maximum strain that can be sustained by a specimen prior to failure.

VDA Video dimension analyzer. An electronic device that uses a video image to measure the strain of soft tissues (such as ligaments) without direct contact with the tissue (Fig. 7-3).

Viscoelastic behavior (properties) The time- and history-dependent mechanical behavior of soft connective tissues such as ligaments. The mechanical properties of such tissues depend upon factors such as the previous strain and loading history, the rate of loading, and the duration of loading. For example, the properties of a ligament tested after one cycle of loading will differ from those of a ligament tested after 10 cycles of loading.

ACKNOWLEDGMENTS

The authors wish to thank the many collaborators and laboratory staff at the Orthopedic Bioengineering Laboratory. We also gratefully acknowledge the financial support of the RR&D Grant A1883RA of the Veterans Administration, NIH Grants AR 14918, AR 33097, and AR 34264, and the Malcolm and Dorothy Coutts Institute for Joint Reconstruction and Research.

REFERENCES

1. Abrahams M. Mechanical behavior of tendon *in vitro. Med Biol Eng* 1967;5:433–443.
2. Ahmed AM, Hyder A, Burke DL, Chan KH. *In vitro* ligament tension pattern in the flexed knee in passive loading. *J Orthop Res* 1987;5:217–230.
3. Allard P, Thirty PS, Bourgault A, Drouin G. Pressure dependence of the "area micrometer" method in evaluation of cruciate ligament cross-section. *J Biomed Eng* 1979;1:265–267.
4. Apter J. Influence of composition on thermal properties of tissues. In: Fung YC, Perrone N, Anliker M, eds. *Biomechanics: its foundations and objectives.* Englewood Cliffs, New Jersey: Prentice-Hall, 1972;217–235.
5. Arms SW, Pope MH, Boyle JB, Davignon PJ, Johnson RJ. Knee medial collateral ligament strain. *Trans Orthop Res Soc* 1982;7:47.
6. Barad S, Cabaud HE, Rodrigo JJ. Effects of storage at −80°C as compared to 4°C on the strength of rhesus monkey anterior cruciate ligaments. *Trans Orthop Res Soc* 1982;7:378.
7. Butler DL, Kay MD, Stouffer DC. Comparison of material properties in fascicle–bone units from human patellar tendon and knee ligaments. *J Biomech* 1986;19:425–432.
8. Cronkite AE. The tensile strength of human tendons. *Anat Rec* 1936;64:173–186.
9. Crowninshield RD, Pope MH. The strength and failure characteristics of rat medial collateral ligaments. *J Trauma* 1976;16(2):99–105.
10. Dorlot JM, Ait ba Sidi M, Gremblay GM, Drouin G. Load–elongation behavior of the canine anterior cruciate ligament. *J Biomech Eng* 1980;102:190–193.
11. Elden HR. Aging of rat tail tendon. *J Gerontol* 1964;19:173–178.
12. Ellis DG. A shadow amplitude method for measuring cross-sectional areas of biological specimens. *21st Annu Conf Eng Med Biol* 1968;51:6.
13. Ellis DG. Cross-sectional area measurements for tendon specimens: a comparison of several methods. *J Biomech* 1969;2:175–186.
14. France PE, Daniels AU, Goble ME, Dunn HK. Simultaneous quantitation of knee ligament forces. *J Biomech* 1983;16:553–564.
15. Frisén M, Mägi M, Sonnerup L, Viidik A. Rheological analysis of soft collagenous tissue. Part I: theoretical considerations. *J Biomech* 1969;2:13–20.
16. Fung YCB. Stress–strain–history relations of soft tissues in simple elongation. In: Fung YCB, Perrone N, Anliker M, eds. *Biomechanics: its foundations and objectives.* Englewood Cliffs, New Jersey: Prentice-Hall, 1972;181–208.
17. Fung YCB. *Biomechanics: mechanical properties of living tissues.* Springer-Verlag, 1981.
18. Gratz CM. Tensile strength and elasticity tests on human fascia lata. *J Bone Joint Surg* 1931;13:334–340.
19. Gupta BN, Subramanian KN, Brinker WO, Gupta AN. Tensile strength of canine cranial cruciate ligaments. *Am J Vet Res* 1971;32:183–190.
20. Haut RC. Age-dependent influence of strain rate on the tensile failure of rat-tail tendon. *J Biomech Eng* 1983;105:296–299.
21. Haut RC, Little RW. Rheological properties of canine anterior cruciate ligaments. *J Biomech* 1969;2:289–298.
22. Henning CE, Lynch MA, Glick KR Jr. Strain gage study of elongation of the anterior cruciate ligament. *Am J Sports Med* 1985;13:22–26.
23. Hunter J, Williams MG. A study of the effect of cold on joint temperature and mobility. *Can J Med Sci* 1951;29:255–262.
24. Iaconis F, Steindler R, Marinozzi G. Measurements of cross-sectional area of collagen structures (knee ligaments) by means of an optical method. *J Biomech* 1987;20:1003–1010.
25. Kennedy JC, Hawkins RJ, Willis RB. Strain gauge analysis of knee ligaments. *Clin Orthop* 1977;129:25–229.
26. Kuei S, Woo SL-Y, Gomez MA, Akeson WH. The viscoelastic, thermoelastic, and time dependent properties of the knee ligaments. *Trans Orthop Res Soc* 1979;4:25.
27. Lee TQ, Woo SL-Y. A new method for determining cross-sectional shape and area of soft tissues. *J Biomech Eng* 1988;110:110–114.
28. Lewis JL, Shybut GT. *In vivo* forces in the collateral ligaments of canine knees. *Trans Orthop Res Soc* 1981;6:4.
29. Lin H-C, Kwan MK-W, Woo SL-Y. On the stress relaxation properties of anterior cruciate ligament (ACL). *Adv Bioeng* [WAM/ASME, BED] 1987;3:5–6.
30. Matthews LS, Ellis D. Viscoelastic properties of cat tendon: effects of time after death and preservation by freezing. *J Biomech* 1968;1:65–71.
31. Meglan D, Zuelzer W, Buck W, Berme N. The effects of quadriceps force upon strain in the anterior cruciate ligament. *Trans Orthop Res Soc* 1986;11:55.
32. Monahan JJ, Grigg P, Pappas AM, et al. *In vivo* strain patterns in the four major canine knee ligaments. *J Orthop Res* 1984;2:408–418.
33. Morein G, Goldgefter L, Kobyliansky E, Goldschmidt-Nathan M, Nathan H. Change in mechanical properties of rat tail tendon during postnatal ontogenesis. *Anat Embryol (Berl)* 1978;154(1):121–124.
34. Nathan H, Goldgefter L, Kobyliansky E, Goldschmidt-Nathan M, Morein G. Energy absorbing capacity of rat tail tendon at various ages. *J Anat* 1978;127:589–593.
35. Neuberger A, Slack HGB. The metabolism of collagen from liver, bones, skin and tendon in the normal rat. *Biochem J* 1953;53:47–52.
36. Njus GO, Njus NM. A non-contact method for determining cross-sectional area of soft tissues. *Trans Orthop Res Soc* 1986;32:126.
37. Noyes FR, DeLucas JL, Torvik PJ. Biomechanics of anterior cruciate ligament failure: an analysis of strain rate sensitivity and mechanisms of failure in primates. *J Bone Joint Surg* 1974;56A:236–253.
38. Noyes FR, Grood ES. The strength of the anterior cruciate ligament in humans and rhesus monkeys: age-related and species-related changes. *J Bone Joint Surg* 1976;58A:1074–1082.
39. Noyes FR, Grood ES, Butler DL, et al. Clinical biomechanics of the knee—ligament restraints and functional stability. In: Funk FJ Jr, ed. *Surgical repair and reconstruction.* American Academy of Orthopaedic Surgeons' Symposium on the Athlete's Knee. St. Louis: CV Mosby, 1980;1–55.

40. Nunley RL. The ligamenta flava of the dog. A study of tensile and physical properties. *Am J Phys Med* 1958;37:256–268.

41. Peterson RH, Woo SL-Y. A new methodology to determine the mechanical properties of ligaments at high strain rates. *J Biomech Eng* 1986;108:365–367.

42. Rigby B, Hirai N, Spikes J, Eyring H. The mechanical properties of rat tail tendon. *J Gen Physiol* 1958;43:265–283.

43. Shrive NG, Lam TC, Damson E, Frank CB. A new method of measuring the cross-sectional area of connective tissue structures. *J Biomech Eng* 1988;110:104–109.

44. Smith JW. The elastic properties of the anterior cruciate ligament of the rabbit. *J Anat* 1954;88:369–380.

45. Stouffer DC, Butler DL. An analysis of crimp unfolding, fluid expulsion and fiber failure in collagen fiber bundles. *Adv Bioeng [WAM/ASME]* 1984:46–47.

46. Tipton CM, Matthes RD, Martin RR. Influence of age and sex on the strength of bone–ligament junctions in knee joints of rats. *J Bone Joint Surg* 1978;60A:230–234.

47. Trent PS, Walker PS, Wolf B. Ligament length patterns, strength, and rotational axes of the knee joint. *Clin Orthop* 1976;117:263–270.

48. VanBrocklin JD, Ellis DG. A study of the mechanical behavior of toe extensor tendons under applied stress. *Arch Phys Med* 1965;46:369–373.

49. Viidik A, Sanquist L, Magi M. Influence of postmortem storage on tensile strength characteristics and histology of rabbit ligaments. *Acta Orthop Scand [Suppl]* 1965;79:1–38.

50. Viidik A, Lewin T. Changes in tensile strength characteristics and histology of rabbit ligaments induced by different modes of postmortal storage. *Acta Orthop Scand* 1966;37:141–155.

51. Walker LB, Harris EH, Benedict JV. Stress–strain relationship in human cadaveric plantaris tendon: a preliminary study. *Med Electron Biol Eng* 1964;2:31–38.

52. Wang C-J, Walker PS, Wolf B. The effects of flexion and rotation on the length patterns of the ligaments of the knee. *J Biomech* 1973;6:587–596.

53. Warren LF, Marshall JL, Girgis F. The prime static stabilizers of the medial side of the knee. *J Bone Joint Surg* 1974;56A:665–674.

54. Wertheim MG. Memoirs sur l'élasticité et la cohésion des principaux tissu du corps humain. *Ann Chim (Phys)* 1847;21:385–414.

55. Woo SL-Y, Akeson WH, Jemmott GF. The measurements of nonhomogeneous, directional mechanical properties of articular cartilage in tension. *J Biomech* 1976;9:785–791.

56. Woo SL-Y, Gomez MA, Akeson WH. The time and history dependent viscoelastic properties of the canine medial collateral ligament. *J Biomech Eng* 1981;103:293–298.

57. Woo SL-Y, Gomez MA, Woo Y-K, Akeson WH. Mechanical properties of tendons and ligaments. I. Quasi-static and nonlinear viscoelastic properties. *Biorheology* 1982;19:385–396.

58. Woo SL-Y, Gomez MA, Seguchi Y, Endo C, Akeson WH. Measurement of mechanical properties of ligament substance from a bone–ligament–bone preparation. *J Orthop Res* 1983;1:22–29.

59. Woo SL-Y, Orlando CA, Camp JF, Akeson WH. Effects of postmortem storage by freezing on ligament tensile behavior. *J Biomech* 1986;19:399–404.

60. Woo SL-Y, Orlando CA, Frank CB, Gomez MA, Akeson WH. Tensile properties of medial collateral ligament as a function of age. *J Orthop Res* 1986;4:133–141.

61. Woo SL-Y, Lee TQ, Gomez MA, Sato S, Field FP. Temperature dependent behavior of the canine medial collateral ligament. *J Biomech Eng* 1987;109:68–71.

62. Woo SL-Y, Gomez MA, Inoue M, Akeson WH. New experimental procedures to evaluate the biomechanical properties of healing canine medial collateral ligaments. *J Orthop Res* 1987;5:425–432.

Knee Ligaments: Structure, Function, Injury, and Repair, edited by D. Daniel, et al.
© 1990 by Raven Press, Ltd. All rights reserved.

CHAPTER 8

Experimental Methods Used to Evaluate Knee Ligament Function

Edmund Biden and John O'Connor

Experiments on whole cadaver joints are often the most direct way of assessing changes in the mechanics of the knee resulting from injury or surgery. Brantigan (9) began the modern era of *in vitro* knee testing by clamping a cadaver femur to a plank and applying loads to the distal tibia. He performed studies to identify the contributions of various ligamentous structures to knee stability. Since then, such tests have become a common method in the study of the mechanics of the knee.

In this chapter we discuss the philosophy behind testing of complete cadaver joints and examine typical types of tests that are used. It is important that the clinician be able to assess the results and conclusions of such tests critically before attempting to apply them in practice. These methods are to be distinguished from tests of individual tissues, such as those described by Woo in Chapter 7. In that approach, tissues are removed from the body and tested in specially designed apparatus in order to determine their elastic or viscoelastic mechanical properties.

One limitation of comparing *in vitro* data to the *in vivo* clinical examination is that the cadaver limb has no muscle tone because the muscle mass that remains is usually almost entirely flaccid. Other limitations may be (a) the change in soft tissue properties that may occur post-mortem and (b) the use of geriatric specimens. Blanton (7), in a study of the ultimate tensile strength of fetal and adult tendons, found that ultimate strength fell with increasing age but that this effect was obscured by the very range of strengths observed. He found that even in fairly homogeneous samples, the ultimate strength could vary by over 100%. Noyes (26) performed a variety of tendon tests including studies of the effects of freezing and thawing. They reported that the elastic properties were not affected by freezing and thawing. Woo (Chapter 7) has reviewed the conflicting evidence in the literature on the effects of post-mortem storage (as well as the effets of aging) on the mechanical properties of ligaments and tendons.

DEFINITIONS

In order to understand the terminology of this and succeeding chapters, it is necessary to define some terms commonly used in the field of mechanics.

Forces and Loads

The soft tissues joining the bones together at a joint apply tension forces along the lines of their fibers

E. Biden: Department of Mechanical Engineering, University of New Brunswick, Fredericton, New Brunswick, Canada E3B 5A3.

J. O'Connor: Department of Engineering Science, University of Oxford, Oxford OX1 3PJ, England.

which resist elongation of the fibers and distraction of the joint. The articular surfaces of the bones apply compressive forces perpendicular to each other to resist indentation of the cartilage layers and interpenetration of the bones. Whenever external load is applied to the body, tension and compressive forces are transmitted by the structures of the joints, the soft tissues, and the articular surfaces.

External loads are forces applied to the body in one of only two possible ways—either throughout its volume or through its surface. There is no other way of applying external loads. Loads such as gravity are body forces, applied throughout the volume of the body. When one stands still, the gravity forces are balanced by the ground reaction (i.e., loads applied by the ground through the soles of the feet). These latter are examples of contact forces (i.e., loads applied over part of the surface area of the body by means of contact pressure or friction). Other examples of contact forces are (a) forces applied through the surfaces of the back, seat, thighs, and feet when sitting and (b) forces applied through the hands when using walking sticks. The gravity loads may be thought of as the primary loads, and the ground forces may be thought of as the external reactions to those loads.

When standing still, the resultant of the ground reaction forces (i.e., the sum of the forces applied through both feet) is exactly equal to the weight of the body. The body is said to be in equilibrium under the action of the weight forces and the ground reactions. When moving, the ground reaction must, in addition to balancing the gravity forces, provide the forces necessary to maintain that movement, so-called inertia forces. When moving slowly, the inertia forces are small in comparison to body weight. When sprinting, they can be quite substantial.

Resultant Force and Moment at a Joint

The forces set up at joints and along the limbs are internal reactions to the external loads. From the point of view of knee mechanics, it is useful to think of the lower leg, from the joint cleft at the knee down to the ground, as being in equilibrium under the action of (a) its own weight (small compared to body weight), (b) the ground reaction, and (c) the forces applied to the lower leg by the structures of the knee.

The simplest way of describing the forces at the knee, requiring no anatomical understanding, is to calculate the resultant force and moment at the joint. Figure 8-1 shows the lower leg loaded by the ground reaction **W**, and it also shows forces applied at the knee. For equilibrium, the sum of the forces acting on the lower leg must be zero; thus the structures of the knee have to combine to provide a force that exactly bal-

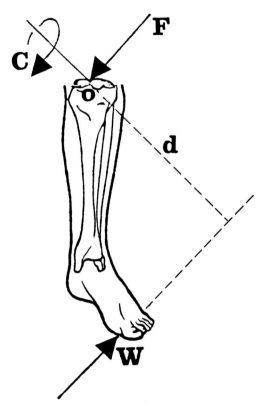

FIG. 8-1. The lower leg in equilibrium under the action of a load **W** applied at the foot. If we neglect the weight of the limb, the resultant force **F** at the knee must be equal and opposite to **W** in order to have balanced vertical, mediolateral, and fore–aft forces. If **F** and **W** do not have the same line of action, then a moment **C** equal to **W**d (d is the perpendicular distance from **W** to **F**) is needed to keep the foot floor force **W** from rotating the leg.

ances the ground reaction. This is the resultant force **F** at the knee which resists translation of the lower leg. It is equal in magnitude and opposite in direction to the load **W**.

In Fig. 8-1, the resultant force **F** at the knee is shown passing through the tibial plateau at the point o. Its line of action does not coincide with that of the ground reaction, although the two forces are parallel. The structures of the knee must therefore also combine to provide a moment (**C** in Fig. 8-1) that resists rotary movements of the lower leg about the point o. The magnitude of the moment **C** must be equal and opposite to the moment of the load about the point o (i.e., the product of the force magnitude **W** times the perpendicular distance d from o to the line of action of the ground reaction).

The forces applied by the structures of the knee therefore reduce to a resultant force through some selected point and a resultant moment about that point. This is the description commonly used in gait analysis (Chapter 14). One of the objects of the study of knee mechanics is to determine how the structures of the knee (the muscles, ligaments, and articular surfaces) are marshaled to provide the resultant force and moment needed to balance various types of load. That study requires anatomical knowledge and is discussed in detail in Chapters 10 and 11.

The resultant force and moment at the knee can be defined with respect to a coordinate system of three mutually perpendicular axes x, y, z meeting at the origin (Fig. 8-2). The x and y axes point in the anterior and medial directions, approximately in the plane of the tibial plateau. The z axis lies perpendicular to that plane, pointing upwards from the tibia. In general, the resultant force at the knee does not coincide with one of the three coordinate directions but has components in each of those directions. The components in the x- and y directions, parallel to the tibial plateau, are called *shear forces* because they resist sliding of the femur on the tibia. The z component is either a tensile or compressive force, resisting distraction or interpenetration of the bones. The sum of the three components, added according to the parallelogram law, is the resultant force, equal in magnitude and opposite in direction to the load applied through the foot.

The external ground reaction does not usually intersect or lie parallel to the x-, y-, or z axes but has a moment about each. The resultant moment at the joint therefore also has three components, one about each axis. The magnitude of each component of the moment is given by the magnitude of the load times the perpendicular distance from the line of action of the load to the corresponding axis. If the load passes posterior to the mediolateral y axis, it tends to flex the knee so that an extending moment about the y axis is required for equilibrium. If the load passes lateral to the anteroposterior x axis, it tends to abduct the knee so that an adducting moment about the x axis is required. If the load does not pass through the z axis, it tends to rotate the tibia internally or externally, and thus a corresponding external or internal twisting moment is required at the knee.

In summary, the resultant force and moment at the knee (i.e., the joint reaction to external load) can be described and specified by a maximum of six components (three of force and three of moment). The coordinate system in Fig. 8-2 is chosen so that the components of force and moment are related to the types of movement that they induce or resist.

Degrees of Freedom

If we were to cut all the soft tissues that hold the bones together at the knee, the tibia would be entirely free to move relative to the femur. We would have given

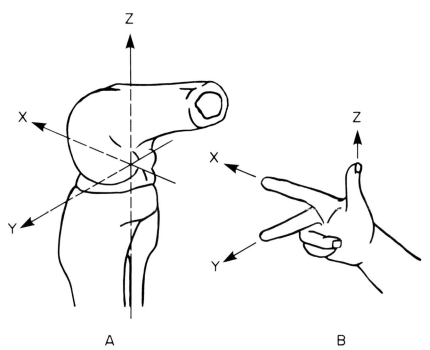

FIG. 8-2. A: Diagram of the knee with axes superimposed. **B**: The axes form a "right-hand" system. The axis system can be thought of as attached or embedded in the tibia. Motion of the femur with respect to the tibia consists of three translations and three rotations. Translation along x is anteroposterior movement, along y is mediolateral inducement, and along z is distraction or interpenetration of the femur; tibia rotation about x is abduction or adduction, about y is flexion–extension, and about z is tibial rotation.

the two bones six degrees of freedom relative to each other. With the femur fixed, the tibia could then slide or translate in each of the three perpendicular directions of Fig. 8-2 and it could spin or rotate about axes in each of those three directions.

Flexion/extension of the knee is a rotation of the tibia relative to the femur about the mediolateral y axis. Abduction/adduction of the knee is a rotation of the tibia about the anteroposterior x axis. Tibial rotation is a rotation about the z axis. Anteroposterior subluxation is a translation along the x axis, mediolateral subluxation is a translation along the y axis, and distraction of the bones is a translation along the z axis.

It is no coincidence that the number of possible degrees of freedom of the tibia—six—is exactly equal to the maximum number of components of force and moment needed to describe the joint reaction. For equilibrium of any body, the sum in each of three directions of all the forces applied to that body must be zero, and so also must the moment of those forces about axes through any point in each of the three directions. There are therefore six mechanical conditions to be satisfied for equilibrium. Six independent forces applied by the muscles, ligaments, and articular surfaces at the knee are therefore sufficient to ensure the equilibrium of the lower leg in the presence of any arbitrary load and to suppress all six degrees of freedom.

Ranges of Movement; Stability

Although the tibia has, in principle, six possible degrees of freedom relative to the femur, the ligaments and other fibers of the capsule, together with the articular surfaces of the knee, allow only a small proportion of that complete freedom of movement, even when the muscles are completely relaxed. The knee can be flexed only through 150° or so out of a possible 360°; the tibia can be rotated internally or externally relative to the femur through a range of about 25°; the range of abduction/adduction is only 5° or so. Only millimeters of translational movements parallel to the three axes are possible.

The bulk of the allowed range of movement at a joint occurs without significant stretch of the ligaments or significant indentation of the articular surfaces of the bones. When the limits to the allowed range of movement are approached, the ligaments and other capsular structures begin to stretch and the articular surfaces begin to indent, offering ever-increasing elastic resistance to further movement. The ligaments and articular surfaces then act together, transmitting the tensile and compressive forces needed to define the limits of the range of allowable movement and to prevent movement beyond that range. In Chapter 9, a review is given of the studies that have attempted to determine the roles of each of the ligaments in limiting movement at the knee. Within the limits of movement, the bones and the ligaments form a linkage that changes its geometry without gross deformation to allow movement of the bones. A detailed description of such a linkage is given in Chapter 10.

The geometry of the ligaments and articular surfaces therefore define the range of allowable movements of the bones. Their combined action in resisting movement beyond that allowable range gives the joint its passive stability. Muscle forces, applied to the bones through their tendons, are used to move the bones actively from one position to another within the allowable range. Even more important, muscle forces are generally necessary to prevent movements within the allowable range in the presence of external loads such as gravity and the ground reaction, to give the joint its active stability. For instance, when the external loads tend to flex the joint, action is needed from the extensors to prevent movement; when the loads tend to extend the joint, action is needed from the flexors.

Coupled Forces, Coupled Motion

It is rare for any anatomical movement to require only one degree of freedom. Knee flexion is associated primarily with rotation about the y axis (Fig. 8-2), but the tibia also translates along the x axis and rotates about the z axis while flexion occurs. Motions such as these are referred to as "coupled motions." Equally, it is rare that the external loads are such that only one component of force or moment is transmitted across the joint. As seen in Fig. 8-3a, an external load that tends to extend the joint and requires a flexing moment at the knee also both pushes the surfaces of the bones together, a movement prevented by a compressive force, and slides the tibia on the femur, a movement resisted by a shear force.

An external load applied parallel to one of the coordinate axes usually produces coupled motion. In Fig. 8-3b, an anteriorly directed force is applied to the tibia lateral to the axis of tibial rotation and produces internal rotation as well as anterior translation of the tibia relative to the femur. In Fig. 8-3d, the force is applied medial to the axis and produces external rotation as well as translation. Only when the load is applied through the axis and has zero moment about the axis is the resulting motion one of pure translation without coupled rotation (Fig. 8-3c).

DESIGN OF WHOLE-JOINT TESTING APPARATUS

Tests on complete joints have been performed for a variety of reasons: to determine the range of move-

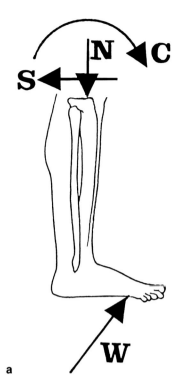

a

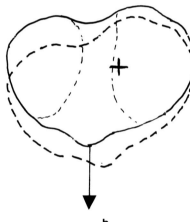

b

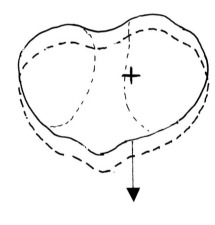

c

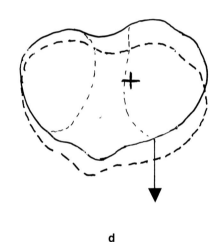

d

FIG. 8-3. (a) An extending load **W** balanced at the knee by a flexing moment **C**, a compressive force **N**, and a shear force **S**. (b) Anterior force applied to the tibia lateral to axis of rotation produces internal rotation as well as anterior translation. (c) Anterior force applied through axis of rotation produces only anterior translation. (d) Anterior force applied medial to axis of rotation produces external rotation as well as anterior translation.

ments of the bones in the presence of various external loads; to determine the roles of the muscles, the ligaments, and the articular surfaces in controlling and limiting the movements of the bones relative to each other; in transmitting load across the joint; and in stabilizing the limb in the presence of external load. If these objectives are to be met fully, it is clearly necessary that the movements of the bones relative to each other should be measured and that the loads applied should be measured in such a way that the resultant force and moment transmitted at the joint can be determined. Only then are the mechanical circumstances of the experiment fully defined.

If, further, the objective is to test the specimen in circumstances approaching the physiological, it is important that the constraints placed on the relative movements of the bones should be those applied by the structures of the joint and not by the apparatus used to hold the specimen or by the devices used to apply load or to measure the movements of the bones.

Restricting naturally occurring motions of the bones (overconstraint) is a common limitation of testing devices. To illustrate the effect, consider the example of a device to test "range of motion" in a door hinge (Fig. 8-4). If we attach a goniometer to the hinge, the combination of the goniometer and the hinge will not move because the axes are not coincident. We have "constrained" the single degree of freedom (namely, rotation) that is available to the hinge and have created a "structure" that will not move. Great care must be exercised in joint testing to ensure that similar effects are not produced and incorrect conclusions drawn.

In a testing device, one must consider how the knee is held and loaded in order to understand the inter-

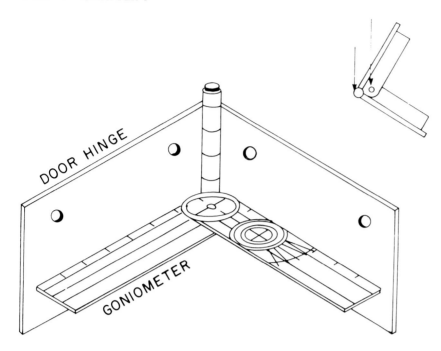

FIG. 8-4. Testing a door hinge. A door hinge allows one degree of freedom, that of rotation about its axis. If a goniometer were attached to the hinge so that the goniometer arms would not slip against the hinge, then because the axis or the hinge isn't aligned with that of the goniometer, neither will move. The testing system constrains the hinge.

action between the testing device and the joint being tested. Figure 8-5 shows a sketch of a knee being tested in compression at a flexion angle of about 60°. The femur and tibia are attached rigidly to the moving and fixed crossheads of a materials testing machine

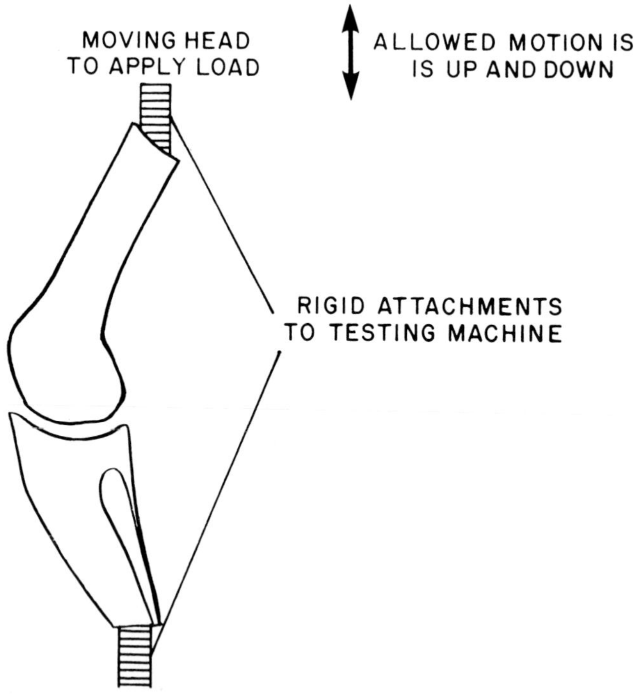

MOVING HEAD
TO APPLY LOAD

ALLOWED MOTION IS
IS UP AND DOWN

RIGID ATTACHMENTS
TO TESTING MACHINE

FIXED BASE OF
TESTING MACHINE

FIG. 8-5. A one-degree-of-freedom rig. Bones can only distract or interpenetrate, and motions involving flexion and rotation are suppressed. Also, the knee is held in flexion without muscle activity, which is not the usual case in a live joint.

which are capable only of translating vertically relative to each other. The apparatus allows only one degree of freedom, that of distraction or interpenetration of the bones. The clamps used to attach the bones to the rig must supply the forces and moments required to suppress flexion, tibial rotation, and anteroposterior displacement. Unless the forces and moments that constrain these motions are measured, the resultant force and moment at the knee are unknown and the test is as likely to reflect the characteristics of the fixation as those of the joint.

Tests on cadaver joints can be put into categories based on how load is applied, how the bones are held, how the measurements are made, and so forth. In this discussion we will consider testing methods on the basis of whether they simulate:

1. clinical tests such as the drawer test;
2. "Life-like" loading; and
3. loads that stretch or compress particular structures.

Simulation of Clinical Tests

In examining a knee, it is common to have the patient lying supine and for the examiner to stabilize the femur and manipulate the tibia. These tests are not easy to interpret quantitatively because the precise nature and magnitudes of the loads applied by the examiner are not known. Tests on cadaver specimens have been used to simulate this condition. The simplest method of testing is to attach the femur to the test bench and to allow the tibia free movement. Loads can then be applied to the tibia (such as one might do in the clinic), and observations can be made of the movements of the tibia allowed by the structures of the knee. This method is the closest to an actual clinical test, and the results are usually such that they relate quite directly to what would be seen in a live patient.

Less constrained testing systems (9) clamped the femur to a plank and applied medially or laterally directed loads to the distal end of the foot (Fig. 8-6). In light of our discussion of coupled motion above, we note that Brantigan's method (9) of loading, intended to apply torque to the tibia, would lead to abduction/adduction and mediolateral subluxation as well as tibial rotation. This is consistent with clinical practice but may obscure the effect of torsion.

Markolf (24) used a similar method of fixing the femur. "Force handles" were used to apply measured loads to the tibia (Fig. 8-7). He measured rotations resulting from applied varus–valgus and axial moments and displacements, elicited by applied antero-posterior forces. He found, in all three test modes, that the load–displacement measurements followed the

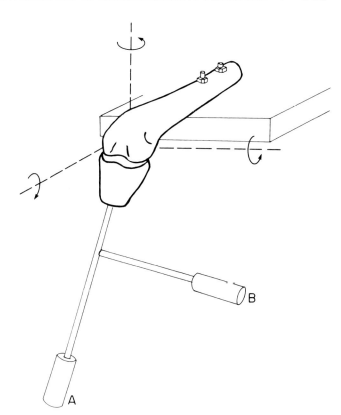

FIG. 8-7. Test rig used by Markolf (24). The force handles at A and B can be manipulated to simulate various clinical tests. Forces are well-defined in this advice, but no muscle action can be simulated.

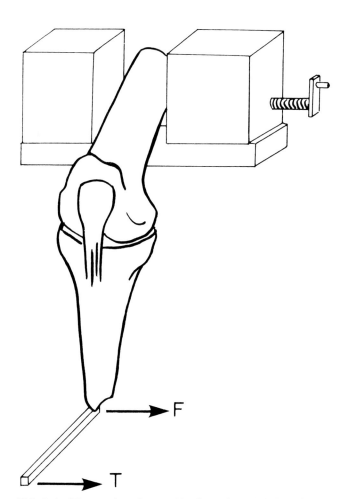

FIG. 8-6. The testing rig used by Brantigan (9). The femur was clamped to a rigid base, and forces at **F** or **T** were applied. Force **F** acts to abduct or adduct the joint. Force **T** is intended to produce tibial torsion.

now familiar pattern of an initially compliant (lax) zone, followed by one of increasing stiffness, as the structures of the knee tightened and the limits of knee motion were approached. He studied the effects on those limits of sectioning various ligaments (Chapter 9). Neilsen (25) used a similar arrangement to measure the response of the knee to sectioning of the medial collateral ligament (MCL) and the anterior cruciate ligament (ACL). Wang (38) used the terms "primary laxity" and "secondary laxity" to distinguish between the compliant and stiff zones. ("Stiffness" in this sense means the change in force per unit change in displacement. It is the inverse of "compliance," i.e., the change in displacement per unit change in force.)

These studies have been criticized because the goniometric system used relies on having the goniometer axes aligned with the "axes" of the joint. One can argue that the error induced by not being perfectly aligned might influence the results. Kinzel (18) developed a method by which the detailed motions of any two bodies in space might be measured with any arbitrary orientation of the measurement axes (Fig. 8-8). Suntay (36) used a similar technique to build a goniometer system which avoids the problems of needing the axes aligned. Results based on testing 15 knees

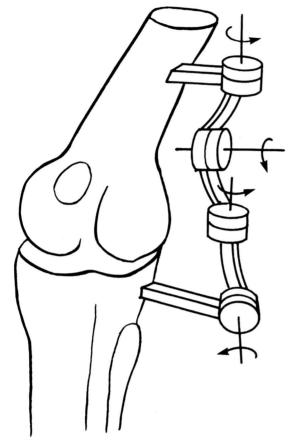

FIG. 8-8. Goniometer system suggested by Kinzel (18) and reported by Suntay (36). Position of the tibia relative to the femur is found by examining the angular displacements of a "chain" of revolute or hinge joints. In practice, the dimensions of each link are known, the orientation of each hinge is sensed with an electrical angle sensor, and relative position is calculated.

using this system were presented by Grood (13). They reinforce the results of Markolf (24), although the amount of displacement in some modes was higher than originally reported.

Fukubayashi (11) and Sullivan (35) also simulated the drawer test. In the apparatus described by Fukubayashi (11) (Fig. 8-9A), the device used to hold the knee between the fixed and moving crossheads of the testing machine allowed the bones 4 degrees of freedom, " . . . preventing unphysiological compression caused by apparatus constraints. . . . " One of his findings was that up to 1.4 N-m of external and 1.2 N-m of internal tibial torque were produced as an adjunct to anteroposterior forces. Sullivan (35), in the follow-up paper that describes a modified rig having 5 degrees of freedom (Fig. 8-9B), found that the lack of allowance for mediolateral motion in the test rig reported in the first paper caused tibial torques considerably different from those observed in the rig with less constraint. In light of our discussion of Fig. 8-3 above, we note that

a coupling between anterior force and internal rotation would be expected only when the line of action of the force passes lateral to the axis of tibial rotation.

The results of these methods of testing are broadly comparable in that they all exhibit zones of laxity surrounded by zones of stiffness, and they reach a broad consensus on the roles of each of the ligaments as primary or secondary stabilizers for different modes of relative movement of the bones. However, qualitative as well as quantitative differences have occurred because of different designs of apparatus. This work points out the importance of recognizing constraint in devices that do not allow completely "free motion" to the joint.

Simulation of "Life-like" Loading

This brings us to the second type of test—namely, that which simulates a life-like loading rather than a clinical test. There is considerable interest in examining the knee under load.

Effects of Tibiofemoral Contact Force

In order to study the contribution of the tibiofemoral contact force to the stability of the knee, a number of studies have used testing machines to apply compressive load between the bones without attempting to simulate muscle action. Wang (38) used a compression/torsion machine, allowing two degrees of freedom, to study the effects of compressive load on the rotatory laxity of the knee. He showed that compressive load decreased the laxity of the knee. In a later paper, Hsieh (16) found a similar influence of compressive load on anteroposterior stability.

A particularly interesting example is the device used by Markolf (23) and Shoemaker (33). This allowed the bones complete freedom of movement, but large loads could be applied across the knee at a variety of flexion angles in such a way that the load always passed through the "center" of rotation of the joint, produced no moment, and hence required no additional muscle forces for stability (Fig. 8-10). They showed that compressive load increased the anteroposterior, mediolateral, varus–valgus, and torsional stiffness and reduced the corresponding laxity of the knee. Blankevoort (6) used a six-degree-of-freedom rig to define the envelope of passive knee joint motion. In the presence of compressive force without simulated muscle action, it was necessary to clamp the bones and remove the freedom to flex or extend to hold different positions of flexion.

In our view, clinical application of the results of such tests is uncertain. In life, large contact forces and large muscle forces occur simultaneously. Large mus-

A

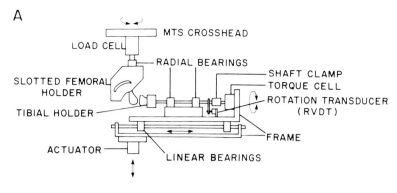

B

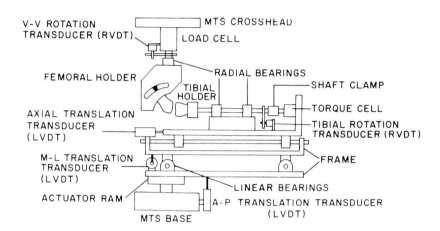

FIG. 8-9. A: A four-degree-of-freedom test rig used by Fukubayashi (11). **B:** A five-degree-of-freedom test rig used by Sullivan (35). The four-degree-of-freedom system suppresses both flexion/extension and mediolateral motion. Significantly different effects between test rigs were observed in experiments. Because most motions consist of a combination of the six basic motions, suppressing one is likely to affect the others. In both rigs, flexion is resisted by the device. No muscle action is simulated.

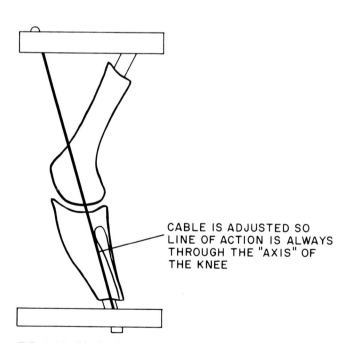

CABLE IS ADJUSTED SO
LINE OF ACTION IS ALWAYS
THROUGH THE "AXIS" OF
THE KNEE

FIG. 8-10. Markolf (23) developed a test rig that allowed considerable freedom of motion to the joint without requiring simulated muscle action. To do this, his rig adjusts so that compression is always applied along the axis of the tibia. Hence, the force has no lever-arm, and the joint does not flex or extend.

cle forces acting through short lever-arms at the knee are needed to balance the rotary effects of relatively smaller external loads, acting through long lever-arms along the leg. Large contact forces pushing the tibia distally are then needed to balance the large muscle forces pulling the tibia proximally and are unlikely to arise in their absence. Studies of active stability are likely to have clinical relevance only if both muscle and contact forces are present simultaneously.

Simulated Muscle Action

The most popular muscle group to simulate has been the quadriceps, both because quadriceps action is important in day-to-day activities and also because the arrangement of the quadriceps, patella, and patellar tendon make it possible to provide reasonably life-like simulation of the effect of muscle action simply by pulling on the stump of the quadriceps tendon.

A number of researchers, including Harding (15), Malcolm (21), and Grood (14), have used this sort of arrangement. Malcolm (21) attached the femur to the test bench and simulated leg lift as did Grood (14) (Fig. 8-11). Using different techniques, they found that the ACL was active in early flexion in association with quadriceps action. Grood (14) showed that ACL sec-

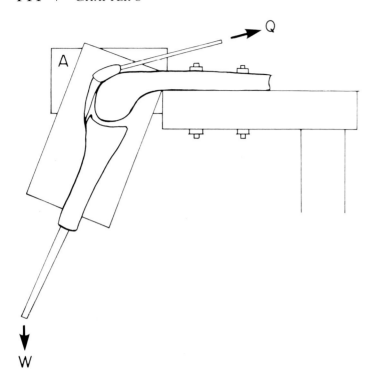

FIG. 8-11. Malcom (21) and Grood (14) used similar test rigs. In both cases the femur is clamped to a table and a weight **W** is applied distal to the joint. The knee is held in equilibrium by a force **Q** applied to the end of the quadriceps tendon. In the Malcom experiment, relative orientation of the femur and tibia was determined by having a plate A attached to the femur and a card attached to the tibia. By marking the card through holes drilled in plate A, the relative orientation of the bones could be documented. This method has some sensitivity to motions outside the sagittal plane, but they are difficult to interpret.

tioning produced additional anterior laxity. Harding (15) attached the tibia vertically to a base, extended the femur using a rod in the medullary canal, and attached a deadweight load to the end. Then he stabilized the knee using a strap attached between the quadriceps tendon and the femur and tracked the movement of the contact areas on the tibial plateau during flexion/extension. Goodfellow (12) used the apparatus to study the kinematics of the patellofemoral joint. Perry (27) placed knees in simulated flexed knee stance, and then she attached a tensile force transducer to the quadriceps tendon and placed a compressive force transducer under the tibial plateau. Vertical load was applied at the hip, and the quadriceps force needed to stabilize the limb in different positions of flexion was measured (Fig. 8-12). She found that both quadriceps force and the compressive force on the tibial plateau were linearly related to load for constant flexion angle and increased in a nonlinear fashion with flexion.

Perry's rig was overconstrained by one degree. The lower tibia was attached to the rig base using a simple hinge that constrained it to move in a plane, without any possibility for tibial rotation. Such constraint is unlikely to affect the relationship between quadriceps force and load, and the results she obtained with this five-degree-of-freedom system are consistent with those found with six-degree-of-freedom devices.

The Oxford Rig

Bourne (8) and Biden (4,5) used a rig that also simulates flexed knee stance (Fig. 8-13). The knee is loaded in flexion, and stability is maintained by pulling on the quadriceps tendon through a load cell. Standing with the knees bent, riding a bicycle, climbing stairs, the early stance portion of gait, and so forth, are examples of conditions that can be simulated in the test rig.

The rig differs from that used by Perry (27) by allowing the bones six degrees of freedom so that their movements upon each other are constrained only by the structures of the knee. We will give a detailed description of this rig here since it has not yet been described extensively elsewhere.

Ankle and Hip Assemblies

The specimen is prepared with about 20 cm of bone above and below the joint cleft, and threaded rods are fixed in the intramedullary cavities of both bones. The threaded rods are used to attach the specimen to the tibial and femoral limbs of the apparatus. The "ankle" assembly comprises three sets of rotary bearings that allow flexion/extension, abduction/adduction, and long axis rotation of the tibial limb. The axes of the three bearings intersect at a fixed point, namely, the center of the ankle. The "hip" assembly comprises two sets of rotary bearings, allowing abduction/adduction and flexion/extension to the femoral limb. The axes of these bearings intersect at a point vertically above the ankle, simulating the center of the hip. Linear bearings running along two vertical rods guide vertical movement of the hip relative to the ankle.

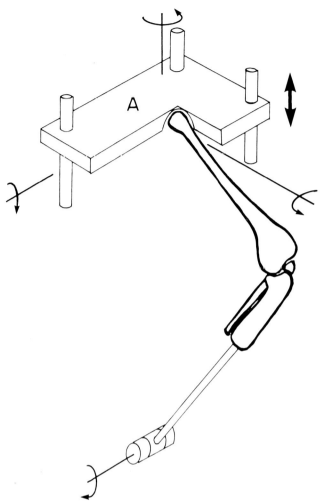

FIG. 8-12. Perry (27) used this rig to measure quadriceps force as a function of flexion angle. Four degrees of freedom (three rotations plus up and down motion) are allowed at the hip, and a fifth degree of freedom (rotation of the ankle) is allowed as well. Equilibrium is maintained by pulling on a strap attached to the quadriceps tendon. This rig appears to have five degrees of freedom, but in fact both tibial rotation and abduction/adduction are suppressed because the tibia is constrained to move in a single plane. Flexed knee stance under a vertical load at the hip involves only minor abduction/adduction or rotatory effects, and these have little effect on quadriceps tension.

Application of Vertical Load

When the moving parts of the apparatus are counterbalanced with the specimen in position, the "leg" can then be placed in any position of flexion and remains there. When vertical load is applied by hanging weights onto the hip assembly, collapse of the system is prevented by means of the tension force in a wire attached to the quadriceps tendon. The specimen is flexed by lengthening the wire. This simulation of muscle force is necessary to stabilize the leg in the presence of vertical load. A strain-gauged proving ring in series with the wire measures the tendon force.

Adjustment in the Coronal Plane

The bearings allowing flexion/extension at the hip are attached to a sliding bar that can be moved mediolaterally on the hip assembly, thus allowing the plane in which the knee flexes and extends to be rotated about the ankle. When the slider is fixed so that the tibia lies in a vertical plane, this arrangement simulates the natural valgus angle of the femur; the plane of the vertical load then coincides with the plane through the so-called mechanical axis of the limb—that is, the plane though the centers of the ankle, knee, and hip (Fig. 8-14A). In other positions, it allows the plane of the limb to be set at any desired angle relative to the vertical load—for instance, to simulate single leg stance (Fig. 8-14B)—when the line of action of the vertical load passes medial to the knee (22, fig. 17).

Measurement of Movement

Five rotary variable differential transformers (RVDTs) (Schaevitz) are used to measure rotations at the five sets of rotary bearings. A linear variable differential transformer (LVDT) (Schaevitz) is used to measure the vertical position of the hip assembly. These transducers give an output voltage proportional to position. The signals are supplied to a microcomputer (Research Machines 380Z) through an analogue/digital converter and are recorded. Records of experiments can then be stored on disk.

Degrees of Freedom

Figure 8-15 shows how the degrees of freedom allowed by the apparatus could be combined to give each of the six possible anatomical movements at the specimen, demonstrating that the apparatus does not restrict any physiologically possible movement of the bones. Distraction of the joint and long axis rotation each require movement at only one of the bearings (Figs. 8-15c and f), but each of the other anatomical movements requires movement at three of the bearings—for instance: flexion of the knee requires flexion and vertical translation at the hip, as well as flexion at the ankle (Fig. 8-15a); and anterior translation of the tibia relative to the femur requires flexion and vertical movement at the hip, as well as flexion at the ankle (Fig. 8-15d). Using Cartesian coordinates, a program was devised to express the measurements in terms of the anatomical movements described in Fig. 8-2.

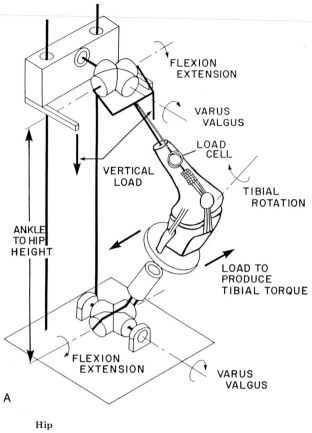

FLEXION EXTENSION

VARUS VALGUS

LOAD CELL

VERTICAL LOAD

TIBIAL ROTATION

ANKLE TO HIP HEIGHT

LOAD TO PRODUCE TIBIAL TORQUE

FLEXION EXTENSION

VARUS VALGUS

A

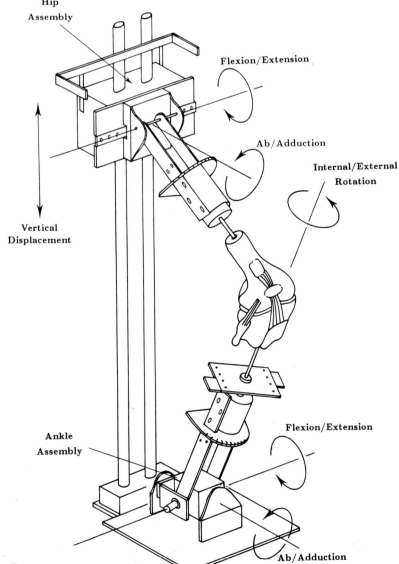

Hip Assembly

Flexion/Extension

Ab/Adduction

Internal/External Rotation

Vertical Displacement

Ankle Assembly

Flexion/Extension

Ab/Adduction

B

FIG. 8-13. A: The original Oxford rig. **B**: The Oxford rig with modification to allow offset of the hip. The Oxford rig allows six degrees of freedom to the knee. The two rotations at the hip and three rotations at the ankle act like a pair of ball-and-socket joints, and the slider allows height to change as the knee flexes. Simulated muscle action is required for equilibrium except at full extension where the load passes down the tibial axis, producing no flexing or extending moment.

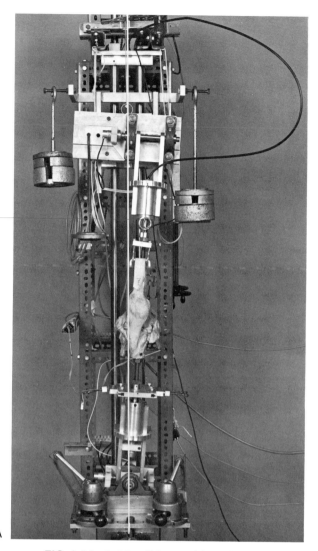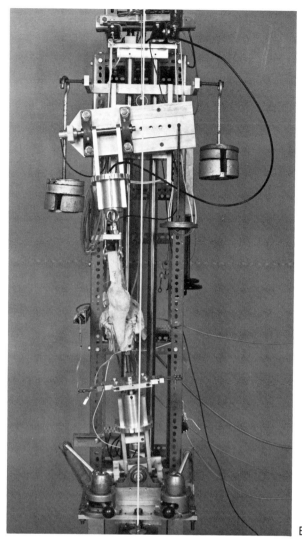

A

B

FIG. 8-14. A: Hip slider positioned so that the vertical plane through hip and ankle passes through the lateral compartment of the knee. **B:** Hip slider positioned so that the vertical plane through centers of hip and ankle passes medial to the knee.

Discussion

Lipke (20) described a similar flexed knee stance device that allows free motion for the bones. Because of the lack of constraint, such apparatuses share with simple arrangements, such as that of Malcolm (21) (Fig. 8-11), the fact that they are "statically determinate." When known loads are applied, the resultant force and moment transmitted by the specimen can be calculated. Together with the displacement measurements from the transducers, this means that the geometrical and mechanical circumstances of the specimen are completely defined. The structures of the knee then combine to transmit that force and moment in a manner that is not determined by the apparatus, and the displacements are the measured responses of the joint to the loading of those structures.

There are some difficulties. In common with the de-

vices used by Markolf (23), Fukubayashi (11), and Blankevoort (6), the arrangement is complicated when compared to the simpler experiments of Harding (15), Malcolm (21), and Grood (14) with one of the bones fixed. When simulating muscle action, the magnitudes of the loads that can be applied are limited by the strength of the attachment to the muscle tendons. The leverage about the knee available to the applied vertical load (Fig. 8-16A) is larger than in life (Fig. 8-16B), where load, applied through the ball of the foot, passes closer to the joint. Indeed, near extension, the load through the foot can pass in front of the knee, requiring flexor action for equilibrium (Fig. 8-16C). The simulated quadriceps forces measured in the rig are therefore larger in proportion to the applied load than is the physiological force.

Results from the Oxford rig are presented elsewhere in this book and won't be discussed here.

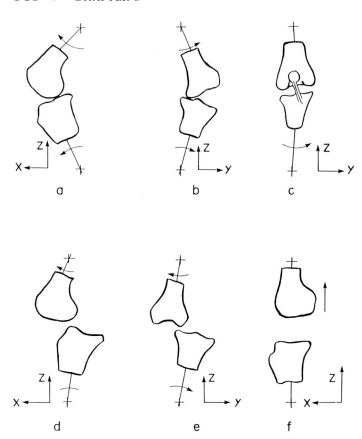

FIG. 8-15. Motions of the Oxford rig to allow six basic degrees of freedom. The six basic degrees of freedom are three rotations and three translations. The Oxford rig allows five rotations and one translation, and thus no simple one-to-one correspondence exists. **a**: Rotation about y flexion is accomplished by the hip flexion axis rotation and the ankle flexion axis rotation. **b**: Rotation about x abduction/adduction causes the hip fore–aft axis to rotate one way while causing the ankle to rotate the other way. **c**: Rotation about z—rotation appears as motion of the tibial rotation of the z ankle axis. **d**: Translation along x occurs when the femur flexes forward and the tibial segment flexes backward, or vice versa. **e**: Translation along y mediolateral motion involves rotation above the fore–aft axis or above the hip and/or the ankle. **f**: Translation along z—distraction of interpenetration is accomplished by movement of the slider. Knee flexion and tibial rotation can be obtained more or less directly. Other motions in this rig usually require mathematical analysis for interpretation.

TESTS OF INDIVIDUAL STRUCTURES

The final category of test is that which is designed to examine the response of a particular structure (or structures) to load or to examine the contribution of that structure to knee stability. Whereas to examine the way the joint responds to load it is usually desirable to have the joint unconstrained, it is possible to take the opposite approach and have a completely constrained rig and then measure all the loads instead of all the motions. Piziali (29,30), Rastager (31), and Seering (32) took this approach. The two bones were each rigidly connected to a six-component dynamometer capable of measuring the three components of the resultant force and the three components of the resultant moment transmitted through it (Fig. 8-17). A cyclic displacement was then applied to one dynamometer relative to the other, and the forces and moments produced at the attachments of the tibia and femur were measured. From these data the "stiffness" of the joint (i.e., the external force or moment required to apply unit displacement) was found. Coupling between movement parallel to or about one axis and the forces and moments required in each of the three coordinate directions was studied (28).

With the joint left in the test machine, ligaments were serially sectioned and the tests repeated. By comparing the external forces between tests, the contri-

bution of each structure cut was determined. Butler (10) also used a fully constrained system when studying the drawer test and reached very similar conclusions about the effects of sectioning the cruciate ligaments. Butler introduced the concept of primary and secondary ligamentous stabilizers, showing how the anteroposterior force needed for a specified anterior or posterior translation of the tibia was much reduced by sectioning of the anterior cruciate ligament (ACL) or posterior cruciate ligament (PCL).

The results of the work of Piziali (29,30), albeit on a very small number of specimens at full extension and at 30° of flexion, showed how medial or lateral translation of the tibia on the femur is restricted and limited by the ligaments. In particular, the ACL (52%) and lateral collateral ligament (30%) were found to mainly restrict medial tibial displacement, whereas the PCL (32–36%) and medial collateral ligament (MCL) (22–42%) were found to mainly restrict lateral tibial displacement.

Using the same apparatus, Seering (32) documented the contributions of the ligaments in resisting varus–valgus and axial tibial rotations. This work demonstrated a possible limitation of such apparatus which defines absolutely the axes about which the bones are made to rotate. The axis of valgus rotation was chosen such that a rotation of 8° was not sufficient to bring the articular surfaces of the lateral compartment into

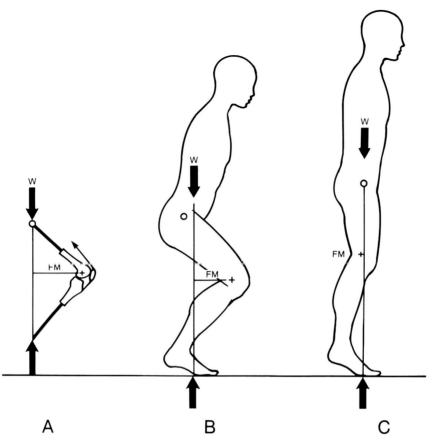

A B C

FIG. 8-16. The Oxford rig simulates flexed knee stance but is not exactly analogous to what occurs in everyday life. For instance, if diagram **A** (representing the rig) and diagram **B** (representing stance) are compared, it is easy to see that shifts in trunk position or where load (**W**) passes through the foot will influence the flexing moment (FM) at the knee. In the Oxford rig, load is applied through the center of the hip, and thus the moment arm is usually longer than normal. Another situation occurring in everyday life is depicted in diagram **C**: When one stands with knees extended and shifts one's weight onto the balls of the feet, body weight passes anterior to the knee fleximaxis (+) and produces an extending moment. This situation cannot occur in the Oxford rig.

contact. Rastager (31) showed how sensitive the load–displacement characteristics are to choice of rotation axis. Coupling was minimized when the axis requiring minimum resisting loads was chosen.

Piziali (28) found that the cruciate ligaments make a large contribution to resisting mediolateral translation of the bones and a small ("but significant") contribution to resisting varus–valgus rotations. In life, these two effects may not be easily separated since loads tending to induce abduction or adduction would also induce mediolateral translation; experiments with fully constrained applied displacement therefore require very careful interpretation in the clinical context.

Tests of Individual Structures Within Intact Joints

A more direct approach to the problem of studying ligament function is to make measurements of the lig-aments themselves, or their attachment areas, rather than infer the actions of the ligaments from the motions of the bones.

A number of techniques have been used for this sort of study. In this section we will discuss five of these techniques: x-ray tracking of marked end points of ligament fibers; the use of mercury strain gauges; the use of Hall Effect strain gauges; the use of a buckle transducer; and digitizing methods.

Wang (37) determined the length changes in ligaments by placing steel pins at the insertions of the ligaments. To determine the coordinates of the pins at various joint positions, the knees were put through a range of motion and biplanar x-rays were taken. Wang calculated the strain patterns induced in various ligament fibers by passive movement of the bones. Neither external loads nor muscle forces were simulated.

A mercury strain gauge consists of a slender elastic tube filled with mercury. The shape of the mercury

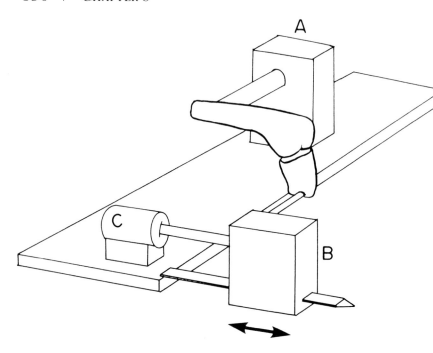

FIG. 8-17. Test device used by Piziali (28,29). This device makes no attempt toward "physiological" loading. Rather, the femur and tibia are attached rigidly to the device (**A,B,C**), which measures the forces and moment needed to maintain equilibrium. One bone is then displaced relative to the other, and the change in forces is noted. Serial sectioning of structures, followed by tests to see how forces and moments change, enables us to determine the contribution of each of these structures.

column changes when the tube is stretched. The change in the electrical resistance of the tube can be related to its extension. Kennedy (17) reports a study in which mercury strain gauges were attached to the ACL, PCL, and MCL in order to record directly the changes in length as the knee was loaded.

Lew (19) reported on the use of a "buckle transducer" (Fig. 8-18) to study forces in the ACL and PCL in cadaver knees with various arthroplasties. The buckle transducer is a small frame that is attached around the ligament in such a way that tension in the ligament deforms the buckle. This deformation is recorded by strain gauges cemented to the buckle itself. By recording data in an intact cadaver specimen and then removing the ligament and testing it in a tension-testing device, the buckle may be calibrated.

Arms (1) "mapped" strain patterns within the MCL using a strain gauge that relies on the "Hall Effect." He applied the same technique to studies of the ACL (2,3). The transducer consists of a very small magnet sliding in a hollow tube (Fig. 8-19). A change in the position of the magnet produces a change in the voltage output from the transducer which may then be recorded. This transducer is very small, is minimally invasive, and is highly accurate for small displacements. The limitations of the transducer are coincident with its strengths. It is so small that it is difficult to handle; it is difficult to find when dropped.

Sidles (34) described the use of a six-degree-of-freedom digitizer to record the positions in space of numerous points on the surfaces of each bone—in particular, the attachment areas of the ligaments. By recording also the movements of the bones relative to each other in a variety of loading conditions, it was

possible to locate the isometric insertions of the ligaments in each knee, using computer search techniques. While he presented a very large body of results, involving the collection of huge numbers of data, the methods of supporting and loading the specimens are described rather briefly.

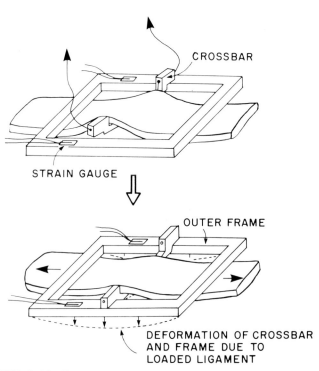

FIG. 8-18. Buckle transducer as used by Lew (19). A ligament is threaded through the buckle as shown. As it tightens, it bends the frame. This bending is sensed by strain gauges, the output from which represents ligament load.

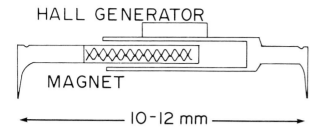

HALL GENERATOR

MAGNET

— 10-12 mm —

FIG. 8-19. Hall transducer as used by Arms (1–3). This device works on the basis of sensing the change in magnetic field as an indication of position as a magnet moves in and out of the Hall generator. The transducer provides a displacement measuring device that is small enough to attach to ligaments inside the knee.

CONCLUSION

We have discussed various types of whole-joint measuring apparatus. The bulk of the work that has been reported has concentrated on simulating clinical tests. There is a need for extensive studies of ligament function during activity; for this purpose, unconstrained rigs stabilized by simulated muscle tension are required.

ACKNOWLEDGMENT

The design and construction of the Oxford rig described in this chapter was supported by a grant from the Arthritis and Rheumatism Council.

REFERENCES

1. Arms S, Boyle J, Johnson R, Pope M. Strain measurement in the medial collateral ligament of the human knee—an autopsy study. *J Biomech* 1983;16:491–496.
2. Arms SW, Pope MH, Johnson R, Fischer RA, Arvideson I, Eriksson E. The biomechanics of anterior cruciate ligament rehabilitation and reconstruction. *Am J Sports Med* 1984;12:8–18.
3. Arms SW, Renstrom P, Stanwyck TS, Hogan M, Johnson RJ, Pope MH. Strain within the anterior cruciate during hamstrings and quadriceps activity. *Trans Orthop Res Soc* 1985;31:139.
4. Biden E. The mechanics of synovial joints. Ph.D. thesis, University of Oxford, 1981.
5. Biden E, O'Connor J, Goodfellow J. Tibial rotation in the cadaver knee. *Trans Orthop Res Soc* 1984;30:30.
6. Blankevoort L, Huiskes R, de Lange A. The envelope of passive knee joint motion. *J Biomech* 1988;21:705–720.
7. Blanton P, Biggs N. Ultimate tensile strength of fetal and adult human tendons. *J Biomech* 1970;3:181–189.
8. Bourne R, Goodfellow JW, O'Connor JJ. A functional analysis of various knee arthroplasties. *Trans Orthop Res Soc* 1978;24:160.
9. Brantigan OC, Voshell AF. The mechanics of the ligaments and menisci of the knee joint. *J Bone Joint Surg* 1941;23A:44–66.
10. Butler DL, Noyes FR, Grood E. Ligamentous restraint to anterior–posterior drawer in the human knee. *J Bone Joint Surg* 1980;62A:259–270.
11. Fukubayashi T, Torzilli P, Sherman M, Warren R. An *in vitro* biomechanical evaluation of anterior–posterior motion of the knee. *J Bone Joint Surg* 1982;64A:258–264.
12. Goodfellow JW, Hungerford D, Zindel M. Patello-femoral joint

13. mechanics and pathology. I. Functional anatomy. *J Bone Joint Surg* 1976;58B:283–287.
13. Grood E, Stowers S, Noyes F. Limits of movement of the human knee. *J Bone Joint Surg* 1988;70A:88–96.
14. Grood E, Suntay W, Noyes F, Butler D. Biomechanics of the knee extension exercise. *J Bone Joint Surg* 1984;66A:725–734.
15. Harding ML, Harding L, Goodfellow JW. A preliminary report of a simple rig to aid the study of the functional anatomy of the cadaver knee joint. *J Biomech* 1977;10:517–523.
16. Hsieh H-H, Walker PS. Stabilising mechanisms of the loaded and unloaded knee joint. *J Bone Joint Surg* 1976;58A:87–93.
17. Kennedy JC, Hawkins RJ, Willis RB. Strain gauge analysis of knee ligaments. *Clin Orthop* 1977;129:225–229.
18. Kinzel G, Hall A, Hillberry B. Measurement of the total motion between two body segments. *J Biomech* 1972;5:93–105.
19. Lew WD, Lewis JL. The effect of knee prosthesis geometry on cruciate ligament mechanics during flexion. *J Bone Joint Surg* 1982;64A:734–739.
20. Lipke J, Janecki C, Neilson C, McLeod P, Thompson C, Thompson J, Haynes D. The role of incompetence of the anterior cruciate and lateral ligaments in anterolateral and anteromedial instability. *J Bone Joint Surg* 1981;63A:954–960.
21. Malcom L, Daniel D. A mechanical substitution technique for cruciate ligament force determinations. *Trans Orthop Res Soc* 1980;26:303.
22. Maquet PGJ. *Biomechanics of the knee.* Berlin: Springer-Verlag, 1976.
23. Markolf K, Bargar W, Shoemaker S, Amstutz H. The role of joint load in knee stability. *J Bone Joint Surg* 1981;63A:570–585.
24. Markolf K, Mensch J, Amstutz H. Stiffness and laxity of the knee. The contributions of the supporting structures. *J Bone Joint Surg* 1976;58A:583–594.
25. Neilsen S, Kromann-Andersen C, Rasmussen O, Anderson K. Instability of cadaver knees after transection of capsule and ligaments. *Acta Orthop Scand* 1984;55:30–34.
26. Noyes R, Grood E. The strength of the anterior cruciate ligament in humans and rhesus monkeys. *J Bone Joint Surg* 1976;58A:1074–1082.
27. Perry J, Antonelli D, Ford W. Analysis of knee joint forces during flexed knee stance. *J Bone Joint Surg* 1975;57A:961–967.
28. Piziali RL, Rastager JC, Nagel DA. Measurement of the nonlinear coupled stiffness characteristics of the knee. *J Biomech* 1977;10:45–51.
29. Piziali RL, Rastager J, Nagel DA, Schurman DJ. The contribution of the cruciate ligaments to the load–displacement characteristics of the human knee joint. *Trans ASME, J Biomed Eng* 1980;102:277–283.
30. Piziali RL, Seering WP, Nagel DA, Schurman DJ. The function of the primary ligaments of the knee in the anterior–posterior and medial–lateral directions. *J Biomech* 1980;13:777–784.
31. Rastager J, Piziali RL, Nagel DA, Schurman DJ. Effect of fixed axis rotation on the varus–valgus and torsional load–displacement characteristics of the *in vitro* human knee. *Trans ASME, J Biomed Eng* 1979;101:134–140.
32. Seering WP, Piziali RL, Nagel DA, Schurman DJ. The function of the primary ligaments of the knee in varus–valgus and axial rotation. *J Biomech* 1980;13:785–794.
33. Shoemaker S, Markolf K. The role of the meniscus in the anterior–posterior stability of the loaded anterior cruciate deficient knee. *J Bone Joint Surg* 1986;68A:71–79.
34. Sidles JA, Larson RV, Garbini JL, Downey DJ, Matson FA. Ligament length relationships in the moving knee. *J Orthop Res* 1988;6:593–610.
35. Sullivan D, Levy M, Sheskier S, Torzilli P, Warren R. Medial restraints to anterior–posterior motion of the knee. *J Bone Joint Surg* 1984;66A:930–936.
36. Suntay W, Grood E, Hefzy M, Butler D, Noyes F. Error analysis of a system for measuring three-dimensional joint motion. *J Biomech Eng* 1983;105:127–135.
37. Wang C-J, Walker PS. The effects of flexion and rotation on the length patterns of the ligaments of the knee. *J Biomech* 1973;6:487–496.
38. Wang C-J, Walker PS. Rotary laxity in the human knee joint. *J Bone Joint Surg* 1974;56A:161–170.

Knee Ligaments: Structure, Function, Injury, and Repair, edited by D. Daniel, et al.
© 1990 by Raven Press, Ltd. All rights reserved.

CHAPTER 9

The Limits of Knee Motion

In Vitro Studies

Stephen C. Shoemaker and Dale M. Daniel

Ligaments function to limit joint motion. Disruption or sectioning of ligaments alone, or in combination, alters the limits of knee motion in a predictable way. The clinical diagnosis of a ligament disruption is based upon the demonstration of pathologic knee motion. This chapter presents a summary of cadaveric ligament sectioning studies that may serve as the basis of interpreting the clinical examination (Chapter 1). A complete description of knee motion must include (a) the translations along three mutually perpendicular axes and (b) rotation about each of the axes (Fig. 8-2). During the clinical examination, joint motions along and about these axes are minimally constrained. Simulation of the clinical examination requires that force application and motion measurements be performed in a manner that does not constrain joint motion and restrict coupled motions. In this chapter the discussion will concentrate on those studies that simulate the conditions under which the clinical knee examination is performed, namely, non-weight-bearing minimally constrained motion. Selected studies have been included (2,5,12,13) in which motion constrained testing systems because results were relevant to this topic. These testing systems are discussed in Chapter 8.

To describe motion limits properly, both the force (or moment) applied to the knee and the displacement (or rotation) that results must be measured and expressed (Chapter 8). Stiffness, by definition, is the slope of the force–displacement curve (change in force per change in displacement) at a given point. The nonlinear relationship between applied force and displacement requires that the measured displacement be described in conjunction with an applied force. Numerous *in vitro* sectioning studies are cited in this chapter. Displacement and rotation values after sectioning a specific ligament often vary considerably. Factors contributing to these discrepancies include level of applied force, testing device, specimen condition, and specimen number. Results from various studies have been normalized in two ways so that a coherent summary can be presented. First, displacement values resulting from similar force levels were chosen. Second, changes in displacement due to ligament section are expressed as a percentage of intact displacements.

S. C. Shoemaker: San Dieguito Orthopedic Medical Group, La Jolla, California 92037

D. M. Daniel: Department of Orthopedic Surgery, University of California, San Diego, School of Medicine, La Jolla, California 92037; and Kaiser Permanente Medical Center, San Diego, California 92120.

In 1980, Butler (2) introduced the concept of primary and secondary restraints to motion in a specific direction. A primary restraint is that structure which accounts for the majority of ligamentous force resisting an externally applied force. A secondary restraint provides a lesser contribution. Sectioning a primary restraint typically results in an increase in joint motion. Isolated disruption of a secondary restraint (in the face of an intact primary restraint) will not result in altering the limits of joint motion, whereas sectioning a secondary restraint in the absence of a primary restraint will alter joint motion. Specific ligaments may be considered in terms of primary and secondary functions. A ligament may function as a primary restraint to motion in one direction and a secondary restraint in another direction. As an illustration, consider the anterior cruciate ligament (ACL) and medial collateral ligament (MCL) in controlling anterior displacement. Sectioning the MCL will not result in detectable anterior tibial displacement if the primary stabilizer (ACL) is intact. However, if the primary stabilizer (ACL) has been sectioned, sectioning a secondary restraint, the MCL, will result in an increase in anterior displacement.

Identification of primary and secondary stabilizers may be surmised by altering the order of ligament section during *in vitro* experiments and measuring the resulting changes in knee motion. Changes in motion limits due to sectioning secondary restraints may be measured *in vitro* and demonstrated to be statistically significant, but they may be clinically undetectable. In this discussion, structures are classified as primary, major secondary, or minor secondary restraints.

ANTERIOR CRUCIATE LIGAMENT

Primary Function

The ACL functions as the primary restraint to limit anterior tibial displacements (3,7,10,12). ACL sectioning results in a greater anterior displacement in 30° of flexion than in 90° of flexion. The ACL offers no restraint to posterior tibial displacements (1–3,9–12,14). In 65 specimens tested with the KT-2000 in our laboratory, sectioning the ACL increased anterior displacement from 2.8 mm to 13.0 mm, with a mean of 6.7 mm (Fig. 9-1). These findings correlate favorably with KT-1000 measurements under anesthesia in ACL-injured patients (Chapter 24).

Secondary Function

The ACL functions as a secondary restraint to tibial rotation. Isolated ACL sectioning increased tibial rotation 38% (3–4°) at full extension (10). Combined MCL–ACL sectioning yielded increases in tibial rotations that were larger than those changes resulting after sectioning these structures individually. Based on available data (9,10,13,14), the ACL probably functions as (a) a major secondary restraint to internal rotation and (b) a minor secondary restraint to external rotation. The relative contribution of the ACL in re-

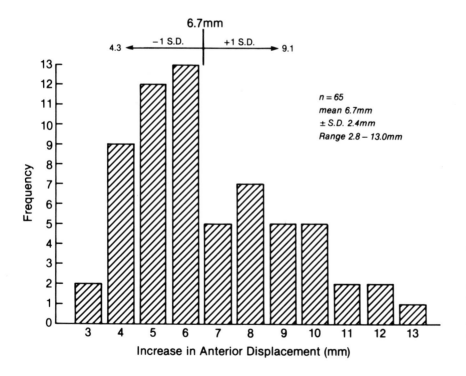

FIG. 9-1. Effect of ACL sectioning on anterior displacement. Anterior displacement measurements with the MEDmetric KT-2000 were performed on 65 fresh cadaveric specimens with the ligaments intact and after sectioning the ACL. The difference between the ligament-intact state and ACL-sectioned state for each specimen is presented.

straining rotation is greater in full extension than it is in early (20–30°) flexion.

The ACL functions as a minor secondary restraint to varus–valgus angulation at full extension. No significant changes were noted from 30° to 90° of flexion with ACL sectioning (10). Changes in stiffness about the neutral position and varus–valgus angulation following combined MCL–ACL section were similar to those changes noted after isolated MCL sectioning. Changes following combined lateral collateral ligament (LCL)–ACL sectioning were moderately larger than those noted following isolated LCL sectioning. Although no breakdown between varus and valgus angulation was reported, these findings suggest that the ACL offers little additional restraint to valgus angulation (and little restraint to varus angulation) beyond that afforded by the primary stabilizers (MCL and LCL) (5,10,13).

POSTERIOR CRUCIATE LIGAMENT

Primary Function

The posterior cruciate ligament (PCL) is the primary restraint to posterior tibial displacement. The increase after PCL sectioning is greater at 90° of flexion than at 30° of flexion (4,6,10).

Secondary Function

The PCL acts as a major secondary restraint to external tibial rotation but does not appear to limit internal rotation (10). Gollehon (4) reported that isolated PCL sectioning did not change external rotation limits. However, PCL sectioning performed after sectioning the LCL and deep posterior capsule increased the limits of external rotation when the knee was flexed more than 30°. Grood (6) substantiated these findings and added that increases in external rotation limits due to sectioning of both PCL and deep posterior lateral structures were largest at 90° of flexion and minimal at 0° and 15° of flexion. The two studies differ slightly in the structures sectioned, but both indicated that the PCL functions as a minor secondary restraint to external rotation at full extension and as a major secondary restraint to external rotation at 90° of flexion.

The PCL offers little (10) to no (4,6) resistance to varus–valgus angulation with the collateral ligaments intact. If the lateral structures are sectioned, sectioning of the PCL does increase the varus angulation (4,6). The most pronounced changes in motion limits are noted in a position of 90° of knee flexion. Based on review of these studies we consider the PCL to be a minor secondary restraint to varus–valgus motion.

MEDIAL STRUCTURES

For the purpose of our discussion, the medial structures of the knee have been divided into superficial MCL and deep medial capsule. The deep medial capsule is further divided into anterior, middle, and posterior thirds. The deep MCL is considered mid-medial capsule, and the posterior medial corner is considered posterior-medial capsule. Difficulty arises in reviewing studies in which authors have not used this convention in devising sectioning protocols. Mention will be made of those studies that depart from this convention.

Primary Function

Medial structures, particularly superficial MCL, act as the primary restraint to limit valgus angulation (5,10,13). As discussed in Chapter 12, the collateral ligaments are better positioned to control rotation than are the cruciate ligaments. Medial structures act as primary restraints to internal tibial rotation. Sectioning of superficial MCL and mid-medial capsule result in increased tibial rotation with the knee in extension and flexion (10,13,15). Definitive comment regarding the relative contributions of individual structures to limiting motion, particularly rotation, is not possible because of differences in sectioning order and flexion position tested. However, it appears that the superficial MCL functions from full extension to full flexion. The posterior medial capsule plays a greater role as the knee approaches extension. The mid-medial capsule acts to limit internal tibial rotation.

Secondary Function

Medial structures act as major secondary restraints to anterior tibial displacement. In two separate studies (10,14), combined section of superficial MCL and mid-medial capsule lead to small or insignificant changes in anterior limits. When MCL sectioning was performed after the ACL (primary restraint) had been divided, the resulting increases in anterior displacement far exceeded those changes seen after individual ligament sectioning.

LATERAL STRUCTURES

The lateral structures restrain varus angulation and external tibial rotation. A major limitation of *in vitro* experiments examining the role of lateral structures is the inability to assess the iliotibial band (ITB) and popliteus properly. Both structures function as dynamic as well as static stabilizers. To date, the relative contributions of each structure have yet to be adequately determined. In addition, the lateral structures function as a complex. With the exception of the LCL, no one structure is responsible for the majority of restraining force in preventing varus angulation.

Primary Function

Several studies (4–6,10,12) indicate that the LCL acts as the primary restraint to limit lateral joint space opening, but discrepancies regarding knee flexion position exist. Markolf (10) reported that LCL sectioning increased varus–valgus angulation 103% at full extension and 30% at 20° and 45° of flexion. Gollehon (4) demonstrated a small but significant increase (1–4°) in varus limit at all flexion positions, but he did not elaborate as to the relative changes from intact values at each flexion position. Grood (6) reported that increases in varus limits due to LCL sectioning in two specimens were greatest at 30° of flexion (5.7°) and smallest at full extension (2.5°). Intact values were not provided for these two specimens. Based on the mean limits of their seven intact specimens, the relative increase in varus limit following LCL sectioning appears to be constant from 0° to 90° of flexion. Grood (6) and Markolf (10) indicated that limits to varus angulation were not significantly altered unless the LCL was cut, whereas Gollehon (4) reported a small but significant increase at 90° of flexion following sectioning of deep posterior lateral structures (DPLS). All three studies found that combined sectioning of LCL and posterior lateral capsule led to an increase in varus limits that was larger than the sum of increases following individual sectioning. Two major conclusions can be drawn from these studies: (i) Although the LCL acts as a primary restraint to limit varus, DPLS provide considerable restraint as a secondary stabilizer. (ii) Increases in varus limit following LCL disruption may be small and difficult to detect clinically, whereas combined injury to LCL and DPLS will result in large changes.

Lateral structures also act as primary restraints to limit external rotation (4,6,10), though relative contributions of individual structures are not as apparent as those for varus limits. Gollehon (4) noted increases in external rotation at all flexion angles after combined sectioning of the LCL and DPLS. When the LCL was left intact and the DPLS were cut, the only increase in external rotation limit observed was at 90° of flexion. The authors attributed the latter finding to contributions of popliteus tendon but did not section this structure separately to confirm this. Grood (6), on the other hand, reported increases in external rotation after division of deep posterior lateral structures, the largest being at 30° of flexion: "Although it appeared that the increased limit to external rotation depended upon which two structures were cut, small numbers of each combination made meaningful statistics impossible." Common to all three studies was the finding that changes in external rotation limits were small after individual structures were cut, yet the limit increases following combined sectioning of LCL and deep lateral structures exceeded the sum of component changes. One interpretation of these findings is that no individual structure acts as the primary restraint to external rotation but that, instead, the posterior lateral corner (LCL, arcuate ligament, posterior lateral capsule, and popliteus tendon) function in concert as a complex to limit external rotation.

Secondary Function

Lateral structures act as secondary restraints to limit anterior and posterior motion. Gollehon (4) demonstrated that isolated sectioning of either LCL or DPLS did not change limits to posterior displacement, yet in combination, small (3 mm) but significant increases resulted. In addition, those changes in posterior limits at 0° and 30° of flexion following combined LCL and DPLS sectioning were comparable to increases seen after the PCL was cut. Grood reported similar findings.

In summary, the LCL and DPLS, when considered individually, act as minor secondary restraints to posterior displacement at full extension. However, in combination, these structures serve as a major secondary restraint from full extension to 30° of flexion. Although data examining effects of lateral structure sectioning on anterior limits is lacking, lateral structures alone or in combination act as minor secondary restraints to anterior displacement (4–6,10,12).

COUPLED MOTION

In vitro testing methods have evolved through various stages. Brantigan (1) secured the femora of cadaveric knees to the bench top and manually applied forces and moments to the tibia before and after ligament sectioning (Fig. 8-6). Motion measurements were crude, imprecise, and basically subjective. Markolf (10) developed a femur-mounted hand-held tibia apparatus and gathered quantitative force and displacement measurements (Fig. 8-7). For the most part, the test system allowed unconstrained motion in planes not being tested but did not measure or record those "incidental movements." The next generation of experiments utilized servohydraulic devices such as the Instron or MTS (2,5,7,9,16). The testing apparatus and data gathering were sophisticated, but sometimes at the expense of constraining motion in planes other than those being tested. It was soon recognized that combined or coupled motions occurred in response to an applied force even if it was applied in a single plane. Thus, efforts were concentrated on devising unconstrained devices (Fig. 8-8). Fukubayashi (3), using an unconstrained test apparatus (Fig. 8-9), reported that an anteriorly applied force resulted in both anterior displacement and internal rotation. If tibial rotation was prevented, anterior displacement was reduced by 30% given the same anterior force. A more complete discussion regarding the theory and practice of documenting coupled motion is presented in Chapter 8. Specific examples of coupled motions are detailed below.

Experiments by Levy (8) and Fukubayashi (3) demonstrated that an anterior force applied to the tibia resulted in a combination of anterior displacement and internal tibial rotation, whereas a posterior force resulted in posterior displacement and external rotation of the tibia. The observed coupled motions in response to a 100-N anterior force were maximal at 30° of flexion (13 mm of anterior displacement and 9° of internal rotation). When a 100-N posterior force was applied, the maximal posterior displacement and external rotation (6 mm and 12; respectively) were seen at 75–90° of flexion. If tibial rotation was constrained, anterior and posterior displacements resulting from a given force were reduced 30%. In addition, a 1.0-N-m internal torque and a 1.0 N-m external torque generated about the tibia were measured in response to a 100-N force applied anteriorly and posteriorly, respectively.

Consistent changes in coupled motion following ligament sectioning have been demonstrated (3,4,8). ACL sectioning increased the limit to anterior displacement by 250% but ablated the coupled internal rotation observed in normal knees. Combined sectioning of the ACL, LCL, and DPLS increased the coupled internal rotation associated with anterior displacement, particularly at 30° of flexion. One explanation for this observation is that the intact ACL provided an axis around which the tibia could rotate. With ACL sectioning, that pivot point was removed. Secondary restraints to anterior displacement are found on both medial and lateral aspects of the knee; therefore, little (if any) rotation occurred in response to anteriorly applied force. Cutting secondary restraints on the lateral side of the knee (LCL and DPLS) allowed the lateral tibial plateau to translate anteriorly more than the medial plateau—in essence, shifting the axis of rotation toward the medial structures. Although this argument seems logical, it is based on data obtained from a small number of specimens. Only three knees in the subgroup with ACL, LCL, and DPLS were tested, and increases in internal rotation ranged from 6° to 17°. A more thorough investigation is indicated.

Division of PCL, LCL, or DPLS, individually or in combination, did not affect the anterior displacement–internal rotation motion couple (4). Similarly, meniscectomy had no effect on any of the motion couples studied. Meniscectomy does have an effect on rotation limits (Chapter 12) and an effect on anterior displacement in the ACL-injured knee (8,15).

Effects of ligament sectioning on the posterior displacement–external rotation motion couple were similar to those seen on its anterior counterpart. Cutting the PCL increased posterior displacement by 300% and ablated coupled external rotation completely (4). Presumably, the PCL serves as an axis around which the tibia rotates in addition to limiting posterior translation. If the LCL and DPLS were sectioned while the PCL was left intact, small changes in posterior limits were observed in conjunction with large increases in coupled external rotation. The lateral tibial plateau apparently translated posteriorly more than the medial did, indicating that the axis of rotation shifted medially with respect to the intact knee. Specimens in which PCL, LCL, and DPLS were divided displayed large increases in both posterior and external rotation limits comparable to the sum of component changes observed after sectioning lateral structures or PCL separately. The number of specimens tested was greater than that for the anterior displacement–internal rotation motion couple, and explanations seem better founded.

Other coupled motions have been observed (4,6). Application of internal torque to the tibia resulted in internal rotation, anterior displacement, and medial translation. Conversely, an external tibial torque resulted in external rotation, posterior displacement, and lateral translation. Isolated sectioning of DPLS, LCL, and PCL had no effect on these coupled motions. When LCL and DPLS were cut, an increase in the posterior limit resulting from applied external torque was observed; combined sectioning of PCL, LCL, and DPLS further increased the posterior limit. The combined sectioning of ACL, LCL, and DPLS increased the anterior displacement resulting from internally applied torque at 30° and 60° of flexion. Because of difficulty in testing rotational limits in vivo, the clinical relevance of these findings has yet to be determined. Findings by Grood (6) regarding varus–valgus limits may provide useful clinical information. Application of a varus moment in intact knees resulted in varus angulation without associated rotation. When DPLS were sectioned and LCL was left intact, applied varus moment led to both external rotation and varus angulation of the tibia. No difference in varus limit was observed. Applied valgus moment resulted in valgus angulation and internal rotation which was not changed by PCL and/or DPLS sectioning.

CLINICAL RELEVANCE

A distillation of those findings considered to be consistently detectable and clinically relevant is provided.

Distinction between isolated ligament disruption and complex ligament tears is made. Certain isolated ligament deficits may be unlikely to occur *in vivo* (i.e., disruption of a minor secondary restraint in the face of an intact primary restraint), and acknowledgment of this will be made. We have also attempted to limit the analysis of complex ligament disruptions to those seen in clinical practice.

Isolated Ligament Disruptions (Tables 9-1 and 9-2)

1. **Anterior cruciate.** Increased anterior limit, most evident at 30° of flexion (Lachman test); decreased anterior stiffness (soft end point).
2. **Posterior cruciate.** Increased posterior limit, most evident at 75–90° of flexion (posterior sag); decreased posterior stiffness (soft end point).
3. **Lateral collateral.** Increased limits to varus and external rotation from 0° to 90° of flexion; small and perhaps difficult to detect.
4. **Deep posterior lateral structures.** Increased limit to varus from 0° to 30° of flexion; small changes and unlikely to occur as an isolated injury without disruption of LCL.
5. **Popliteus.** Increase external rotation limit at 90° of flexion; unlikely to occur in isolation and not easily detected clinically.
6. **Superficial medial collateral.** Increased limits to valgus and internal rotation from 0° to 90° of flexion; small and perhaps difficult to detect.
7. **Mid-medial capsule (deep MCL).** Increased limits to valgus and internal rotation; unlikely to occur

TABLE 9-1. *Primary and secondary restraints to limits of knee motion based on quantitative in vitro studies—ACL/PCL*

	Anterior cruciate ligament	Posterior cruciate ligament
Anterior displacement	Primary	0
Posterior displacement	0	Primary
Varus	Minor secondary (full ext)	Minor secondary
Valgus	Minor secondary (full ext)	Minor secondary
Internal rotation	Major secondary	0
External rotation	Minor secondary	Major secondary (90°)/minor secondary (full ext)

as an isolated injury without disruption of superficial MCL.

Complex Ligament Disruptions

Medial Structure–ACL (Fig. 9-2)

Isolated sectioning of superficial MCL or mid-medial capsule will result in small, perhaps clinically imperceptible increases in valgus and internal rotation limits. Disruption of either structure individually may very well go undetected if the diagnosis were to be made strictly on the basis of motion limits. Injury to both superficial MCL and mid-medial capsule leads to clinically obvious increases in valgus limits; however, associated changes in internal rotation and anterior translation are small. Because the MCL provides restraint to both valgus and internal rotation from full extension to beyond 90° of flexion, disruption of the mid-medial capsule without injury to the MCL would be unlikely. It is theoretically possible to disrupt the mid-medial capsule without disturbing the superficial MCL if the mechanism of injury involves pathologic anterior tibial translation (i.e., concomitant ACL tear). This combination of ligament deficit (ACL and mid-medial capsule tears) would increase the anterior limit and produce small changes in valgus and internal rotation.

In isolation, ACL sectioning results in variable amounts of pathologic motion that is best demonstrated at 30° of flexion. No clinically detectable changes in rotational limits are noted, but there is a loss of the anterior displacement–internal rotation motion couple found in intact knees. Disruption of ACL, MCL, and mid-medial capsule results in large increases in anterior displacement, valgus angulation, and internal rotation.

Lateral Structure–ACL (Fig. 9-3)

Isolated injury of either LCL or DPLS will lead to subclinical limit increases in external rotation and varus angulation. However, isolated capsular injury in the face of intact LCL is unlikely to occur with a varus and/or external rotation mechanism because the LCL functions as primary restraint to those motions. Combined disruption of LCL and DPLS will yield noticeable increases in varus and external rotation. In addition, an increase in posterior limit and an accentuation of the posterior displacement–external rotation motion couple may be evident between 0° and 30° of flexion. Because lateral structures function as secondary anterior restraints, increases in anterior limits following LCL and/or DPLS sectioning are small

TABLE 9-2. *Primary and secondary restraints to limits of knee motion based on quantitative in vitro studies—medial/lateral structures*

	Medial structures				Lateral structures		
	Superficial medial collateral	Anterior medial capsule	Middle medial capsule	Posterior medial capsule	Lateral collateral	Posterior lateral capsule (DPLS)	Popliteus tendon
Anterior displacement	Minor secondary	0	Major secondary (full ext)	?	Minor secondary	Minor secondary	?
Posterior displacement	Minor secondary	0	0	0	Minor secondary (full ext)	Minor secondary (full ext)	?
Varus	0	0	0	0	Primary	Major secondary	?
Valgus	Primary (full ext to 90°)	?	Primary (full ext to 30°)	?	0	0	0
Internal rotation	Primary (full ext to 90°)	?	Primary (full ext to 30°)	?	0	0	0
External rotation	0	0	0	0	Primary (full ext to 90°)	Primary (full ext to 45°)	90°

and probably not detectable on clinical exam. Combined disruption of ACL and DPLS without injury to LCL may occur with a purely anteriorly directed force. In this situation, the intact LCL would restrain external rotation and varus angulation, leaving an increase in anterior limit as the only clinically evident finding. The patient with an "isolated" ACL tear, stable varus–valgus limits, and a marked pivot shift due to "stretching" of the lateral structures may exemplify this situation. When the ACL, LCL, and DPLS are rendered incompetent, anterior and varus limit increases become clinically obvious. In addition to increases in external rotation limits, the anterior displacement–internal rotation motion couple is accentuated between 30° and 60° of flexion.

Lateral Structure–PCL (Fig. 9-4)

The findings of disrupted LCL and DPLS alone or in combination are discussed above.

As discussed in the previous section, the hallmark of an isolated PCL disruption is an increased posterior displacement most evident between 75° and 90° of flexion (posterior sag). No increase in external rotation or varus is noted, but there is a loss of the posterior displacement–external rotation motion couple.

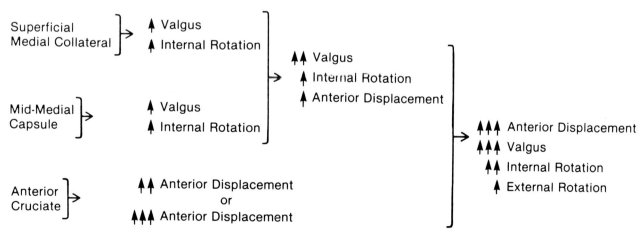

FIG. 9-2. Combined medial structure–ACL disruption. (▲▲▲) Clinically apparent, large increase; (▲▲) clinically apparent, small increase; (▲) demonstrable increase *in vitro* but probably too small to detect clinically. See text for further information.

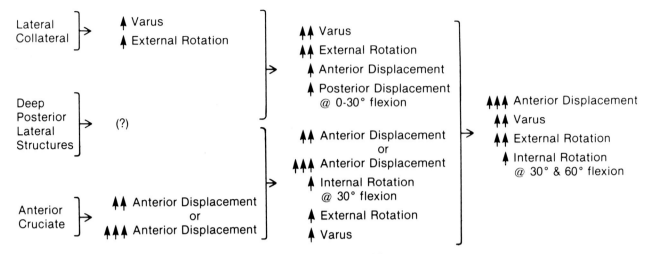

FIG. 9-3. Combined lateral structure–ACL disruption. (▲▲▲) Clinically apparent, large increase; (▲▲) clinically apparent, small increase; (▲) demonstrable increase *in vitro* but probably too small to detect clinically. See text for further information.

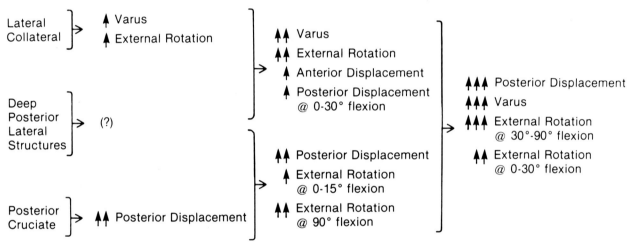

FIG. 9-4. Combined lateral structure–PCL disruption. (▲▲▲) Clinically apparent, large increase; (▲▲) clinically apparent, small increase; (▲) demonstrable increase *in vitro* but probably too small to detect clinically. See text for further information.

Combined injury of PCL, LCL, and DPLS results in (a) large limit increases in posterior displacement and (b) varus angulation from full extension to 90° of flexion. Similar increases in external rotation are noted from 30° to 90° flexion, whereas slightly more modest changes are seen from full extension to 30° of flexion.

ACKNOWLEDGMENT

Support from the following sources is gratefully acknowledged: Baxter Health Care Corporation, Santa Ana, California 92711 and the Southern California Kaiser Permanente Research Program, San Diego, California 92120.

REFERENCES

1. Brantigan OC, Voshell AF. The mechanics of the ligaments and menisci of the knee joint. *J Bone Joint Surg* 1941;23:44–66.
2. Butler DL, Noyes FR, Grood ES. Ligamentous restraints to anterior–posterior drawer in the human knee. A biomechanical study. *J Bone Joint Surg* 1980;62A:259–270.
3. Fukubayashi T, Torzilli PA, Sherman MF, Warren RF. An *in vitro* biomechanical evaluation of anterior–posterior motion of the knee. Tibial displacement, rotation, and torque. *J Bone Joint Surg* 1982;64A:258–264.
4. Gollehon DL, Torzilli PA, Warren RF. The role of the posterolateral and cruciate ligaments in the stability of the human knee. A biomechanical study. *J Bone Joint Surg* 1987;69A:234–242.
5. Grood ES, Noyes FR, Butler DL, Suntay WJ. Ligamentous and capsular restraints preventing straight medial and lateral laxity in intact human cadaver knees. *J Bone Joint Surg* 1981;63A:1257–1269.

6. Grood ES, Stowers SF, Noyes FR. Limits of motion in the human knee. Effect of sectioning the posterior cruciate ligament and posterolateral structures. *J Bone Joint Surg* 1988;70A:88–97.

7. Hsieh HH, Walker PS. Stabilizing mechanisms of the loaded and unloaded knee joint. *J Bone Joint Surg* 1976;58A:87–93.

8. Levy IM, Torzilli PA, Warren RF. The effect of medial meniscectomy anterior–posterior motion of the knee. *J Bone Joint Surg* 1982;64A:883–888.

9. Markolf KL, Bargar WL, Shoemaker SC, Amstutz HC. The role of joint load in knee stability. *J Bone Joint Surg* 1981;63A:570–585.

10. Markolf KL, Mensch JS, Amstutz HC. Stiffness and laxity of the knee—the contributions of the supporting structures. A quantitative *in vitro* study. *J Bone Joint Surg* 1976;58A:583–594.

11. Nielsen S, Helmig P. Instability of knees with ligament lesions. Cadaver studies of the anterior cruciate ligament. *Acta Orthop Scand* 1985;56:426–429.

12. Piziali RL, Seering WP, Nagel DA, Schurman DJ. The function of the primary ligaments of the knee in anterior–posterior and medial–lateral motions. *J Biomech* 1980;13:777–784.

13. Seering WP, Piziali RL, Nagel DA, Schurman DJ. The function of the primary ligaments of the knee in varus–valgus and axial rotation. *J Biomech* 1980;13:785–794.

14. Shoemaker SC, Markolf KL. Effects of joint load on the stiffness and laxity of ligament-deficient knees. An *in vitro* study of the anterior cruciate and medial collateral ligaments. *J Bone Joint Surg* 1985;67A:136–146.

15. Shoemaker SC, Markolf KL. The role of the meniscus in the anterior–posterior stability of the loaded anterior cruciate-deficient knee. *J Bone Joint Surg* 1986;68A:71–79.

16. Wang CJ, Walker PS. Rotatory laxity of the human knee joint. *J Bone Joint Surg* 1974;56A:161–170.

Knee Ligaments: Structure, Function, Injury, and Repair, edited by D. Daniel, et al.
© 1990 by Raven Press, Ltd. All rights reserved.

CHAPTER 10

Geometry of the Knee

John O'Connor, Tessa Shercliff, David FitzPatrick, John Bradley, Dale M. Daniel, Edmund Biden, and John Goodfellow

Ligaments are the tough fibrous tissue structures that hold our bones together. The words *ligament* and *ligature* share a common Latin root, the verb *ligare*, meaning to bind or to tie. Although this book deals with the ligaments of the knee, it is impossible to discuss their function without including as equal partners the other structures of the joint. The articular surfaces hold the bones apart. The muscles with their tendons stabilize the skeleton in the presence of gravity and other loads; they also initiate and maintain movements. In this and the following chapter, we seek to explain the geometric and mechanical relationships between the ligaments, the articular surfaces, and the muscle tendons at the knee. In this chapter, dealing mainly with the geometry of the joint, we show how the ligaments of the knee guide the movements of the bones upon each other, within their allowable range of movement. In the next chapter, dealing mainly with the mechanics of the joint, we will show how the ligaments can act with the muscles and the articular surfaces to transmit load from one bone to the other within the allowable range of movement and how they combine with the articular surfaces to define that range of movement. The study of the geometry of the joint has

J. O'Connor, T. Shercliff, and D. FitzPatrick: Department of Engineering Science, University of Oxford, Oxford, OX1 3PJ, England.
J. Bradley: Department of Orthopaedic Surgery, Colchester General Hospital, Colchester, Essex CO4 5JL, England.
D. Daniel: Department of Orthopedic Surgery, University of California, San Diego, School of Medicine, La Jolla, California 92037; and Kaiser Permanente Medical Center, San Diego, California 92120.
E. Biden: Department of Mechanical Engineering, University of New Brunswick, Fredericton, Canada E3B 5A3.
J. Goodfellow: Department of Orthopaedic Surgery, Nuffield Orthopaedic Centre, Oxford OX3 7LD, England.

intrinsic interest but is also a necessary precursor to the study of the mechanics. We shall discuss first the relationship between geometry and mechanics.

JOINT CENTERS, LEVER-ARMS

At the outset, it is interesting to compare the knee with a closely fitting congruous joint like the hip. The geometric center of the hip lies at the center of the femoral head, with its position defined by the geometry of the articular surfaces of the bones. The femur and the pelvis rotate relative to each other about axes through that center.

The center of the femoral head is not only the geometric center of the hip, but it is also the mechanical center, the fulcrum about which the muscles exert their leverage. This can be seen by considering first the effect of a load applied to the leg with a line of action passing through the center of the femoral head (Fig. 10-1), analogous to the effect of a load that passes through the axle of a wheel. A purely radial load rotates the wheel neither clockwise nor anticlockwise; the length of the lever-arm of the load about the axis of rotation is zero.

Likewise, a radial load passing through the center of the femoral head tends neither to extend nor to flex the hip, nor does it tend to abduct or adduct the hip. It merely compresses the articular surfaces together and can be balanced by the intraarticular compressive force, without muscle or ligament action. If the line of

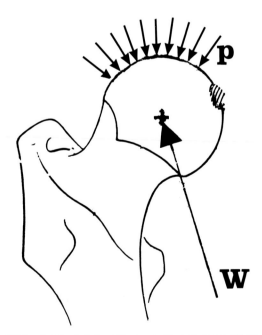

FIG. 10-1. A hip joint with an external load *W* passing through the center of the femoral head. The load is balanced by radial pressure *p* on the articular surface of the femoral head and does not induce rotatory movements.

action of the load does not pass through the center of the femoral head, flexion/extension, abduction/adduction, or rotation will occur unless prevented by muscle action (Fig. 10-2). The precise line of action of the load in relation to the center of the hip determines which muscle group is mechanically necessary to stabilize the joint. The perpendicular distance from the center of the hip to the line of action of the load, the extrinsic lever-arm of the load, is a direct measure of the flexing/ extending, abducting/adducting, or rotating effect of the load. The intrinsic lever-arm of the muscle, the perpendicular distance from the hip center to the line of action of its tendon, is a measure of its ability to stabilize the limb and to induce movement.

The triangles of forces in Fig. 10-2 show that nonradial loads can be transmitted across the hip by a combination of muscle and compressive contact forces without ligament action. The muscle forces are larger than the load whenever their intrinsic lever-arms are shorter than the extrinsic lever-arms of the load. The contact forces between the bones are larger still whenever the component of the load parallel to the muscle force acts in the same direction as the muscle force.

The position of the center of the hip, defined by the geometry of the articular surfaces, therefore controls not only the possible movements of the bones relative to each other but also the mechanics of the joint, the muscle action necessary to stabilize the limb, and the values of the muscle and contact forces.

The considerations that determine the center of the knee are in complete contrast to those of the hip. The surfaces of the femur and tibia do not fit together, particularly when seen from the side, and do not define any obvious geometric or mechanical center. We shall show that the center of the knee, about which muscles and loads exert their leverage, is defined by the geometry of the ligaments. Because the geometry of the ligaments changes as the joint flexes and extends, the center of the knee moves relative to both bones. We shall show that the relationship of the line of action of a load to the geometry of the ligaments determines whether it tends to extend or flex the joint and whether flexor or extensor muscle action is necessary for stability.

THEORETICAL STUDIES OF LIGAMENT FUNCTION AND JOINT STABILITY

When compared to the huge bulk of experimental work on the knee, there has been very little theory, especially with regard to ligament function. One train of thought, which we shall develop in detail in this and the next chapter, follows from the work of Strasser (41), who studied the geometry of a four-bar linkage model of the knee comprising the femur, the tibia, and the two cruciate ligaments (Fig. 10-3). The develop-

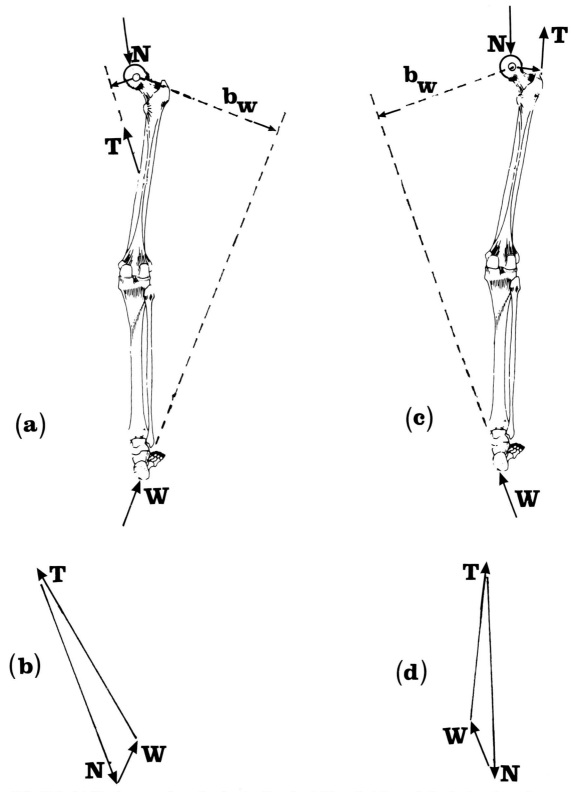

FIG. 10-2. (a) The leg seen from the front with a load *W* applied through the foot and passing lateral to the femoral head. Abduction is prevented by an adductor muscle force *T*. The lever-arm available to the load is the distance b_w. Similarly, the lever-arm available to the muscle is the perpendicular distance from the center of the hip to the line of action of the muscle force. The relationships between load, muscle force, and the intraarticular contact force *N* are indicated by the triangle of forces (**b**). (**c,d**) Abductor response to an adducting load passing medial to the femoral head. In both examples, the muscle force is larger than the load because the muscle lever-arm is shorter than that of the load.

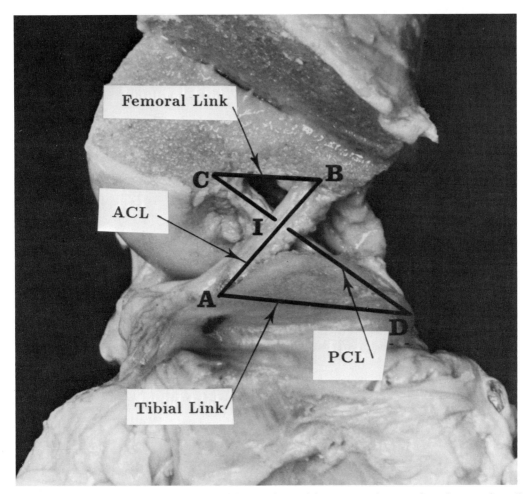

FIG. 10-3. A human knee with the lateral femoral condyle removed, exposing the cruciate ligaments. Superimposed is a diagram of a four-bar linkage comprising the anterior cruciate ligament *AB*, the posterior cruciate ligament *CD*, the femoral link *CB* joining the ligament attachment points on the femur, and the tibial link *AD* joining their attachment points on the tibia. (Courtesy of Institution of Mechanical Engineers, London.)

ment leads to a theory of the geometry and mechanics of the knee in the sagittal plane. The model does not take account of rotations about the tibial axis or about an anteroposterior axis. While this is clearly a shortcoming, it is also a simplification. It makes it possible to explain in elementary terms the relationships between the geometry and mechanics of the ligaments, the articular surfaces, and the muscle tendons.

It is profitable to start with the simplest possible model, to validate the model by comparing its predictions with experimental measurements, and only to admit further complication when the results of that comparison are unsatisfactory. A successful mathematical model not only can describe what happens but can sometimes explain why. It can be used to calculate values of quantities that are not easily measured. It can help in the design and interpretation of experiments.

Although our account is based on a mathematical analysis, the reader should not immediately be fright-

ened, since we shall present none of the mathematical formulae here but shall, instead, describe only the arguments and the conclusions. It is assumed that the reader is familiar with the anatomy of the knee, its ligaments, capsule, and articular sufaces, as described in Chapter 4. The mathematical model, developed from first principles, formed the basis of a computer program that was used to draw many of the diagrams in this and later chapters. Where we can, we shall provide collaborative experimental evidence to support the results derived from the computer model. Further evidence is described in Chapter 12. We shall draw particular attention to those results and conclusions which may have application to ligament surgery.

THE FOUR-BAR CRUCIATE LINKAGE

The bones that meet at a joint, as well as the ligaments that hold the bones together, can be analyzed as a me-

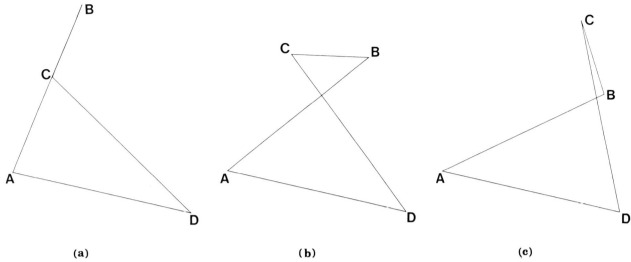

(a)   **(b)**   **(c)**

FIG. 10-4. The cruciate linkage *ABCD* drawn by the computer at full extension and at 70° and 140° of flexion. Between (**a**) and (**c**), the femoral link *CB* rotates through 140° relative to the tibial link *AD*, and the cruciate ligaments *AB* and *CD* rotate through 40° about their tibial attachments *A* and *D* and through 100° about their femoral attachments *B* and *C*. (Courtesy of Institution of Mechanical Engineers, London.)

chanical linkage. Since the movements allowed to the bones at the human knee occur mainly in the sagittal plane, much can be learned by treating the knee as a two-dimensional single-degree-of-freedom linkage moving in a single plane. Following Strasser (41), Kapandji (21), Huson (20), and Menschik (29),[1] we start by assuming that the main ligamentous elements of the linkage are the cruciates. Our first purpose is to describe the geometric relationships between the ligaments and the articular surfaces of the tibiofemoral joint during flexion and extension.

Figure 10-3 shows a human knee from which the lateral femoral condyle has been excised, exposing the cruciate ligaments. The ligaments, together with the two bones, form the "cruciate" linkage *ABCD*. *AD* will be called the *tibial link,* the line joining the attachment points of the two ligaments to the tibia. *BC* is the *femoral link.* The tibial link is more or less parallel to the tibial plateau of the joint, and the femoral link more or less coincides with the roof of the femoral intercondylar notch. The tibial and femoral links are rigidly attached to the two bones and move with them, with any change in the flexion angle resulting in an equal change in the angle between them. The lines *AB* and *CD* represent the anterior and posterior cruciate ligaments, respectively. *AB* and *CD* may be considered to be neutral fibers within the two cruciates, which remain isometric during passive flexion.

Ligament Angles

During flexion and extension of the knee, the shape of the cruciate linkage changes. As the two bones rotate

relative to each other about the flexion axis, the angle between the tibial and femoral links changes as do the angles between the tibial and femoral links and each of the ligaments. Algebraic formulae for the values of the ligament angles at each position of flexion were obtained by applying trigonometry to the geometry of Fig. 10-3. The formulae were given by O'Connor (34) and were used as the basis of a computer program that can draw the linkage in any position of flexion. Three examples are shown in Fig. 10-4; at full extension and at 70° and 140° of flexion.

During 140° of flexion, the anterior cruciate ligament (ACL) rotates through an angle of about 40° around its tibial attachment towards the tibial plateau. It rotates through 100° about its femoral attachment and away from the femoral link. The posterior cruciate ligament (PCL) rotates through 40° about its tibial attachment and away from the tibial plateau. It rotates through 100° about its femoral attachment and, in flexion, approaches the roof of the intercondylar notch. The rotations of the ligaments about their attachment points on the two bones are further illustrated in Fig. 10-5.

Ligament Isometry

In Fig. 10-5, the three diagrams of Fig. 10-4 are superimposed in two ways. In Fig. 10-5a, the tibial link *AD* is held stationary and the femur may be considered to be moving from full extension in the position AB_1C_1D to full flexion AB_3C_3D. The femoral link *BC* is rotated through 140° between the two extreme positions. The point *B* on the femur moves along a circular arc centered at *A*. The point *C* moves on a

[1] Menschik's work has been described in English by Müller (31).

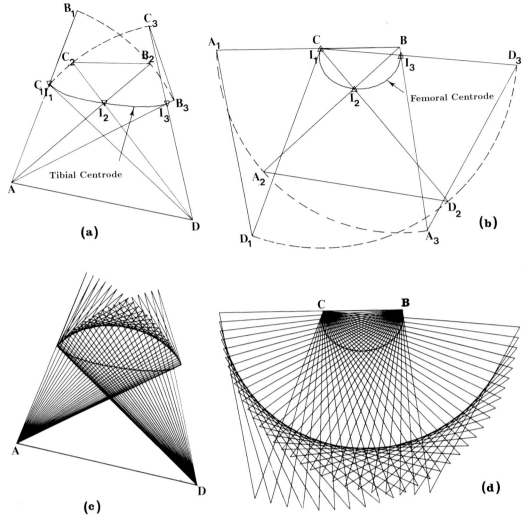

FIG. 10-5. The cruciate linkage drawn by the computer with the tibial link fixed, (**a**) and (**c**), and with the femoral link fixed, (**b**) and (**d**). The *relative* positions of the links are the same in the pair of diagrams (**a**) and (**b**) for each of the corresponding three configurations and in (**c**) and (**d**) for each of the corresponding 30 configurations. In (**a**) and (**c**), the femoral attachments of the ligaments move on circular arcs about their tibial attachments, and in (**b**) and (**d**) the tibial attachments move on circular arcs about the femoral attachments. The curves marked "Tibial Centrodes" and "Femoral Centrodes" are the tracks of the flexion axis of the joint on the tibia and femur, respectively, and are drawn through the successive intersections of the cruciates. (Courtesy of Institution of Mechanical Engineers, London.)

circular arc centered at *D*. These movements demonstrate that changes in the geometry of the linkage allow flexion and extension of the bones while the neutral fibers *AB* and *CD* remain isometric. They show why the bones can move relative to each other within the allowable range without ligament strain or cartilage indentation.

In Fig. 10-5b, the femoral link *CB* is held fixed and the tibia is moved from full extension A_1BCD_1 to full flexion A_3BCD_3. The point *A* on the tibia moves on a circular arc centered at *B* on the femur; *D* moves on a circular arc about *C*, a further demonstration of the isometry of the neutral fibers.

Similar constructions are shown in Fig. 10-5c and d, but for 30 superposed configurations of the linkage. These figures demonstrate the rotations of the ligaments about their tibial and femoral attachments.

Parameters of the Model

The shape of the cruciate linkage at any position of flexion depends only on the lengths of the ligaments and the distances apart of their attachment points on the bones, that is, on the lengths on the four links *AB*, *BC*, *CD*, and *DA*. These distances are the parameters of the linkage. A further parameter implied in Figs. 10-4 and 10-5 is the angle between the tibial and femoral links at full extension. When the values of the parameters have been specified, the shape of the linkage at any flexion position is completely defined. Values of the parameters used to draw the diagrams and graphs for this and subsequent chapters were obtained from anthropometric studies on cadaver knee specimens (6). The technique of measurement and the full list of parameter values are given in the appendix to this chapter.

The angles between the cruciate ligaments and the bones depend only on the values of the parameters and on the flexion angle. Apart from the effects of elastic deformations, the angles of the ligaments are independent of the values of the forces that the ligaments may be transmitting.

Implantation of a Ligament Prosthesis

The rotations of the ligaments about their attachment points on the bones, as indicated in Fig. 10-5, have important implications for the design and implantation of artificial ligaments. Ligaments bend about their attachment points, and a prosthesis must be strong enough to withstand such bending. To minimize bending, the bone tunnels through which the prosthesis is introduced should enter the joint space at the appropriate angle for each ligament on each bone, that is, the angle of entry bisecting the extreme positions of the neutral fibers in Fig. 10-5. In Fig. 10-6, the appropriate angles of entry are shown for the ACL on both femur and tibia.

The largest bending of the ligament occurs at its femoral attachment. Mechanical testing should be carried

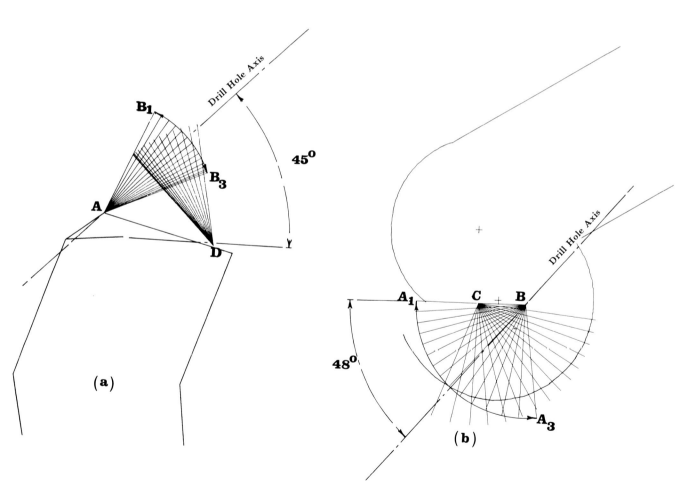

FIG. 10-6. Diagrams of the tibia (**a**) and the femur (**b**) with the range of positions occupied by the ACL from full extension to 140° of flexion when the ligament moves (**a**) from AB_1 to AB_3 relative to the tibia and (**b**) from A_1B to A_3B relative to the femur. The drill hole axes suggest appropriate angles for bone tunnels so as to minimize bending of a ligament prosthesis. These diagrams are diagrammatic; exact values of the appropriate angles should be deduced from x-ray analysis of each individual knee.

out to ensure that a ligament prosthesis can be bent repeatedly through ±50° at a clamped end.

THE INSTANT CENTER OF THE JOINT; THE FLEXION AXIS

An important property of the cruciate linkage, on which much geometric and mechanical theory depends, is that the point *I* (Fig. 10-3) at which the ligaments cross is the *instant center* of the joint (its full name is the *instant center of zero velocity* of the femur relative to the tibia). It is the point at which the flexion axis intersects the parasagittal plane through the knee. The instant center is the geometric center of the knee in the sagittal plane, but we shall refer to it mainly as the *flexion axis*.

Figure 10-5 shows that the flexion axis moves relative to both bones during flexion/extension because of the changing shape of the cruciate linkage. It moves backward on both bones, relative to the tibia along a path more or less parallel to the tibial plateau (Fig. 10-5a and c), relative to the femur along an elliptical path (Fig. 10-5b and d). These paths are called the tibial and femoral *centrodes*. In the introduction above, we contrasted the hip (with its center defined by the geometry of the articular of the bones and fixed relative to them) and the knee (with its center defined by the geometry of the ligaments). Figure 10-5 shows that the center of the knee moves relative to both bones.

GEOMETRY OF THE ARTICULAR SURFACES[2]

The shapes of the articular surfaces of the bones must fulfill the requirement that they move in contact with one another while maintaining the neutral fibers of the cruciate ligaments at constant length. Such surfaces may be said to be compatible with the ligaments. We now show that there is not a unique pair of surface shapes that can fulfill this requirement; if the shape of one articular surface is given, the shape of the complementary surface of the other bone can be deduced. In order to avoid interpenetration or separation of the bones, the construction of the complementary surface

depends on the principle, illustrated in Fig. 10-7, that the common normal to the articular surfaces at their point of contact must pass through the flexion axis.

Using this principle, the shape of the femoral surface complementary to a flat tibial plateau has been deduced and is shown in three positions of flexion in Fig. 10-8. The model tibial plateau has been positioned (as in life) slightly distal to the tibial attachment *A* of the ACL and slightly proximal to the attachment *D* of the PCL. The dashed line is the perpendicular to the tibial plateau at the contact point (the common normal of the previous paragraph), passing through the flexion axis, *I*. The movement of the contact point *X* on the tibia illustrates the rolling component of the movement of the femur on the tibia, caused by the changing position of the flexion axis. Five pairs of contact points are included on each articular surface, corresponding to flexion angles of 0°, 35°, 70°, 105°, and 140°. There is a larger distance between successive points on the femur than between those on the tibia, demonstrating that the femur must slide forward on the tibia while rolling backward during flexion and must slide backward while rolling forward during extension.

The contrary pattern of rolling and sliding of the femur on the tibia was attributed by Weber (45) to the geometry of the articular surfaces. In fact, it occurs because contact between the bones lies distal to the flexion axis. It makes necessary more extensive articular surfaces on the femur than on the tibia. The distance between successive contact points on the femur is three to four times greater than the corresponding distance on the tibia.

The femoral surfaces complementary to slightly concave and to slightly convex tibial plateaus, as found in the medial and lateral compartments of the human knee, were also calculated using the principles of Fig. 10-7. Figure 10-9 shows parasagittal sections taken through the medial and lateral femoral condyles of a human knee. Superimposed on the posterior aspects of these condyles are the shapes calculated by the method just described. The calculated shapes' close approximation to the shapes of the natural condyles suggests that although the articular surfaces in the two compartments are different, the shapes of both pairs are ordained by their need to be compatible with the one cruciate linkage. Figure 10-9 meets the objection by Rehder (38) to the application of the theory of the four-bar linkage to the human knee.

The different pairs of calculated surface shapes of Figs. 10-8 and 10-9, as well as the surfaces defined by the envelopes of Fig. 10-5c and d, are illustrations of the fact that there is an infinite number of possible pairs of articular surface shapes, all compatible with the same cruciate linkage. The shape of one of the surfaces can be calculated using the methods just described following arbitrary choice of the shape of the other. Each

---

[2] The tibial plateau used by Menschik (29) in his drawings coincided with the tibial link *AD* of the cruciate linkage. He deduced the shape of the complementary femoral condyle by drawing the linkage superposed in successive positions with the femoral link fixed, as in Fig. 10-5d. The shape of the femoral condyle is that of the envelope defined by the successive positions of the tibial link. By the same argument, the envelope defined by the successive positions of the femoral link in Fig. 10-5c is the shape of a tibial articular surface that would be complementary to a flat femoral condyle coincident with the femoral link *BC* of the linkage. In the articulation of Fig. 10-5c, the tibial surface is longer than the femoral surface because the articulation lies proximal to the flexion axis so that, during flexion and extension, the directions of rolling and sliding of the femur and the tibia are the same.

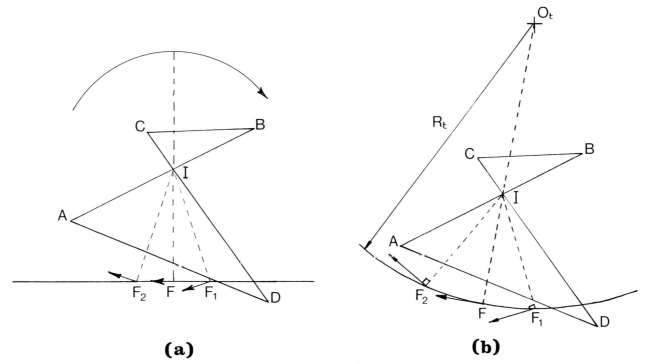

(a) **(b)**

FIG. 10-7. Demonstration that contact between the femur and (a) a flat tibial plateau or (b) a concave tibial plateau occurs at the point *F* where the common normal to the articular surfaces at their point of contact passes through the flexion axis at *I*. In (b), the tibial plateau is a circle of radius R_t centered at O_t. With the surface of the tibia fixed, all points on the femur move on circular arcs centered on the flexion axis. Contact between the bones at F_1 would lead to interpenetration and at F_2 to separation of the bones. Contact at *F* allows the bones to slide upon each other without interpenetration or separation. If the surface of the tibia is flat (a), the perpendicular to that flat surface at the contact point must pass through the flexion axis.

such pair exhibits a unique combination of rolling and sliding. We have shown elsewhere (36) that the only pair of surfaces that would roll upon each other without slip, so-called pure rolling, would be coincident with the centrodes of Fig. 10-5.

There is an obvious application of these ideas to the design of a surface replacement knee prosthesis that allows retention of all the ligaments (16,17), but that topic will not be pursued here.

Movement of the Tibial Contact Point; Roll-Back

Rolling movement of the femur on the tibia during flexion/extension has long been observed in the human knee. Backwards movement of the menisci on the tibia during flexion was described by Borelli (5) and by Brantigan (7); occurring "a few millimeters medially and at least one centimeter laterally." Kapandji (21) attributed the movement to the action of the cruciate linkage and reported that it occurred "6 mm medially and 12 mm laterally." Walker (42) removed the menisci and used a casting technique to locate the contact areas over the flexion range in the presence of com-

pressive load applied along the axis of the tibia. He showed a posterior excursion on the medial plateau which was larger than the one on the lateral. Harding (18) also removed the menisci when using a dye exclusion technique developed by Deane (11) to demonstrate the movement of the contact areas in the presence of simulated quadriceps action. Maquet (28) examined x-ray pictures of loaded intact specimens injected with barium sulfate and deduced the contact areas from the radiolucent regions from which the opaque material had been expelled. He found contact in both compartments over the bulk of the tibial plateau in extension but limited to the posterior regions in flexion. The posterior movement of the contact areas has been confirmed by Draganich (12), who, in addition, demonstrated that the pattern of movement of the contact areas was altered by division of the cruciate ligaments. Kurosawa (23), however, suggested that the medial femoral condyle rolls forward on the tibia during flexion while the lateral compartment rolls backward. The precise relationship between movements medially and laterally depends on the amount of axial rotation allowed or imposed during the experiment.

We have studied rolling of the femur on the tibia in

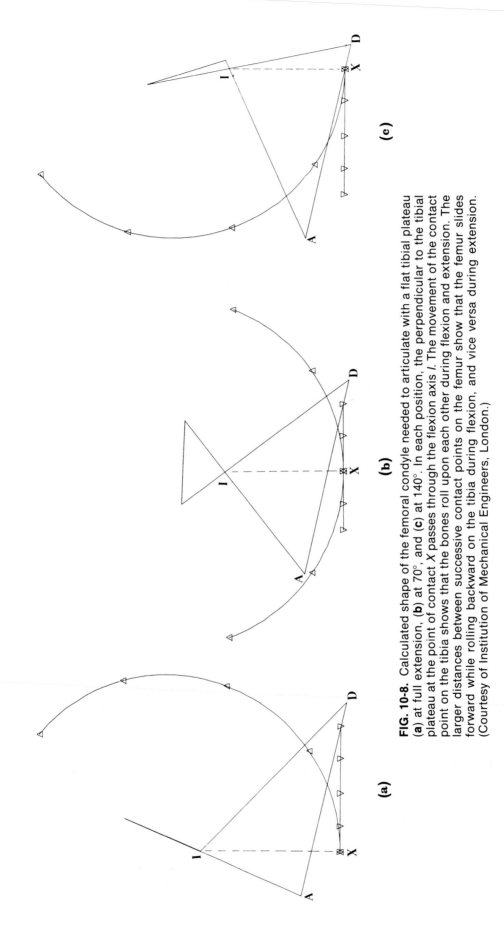

FIG. 10-8. Calculated shape of the femoral condyle needed to articulate with a flat tibial plateau **(a)** at full extension, **(b)** at 70°, and **(c)** at 140°. In each position, the perpendicular to the tibial plateau at the point of contact *X* passes through the flexion axis *I*. The movement of the contact point on the tibia shows that the bones roll upon each other during flexion and extension. The larger distances between successive contact points on the femur show that the femur slides forward while rolling backward on the tibia during flexion, and vice versa during extension. (Courtesy of Institution of Mechanical Engineers, London.)

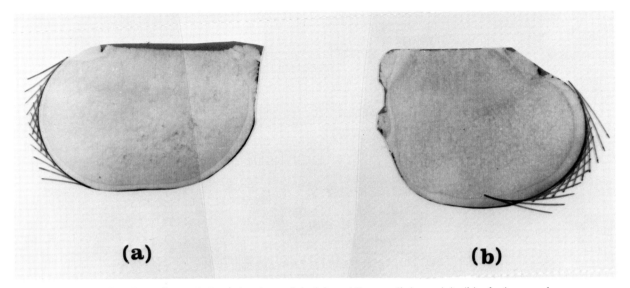

FIG. 10 9. Sections through the lateral condyle (**a**) and the medial condyle (**b**) of a human femur. The calculated shapes of the femoral condyles compatible with a convex tibial plateau (**a**) and a concave tibial plateau (**b**) are superimposed on (**a**) and (**b**), respectively. Emphasis is given to the comparison by including the corresponding tibial plateau drawn in each of 15 positions of flexion, with the envelopes in each case outlining the shape of the femoral condyle. (Courtesy of Institution of Mechanical Engineers, London.)

the cadaver in a different way, using prosthetic components separated by freely sliding prosthetic meniscal bearings (16,17), the movements of which can readily be measured. Spherical metal components were applied to the femoral condyles, and flat metal components were applied to the tibial plateaus. Unconstrained polyethylene bearings, spherical above and flat below, simulated the menisci. The backward movements of the bearings relative to the tibia were measured in four cadaveric specimens, using a micrometer reading to 0.01 mm. The lateral bearing moved, on average, 2.25 mm more than the medial over 90° of flexion.

In Fig. 10-10, the measured movements are plotted against flexion angle. The figure also includes three lines that represent the calculated movements of the contact point on the tibia for convex, flat, and concave tibial surfaces. The line for the flat tibial plateau describes the average movements of the bearings quite well, but those for the curved tibial plateau reveal a limitation of the sagittal plane theory. Whereas the movement of the contact point in the lateral compartment of the human knee was usually observed to be larger than that in the medial, the calculations suggest the reverse. This discrepancy is almost entirely explained by the fact that the calculation takes no account of rotation about the long axis of the tibia. Twenty-five degrees of external rotation of the femur on the tibia occurs during 90° of flexion and would increase the calculated lateral movement and decrease the calculated medial movement by about 6 mm. The

calculations would then fit the observed movements of the meniscal bearings very closely.

Centers of Curvature of the Femoral Condyles

A curve is polycentric (many centered) if it is drawn about a series of centers of curvature. It is polyradial if the radius of curvature varies from center to center. The polycentric and polyradial nature of the femoral condyles of the human knee was described by Strasser (41). The radius of curvature and the position of the center of curvature vary for different points along the articular surface. Rehder (38) fitted involutes, logarithmic spirals, and Archimedean spirals to parasagittal sections like those in Fig. 10-9. Kapandji (21) showed diagrams of the femoral condyles with radii of curvature varying from 3.8 to 1.7 cm medially and from 6.0 to 1.2 cm laterally.

We have analyzed the curvature of the theoretical femoral surfaces of Figs. 10-8 and 10-9. The result for the condyle compatible with a flat tibial plateau is shown in Fig. 10-11, with the articular surfaces drawn in the configuration of full extension. Contact points corresponding to five equispaced positions of flexion are shown. The straight lines are the radii of curvature at the various contact points on the femur. Although the calculated shape of the femoral condyle is undoubtedly polycentric and polyradial, the resulting curve differs little from one drawn from a fixed center at constant radius, that is, a circle. Such a circle is

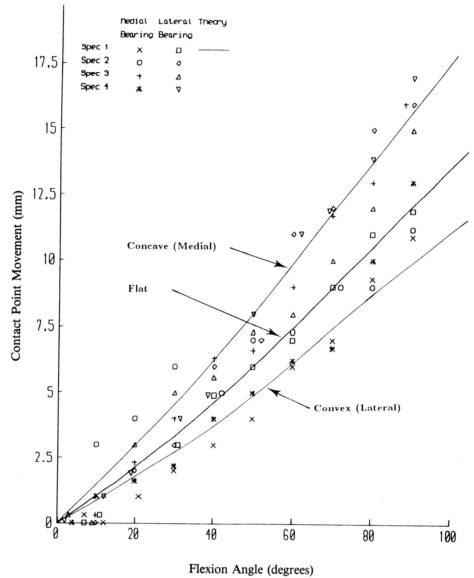

FIG. 10-10. Measured movements of meniscal bearings in four cadaver specimens into which Oxford meniscal arthroplasties had been implanted bicompartmentally. The curves represent the calculated movement of the contact point on concave (medial), flat, and concave (lateral) tibial plateaus. (Courtesy of Institution of Mechanical Engineers, London.)

shown, with its center at the center of curvature of the polycentric condyle at full extension. The circle (which is drawn with a slightly smaller radius to allow it be distinguished from the profile of the femoral condyle) fits the polycentric surface quite well.

Parasagittal sections of a human knee are shown in Fig. 10-12a and b. A single circle is included on each photograph. The circle follows the outline of the lateral section very closely over the full extent of the tibio-femoral facet; the fit on the medial side is equally good, except where the drawn circle intersects the medial flange of the patellar facet of the femur. Sections from five human knees have been examined in the same way and have been found to be effectively circular over most of their posterior aspects. Kurosawa (23) digi-

tized the shapes of sections of human knees, and "the posterior femoral condyles were shown to closely fit spherical surfaces."

Figure 10-13 shows a sagittal section through the sulcus of the trochlear groove of a human femur. It shows that the patellar facet and tibial facets of the femur are geometrically distinct and discontinuous from each other. The distal end of the femur is polycentric, mainly in the sense that the centers of its tibial and patellar facets are quite distinct and separate.

Slip Ratio

Figure 10-8 demonstrated that the femoral condyle of the knee is longer than the tibial plateau. The distances

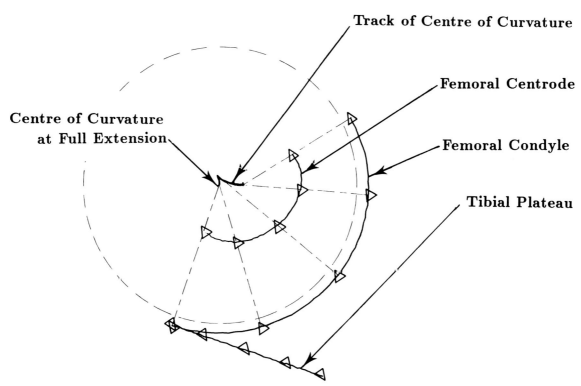

FIG. 10-11. The calculated shape of the femoral condyle compatible with a flat tibial plateau, shown touching at full extension, as in Fig. 10-8a. The calculated track of the center of curvature of the femoral condyle is included, together with the femoral centrode from Fig. 10-5b and 5d. Radii corresponding to the contact points at 0°, 35°, 70°, 105°, and 140° of flexion connect each contact point to its corresponding center of curvature. Each radius necessarily passes through the flexion axis at its position on the femoral centrode appropriate to the corresponding flexion angle. The dashed circle, centered on the center of curvature of the full extension contact point, demonstrates that the femoral condyle is approximately circular. (Courtesy of Institution of Mechanical Engineers, London.)

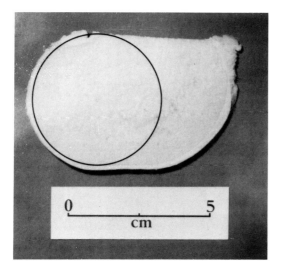

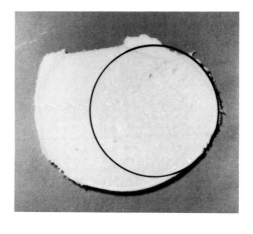

(a)   (b)

FIG. 10-12. Parasagittal sections through the lateral condyle (a) and the medial condyle (b) of a human knee, with circles of radius 24 mm superimposed. (Courtesy of Institution of Mechanical Engineers, London.)

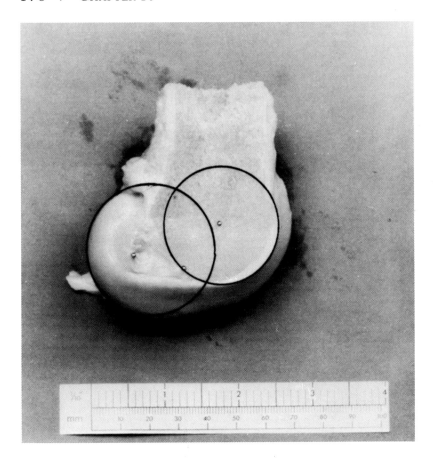

FIG. 10-13. Section through the sulcus of the trochlear groove of a human femur. The anterior circle outlines the articular surface at the base of the trochlear groove, the surface that guides the patella over the femur. The posterior circle outlines the tibial facet of the femoral condyle. Functionally, the distal end of the femur is like a bicircular cam, with the circles joined by the flanges of the trochlear groove. (Courtesy of Institution of Mechanical Engineers, London.)

between successive points of contact on the femur are larger than on the tibia so that the femur slides as well as rolls on the tibia during flexion/extension. The proportion of sliding and rolling depends on the shapes of the articular surfaces and on the flexion angle. Walker (43) found considerable variation in the proportions of rolling and sliding in different specimens, but the method used—that of Rouleux—is known to be fundamentally inaccurate.

We define the *slip ratio* as the ratio of the length of the femoral articulation between two successive contact points and the length of the tibial articulation between the corresponding contact points. Figure 10-14 shows how the calculated slip ratio varies with flexion angle for articulations in which the tibial plateau is flat, convex, and concave; the latter two are of dimensions compatible with the condyles of a human femur, which are shown in Fig. 10-9. It will be seen that the three pairs of articular surfaces, all of them compatible with the same cruciate linkage, exhibit different values of the slip ratio over the flexion arc. Nowhere is the slip ratio equal to unity, corresponding to pure rolling. Different pairs of articular surfaces can be compatible with the same cruciate linkage by exhibiting different values of the slip ratio.

These results do not support the view that the articular surfaces of the knee can exhibit pure rolling in some positions. Were they to do so, the flexion axis would have to lie at the level of the articular surfaces which would have to coincide with that of the centrodes of Fig. 10-5.

The Bones

The modeling of the geometry of the knee in the sagittal plane is further developed (Fig. 10-15) by adding the bones to the articular surfaces of Fig. 10-8. The model bones are shown with the knee at 45° of flexion. The tibial plateau is taken to be flat, as in Fig. 10-8. To add the tibia to its flat plateau, some further parameters had to be defined, but only three of them have functional significance from the point of view of the geometry and mechanics of the knee. The plateau is shown to slope backward relative to the axis of the proximal tibia at an angle of 13°. This fits within the range 10–15° cited by Moore (30). The position of the tibial tubercle is included amongst the model parameters in the appendix. Other features of the top of the tibia are sketched in Fig. 10-15 but do not affect the geometry or mechanics of the knee and are not intended to be anatomically precise.

The modeled shape of the patellar facet of the femur in Fig. 10-15 is based on the shape of the sulcus of the

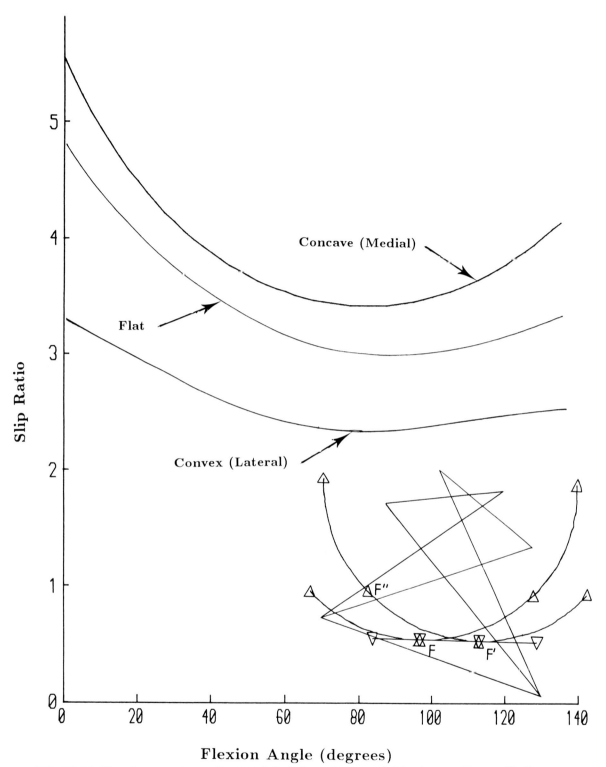

FIG. 10-14. The diagram shows the cruciate linkage in two neighboring positions with the corresponding femoral surface touching a flat tibial plateau at F and F'. F'' is the point on the femoral surface which makes contact with F. The slip ratio is the distance $F'F''$ measured along the femur, divided by the distance FF' measured along the tibia. The graphs show the variation with flexion angle for convex, flat, and concave tibial plateaus.

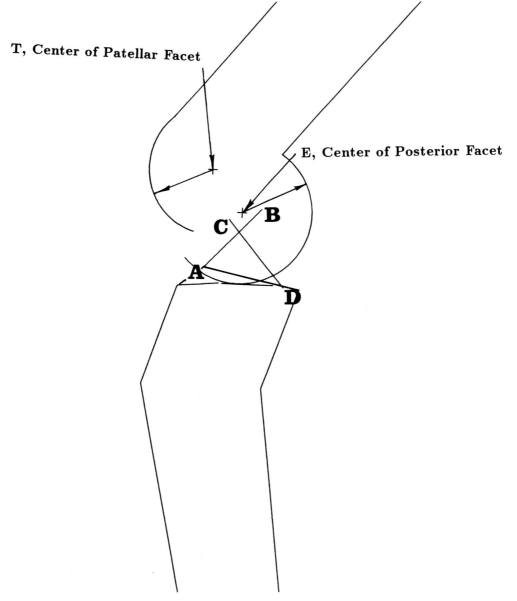

FIG. 10-15. The model bones with the cruciate linkage of Fig. 10-3 and the articular surfaces of Fig. 10-8. The patellar facet of the femur is a circle centered at *T*, the posterior face of the femoral condyle is a circle centered at *E*, and the center of curvature of the femoral condyle is at the 140° contact point.

trochlear groove (Fig. 10-13) and is taken to be a circle. The radius and the coordinates of its center are given in the appendix and are the only femoral parameters of functional significance to the geometry of the knee in the sagittal plane. The remainder of the drawing of the distal femur in Fig. 10-15 is purely diagrammatic.

Figure 10-16 shows the model femur superposed in 30 positions on a fixed tibia. It illustrates the rolling movement of the femur on the tibia during flexion/extension. It shows the tracks (relative to the tibia) of the centers of the patellar and tibial facets (as defined in Figs. 10-15 and 10-11, respectively). Both centers move backward during flexion, a fact that will be seen to have significance when we come to consider the mechanical interactions between the quadriceps and the cruciates. The distance of the center of curvature of the femoral condyle from the tibial plateau remains almost constant during flexion, a further illustration of the fact that the tibial facet of the femoral condyle is almost circular. In contrast, the center of the patellar facet moves proximally as well as posteriorly during flexion. Although the shape of the end of the femur is like that of a bicircular cam (Fig. 10-13), its movement is more complex, since it rolls as well as slides on the

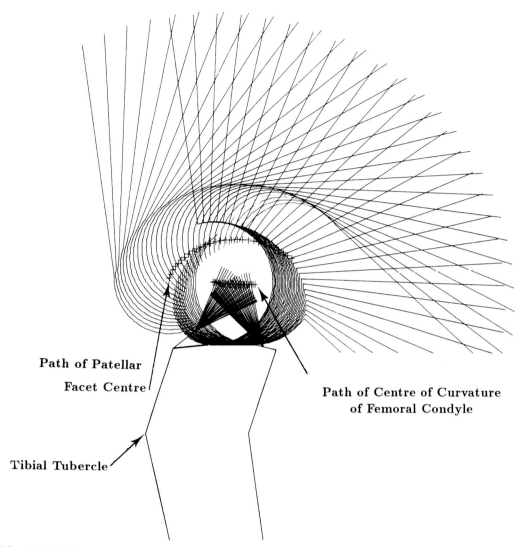

Path of Patellar
Facet Centre

Path of Centre of Curvature
of Femoral Condyle

Tibial Tubercle

FIG. 10-16. Thirty images of the model femur flexing/extending on a fixed tibia with superimposed images of the cruciate ligaments (Fig. 10-5c), demonstrating the rolling component of the movement of the femur on the tibia. The tracks of the center of the patellar facet (point *T*, Fig. 10-15) and of the center of the posterior facet (point *E*, Fig. 10-15) of the femoral condyle are included.

tibial plateau. In engineering, a cam usually rotates about a fixed center.

LIGAMENT ANISOMETRY

Discussions of ligament surgery place much emphasis on the idea of ligament *isometry,* the assumption that a ligament fiber does not change its length when the joint is passively extended or flexed in the absence of external load and muscle action. There is a huge literature describing the changing length patterns of ligament fibers, starting with Fick (14). Brantigan (7) summarized the many contradictory statements in the

literature prior to 1941. Since then, more quantitative methods of measurement have been developed and have produced a broader consensus. Ligament attachment areas have been marked with pins, and their relative movements have been calculated from measured movements of the pin heads (44). Mercury strain gauges (22), buckle transducers (24), and Hall effect transducers (1,2) have been used to give more direct measurements of ligament fiber strain. Recently, methods of digitizing surfaces developed for the aerospace industry have been applied to determine the length-change patterns of the ligaments of the knee (39).

In describing the development of the model of the knee, we have assumed so far that the movements of the bones upon each other in the sagittal plane are controlled entirely by the neutral fibers of the cruciate ligaments, which remain isometric during passive extension and flexion. We will now consider the extent to which that assumption is consistent with the presence of other ligament fibers, both in the cruciate and the collateral ligaments.

Figure 10-17 shows the following: A ligament fiber that lies in front of the flexion axis in any position of the joint must instantaneously stretch as the joint flexes; a fiber that passes through the flexion axis is instantaneously isometric; and a fiber lying behind the flexion axis instantaneously shortens. This *principle of ligament strain* explains much of the observations on length-change patterns of ligament fibers which have been reported in the literature. It was mentioned in passing by Steindler (40). Menschik (29) and Müller (31) have shown how ligament fibers that are attached to the bones along the Burmester curves of the four-bar cruciate linkage pass through the flexion axis in all positions of the joint and therefore remain isometric.

It is clear that all the fibers of all the ligaments cannot always pass through the flexion axis, so that some fibers must be expected to slacken and others to stretch during passive flexion. The typical ligament fiber is therefore likely to exhibit anisometry rather than isometry.

The Collateral Ligaments

Figure 10-18 shows the model bones with the neutral fibers of the cruciates, *AB* and *CD*. It includes also a pair of lines *LL* and *MM*, intended to represent the central fibers of the collateral ligaments. The anthropometric studies referred to in the appendix to this chapter included definition of the attachment areas of both collaterals on both bones. The lines *LL* and *MM* in Fig. 10-18 join the centers of those areas of attachment. The succession of diagrams (Fig. 10-18a, b, and c) shows how the points *L* and *M*, fixed in the femur, move relative to the tibia during flexion/extension under the control of the cruciate linkage.

Comparison of the positions of the collateral ligament fibers in Fig. 10-18a, b, and c shows that both lie in front of the flexion axis *I* in extension and move progressively backward relative to that axis as the joint flexes, the lateral fiber *LL* more rapidly than the medial fiber *MM*. In consequence, one would expect the medial fiber to lengthen initially and then to shorten. The lateral fiber would be expected to shorten almost as soon as flexion commences. These phenomena can be seen in Fig. 10-18d, where the two fibers are drawn by the computer in 30 successive positions on a fixed tibia as the joint flexes in the sagittal plane from full extension to 140° of flexion. The medial fiber appears to stretch during early flexion as its points of attachment

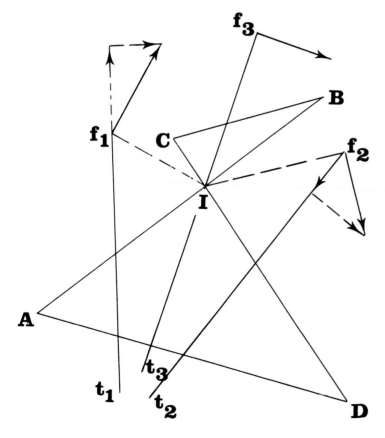

FIG. 10-17. Principle of ligament fiber strain. The fiber $f_1 t_1$ lies in front of, $f_2 t_2$ lies behind, and $f_3 t_3$ passes through the flexion axis. Considering the femur to be flexing on a fixed tibia, the points f_1, f_2, and f_3 move perpendicular to their radii from the flexion axis. The component of the displacement of f_1 parallel to $f_1 t_1$ is directed away from t_1, and the fiber $f_1 t_1$ instantaneously extends. f_2 has a component of displacement toward t_2, and the fiber $f_2 t_2$ contracts. The displacement of f_3 is perpendicular to the fiber $f_3 t_3$, which remains instantaneously isometric.

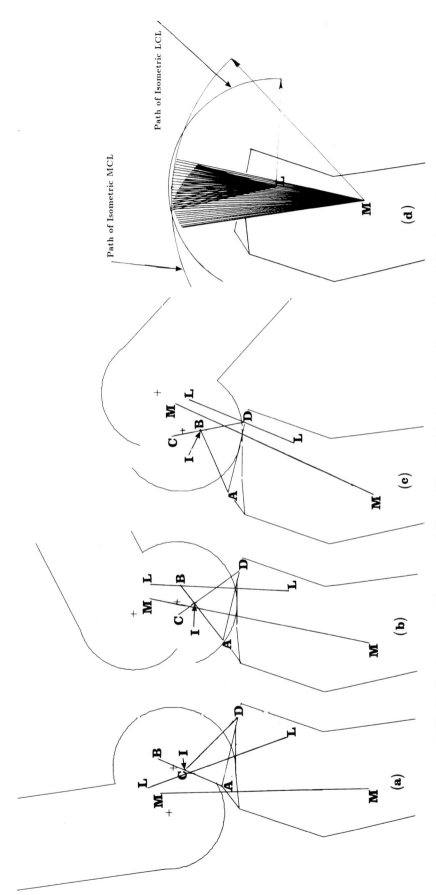

FIG. 10-18. Computer diagrams of fibers *MM* and *LL* drawn from the centers of the femoral attachment areas of the MCL and LCL to the centers of the tibial attachment areas at full extension (**a**), at 70° of flexion (**b**) and at 140° of flexion (**c**). These "anatomic" fibers lie in front of the flexion axis *I* in extension and behind *I* in flexion. In (**d**), the anatomic fibers are drawn on a fixed tibia in 30 positions ranging from full extension to 140° of flexion, controlled by the cruciate linkage. Patterns of length change may be visualized by comparing the femoral ends to circular arcs centered on the tibial attachments. The medial fiber appears to extend as its attachment points move apart, whereas the lateral fiber appears to shorten as its attachment points move together.

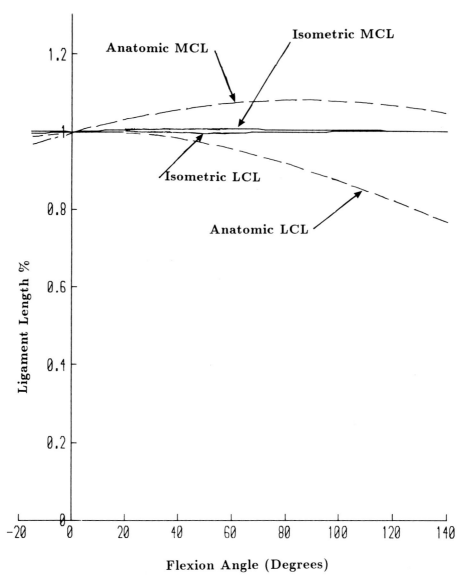

FIG. 10-19. Fiber strain (ligament length, %) plotted against flexion angle for the anatomic fibers of Fig. 10-18 and the isometric fibers of Fig. 10-20. Fiber length is expressed as a proportion of the length at full extension.

on the two bones move apart; the lateral fiber appears to shorten as its points of attachment move toward each other. This pattern of behavior illustrates the principle of the previous paragraph. A more precise view of the strain in these fibers during passive flexion is given in Fig. 10-19, where fiber length, expressed as a proportion of length at full extension, is plotted against flexion angle. Strain patterns are given for the "anatomic" collateral fibers of Fig. 10-18, connecting the centers of the attachment areas on the bones. The medial fiber *MM* reaches its maximum length at about 80° of flexion and shortens slowly with further flexion. The lateral fiber shortens rapidly with flexion to less than 80% of its initial length at 140° of flexion.

In contrast, Fig. 10-20 shows a similar pair of fibers,

which were chosen because they remain isometric to within 0.5%. The lateral fiber *LL* passes precisely through the flexion axis *I* in Fig. 10-20a, b, and c; the medial fiber lies slightly in front of *I* in Fig. 10-20a and slightly behind in Fig. 10-20c. The pattern of strain of these "isometric fibers" is compared with that of the anatomic fibers in Fig. 10-19. Figure 10-20d shows that the femoral ends of the isometric fibers lie very close to the isometric circle centered at the tibial attachments, in contrast to what is shown Fig. 10-18d.[3]

As an indication of the sensitivity of fiber strain to attachment position, we note that the tibial attach-

---

[3] The points of attachment of the isometric fibers in Fig. 10-20 lie close to the Burmester curves of the cruciate linkage [cf. Menschik (29) and Müller (31)].

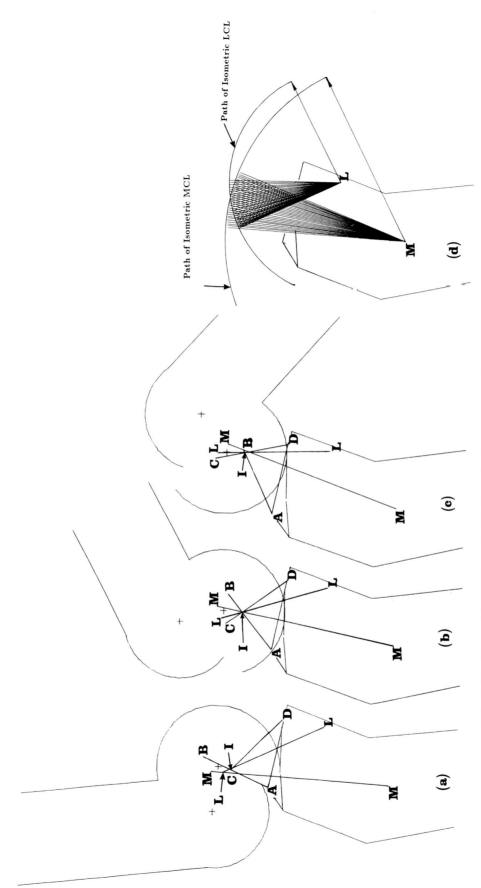

FIG. 10-20. "Isometric" MCL and LCL fibers in the same positions as Fig. 2-15. The fibers pass close to the flexion axis over the flexion range (**d**). The isometric fibers drawn on a fixed tibia in 30 positions of flexion. Their lengths remain constant within 0.5%.

ments of the anatomic fibers of Fig. 10-18 and the isometric fibers of Fig. 10-20, as well as the femoral attachments of the medial fibers in the two figures, are no more than 1 cm apart. The femoral attachments of the two lateral fibers are 2.05 cm apart.

Before attempting to apply the results of Figs. 10-18, 10-19, and 10-20 to the human knee, it is necessary to take account of the effects of tibial rotation. In the flexed knee, internal rotation of the tibia on the femur during flexion tends to slacken the fibers of the medial collateral ligament (MCL) and tighten those of the lateral collateral ligament (LCL), so that the sagittal plane theory probably exaggerates the strain of the central fiber of the MCL and underestimates that of the LCL. However, direct observation of strain in various fibers of the MCL (1) shows that its anterior fibers tighten and its posterior fibers slacken during passive flexion and suggests, as does Fig. 10-10, that the movements of the bones in the sagittal plane during flexion dominate the effects of tibial rotation.

This is further confirmed by observation (44) of the fibers of the LCL of the human knee, all of which slacken during passive flexion; thus the tightening effect of tibial rotation does not compensate for the slackening due to sagittal plane movements.

Observations that the anterior fibers of the ACL, PCL, and MCL tighten and posterior fibers slacken during passive flexion can then be interpreted in terms of the principle of ligament strain to imply that the flexion axis of the human knee penetrates the ACL, PCL, and MCL and lies wholly in front of all the fibers of the LCL. This pattern of ligament strain is predicted by the sagittal plane theory, although that theory probably overestimates the strain in the anterior fibers of the MCL.

Strain Patterns Within the Cruciate Ligaments

Figure 10-21 shows a computer-drawn diagram of the knee with the neutral fibers of the cruciates. We will now consider the pattern of strain within each of the cruciates on the assumption that all their fibers do not pass through the flexion axis at the intersection of the neutral fibers. The ligaments are attached to each bone over a finite area. For each cruciate, Fig. 10-21 also contains a line joining the anterior edge of the femoral attachment area to the anterior edge of the tibial attachment area; similar lines join the posterior edges. If these lines represent the anterior and posterior fibers of the two ligaments, it is clear that the anterior fibers lie in front of the flexion axis in all positions and the posterior fibers lie behind. By the principle of ligament strain, the anterior fibers should stretch and the posterior fibers should slacken during passive flexion.

Figure 10-22 shows the model bones and contains lines for each ligament; one of these lines joins the anterior edge of the tibial attachment to the posterior edge of the femoral attachment (the anteroposterior fibers), and the other joins the posterior edge of the tibial attachment to the anterior edge of the femoral attachment (the posteroanterior fibers). In comparison with the anterior and posterior fibers of Fig. 10-21, it will be seen that the crossed fibers of Fig. 10-22 pass much closer to the flexion axis and might then be expected to be more nearly isometric.

Figure 10-23 shows the calculated length-change patterns of the two groups of fibers in the ACL plotted against flexion angle. Whereas the anterior fibers of Fig. 10-21 stretch and the posterior fibers contract by more than 20%, the length changes of the crossed fibers of Fig. 10-22 are very much less; the anteroposterior fiber lengthens initially and shortens later, to remain effectively isometric over the flexion range. This analysis may explain Norwood's (32) observations that the fibers within the cruciate ligaments of the human knee are twisted upon each other, one effect of which is that a ligament, although of finite cross-sectional area, can nonetheless approach the ideal of isometry during passive flexion. Müller (31) demonstrated a similar twist in the fibers of the MCL, with a similar interpretation.

Cruciate Neutral Fibers

This analysis then explains what is meant by the neutral fibers of the cruciate linkage. Comparing parts a and b of Fig. 10-21, it will be seen that the attachment areas of the ligament on the two bones rotate relative to each other during flexion/extension, changing the shapes of the ligaments when seen from the side. The femoral attachment area of each ligament may be considered to rotate relative to the tibial attachment area about a point, and vice versa. During flexion, points in front of the centers of rotation of the attachment areas move away from each other while points behind approach each other. The neutral fibers are lines joining the centers of rotation and remain isometric during passive flexion and extension. There may well be no physical fibers joining the centers of rotation. The complex bundles of fibers within the ligaments behave as though there were.

Sidles (39) has mapped out contours within the attachment areas of each bone, along which attached fibers exhibit mean axial strains (MAS) of various values. These contours appear to enclose a very small area on each bone, upon which attached fibers remain isometric. O'Brien (33) has recently shown sections of human knees which suggest that the neutral fibers of the human cruciate ligaments may lie close to the front of the ACL and near the back of the PCL. This would

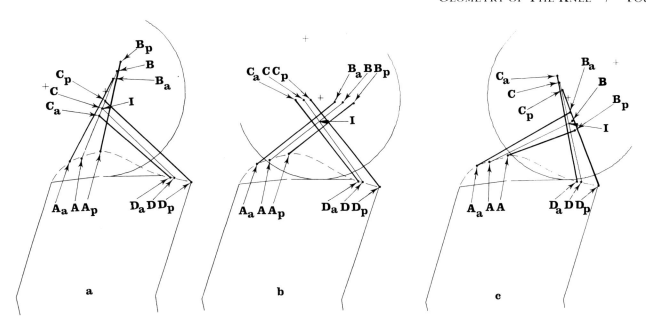

FIG. 10-21. Finite cruciate ligaments with "parallel" fibers. The model bones with the neutral fibers AB and CD of the cruciate linkage (Fig. 10-3). The lines A_aB_a and C_aD_a joining the anterior edges of the attachment areas represent anterior fibers of the cruciate ligaments. A_pB_p and C_pD_p joining the posterior edges of the attachment areas represent the posterior fibers of the cruciates. As the attachment areas rotate relative to each other during flexion, the shapes of the ligaments change, points on the attachment areas in front of the neutral fibers move apart, and points behind them move together. The anterior fibers stretch, whereas the posterior fibers shorten.

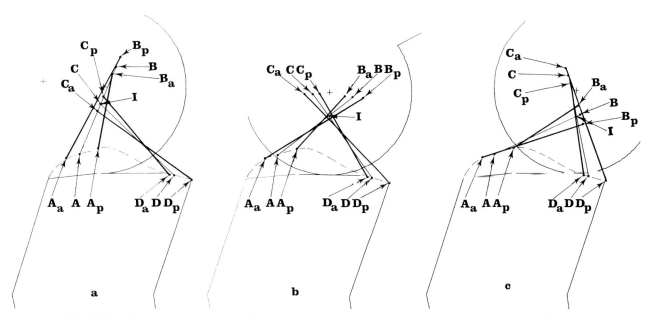

FIG. 10-22. Cruciate ligaments with crossed fibers. The model bones with the neutral fibers AB and CD of the cruciate linkage. "Anteroposterior" fibers A_aB_p and D_aC_p join the anterior edges of the tibial attachment areas to the posterior edges of the femoral attachments. "Posteroanterior" fibers A_pB_a and D_pC_a join the posterior edges of the tibial attachments to the anterior edges of the femoral attachments. During flexion/extension, the crossed fibers remain close to the flexion axis I and remain approximately isometric.

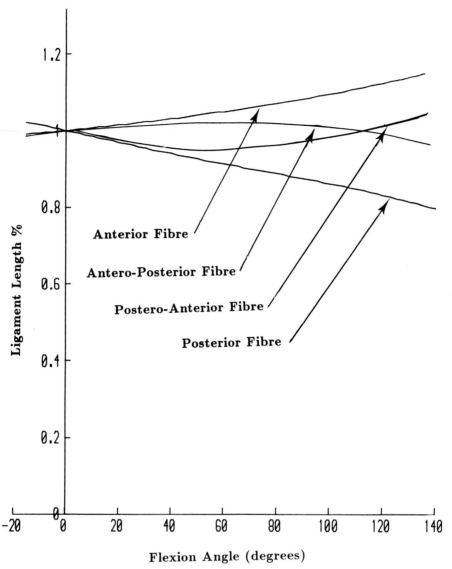

FIG. 10-23. Change in length per unit length of the "parallel" cruciate fibers of Fig. 10-21 and the crossed cruciate fibers of Fig. 10-22.

suggest that all the fibers of the ACL are tight in extension and that all the fibers of the PCL are tight in flexion.

The change with flexion/extension of the shapes of the ligaments implies that the relative directions of the fibers within a single ligament also change with position, as does the cross-sectional area at any site along a ligament. The concept of the force per unit fiber may then be of more utility than the common concept of stress (force per unit area). Likewise, it may be more realistic to think of fiber strain rather than average ligament strain.

Sensory Function of the Ligaments

Barrack and Skinner (Chapter 6) described the possible role of the ligaments as mechanoreceptors, distinguish-ing between (a) rapidly adapting receptors stimulated by rapid loading and (b) slowly adapting receptors giving steady-state information on joint position and motion. We speculate here that the pattern of strain within individual ligaments may provide a means of discriminating between these various types of signal.

As the joint flexes, the anterior fibers lengthen and the posterior fibers shorten. Let us assume that the mechanoreceptors are sensitive to strain (change of length per unit length, as in Figs. 10-19 and 10-23 and that the anterior signal increases and the posterior signal decreases at the same rate with change in position. The algebraic sum of the signals would then remain constant, but the algebraic difference between the signals would increase as the joint flexes; the value of the difference at any position would be a function of that position. The difference would increase as the joint flexes and decrease as the joint extends, sensing the direction of motion. Elementary neural circuits designed to sense the difference between the signals would then give a direct measure of position and direction of motion. Rate-sensitive circuitry would sense velocity.

At any position, the signals from the receptors would also respond to slowly applied load. Strain signals from both anterior and posterior fibers would increase with increasing load. If both increase at the same rate, their difference would remain constant, indicating constant position. The sum of the signals would be a direct measure of the force in the ligament and, for a constant force, would remain constant as the joint flexes and extends. Thus, by determining simultaneously the difference and the sum of the signals, a simple neural network could discriminate between position-dependent signals and force-dependent signals.

ATTACHMENT OF LIGAMENT GRAFTS OR REPLACEMENTS

Ligament injury is increasingly recognized as one of the significant causes of instability and long-term morbidity of the knee. As a consequence, ligament repair and reconstruction has become more commonplace. In this section, we will apply sagittal plane modeling to discuss placement of the attachments (to bone) of ligament grafts or replacements.

Theory

Ligament fibers that lie in front of the flexion axis lengthen as the knee is flexed, and fibers lying posterior to the flexion axis shorten (Figs. 10-19 and 10-23). Coupled with experimental observations of strain patterns within the ligaments during passive extension and flexion, we deduced that the flexion axis of the human knee penetrates the MCL, ACL, and PCL but lies in front of the LCL. The evidence justifies the assumption of neutral fibers within the ACL, PCL, and MCL that pass through the flexion axis and stay isometric throughout the flexion arc. The attachment points of the neutral fibers are referred to below as the *isometric sites*.

The object of ligament repair/reconstruction is to reestablish normal joint kinematics by restoring the relationship between the joint surfaces and the ligament system. When repair is not possible, the surgeon attempts to replace the ligament with a structure of comparable mechanical properties along the line of the neutral fiber of the original ligament such that the substitute remains approximately isometric over the flexion range.

The positioning of the attachments of a single ligament fiber can have five possible outcomes in terms of length change during passive flexion:

1. No length change; the ideal isometric position.
2. Increase in length; the fiber passes wholly in front of the flexion axis throughout the flexion range.
3. Decrease in length; the fiber passes wholly behind the flexion axis throughout the flexion range.
4. Shortens initially and then lengthens; at extension the fiber lies behind the flexion axis, but with flexion it moves to lie in front. The overall length change will depend on the arc of flexion where the replacement lies behind the flexion axis relative to the arc where it lies in front.
5. Lengthens initially and then shortens; the converse of condition 4.

The first of these possibilities is demonstrated in Figs. 10-4 and 10-5. The other four possibilities are demonstrated in Figs. 10-21 and 10-22. It is possible that a ligament or a graft may contain fibers that exhibit each of these five patterns of behavior.

We have used the computer model to examine the length change with flexion that results from positioning a ligament or graft fiber other than in the isometric attachment sites (e.g., conditions 2 to 5). In the calculations, it is assumed that the bones move relative to each other under the control of the cruciate linkage. The parameters of the model used were measured from the lateral x-rays of four cadaver knees in full extension with markers placed at the centers of the attachment sites, as described in the appendix to this chapter. Calculations were performed for parameters appropriate to each of the four specimens.

Shown in Table 10-1 are (a) the parameters of the four-bar linkage in the four specimens and (b) the angle between the femoral link and the roof of the femoral notch. On the bottom line, values are given for the distance γ as described by Odensten (37). This is the distance measured on the specimens from the center of the femoral insertion of the ACL posteriorly and superiorly to the point where the femoral shaft meets the lateral femoral condyle (Fig. 10-24). It is of interest in the "over-the-top" method of reconstruction of the ACL.

Cruciate Ligaments

Examples of the length changes consequent on moving the femoral attachment of the ACL (including the "over-the-top" position), moving the femoral attachment of the PCL, and moving the tibial attachment of the ACL are shown, respectively, in Fig. 10-25a, b, and c.

By performing numerous calculations, it was possible to define zones around the isometric point of attachment where the length change of the replacement

TABLE 10-1. *Results of radiographic measurement of the parameters for the sagittal view of the four-bar linkage in four cadaveric knees*

	Specimens			
	1	2	3	4
Length of anterior cruciate (mm)	30	33	32	33
Length of posterior cruciate (mm)	28	29	24	33
Length of tibial link (mm)	28	31	29	34
Length of femoral link (mm)	12	16	15	15
Angle between femoral link and the roof of the notch (degrees)	10	5	6	7
(gamma) displacement of "over-the-top" femoral attachment (Fig. 10–24) (mm)	11	12	14	10

could be predicted. Figure 10-26 shows the ACL femoral attachment zones, assuming that the tibial attachment is in the normal isometric position. Figure 10-27 shows the similar zones for the PCL femoral attachment, assuming that the tibial attachment is in the normal isometric position. When the surgeon finds, at first attempt, that exploratory bone tunnels have been drilled to sites that prove to be nonisometric, the zones in Figs. 10-26 and 10-27 guide remedial action.

Figure 10-28 plots the percentage length change at 90° of flexion and at 140° of flexion against fiber attachment position for the mean dimensions of the four-bar linkage of the four specimens. Figure 10-28A shows the effect of movement of the femoral attachment of an ACL fiber anteriorly and posteriorly along the line of the femoral link; in Fig. 10-28B, the same attachment is moved superiorly and inferiorly (i.e. perpendicular) to the femoral link; Fig. 10-28C shows the effect of moving the tibial attachment of an ACL fiber anteriorly and posteriorly along the line of the tibial plateau.

Figure 10-29 shows the effect of changing the femoral attachment of a PCL fiber relative to the line of the femoral link.

Isometric positioning of a cruciate replacement will allow the knee to be put through a full range of flexion without excessive tension on the graft. If successfully achieved, the risk of graft disruption during an early passive and assisted active motion program is reduced.

The consequences of nonisometric graft positioning are as follows: If a graft has been placed in a position where it lengthens as the knee is passed from flexion to extension and is fixed with the knee in flexion, then either a flexion contracture results or, if the knee does manage to extend fully, the graft will be stretched and is at risk of rupture. If the same graft is fixed at full extension, it will be flaccid during the rest of the range of flexion and therefore will not contribute to the normal guidance of the joint motion.

At surgery, correct positioning of the tibial attachments for both anterior and posterior ligaments is relatively straightforward. Finding the isometric points for the femoral insertions is more difficult. It is unfortunate, therefore, that for a given error in positioning the attachments, the percentage length change in the replacement over the flexion range is proportionately greater for malpositioning the femoral site than for malpositioning the tibial site (Fig. 10-28). As a result, the technically more difficult site to position is also the more critical in achieving isometric graft length. Indeed, these results narrow things down, further show-

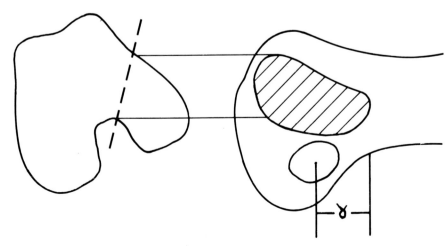

FIG. 10-24. Diagram adapted from Odensten (37) (see Fig. 10-3) to show the dimension "γ." Drawing of the medial surface of the right lateral femoral condyle (with the medial femoral condyle removed as shown by hatched area) outlining the femoral attachment of the ACL.

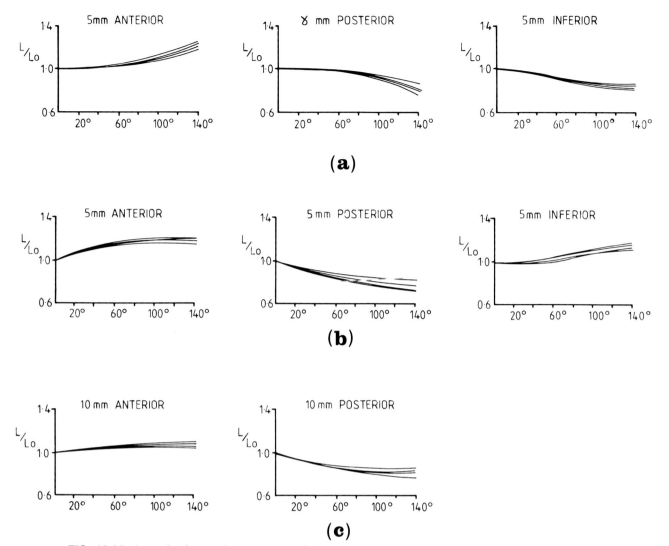

FIG. 10-25. Length change between attachment sites versus flexion angle. The length L at any flexion angle is expressed as a ratio of the length L_0 at full extension. (**a**) Movement relative to the femoral link of an ACL fiber attachment anteriorly 5 mm, posteriorly γ, and inferiorly 5 mm. Tibial attachment in the normal isometric site. (**b**) Movement relative to the femoral link of a PCL fiber attachment anteriorly, posteriorly, and inferiorly 5 mm. Tibial attachment at the isometric site. (**c**) Tibial attachment of an ACL fiber moved 10 mm anteriorly and posteriorly, parallel to the tibial plateau. Femoral attachment at the isometric site.

ing that variation anteriorly and posteriorly along the line of the femoral link is more important than superiorly and inferiorly for the ACL, though this observation is less marked for the PCL (Figs. 10-28 and 10-29). For practical purposes, the line of the femoral link of the cruciate linkage may be taken as the line of the notch roof as can be seen from the penultimate line in Table 10-1.

When a cruciate ligament is reconstructed, placing the center of the graft at the isometric point will minimize the length change of the anterior and posterior fibers of the graft. The surgical technique of graft placement is discussed in Chapter 2. A popular orientation of an ACL graft is the "over-the-top" position described by MacIntosh (25). This orientation is non-

isometric and results in a decrease in the attachment site distance as the knee is flexed (Fig. 10-26). However, the length change with flexion can be reduced by moving the tibial attachment site anteriorly and/or by changing the value of γ to simulate the effect, making a bone trough in the superolateral corner of the notch at the back of the lateral femoral condyle. This agrees with cadaveric studies (10) of graft length changes in these configurations.

Medial Collateral Ligament

In Figs. 10-18 and 10-19, we discussed strain patterns in a fiber joining the centers of the attachment areas

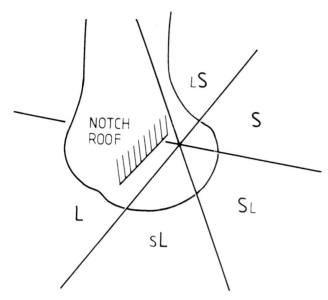

FIG. 10-26. Zones around the isometric ACL fiber femoral attachment. Medial aspect of lateral femoral condyle. *L*, lengthening; *S*, shortening. Capital lettering indicates the overall effect over 140°. The first letter indicates the initial effect as the knee is flexed from full extension. Thus, *SL* indicates initial shortening followed by lengthening, the overall effect being lengthening. If, at surgery, initial test reveals one of these four patterns of behavior, appropriate movement of the attachment site might be attempted.

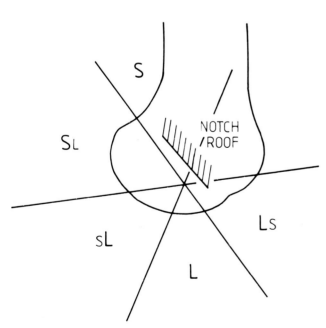

FIG. 10-27. Zones around the isometric PCL fiber femoral attachment. Lateral aspect of medial femoral condyle. Labeling of zones as in Fig. 10-26.

of the MCL. The attachment centers were based on the mean values of measurements made on the four specimens (see appendix to this chapter). Figure 10-30 gives length-change patterns for the anterior and posterior fibers of an MCL 12 mm wide. In Fig. 10-30A the fibers are attached symmetrically with respect to the mean attachment centers. As in previous examples, the anterior fiber lengthens and the posterior fiber shortens with flexion. Figure 10-30B shows how these fibers fare when the tibial attachment of the ligament is moved 30 mm proximally up the tibia. Clinically, this situation may be encountered after a distal avulsion of the ligament and represents an attempt to obtain secure fixation by reattaching it more proximally. It is important to realize that the normal attachment site lies about 6 cm distal to the joint line. In comparison with Fig. 10-30A, proximal reattachment results in considerable increase in the strain in the anterior fibers of the ligament. Figure 10-30C shows the effect of moving the tibial attachment 10 mm distally. This is analogous to a distal advancement of a chronic MCL laxity. The length-change patterns do not differ significantly from Fig. 10-30A. Figure 10-30D shows the effect of transferring the femoral attachment 10 mm distally (i.e., toward the joint line), analogous to the repair of an acute proximal avulsion. This causes a marked overall lengthening of the entire width of the ligament.

The results for the MCL show the need to maintain the attachment sites out to length when repairing the structure. This is of particular relevance when repairing a ligament ruptured at, or near, the attachment sites where the temptation is to staple or fix the ligament back to bone through a relatively undamaged portion of ligament. Such a repaired ligament lengthens with flexion and therefore is at risk of recurrent rupture or, at best, at risk of being stretched (with resulting instability). If the tibial attachment is moved distally or anteriorly, the length change in the anterior and posterior fibers differ little from that observed when the attachments are in their normal positions.

Conclusions

Modeling the knee in the sagittal plane as a four-bar linkage based on the neutral fibers of the cruciate ligaments makes it possible to demonstrate the theoretical changes in length which occur when "replacement" ligament fibers are attached at different sites. The model predicts length changes that are in good qualitative agreement with *in vitro* measurements by other authors. Zones have been identified around the isometric femoral attachment sites of the ACL and PCL where this length change may be predicted.

In trying to achieve an isometric graft, the correct

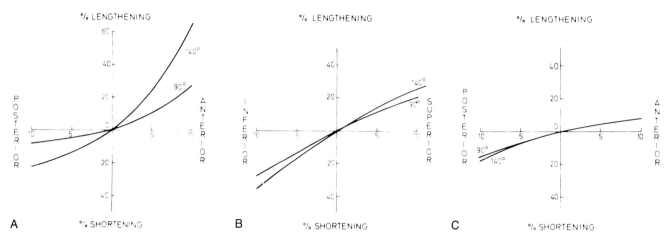

FIG. 10-28. Percentage length change versus ACL fiber attachment position (relative to the isometric site) in millimeters. (**A**) ACL fiber femoral attachment moved along the line of the femoral link, with the tibial attachment being at the isometric position. (**B**) ACL fiber attachment moved perpendicular to the femoral link, with the tibial attachment being at the isometric site. (**C**) ACL fiber tibial attachment moved anteriorly and posteriorly along the tibial eminence, with the femoral attachment being at the isometric site.

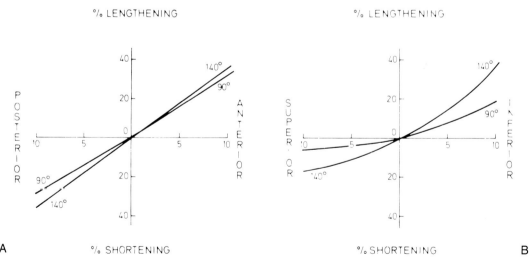

FIG. 10-29. Percentage length change versus PCL fiber attachment position (relative to the isometric site) in millimeters. (**A**) PCL fiber femoral attachment moved along the line of the femoral link, with the tibial attachment being at the isometric site. (**B**) PCL fiber femoral attachment moved perpendicular to the femoral link, with the tibial attachment being at the isometric site.

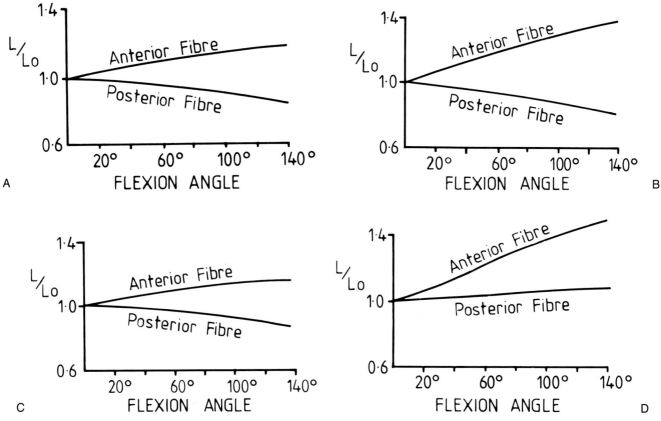

FIG. 10-30. Length change versus flexion angle for the 12-mm-wide MCL. **(A)** Attachment sites are anatomic, as in Fig. 10-18. **(B)** Tibial attachment moved 30 mm proximally, the femoral attachment being anatomic. **(C)** Tibial attachment moved 10 mm distally, the femoral attachment being anatomic. **(D)** Femoral attachment moved 10 mm distally, the tibial attachment being anatomic.

positioning of the femoral attachment sites is more critical than that of the tibial sites. Variation along the line of the femoral link/notch roof has more an effect on graft strain than does movement superior or inferior to this line. The observed change in length of a nonisometrically placed graft may be proportionally greater from 90° to 140° than from extension up to 90°.

In repairing the MCL, it is important that the structure is not reattached to either femur or tibia short of its normal insertion site, since this may result in considerable lengthening with flexion.

GEOMETRY OF THE MUSCLE TENDONS

To investigate the mechanics of the knee and thus describe the loads that individual ligaments have to carry, it is necessary to study the geometry of the muscle tendons in addition to studying the geometry of the ligaments and articular surfaces just described. We have seen that the directions of the ligaments change systematically and predictably during flexion/extension (Figs. 10-4 and 10-5). So also do the lines of action

of the forces that they transmit. The point of contact between the femur and the tibia moves backward on the tibia during flexion (Figs. 10-8, 10-9, and 10-16). So also does the line of action of the tibiofemoral contact force. For the mechanical analysis of the joint we also need to describe the way in which the lines of action of the extensor and flexor muscles at the knee move with flexion.

To keep the description as simple as possible, we shall combine the separate heads of quadriceps, gastrocnemius, and hamstrings, the main muscle groups that span the knee. Each of the three muscle groups is represented by a single line, namely, the line of action of the resultant force which it transmits across the knee. Models of the tendons are shown in the computer-drawn diagrams of the knee in Figs. 10-31 and 10-32 and will each be described separately.

The Hamstrings Tendon

Figure 10-31 shows the model bones of Figs. 10-15 and 10-16 in three positions, with the addition of lines rep-

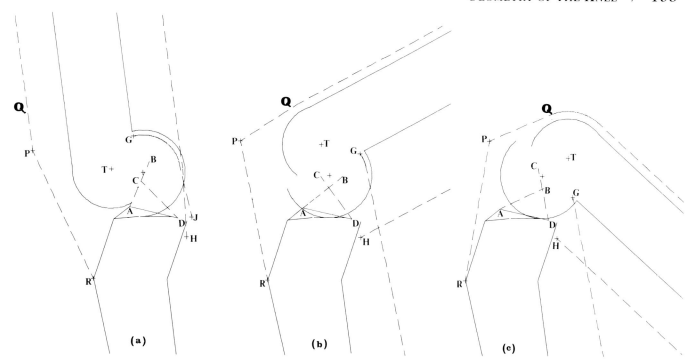

FIG. 10-31. Models of the muscle tendons added to the model bones of Fig. 10-15 and to the cruciate ligaments of Fig. 10-3. Details are described in the text.

resenting the muscle tendons. The hamstrings tendon is attached to the model tibia at a point *H* posteriorly and distally from the plateau. The point *H* was taken as a compromise between the attachments of semimembranosis and biceps. Its coordinates are parameters of the model, given in the appendix to this chapter. The tendon is taken to lie parallel to the femur over the range of flexion. The direction of the hamstrings force applied to the tibia changes over the flexion arc, as indicated by the three diagrams of Fig. 10-31 and the superposed diagrams of Fig. 10-32. Near full extension (Fig. 10-31a), the model tendon makes contact with the back of the femoral condyle, like semimembranosis, rather than running forward along the outer edge of the femoral condyle, like biceps. In Fig. 10-31a, the tendon therefore changes its direction slightly as it passes over the back of the condyle. It lies within the outline of the femoral condyle (the effective tendon thickness parameter is therefore given as negative in the appendix).

The Gastrocnemius Tendon

The gastrocnemius tendon is shown in Figs. 10-31 and 10-32 as a single line connecting the point *G* at the back of the femoral condyle to a point (off the diagram) representing the attachment of the Achilles tendon to the heel. The tendon is shown, within the outline of the model femoral condyle in Figs. 10-31a and b, to represent a line of action of the resultant gastrocnemius force passing between the two femoral condyles of the human knee. (The tendon thickness is given a negative value in the appendix.) Near extension (Fig. 10-31a), the line of action of the tendon passes through the point *J*, where it touches the back of the tibial plateau. At high flexion angles (Fig. 10-31c) the tendon loses contact with the back of the femoral condyle and passes directly from its femoral attachment to the heel.

Although the gastrocnemius muscles lie more or less parallel to the back of the tibia, the diagrams of Figs. 10-31 and 10-32 suggest a small but significant change in direction during flexion/extension, due in part to the rolling movement of the femur on the tibia (Fig. 10-16).

The coordinates of the attachment of the tendon to the back of the foot are parameters of the model. Values are given in the appendix.

The Quadriceps Mechanism and the Patellofemoral Joint

Based on Fig. 10-13, the sulcus of the trochlear groove, which guides the patella over the femur in the sagittal plane, is taken to be circular. In the simplest model of the quadriceps mechanism in Figs. 10-31 and 10-32, the patella is taken to be a single point, *P*, at which the patellar tendon *RP* intersects the quadriceps tendon *QP*. It moves on a circular arc about the center, *T*, of the circle representing the trochlea. *P* is the point at which the forces applied to the patella by the quadriceps and patellar tendons intersect. The only other significant force applied to the patella in the sagittal

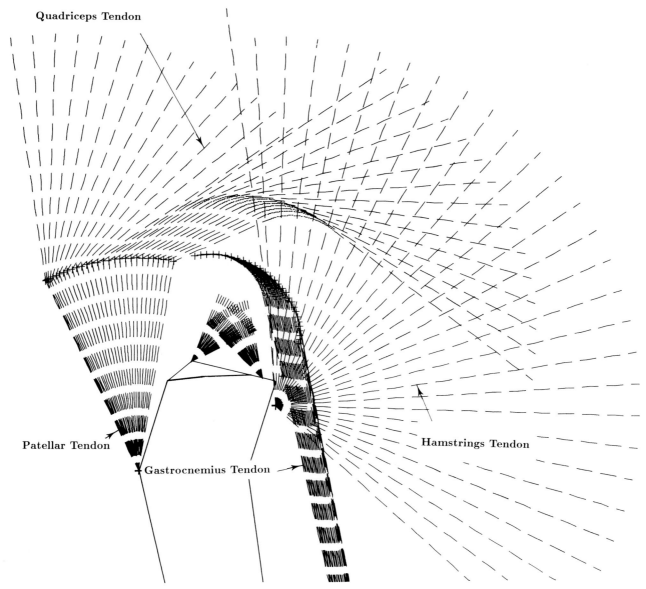

Quadriceps Tendon

Patellar Tendon

Gastrocnemius Tendon

Hamstrings Tendon

FIG. 10-32. The model tibia with superimposed images of the cruciate ligaments and muscle tendons during flexion ranging from 0° to 140°, demonstrating the changing directions of the tendons during flexion/extension.

plane is the patellofemoral force, which, for equilibrium of the patella, must also pass through the point of intersection of the two tendon forces. The radial line *PT* is taken to be the line of action of the patellofemoral contact force, always perpendicular to the trochlea.

The point *P* in the model should be interpreted as the "center of force" of the patella. It is connected to the tibia through the patellar tendon, attached at the tibial tubercle *R*. Near extension (Fig. 10-31a), the quadriceps tendon *QP* leaves the patella parallel to the femur. At about 70–80° (Fig. 10-31b), such a line of action begins to intersect the femur; at higher flexion angles (Fig. 10-31c), the tendon wraps around the surface of the trochlea to form the "tendofemoral" joint.

Although the importance of the tendofemoral joint was stressed by Goodfellow (15) and by Bishop (3), it does not appear to have been considered in subsequent analyses of patellofemoral mechanics.

The coordinates of the tibial tubercle on the tibia, the length of the patellar tendon, the thickness of the quadriceps tendon where it contacts the front of the femur, the coordinates of the center of the trochlea and the radii of the trochlea, and the patellar force center are parameters of the model. Values are given in the appendix.

This model of the quadriceps mechanism is not intended to describe the details of the mechanics of the patella, but, from the point of view of the mechanics of the knee, it reproduces two important features of the natural joint. Because the angle *QPT* between the quadriceps tendon and the line of action of the patellofemoral force is not equal to the angle *RPT* between the patellar tendon and the patellofemoral force, the two tendon forces cannot be equal and the patellofemoral joint does not behave like a simple frictionless pulley. Maquet (27,28) came to this conclusion by arguing that the lever-arms available to the quadriceps and patellar tendon forces are not equal. The deduction has been confirmed experimentally by Bishop (3), Ellis (13), Huberti (19), and Buff (8). In Fig. 10-33a, we plot our calculated patellofemoral/patellar tendon angle (angle *RPT* in Fig. 10-31) and patellofemoral/quadriceps tendon angle (*QPT*, Fig. 10-31) against flexion angle. The total included angle *QPR* between the tendons [called by Buff (8) the patellar mechanism angle] is also plotted against flexion angle and compared with direct measurements made on cadaver specimens by Buff (8). The discontinuity in slope of the graph, reproducing the experimental data, arises because the angle between the quadriceps tendon and the line of action of the patellofemoral force remains constant

with increasing flexion once the tendofemoral joint is formed. The angle subtended by the quadriceps tendon at the center of the trochlear groove, the angle of wrap of the tendon around the front of the femur, was calculated from the computer model and is also plotted against flexion in Fig. 10-33a.

In Fig. 10-33b, we plot our calculated values of the ratio of patellar tendon to quadriceps tendon forces against flexion. The graph includes data extracted from the four references just cited. The calculated result agrees well with the experimental data.

A second feature of quadriceps geometry reproduced by the model which has important mechanical implication is that the patellar tendon rotates about the tibial tubercle during flexion and extension, due in part to the rolling of the femur on the tibia and in part to the cam-like action of the trochlea as it rotates about the flexion axis. Malcolm (26) and O'Connor (34–36) have shown that the changing directions of the muscle tendons determine which of the cruciate ligaments is loaded during active extension/flexion. Blick (4) measured the backward movement of the patella relative to the tibia over 90° of flexion in specimens stabilized

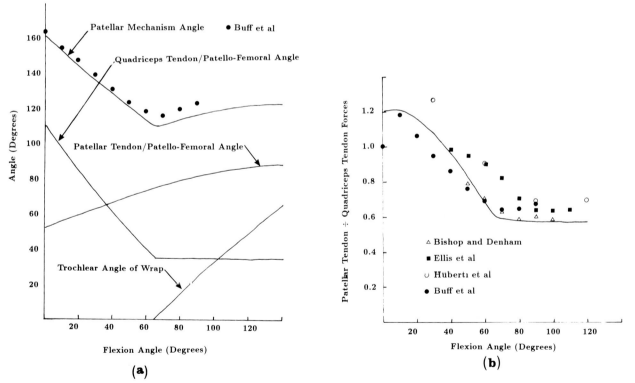

FIG. 10-33. (a) Flexion angle plotted against the angles between the line of action of the patellofemoral contact force and the patellar and quadriceps tendons, as well as against the total patellar mechanism angle and against the angle of wrap of the tendofemoral joint. Experimental measurements of the patellar mechanism angle were extracted from Buff (8). (b) Ratio of the patellar tendon to quadriceps forces plotted against flexion angle. Solid line is calculated from the computer model. Experimental points were obtained from Bishop (3), Ellis (13), Huberti (19), and Buff (8). The tendon forces can be equal only when the tendon angles are equal, that is, at about 37°.

by tension in the quadriceps tendon. He reported a movement of 40 mm as compared with the movement of 35 mm indicated by the computer model in Figs. 10-31 and 10-32.

Limitation of Extension

Finally, it is necessary to take explicit account of the action of the posterior capsule in limiting extension. It was modeled as a single line element connected to the back of the tibia at *J* and passing over the rear of the femoral condyle to its attachment at *G* (Fig. 10-34). In

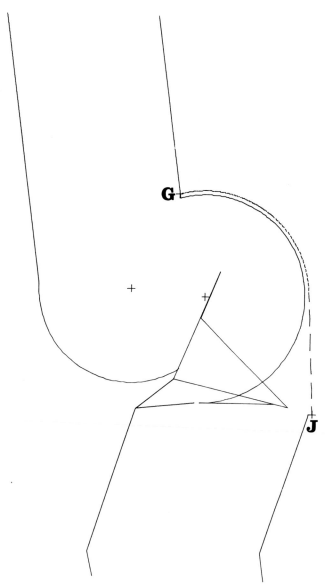

FIG. 10-34. Model of the posterior capsule. The capsule is attached to the back of the femur at *G* and to the back of the tibia at *J*. It is taken to be nonlinearly elastic. It begins to tighten when extension is approached and offers infinite resistance to stretching (i.e., becomes rigid) in hyperextension.

the mechanical analysis described in the next chapter, the capsule is taken to be slack in flexion. As extension is approached, it begins to tighten, offering increasing resistance to extension. The addition of the link representing the tight capsule converts the mobile cruciate linkage of Figs. 10-4 and 10-5 into a rigid structure incapable of further gross movement into extension. This structure allows further movements of the bones into hyperextension only to the extent permitted by indentation of the articular surfaces and/or stretching of ligaments and capsule. The angles at which the capsule begins to tighten and at which it becomes effectively rigid are parameters of the model. This model of the posterior capsule is a good demonstration of the way in which the ligaments can limit the range of allowable movements of the bones.

VALIDATION OF THE MODEL AND ITS PARAMETERS

In the description of the development of the model of the knee, certain quantities were called *parameters*. The lengths of the ligaments, the positions on each bone of their attachments, the positions of the point of insertion of the muscle tendon, and so on, are parameters of the model. A complete list of the 49 parameters needed to draw the various diagrams of the model knee is given in the appendix.

How were the values of the parameters chosen? An initial set of parameters was based on measurements made on cadaver specimens, as described in the appendix. The computer model was then used to calculate the values of other variables. We have already described the results of some of these calculations: the shape of the femoral condyle (Figs. 10-8 and 10-9), movements of the femur on the tibia (Fig. 10-10), strain patterns within individual ligaments (Figs. 10-19 and 10-23), patellar mechanism angle, and the ratio of patellar tendon to quadriceps tendon forces (Fig. 10-33). In the next chapter we shall report the results of calculations of muscle and ligament forces in a number of configurations, and those calculations are compared with measurements in Chapter 12. The parameters of the model were adjusted until ʾsonable agreement was obtained between calculations and the wide variety of measurement just described, both geometrical and mechanical.

The final values of the 49 parameters listed in the appendix therefore encapsulate a large body of experimental observation on the cadaver human knee. This method of validation of the model demonstrates the essential role of experiment in the development of a theory. The discussion of Fig. 10-10 above also demonstrates the insight to be gained even from the shortcomings of a theoretical model. We have used the theory to interpret the very large body of experimental work on strain patterns within individual ligaments, and, in describing measurements of muscle and ligament forces in Chapter 12, we shall use the theory to help interpret the results of experiments. Theory feeds on experiment and experiment feeds on theory.

However, Table 10-1 shows the values the basic cruciate linkage parameters as measured on each of four specimens. It will be seen that there is significant variation from specimen to specimen. It is therefore unlikely that a single set of parameters would fit every specimen. In order to make predictions for a particular knee, it would be necessary to measure the parameters directly for that knee. The list given in the appendix represents a set of values that yield qualitative predictions of the behavior of the knee, with some quantitative validity.

Once the model is validated, and its limitations clearly defined, it can be used with some confidence to calculate quantities not directly measurable. In Chapter 14, we describe the use of the model to calculate the values of ligament forces during level walking. The model has clinical application: the discussion of the relationship between ligament and articular surface geometry has clear application to prosthesis design, which cannot be developed further in this book; moreover, the discussion of ligament anisometry can be used to guide the ligament surgeon in the optimal placement of grafts or ligament prostheses.

DISCUSSION

A two-dimensional model of the knee must suffer from the defect that it fails to account for the obligatory axial rotations which always accompany flexion/extension and which cannot fail to influence the tensions in all the ligamentous structures that cross the joint cleft. However, apart from the discrepancies noted in the discussion of Figs. 10-10, 10-18, 10-19, and 10-20 above, it appears that the influence of these rotations is, in fact, secondary to the geometry and mechanics of the knee in the sagittal plane. The primary determinant of sagittal plane geometry and movement is the cruciate linkage of Fig. 10-3. It is remarkable that a process of logic which requires as its predicates only the dimensions of the straight-line planar cruciate linkage (the parameters) can be used to deduce the shapes of the femoral and tibial articular surfaces, predict the pattern of their rolling and sliding movements upon each other, and even foretell the changing pattern of strain within all the ligaments that span the joint.

Of course, there is a circularity in the argument. If we were given the shapes of the natural articular surfaces and the pattern of their rolling and sliding relative movements, then the parameters of the cruciate linkage which would match them could be deduced. This was, to some extent, the approach taken by Crowninshield (9) and Wismans (46). Why, then, do we stress the overriding importance of the design of the cruciate linkage and regard the articular surface shapes as secondary and dependent? The reason is that nothing very useful can be deduced from the description of the shapes of the surfaces unless one also knows the pattern of their movements (the slip ratio, Fig. 10-14). The shapes of the articular surfaces do not determine the slip ratio any more than they determine the axis of flexion. They represent nothing more than one solution to the problem of keeping the neutral fibers of the cruciate ligaments uniformly tight over the range of movements, a problem that could be solved by any of an infinite number of pairs of surfaces.

Within its obvious limitations, the results of theoretical modeling have demonstrated how, with a minimum of anatomical measurement (49 parameters), it is possible to gain insight into the relationship between the geometry of the ligaments, the geometry of the articular surfaces, and the geometry of the muscle tendons. A purely experimental descriptive approach, which can involve the acquisition of thousands of pieces of data (39), may give a more precise picture of the behavior of an individual specimen but does not yield reasons for that behavior.

Our study of the geometry of the knee in the sagittal plane has demonstrated the central role of the ligaments. In the next chapter, we shall show that the ligaments are also the key to understanding the mechanics of the joint.

APPENDIX: PARAMETER VALUES

The values of the parameters used in the calculations were based on anthropometric studies on four cadaver knees (6). Some of these measurements have been given in Table 10-1. Figures 10-25 through 10-30 were based directly on those measurements. A computer experiment was then performed, starting with the average values of the measurements. The values of the parameters were then adjusted until the results of calculations agreed reasonably well with further independent measurements on cadaver specimens, such as those in Figs. 10-9, 10-10, and 10-33. The final values of the parameters also reflect comparisons between calculations and measurements of muscle and ligament forces (35), as will be described in Chapters 11 and 12.

Specimens

Four fresh cadaveric adult male knee specimens were kept frozen until the time of dissection. The skin and soft tissues were removed down to the joint capsule and ligamentous structures, retaining the muscle tendons. With the exception of some minor degenerative changes in the patellofemoral joints of two of the specimens, there was no evidence of joint pathology. Anterior and posterior arthrotomies were performed to identify the cruciate ligaments that were stripped of their synovial covering. The femur was then sectioned sagittally through the intercondylar notch with a fine blade saw without injury to the cruciate attachments. The centers of the origins and insertions of the cruciates were each marked with a metal tack with a 2-mm head. The osteotomized femur was anatomically reduced and held with cross bolts. Metal tacks were also used to mark the attachment sites of the MCL and LCL and the insertions of the muscle tendons. A 5- to 6-N load was applied to the quadriceps tendon to place the knee in extension. Then x-rays of the specimens were taken, with one view containing a radio-opaque metal rule at the level of the intercondylar notch to assess magnification of the image. The specimens were disarticulated and the ligament and tendon attachments dissected to check the positions of the markers relative to centers of the attachment sites. Measurements were made if, on dissection, a tack was not centrally located within the bony attachment site of the ligament.

In the list that follows, lengths are given in centimeters and angles are given in degrees. Coordinates of points are quoted as pairs of numbers, measured in centimeters. On the tibia, distances are measured from an origin at the tibial attachment of the ACL (point A in Figs. 10-3 through 10-8). The first coordinate is the distance from the origin along an axis parallel to the tibial plateau (positive distances measured toward the back of the joint). The second coordinate is the distance perpendicular to the tibial plateau (positive distances measured upward). On the femur, distances are measured from an origin at the femoral insertion of the PCL (point C in Figs. 10-3 through 10-8). The first coordinate is the distance (cm) along the femoral link toward B, and the second coordinate is the distance perpendicular to CB, measured positively upward.

The cruciate linkage and the articular surfaces (Figs. 10-3 through 10-8)

Length of tibial link, AD:	3.05
Length of ACL AB:	2.99
Length of femoral link BC:	1.28
Length of PCL CD:	3.22
Distance of flat tibial surface below origin A (Fig. 10-8):	0.60

Angle of femoral link at full extension (Fig. 10-4a):	80.00
Inclination of tibial link to tibial plateau (Fig. 10-8):	13.00
Radius of convex tibial plateau (Fig. 10-9a):	7.50
Center of convex tibial plateau:	0.93, −7.80
Radius of concave tibial plateau (Fig. 10-9b):	8.75
Center of concave tibial plateau:	1.50, 8.10
Tibial attachment of "anatomic" MCL (Fig. 10-18):	1.30, −5.75
Femoral attachment of "anatomic" MCL (Fig. 10-18):	0.33, 0.69
Tibial attachment of "anatomic" LCL (Fig. 10-18):	1.90, −1.90
Femoral attachment of "anatomic" LCL (Fig. 10-18):	1.11, 0.20
Tibial attachment of "isometric" MCL (Fig. 10-20):	0.30, −5.40
Femoral attachment of "isometric" MCL (Fig. 10-20):	0.70, 0.40
Tibial attachment of "isometric" LCL (Fig. 10-20):	2.70, 2.50
Femoral attachment of "isometric" LCL (Fig. 10-20):	0.20, 0.20

Models of bones (Fig. 10-15):

Diameters of femoral and tibial shafts:	3.35
Radius of patellofemoral facet:	2.40
Center of patellofemoral facet on femur:	−0.05, 1.95
Posterior edge of tibial plateau:	3.50, −0.85
Intersection of tibial axis and plateau:	0.00, 0.00
Anterior edge of tibial plateau:	−1.00, −0.75
Tibial tubercle:	−2.20, −4.40

Muscle tendons (Fig. 10-31)

Radius of patellar force center:	5.00
Insertion of hamstrings on tibia:	3.50, −1.80
Insertion of gastrocnemius on calcaneous:	12.30, −38.70
Thickness of quadriceps tendon:	0.47
Thickness of hamstrings tendon:	−0.15
Thickness of gastrocnemius tendon:	−0.30

ACKNOWLEDGMENT

The work reported here was supported by the Arthritis and Rheumatism Council, 41 Eagle Street, London. J. Bradley was supported by a one-year fellowship from the Leverhulme Trust.

REFERENCES

1. Arms S, Boyle J, Johnson R, Pope M. Strain measurement in the medial collateral ligament of the human knee—an autopsy study. *J Biomech* 1983;16:491–496.
2. Arms SW, Renstrom P, Stanwyck TS, Hogan M, Johnson RJ, Pope MH. Strain within the anterior cruciate during hamstrings and quadriceps activity. *Trans Orthop Res Soc* 1985;31:139.
3. Bishop RED, Denham RA. A note on the ratio between tensions in the quadriceps tendon and infra-patellar ligament. *Eng Med* 1977;6:53–54.
4. Blick SS, personal communication.
5. Borelli GA. *De motu animalium.* Lugdunic Bavorum, 1679. P. Marquet, translator. *On the movement of animals.* Berlin: Springer-Verlag, 1989.
6. Bradley J, FitzPatrick D, Daniel D, Shercliff T, O'Connor J. The evaluation of cruciate ligament orientation in the sagittal plane—a method of predicting length change vs. knee flexion. *J Bone Joint Surg [Br]* 1988;70B:94–99.
7. Brantigan OC, Voshell AF. The mechanics of the ligaments and menisci of the knee joint. *J Bone Joint Surg [Am]* 1941;23A:44–66.
8. Buff H-U, Jones LC, Hungerford DS. Experimental determination of forces transmitted through the patello-femoral joint. *J Biomech* 1988;21:17–23.
9. Crowninshield R, Pope MH, Johnson RJ. An analytical model of the knee. *J Biomech* 1976;9:397–405.
10. Daniel D, Penner D, Burks R. Anterior cruciate graft isometry and tensioning. In: Friedman M, Ferkel R, eds. *Prosthetic knee ligament reconstruction.* New York: Grune and Stratton, 1987.
11. Deane G. Contact print studies in the human knee joint. M.Sc. thesis, University of Surrey, 1970.
12. Draganich LF, Andersson GBJ, Andriacchi TP, Galante JO. The influence of the cruciate ligaments on femoro-tibial contact movement during knee flexion. *Trans Orthop Res Soc* 1984;30:29.
13. Ellis MI, Seedhom BB, Wright V, Dowson D. An evaluation of the ratio between the tensions along the quadriceps tendon and the patellar ligament. *Eng Med* 1981;9:189–194.
14. Fick R. Anatomie und mechanic der gelewke unter berucksichtigung der bewengenden mulken. In: von Berdeleken K, ed. *Handbuck der anatomie des munschen,* Bd. 11, Teil III. Jena: Fisher, 1911.
15. Goodfellow JW, Hungerford D, Zindel M. Patello-femoral joint mechanics and pathology. I. Functional anatomy *J Bone Joint Surg [Br]* 1976;58B:283–287.
16. Goodfellow J, O'Connor J. The mechanics of the knee and prosthesis design. *J Bone Joint Surg [Br]* 1978;60B:358–369.
17. Goodfellow JW, O'Connor JJ. Clinical results of the Oxford Knee. *Clin Orthop* 1986;205:21–42.
18. Harding ML, Harding L, Goodfellow JW. A preliminary report of a simple rig to aid the study of the functional anatomy of the cadaver knee joint. *J Biomech* 1977;10:517–523.
19. Huberti HH, Hayes WC, Stone JL, Shybut GT. Force ratio in the quadriceps tendon and ligamentum patellae. *J Orthop Res* 1984;2:49–54.
20. Huson A. Biomechanische probleme des kniegelenks. *Orthopade* 1974;3:119–126.
21. Kapandji I. *The physiology of the joints,* vol 2. Edinburgh: Churchill Livingstone, 1970.
22. Kennedy JC, Hawkins RJ, Willis RB. Strain gauge analysis of knee ligaments. *Clin Orthop* 1977;129:225–229.
23. Kurosawa H, Walker PS, Abe S, Garg A, Hunter T. Geometry and motion of the knee for implant and orthotic design. *J Biomech* 1985;18:487–499.
24. Lew WD, Lewis JL. The effect of knee prosthesis geometry on cruciate ligament mechanics during flexion. *J Bone Joint Surg [Am]* 1982;64A:734–739.
25. MacIntosh DL, Tregonning RJ. A follow-up study and evaluation of "over-the-top" repair of acute tears of the anterior cruciate ligament. *J Bone Joint Surg [Br]* 1977;59B:511.
26. Malcolm L, Daniel D. A mechanical substitution technique for cruciate ligament force determinations. *Trans Orthop Res Soc* 1980;26:303.
27. Maquet P. Advancement of the tibial tuberosity. *Clin Orthop* 1969;115:225–230.
28. Maquet PGJ. *Biomechanics of the knee.* Berlin: Springer-Verlag, 1976.
29. Menschik A. Mechanik des knielgelenks, Teil 1. *Z Orthop* 1974;113:481–495.
30. Moore TM, Harvey JP. Rheontgenographic measurement of tibial plateau depression due to fracture. *J Bone Joint Surg [Am]* 1974;56A:155–160.
31. Müller W. *The knee: form, function and ligament reconstruction.* Berlin: Springer-Verlag, 1983.
32. Norwood LA, Cross MJ. Anterior cruciate ligament: functional anatomy of its bundles in rotary instabilities. *Am J Sports Med* 1979;7:23–26.
33. O'Brien WR, Friederich NF, Müller W, Henning CE. Functional anatomy of the cruciates and their substitutes. Scientific basis for clinical application. To be published, 1990.
34. O'Connor J, Goodfellow J, Biden E. Designing the human knee. in: Stokes IAF, ed. *Mechanical factors and the skeleton.* London: John Libbey, 1981;52–64.
35. O'Connor JJ, Goodfellow JW, Young SK, Biden E, Daniel D. Mechanical interactions between the muscles and the cruciate ligaments in the knee. *Trans Orthop Res Soc* 1985;31:140.
36. O'Connor J, Shercliff T, Goodfellow J. Mechanics of the knee in the sagittal plane—mechanical interactions between the muscles and the ligaments. In: Müller W, Hackenbruch W, eds. *Surgery and arthroscopy of the knee.* Berlin: Springer-Verlag, 1988;12–30.
37. Odensten M, Gillquist J. Functional anatomy of the anterior cruciate ligament and a rationale for reconstruction. *J Bone Joint Surg [Am]* 1985;67A:257–262.
38. Rehder U. Morphological studies on the symmetry of the hman knee joint: femoral condyles. *J Biomech* 1982;16:351–361.
39. Sidles JA, Larson RV, Garbini JL, Downey DJ, Matson FA. Ligament length relationships in the moving knee. *J Orthop Res* 6:593–610.
40. Steindler A. *Kinesiology of the human body under normal and pathological conditions.* Springfield, IL: Charles C Thomas, 1955.
41. Strasser H. *Lehrbuch der muskel und gelenkmechanik,* III. Berlin. Springer, 1917.
42. Walker PS, Hajek JV. The load bearing area in the knee joint. *J Biomech* 1972;5:581–589.
43. Walker PS, Shoji H, Erkman MJ. The rotational axis of the knee and its significance to prosthesis design. *Clin Orthop* 1972;89:160–170.
44. Wang C-J, Walker PS. The effects of flexion and rotation on the length patterns of the ligaments of the knee. *J Biomech* 1973;6:487–496.
45. Weber W, Weber E. *Mechanik der menschlichen genverkzenge.* Gottingen, 1836.
46. Wismans J, Veldpaus F, Janssen J, Huson A, Struben P. A three-dimensional mathematical model of the knee joint. *J Biomech* 1980;13:677–685.

CHAPTER 11

Mechanics of the Knee

John O'Connor, Tessa Shercliff, David FitzPatrick, Edmund Biden, and John Goodfellow

Our purpose in this chapter is to discuss the forces transmitted by the ligaments of the knee when the leg is subjected to external loads (e.g., those applied by gravity and the reaction force between the foot and the ground) while the knee is being stabilized by one of the three main muscle groups: quadriceps, hamstrings, or gastrocnemius. The bulk of the discussion is con-

cerned with sagittal plane mechanics, but an introduction to coronal plane mechanics is given at the end.

In Chapter 10, we have seen something of the geometric relationships between muscles and ligaments. In this chapter, we will show that mechanical interactions between muscles and ligaments occur for a number of reasons (28). In the sagittal plane, the geometry of the ligaments defines not only the geometric center but also the mechanical center of the joint, the point about which both muscle forces and external loads exert their leverage. The geometry of the ligaments therefore determines whether flexor or extensor action is necessary to balance any given external load. The direction of the force applied by each muscle group changes during flexion (Fig. 10-32), so that the

J. O'Connor, T. Shercliff, and D. FitzPatrick: Department of Engineering Science, University of Oxford, Oxford OX1 3PJ, England.
E. Biden: Department of Mechanical Engineering, University of New Brunswick, Fredericton, New Brunswick, Canada E3B 5A3.
J. Goodfellow: Department of Orthopaedic Surgery, Nuffield Orthopaedic Centre, Oxford OX3 7LD, England.

balance of forces between external loads and muscles can require loading of different ligaments in different positions. The direction of the external load also influences the loading of the ligaments.

LOADS

The main mechanical function of the musculoskeletal system is to support its own weight. Muscle action is necessary for such support. Muscle action is also necessary to initiate or maintain movement. Loading of the joints of the leg is largest when that leg is in contact with the ground.

During ground contact, the forces applied to the foot by the ground (the ground reaction) serve mainly to balance the weight of the body, but they also serve to accelerate and decelerate the body. If the ground reaction is known (i.e., from force plate measurements; see Chapter 14), the forces transmitted across the knee can be analyzed by considering the mechanics of the lower leg, from the joint cleft of the knee down to the ground. We then regard the ground reaction as the main load applied to the shank through the sole of the foot. We then have to consider the response at the joint in the form of forces transmitted by the ligaments, by contact between the articular surfaces of the bones, and by the muscles and their tendons.

CRUCIATE LIGAMENT FORCES

In Chapter 10, we based the computer model of the knee on the four-bar linkage comprising the femur, the tibia, and the neutral fibers of the cruciate ligaments. We shall now assume that the directions of those neutral fibers define the lines of action of the tension forces transmitted by the cruciate ligaments. We note therefore that the directions of the cruciate forces change during flexion/extension in a systematic and calculable way (Figs. 10-4 and 10-5). Because the cruciate ligaments intersect at the flexion axis of the joint (Fig. 10-5), so also do the lines of action of the forces that they transmit. Forces that pass through the flexion axis cannot, by themselves, induce or resist extension or flexion. In the language of mechanics, such forces have no moment or turning effect about the flexion axis.

TIBIOFEMORAL CONTACT FORCE

In Fig. 10-7, we showed that the line perpendicular to both articular surfaces at their point of contact, the common normal, also passes through the flexion axis. Since there is negligible friction between the articular surfaces (9), the resultant contact force transmitted between them must be purely compressive, with its line

of action lying along that common normal and therefore passing through the flexion axis, where it intersects the lines of action of the cruciate forces. The contact force also has no moment about the flexion axis. It moves backwards and forwards on the tibial plateau as the femur rolls on the tibia during flexion/extension (Figs. 10-8 and 10-16).

NON-TURNING LOADS

The tibiofemoral contact force and the cruciate forces therefore all intersect at the flexion axis (Fig. 11-1). They have no turning moment about that axis and cannot by themselves induce or resist flexion or extension. On the other hand, they are sufficient in themselves to balance a "non-turning" load, a load applied to the leg in the sagittal plane whose line of action also passes through the flexion axis. Just like the effect of a load passing through the center of the femoral head at the hip (Fig. 10-1), such a load can cause neither flexion nor extension. At the knee, a non-turning load can be balanced by some combination of cruciate and tibiofemoral contact forces, without muscle action. Mus-

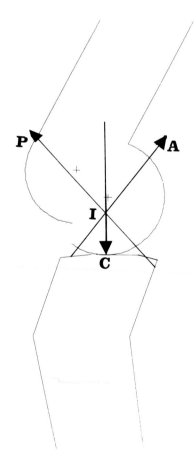

FIG. 11-1. The cruciate ligament forces **A** and **P** and the tibiofemoral contact force **C** intersect at the flexion axis **I**. They have no moment about that axis.

cle action is necessary only if the line of action of the load does not pass through the flexion axis.

THE MECHANICAL CENTER OF THE KNEE

The intersection of the cruciates, through which the flexion axis of the knee passes, therefore defines the mechanical center of the joint in the sagittal plane. If the line of action of the foot/ground reaction passes anterior to the flexion axis, it tends to extend the knee; flexor action, from the hamstrings or the gastrocnemius muscles, is necessary to stabilize the limb. If the line of action of the foot/ground reaction passes posterior to the flexion axis, it tends to flex the knee; extensor action, from the quadriceps muscles, is necessary for equilibrium. The perpendicular distance of the line of action of the load from the flexion axis is a direct measure of its tendency to extend or flex the joint and defines the length of the lever-arm of the load. The lever-arm of the load is zero when the load passes through the flexion axis, and the load then has neither a flexing nor an extending effect.

We showed in Chapter 10 that the mechanical center of the hip is defined by the geometry of the bones and remains fixed relative to them. The knee is more complicated because its mechanical center is defined by the geometry of the ligaments and moves, during flexion and extension, relative both to the bones and to the ligaments.

MUSCLE LEVER-ARMS

Having established that an external load can induce flexion or extension at the knee only if its line of action does not pass through the flexion axis, we can argue in the same way that a muscle can induce or resist flexion or extension at the knee only if its line of action does not pass through the flexion axis. The intrinsic lever-arm or moment-arm of a muscle is the distance perpendicular to its line of action from the intersection of the cruciates, as indicated in Fig. 11-2. Figure 11-3 shows the lengths of the lever arms of the quadriceps tendon, the patellar tendon, and the tendons of hamstrings and gastrocnemius, as calculated from the computer model of Chapter 10, plotted against flexion angle. The lever-arm lengths vary with flexion because the flexion axis moves and because the directions of each of the tendons change. Since the geometry of the ligaments defines the position of the flexion axis and to some extent controls the directions of the muscle tendons as they span the knee, it can be said that the geometry of the ligaments defines the leverage available to the muscles.

Grant (15) pointed out the mechanical significance of the instant center of the temporomandibular joint.

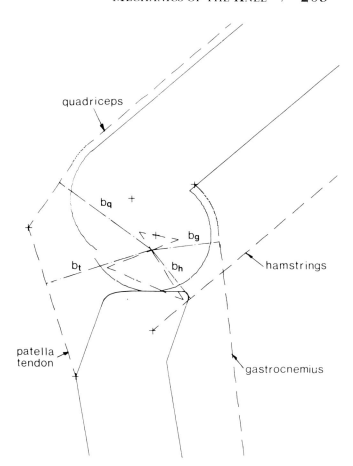

FIG. 11-2. The lever-arms b_q of the quadriceps, b_t of the patellar tendon, b_g of the gastrocnemii, and b_h of hamstrings—the perpendicular distances from the instant center to each of the muscle tendons.

He measured the lever-arms of the muscles with respect to the instant center, which moves with respect to the bones in such a way that "each muscle has its greatest effectiveness in the position in which it is known to function." Smidt (33) defined the lever-arms of the extensors and flexors at the knee to be the perpendicular distances from the instant center of joint to the tendons. To find the instant center in a number of positions of flexion in living patients, he used the method of Rouleaux described by Frankel (13); he then measured lever-arms from x-ray pictures. His analysis of eccentric, isometric, and concentric contractions of quadriceps and hamstrings threw much light on the mechanics of the joint. He did not, however, relate the instant center to the geometry of the ligaments or discuss their role in load-bearing.

Baratta (2, fig. 3) plotted quadriceps and hamstrings lever-arms against flexion angle, using data from others (18,20,32). Our calculation of the lever-arm of the hamstrings is in close accord with his results, and our quadriceps lever-arm follows a similar variation with flexion angle; however, our values near extension are about 10% higher.

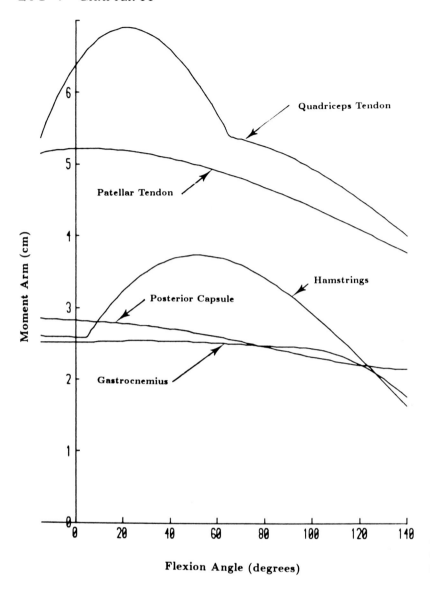

FIG. 11-3. Variation of the lever-arms of the muscle tendons with flexion angle. Also included is the lever-arm of the posterior capsule, the perpendicular distance from the instant center to the capsule (Fig. 10-34).

Grood (16) attempted to determine the length of the quadriceps lever-arm experimentally by dividing the measured flexing moment (product of the measured applied load times its lever-arm from the tibiofemoral contact point) by the measured quadriceps force. As we shall show, this approach cannot take account of the increasing antagonistic effect of the posterior capsule as extension is approached. His values near extension were as low as 1.5–2.5 cm. He quoted (16, fig. 8) Bandi (1), who found values of the quadriceps lever-arm varying from 5 cm at extension and 90° to 6 cm at 30°, much closer to our calculated values.

Despite Smidt's lead, others (4,5,8,11,16,24) defined the lever-arms of the muscles to be the perpendicular distances from the tibiofemoral contact point to the muscle tendons and they estimated those distances from x-ray pictures. Draganich (10) measured patellar tendon leverage from the center of pressure of the tibiofemoral contact areas on the tibial plateau, detected in each position using pressure-sensitive film. His methods of measurement took explicit account of the movement of the contact areas and the changing directions of the muscle tendons but, although the errors involved are not likely to be large, they ignored the moments of the ligament forces about the contact point. Some authors (4,24,33) calculated the values of the resultant shear forces parallel to the tibial plateau which they assumed to be carried by the ligaments. This approach ignores the components of the ligament forces perpendicular to the tibial plateau and therefore underestimates the value of the tibiofemoral contact force.

THE DRAWER TEST

From the point of view of the clinical testing of ligament integrity, the non-turning loads described above have an important application, namely, the drawer test or anteroposterior laxity test. We defined a non-turning load as a load with a line of action passing through the flexion axis and therefore not requiring muscle action.

In performing the drawer test, the leg is placed with the knee flexed to 90° and the muscles relaxed. Holding the top of the tibia in such a way as to maintain the flexion angle at 90°, the clinician slides the tibia backwards and forwards relative to the femur, sensing the range of anteroposterior movement allowed by the ligaments. Any increase from the normal range is usually attributed to ligament injury. In the Lachman test, the same procedure is followed but with the joint flexed to about 20°, sufficient to relax the posterior capsule.

Loads Applied in the Drawer Test

It is not easy to say precisely what loads are applied during this test. Piziali (29, fig. 5) found that, apart from an anteroposterior force, mediolateral and axial forces and moments about all three axes were necessary to achieve a pure anteroposterior translation of the tibia relative to the femur. We shall present here an analysis of the drawer test, which considers only the most important of these effects. In addition, our analysis does not account for the loads that the clinician has to apply to overcome the posterior subluxation of the tibia due to its own weight.

Figure 11-4a is a simple view of the forces applied to the tibia in the anterior drawer test. A force F pulls the tibia forward. Since the force is applied distal to the flexion axis of the knee, it tends to extend the joint. To maintain the flexion angle at 90° without muscle action, the clinician also has to apply a flexing moment M to the tibia. The combined effect of the force and the moment is equivalent to a force of the same magnitude and direction as F applied through the flexion axis (Fig. 11-4b), a non-turning force.

Ligament and Contact Forces; Inextensible Ligaments

The triangles of forces in Figs. 11-5a and b demonstrate that anterior and posterior drawer loads can be bal-

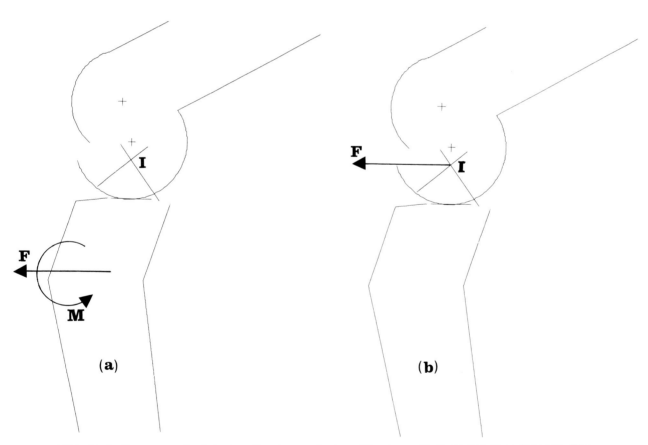

FIG. 11-4. Forces applied during the drawer test. **a:** The force **F** slides the tibia forward. The couple **M** is required to maintain the angle of flexion constant. **b:** The force and couple in part A are statically equivalent to a force **F** through the flexion axis **I**. (In the language of mechanics, the force **F** and the moment **M** applied to the tibia in Fig. 11-4a are "statically equivalent" or "equipollent" to a force of the same magnitude **F** applied at a distance *d* through the flexion axis (Fig. 11-4b), provided that **M** = **F***d*. The two systems of forces shown in Fig. 11-4a and b then have the same effect on the equilibrium of the tibia.)

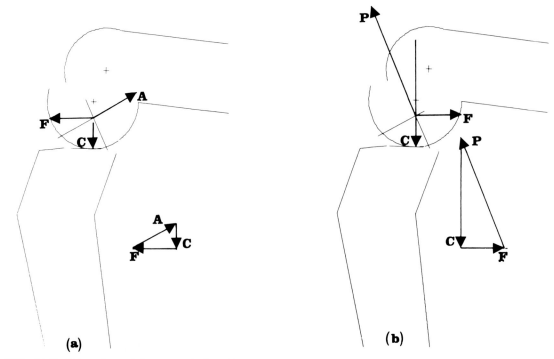

FIG. 11-5. Triangles of forces relating ligament and contact forces to applied load **F** for (**a**) anterior and (**b**) posterior tibial displacement tests.

anced at the knee by forces **A** or **P** [in the anterior cruciate ligament (ACL) or posterior cruciate ligament (PCL), respectively] plus a tibiofemoral contact force **C**. The components of the ligament forces parallel to the tibial plateau are, in both diagrams, equal to the applied drawer load **F**. However, since the ligaments do not lie exactly parallel to the plateau, they pull the tibia upwards against the femur. The contact force is then needed to push the tibia downwards, and in both pictures it has a value equal to the upwards pull of the ligament.

The directions of the ligaments change with flexion (Figs. 10-4 and 10-5), so that the relationships between the drawer load and the ligament and contact forces implied by Fig. 11-5 also depend on flexion angle. In calculating the ligament and contact forces, we start by using the ligament directions calculated at each position from the four-bar linkage of Chapter 10, assuming the ligaments to be inextensible. Although this calculation cannot account for joint laxity, it gives insight into the forces transmitted by the knee structures in the drawer test.

Results

The triangles of forces in Fig. 11-5 imply that the ligament and contact forces are each proportional to the

load: the bigger the load, the bigger the ligament and contact forces. It is therefore convenient to express the results nondimensionally and to plot ligament and contact forces per unit applied load against flexion angle (Fig. 11-6).

Ligament Forces

Figure 11-6 shows plots of the values of the anterior cruciate force per unit load and the contact force per unit load in the anterior drawer test, and the posterior cruciate and contact forces per unit load in the posterior drawer test. The forces vary with flexion angle because of the changing directions of the ligaments. In the fully flexed joint, the ACL is most nearly parallel to the tibial plateau (Fig. 10-8c). It is then nearly ideally aligned to resist forward displacement of the tibia; moreover, its upwards component, pulling the tibia against the femur, is small. The ACL force is virtually equal to the applied load, the ligament force per unit load is almost unity, and the contact force diminishes to zero. As extension is approached, the direction of the ligament becomes less ideal and the total ligament force has to grow to ensure that its component parallel to the plateau is equal to the applied load. The contact force also has to grow to balance the increasingly upwards component of the ligament force.

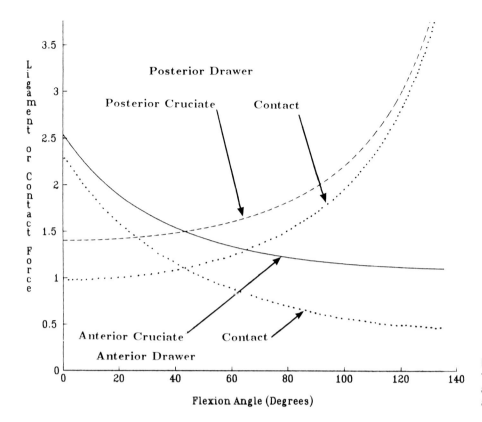

FIG. 11-6. Ligament and contact forces per unit applied load, plotted against flexion angle, for anterior and posterior drawer tests.

Almost the opposite considerations apply to the posterior drawer test. In the highly flexed joint, the PCL is almost perpendicular to the tibial plateau (Fig. 10-8c), a direction least ideal to resist posterior translation of the tibia. The PCL and contact forces are therefore very large in flexion but diminish as extension is approached because the PCL rotates towards the tibial plateau.

Using buckle transducers (Fig. 8-18), Hanley (17) measured the forces in the ACL during anterior drawer. Although the general shape of the measured force–flexion-angle curve was similar to that of Fig. 11-6, his ACL forces at higher flexion angles were substantially less than the applied load. In our view, his finding implies either that the collateral ligaments carry a much higher proportion of the applied anterior force than the values 15% (6) and 25% (30) previously estimated or that the transducer measures changes in values of the ligament force more accurately than it measures absolute values.

Clinical practice seems to have established the Lachman test, at 20° of flexion, as the more sensitive way of detecting ACL deficiency, whereas the posterior drawer test, at 90° of flexion, most sensitively detects PCL deficiency. These are the positions in which, in the intact joint, the ligament forces applied by the test would be expected to be largest (Fig. 11-6).

Contact Forces

We note that both forward and backward loading of the tibia in these tests involves the development of contact forces between the femur and the tibia. This may be why the results of the drawer test in arthritis can be misleading. Erosion of the articular surfaces by the disease process can render the ligaments slack, and the relationship implied by Fig. 10-7 between ligament geometry and articular surface shape is lost. Thus, in early arthritis before the ligaments have been damaged, a knee may exhibit increased anteroposterior translation because the ligaments are slack. In advanced arthritis, after the ligaments have been disrupted, osteophytes may inhibit anteroposterior movement of the bones and the joint might exhibit a normal range (or less) of anteroposterior translation. This interpretation may explain why no correlation was found between the results of the drawer test and the presence or absence of the ACL in arthritic knees (14). Laxity tests can be accurate tests of ligament integrity only if the articular surfaces are intact.

Shortcomings of the Inextensible Ligament Model

Our analysis of ligament and contact forces in the drawer test neglected the elastic nature of ligaments. We considered the static equilibrium of an inextensible ligament under the action of an applied load. Although this method gives some understanding of the mechanics of the drawer test and some idea of the magnitude of the ligament and contact forces, it is unable to provide any information about joint laxity. If we are to model the drawer test adequately, then the effect of ligament elasticity must also be included.

Furthermore, Piziali (30) and Butler (6) have shown that the ACL provides most (but not all) of the ligamentous restraint to anterior translation of the tibia. Our previous analysis could account for the contribution of only one ligament. To calculate the contribution of more than one ligament, the added complication of statical indeterminacy is introduced. The number of unknown forces exceeds the number of equilibrium equations available for their determination. A further complication is that the angles of the ligaments change significantly during anteroposterior movement of the tibia, influencing the values of the forces that they transmit. To overcome these deficiencies in the theory, we now take account of the elasticity of the ligaments.

Method of Analysis; Elastic Ligaments

In this analysis of the anterior drawer test, we consider the system of Fig. 10-20 and evaluate the contributions of the ACL and the isometric medial collateral ligament (MCL) of that figure. In the unloaded state, the isometric MCL fiber passes through the flexion axis (Fig. 10-20b); furthermore, the concept of a non-turning load, intersecting the lines of action of the ligament and contact forces at the flexion axis, still applies.

As the knee flexes, the angles between the tibial plateau and the ACL and MCL change. Using the four-bar linkage model, these angles were determined for any flexion angle (Fig. 10-20), giving the initial unstretched orientation of each ligament (Fig. 11-7).

When the tibia is displaced anteriorly by a distance x, the length of the ligament increases while the angle between the ligament and the plateau decreases. From the geometry of Fig. 11-7a, the change in length of the ligament for any tibial displacement x was calculated, leading to the value of the ligament strain. The value of the ligament force required was then calculated from knowledge of the elastic properties (Young's modulus and Poisson's ratio) and cross-sectional area of the ligament. This method gives a relationship between ligament force and tibial displacement.

The associated contact and drawer forces were calculated using triangles of forces (Fig. 11-5). By basing this calculation on the geometry of the stretched ligament, account was taken of the effects of elastic changes of ligament orientation. Since the change in orientation can be 10° or more, a calculation of the

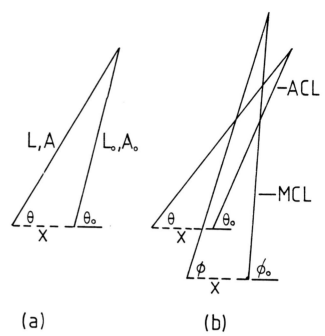

FIG. 11-7. a: The ligament increases in length from L_0 to L, and its inclination decreases from θ_0 to θ, when the tibia moves forward a distance x. The total cross-sectional area of the fibers of the ligament decreases from A_0 to A. **b**: Geometrically compatible extensions of the ACL and MCL (in the manner of diagram a) when the tibia moves forward a distance x.

drawer forces must take account of that change. Since the relationship between the ligament forces and the drawer force changes with ligament orientation, an incremental analysis is necessary (12).

In determining the relative contributions of the ACL and MCL, we used the ideas of geometric compatibility to circumvent the problem of statical indeterminacy by calculating the strains in different ligament fibers compatible with a shared forward movement of the tibia (Fig. 11-7b). We then used the method described in the previous two paragraphs to calculate the values of the ligament forces compatible with that shared movement. For each ligament, triangles of forces based on the deformed geometry were used to determine its contribution to the overall contact force and drawer force. The total contact force and drawer force were then calculated by summing the contributions of each of the ligaments. Since each ligament force was calculated in terms of a specified tibial displacement, this method yields a relationship between the drawer force and the anterior tibial displacement. The relationship between drawer force and displacement for the MCL alone is also the relationship for the ACL-deficient joint, and vice versa.

Calculations were carried out over the range of flexion. At each flexion angle, the drawer, contact, and ligamentous forces were calculated for 0.2-mm steps in tibial displacement from 0.0 to 10.0 mm.

A more complete description of the analysis and the associated algebraic formulae was given by FitzPatrick (12).

Parameters

The unstretched configuration of the ligaments in each flexion position was calculated from the cruciate linkage, using the parameters given in Chapter 10, Appendix. Cross-sectional areas for both ACL and MCL were found to be 40.0 mm². The equality of areas is based on the findings of Crowninshield (7). The resting length of the MCL was found by calculating the distance between the isometric attachment sites on the femur and tibia (Fig. 10-20b). This gave a value of 77.6 mm for attachment sites within the areas of attachment of the superficial MCL.

A value of 80.0 N/mm² for Young's modulus was within the range given by Noyes (25). Poisson's ratio, the ratio between radial and longitudinal strain of the collagen fibers, was taken to be 0.4.

Results

Figure 11-8a shows values of the ligament forces per unit applied load plotted against flexion angle. For the intact joint (when the contributions of the ACL and MCL are added together), the calculated ACL force given by the inextensible ligament theory of Fig. 11-6, included for comparison, only slightly overestimates the ACL force for an anterior tibial displacement of 0.2 mm; for a displacement of 5.0 mm, the inextensible theory overestimates the ACL force near extension by about 30% but is much closer to the elastic theory in high flexion. At 5.0 mm displacement, the calculated MCL force in the intact joint varies from 25% of the ACL force near extension to 38% at 120° of flexion. In proportion to the applied load, very much larger forces are required in the MCL when it alone resists anterior displacement.

Figure 11-8b shows the calculated variation in anterior joint laxity with flexion angle for an applied anterior force of 89 N. In the intact joint, the calculated anterior laxity decreases from 3.1 mm at 10° of flexion to 1.1 mm at 90° of flexion. In the ACL-deficient joint (i.e., when the contribution of the MCL alone is considered), the calculated total laxity is much greater but also decreases with flexion angle, from 11.8 mm at 20° to 4.5 mm at 90° of flexion.

Figure 11-8c shows the calculated ligament forces plotted against tibial displacement, and Fig. 11-8d shows the relationship between the applied drawer force and tibial displacement. The families of curves

for different flexion angles included in Fig. 11-8d imply that the joint becomes more stiff and the force required for a given displacement increases as the flexion angle increases and both ACL and MCL come to lie more nearly parallel to the tibial plateau. The larger contribution of the ACL arises because the MCL lies more perpendicular to the direction of tibial movement and is more than twice the length of the ACL.

Discussion

In the clinical test with a KT-2000, Daniel and Stone (Chapter 24) report a mean anterior displacement in 338 normal subjects of 5.7 mm under an anterior load of 89 N at flexion angles between 20° and 35°. Piziali (30, fig. 2), with one specimen at full extension, found that an anterior displacement of 5.7 mm required an anterior force which we estimate from their graph to be about 240 N, nearly three times that of the clinical test. Butler (6) found the knee to be stiffer still, with an anterior displacement of 5 mm requiring a mean anterior force of 292.3 N for three knees at 30° and 374.9 N for 11 knees at 90° of flexion. Both sets of experiments used fully constrained rigs in which all motions other than anterior displacement were suppressed, as we have discussed in Chapter 8. In the clinical test, long axis rotation is not restrained and could account for the significantly smaller force than required to induce anterior displacement (Fig. 23-2).

A further reason why greater anterior laxity is observed in the clinical test is that measurement is made from the neutral position in which the weight of the lower leg is balanced partly by the foot and partly by the PCL of the knee (Fig. 23-3). The neutral position from which anterior laxity is measured is further posterior in the clinical test than in the experiment.

Our theoretical study is therefore best compared with the fully constrained experiment, since it considers the effect of an anterior translation of the tibia with no change in flexion angle and no tibial rotation. The calculated forces required for an anterior displacement of 5 mm are 269 N at 30° and 490 N at 90° (Fig. 11-8c), compared with Butler's (6) 333 N and 440 N, respectively.

At 5-mm anterior displacement, the calculated ACL force varies from about four times the MCL force in extension to 2.7 times at 90° (Fig. 11-8c). The ACL accounts for 84.2% of the applied anterior load at 30° and 77.1% at 90° (Fig. 11-8c). The corresponding percentages obtained experimentally by Butler (6) were 87.8% and 85.2%, respectively. Piziali's (30) value at full extension was 75%. Reasonable correspondence between calculated and measured percentages indicates that the mechanism of load-sharing between lig-

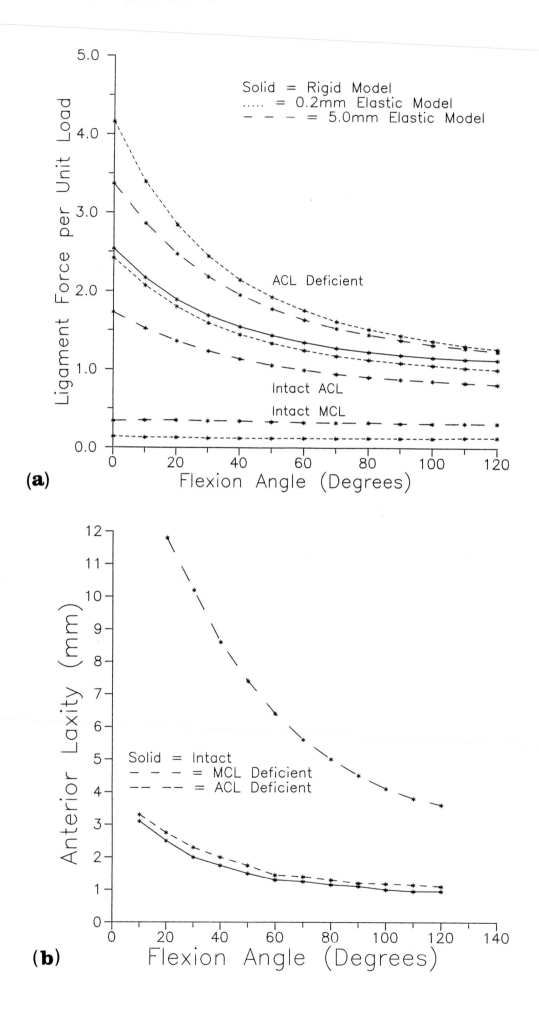

(a)

(b)

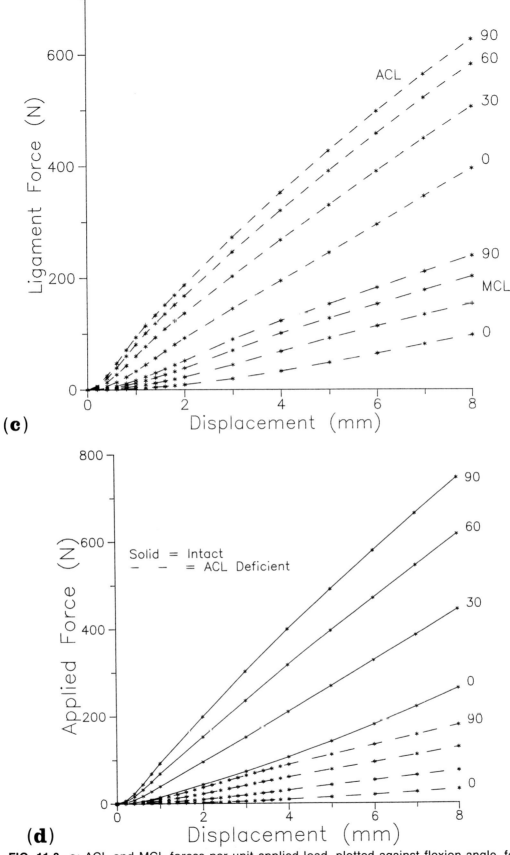

FIG. 11-8. a: ACL and MCL forces per unit applied load, plotted against flexion angle, for 0.2 and 5 mm anterior tibial displacement. The ACL force, on the basis of the inextensible ligament analysis, is included for comparison. The large increase in MCL force required in the ACL-deficient knee is indicated. **b**: Anterior tibial displacement (laxity) under a load of 89 N, plotted against flexion angle, for intact and ACL- and MCL- deficient knees. **c**: Ligament forces plotted against anterior tibial displacement at four flexion angles. **d**: Required anterior force plotted against tibial displacement at four flexion angles for intact and ACL-deficient knees.

aments is governed by the geometric compatibility condition suggested by Fig. 11-7b.

Partly for the reasons stated in relation to the experiments, the calculated anterior displacement under an 89-N load at 30°, 1.9 mm, is smaller than the mean value of 5.7 measured by Daniel and Stone (Chapter 24). Using the same methods of analysis, we have estimated that the posterior displacement of the tibia under its own weight would be about 1 mm, reducing the discrepancy somewhat. The theory reproduces the clinical observation that the increase in laxity due to ACL rupture is much larger near extension than in flexion (Fig. 11-8b).

The results of the calculations are very sensitive to the choice of material and geometric parameters for the ligaments; thus for the crudely chosen values used in this chapter, we consider that agreement with published measurements is reasonable.

It can be seen from Fig. 11-8a that ignoring the elasticity of the ACL and ignoring the contribution of the MCL results in an overestimate of the ACL force. In other words, the inextensible ligament theory provides an upper bound to the value of the ligament force but becomes increasingly more accurate as the joint is flexed.

Further work required includes a parametric study to determine more thoroughly the effects of ligament elasticity and cross-sectional area. Account should be taken of (a) the nonlinear nature of the stress–strain relationships of collagenous materials and (b) the recruitment into load-bearing of ligament fibers, lax due to their position behind the flexion axis of the joint (Fig. 10-23). These are matters currently under study.

MUSCLE, LIGAMENT, AND CONTACT FORCE INTERACTIONS (3,26)

Since the lines of action of the ligament, contact, and muscle forces all change continuously as the joint flexes, the relationships in mechanics between those forces vary with flexion angle. This is true even in the unlikely event that the lines of action of the external loads remain fixed relative to the tibia or the femur. During walking and other activities, the leg moves and changes its direction in space. The flexion axis of the knee therefore moves in relation to the line of the foot/ground reaction both because the axis moves in relation to the bones and because the bones move in relation to the ground reaction. Because of these movements, the demand for muscle or ligament action changes. We shall explain muscle–ligament interactions in terms of a few simple examples. In Chapter 14, the ideas developed here are applied to an analysis of knee ligament forces during gait.

Passive and Active Muscle Forces

It is usual to think of muscles as the initiators of movement. In fact, their most important role is to stabilize the skeleton and to hold it still in the presence of gravity forces and in the presence of the reactions to gravity forces such as the foot/ground reaction. For all but the most strenuous activities, the so-called transmitted forces needed to stabilize the skeleton are much larger than the so-called inertia forces needed to initiate and maintain motion.

We shall treat muscle forces (in the same way as ligament and intraarticular contact forces) as though they were passive reactions to external loads rather than being active forces, which are applied consciously or subconsciously by the individual to achieve stability or motion. The relationships in geometry and mechanics between muscle, ligament, and contact forces hold whether we think of muscle forces as active or passive. We shall consider first those circumstances in which a single muscle group (either quadriceps, gastrocnemius, or hamstrings) is used to balance extending or flexing loads.

Quadriceps–Cruciate Interactions

Figure 11-9 shows a load **W** is applied by the ground through the foot parallel to the tibial plateau. Because the force is directed backwards, it tends to flex the knee. We call it a flexing load. Its flexing effect is balanced by the extending effect of a force, **T**, in the patellar tendon.

In Figs. 11-9b,c, and d the lower leg is in mechanical equilibrium under the action of the external load and three forces applied to the tibia at the knee. These comprise the muscle force **T**, a ligament force **A** or **P**, and the tibiofemoral contact force **C**. The three forces applied at the knee are sufficient to suppress the three degrees of freedom of the lower leg in the sagittal plane. The ligament and contact forces intersect at the flexion axis so that the muscle force alone balances the flexing effect of the load; the value of this force is determined by this condition alone. Ligament and contact forces are needed to prevent movement parallel and perpendicular to the tibial plateau. However, the direction of the patellar tendon changes during flexion (Figs. 10-31 and 10-32), so that the requirement for associated ligamentous action changes with flexion. We will show now that, near extension, ligament action is needed to pull the tibia backwards and that, in the highly flexed joint, ligament action is needed to pull the tibia forwards. In the simplest model, it is assumed that the ligament forces are applied by the ACL and PCL, respectively.

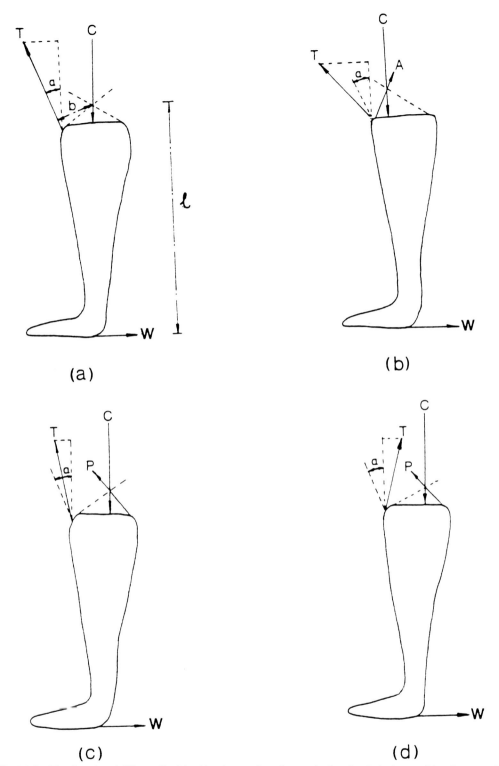

FIG. 11-9. Flexing load **W** applied to the lower leg through the foot, balanced by forces at the knee. **a**: Tendon force **T** and contact force **C** sufficient for equilibrium if tendon angle has its critical value *a*, where sin *a* = *b/l* = **W/T**. **b**: Tendon angle greater than *a*; a force **A** is also required in the ACL. **c**: Tendon angle less than *a*; a force **P** is required in the PCL. **d**: In opposite direction to *a*; a force **P** is required in the PCL.

The Critical Angles

A special case occurs in Fig. 11-9a and is discussed first. There, the component of the tendon force parallel to the plateau pulling the tibia forward is precisely equal to the component of the load parallel to the plateau pushing the tibia backwards. The tibiofemoral contact force **C** acting downwards balances the upward pull of the muscle perpendicular to the tibial plateau. Mechanical equilibrium can therefore be achieved without ligamentous action but only for a particular direction of the patellar tendon, defined by the formula in the caption to Fig. 11-9. We call the angle of the tendon in Fig. 11-9a the *critical tendon angle*. The corresponding flexion angle is the *critical flexion angle*.

Loading of the Cruciate Ligaments

In Fig. 11-9b, at flexion angles less than the critical angle, the angle of the patellar tendon is greater than the critical tendon angle, the component of the muscle force parallel to the plateau is greater than the corresponding component of the load, and ligament tension is needed to help pull the tibia backward. For our present purposes, we assume that ligament tension is provided entirely by the force **A** in the ACL. In Fig. 11-9c, at flexion angles somewhat greater than the critical angle, the angle of the patellar tendon is less than the critical tendon angle, the component of the muscle force parallel to the plateau is less than that of the load, and ligament tension is needed to prevent the tibia from sliding backwards. It can be provided by the force **P** in the PCL. In Fig. 11-9d, at high angles of flexion, the patellar tendon now points somewhat posteriorly so that the component of its force parallel to the plateau pulls the tibia backwards, in the same direction as the load. The forwards component of the PCL force has to balance the combined effects of muscle and load.

Similar arguments apply when loads tending to extend the joint are balanced by flexor muscles, either hamstrings or gastrocnemius. In each case, the ACL is needed for equilibrium near full extension, whereas PCL is required at high angles of flexion. The critical flexion angle at which no ligamentous action is needed lies near mid-range for the quadriceps, near extension for the hamstrings, and in high flexion for the gastrocnemius, but the precise values also depend on the direction and line of action of the load.

Quadriceps-Strengthening Exercises

As an example of the way the cruciate ligaments exchange roles in the muscle-stabilized knee, let us consider the configuration of Fig. 11-10, where the quadriceps are being used to lift a weight suspended from the end of the tibia with the femur fixed at 45° to the horizontal and the flexor muscles relaxed.

Results

As in our analysis of the drawer test above, muscle ligament and contact forces should be proportional to load, shown in Fig. 11-10 as a force **W** suspended from the tibia. In presenting the values of the forces at the knee, it is again economical to plot knee forces against flexion angle in nondimensional form, as muscle, ligament, and contact force per unit load, in a manner similar to that shown in Fig. 11-6. The results of the mechanical analysis of Fig. 11-10 are shown in Figs. 11-11 and 11-12. The quadriceps and patellar tendon forces per unit load are plotted against flexion angle in Fig. 11-11a, and the tibiofemoral contact force and the cruciate ligament forces are plotted against flexion angle in Fig. 11-11b. For purposes of comparison, Fig. 11-12 is an amalgam of these graphs.

As the leg is lifted from vertical at 135°, the quadriceps force required increases rapidly to reach a value of nearly 15 times the applied load at 70° of flexion (Fig. 11-11a). These large muscle forces, acting through small lever-arms, are required to balance small loads, acting through lever-arms as large as the length of the leg. The quadriceps force then falls as the knee is further extended, to reach a minimum of seven times the applied load at 20°; thereafter it increases rapidly as the posterior capsule offers increasing resistance to hyperextension. Near extension, the quadriceps not only has to lift the tibia but also has to strain the posterior capsule.

It should be noted that the maxima in the quadriceps and patellar tendon forces do not occur at 45° of flexion, where the tibia is horizontal and the lever-arm available to the external load is largest. The patellar tendon force reaches its maximum at about 55°. The lever-arm of the patellar tendon diminishes with flexion angle (Fig. 11-3). The patellar tendon force in Fig. 11-11a would be expected to peak at 45° only if its lever-arm were constant. For the quadriceps force, there is the additional factor that it does not change with flexion angle in proportion to the patellar tendon force for reasons given in the discussion of Fig. 10-33 above.

The cruciate ligament forces are shown in Fig. 11-11b. Tension in the ACL is required from full extension to 85° of flexion, the critical flexion angle. The PCL is loaded thereafter. The largest ligament forces are those in the ACL near extension, where all the joint forces are increased by the intervention of the posterior capsule. Although the ligament forces are smaller than the quadriceps or contact forces (Fig. 11-12), they can be

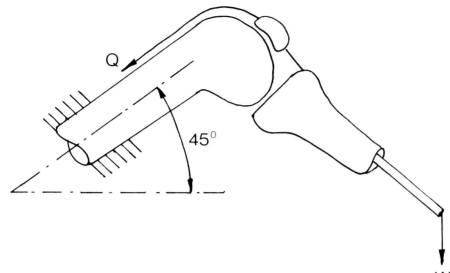

FIG. 11-10. Simulation of the quadriceps-strengthening exercise, where quadriceps force **Q** is used to balance the weight **W**.

several times larger than the applied load. The calculated values of the ACL forces are in reasonable agreement with measurements by Malcolm (22).

The mechanical disadvantage of the muscles relative to the load has consequences for the contact force (Fig. 11-11b), which increases steadily as extension is approached and at an even more rapid rate once the posterior capsule begins to tighten, in this example at 15°

of flexion. The large contact forces are required to balance the large proximal pull of the patellar tendon and the ligaments.

The implications of Fig. 11-11b for the ligament surgeon are clear. During rehabilitation, quadriceps exercises such as that shown in Fig. 11-10 may be considered. Following an ACL enhancement or replacement, the new structures are placed under max-

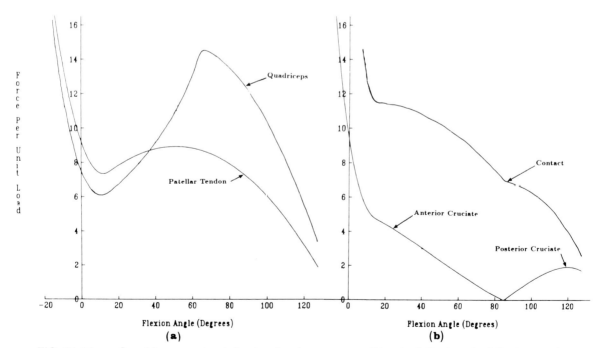

FIG. 11-11. a: Quadriceps and patellar tendon forces per unit load, plotted against flexion angle, for the configuration of Fig. 11-10. **b**: Cruciate ligament and tibiofemoral contact forces, plotted against flexion angle, for the configuration of Fig. 11-10. The critical flexion angle is 85° where no ligament forces are required. Large forces near extension occur as a result of intervention of the posterior capsule, thereby limiting extension.

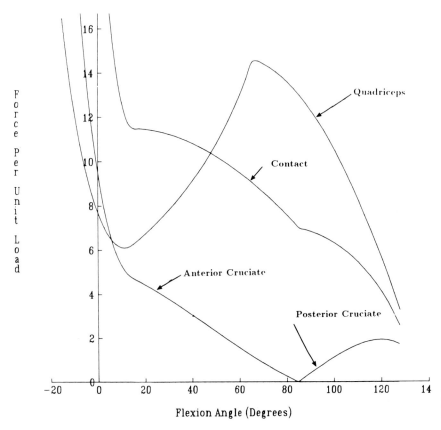

FIG. 11-12. The forces of Fig. 11-11 superposed on one diagram for comparison of their magnitudes.

imum strain near extension. Quadriceps exercises from extension to 70–80° should be avoided. Similar advice would apply to the conservative management of an ACL injury.

Comparison with Published Data

The reader is reminded that the results described in Figs. 11-11 and 11-12 are purely theoretical estimates from the computer model. In Chapter 12 we shall present measurements of ligament and muscle forces which agree quite well with and validate the conclusions of the theoretical model. The plots of quadriceps force versus flexion angle are very similar to measurements made by Hungerford (19) and Grood (16) for loading configurations similar to that of Fig. 11-10 but with the femur horizontal.

Figure 11-13 is a plot of Grood's results, estimated from ref. 16 (16, fig. 3), for a lower leg loaded by its own weight compared with our calculations for the same configuration. He plotted quadriceps force per unit leg weight against flexion but showed a separate family of curves for tests in which, in addition, a 31-N weight was hung from the foot. The curve in Fig. 11-13 was calculated on the assumption that the external load acted at a distance of 30 cm from the tibial plateau. Except at high flexion angles, the theoretical curve intersects the bars indicating the range of Grood's data.

The peak quadriceps force in mid-range of Fig. 11-11a was not found in Fig. 11-13 for a horizontal femur when the leverage available to the external load is largest at extension, making the point that the relationship of the line of action of the external load to the limb is one of the factors determining the values of the joint forces.

Hamstrings-Strengthening Exercises

For comparison, consider the configuration of Fig. 11-14, where the hamstrings are used to lift a weight **W** hung from the end of the tibia with the femur fixed at 45° and the other muscles relaxed.

The results of a mechanical analysis of this configuration using the computer model are presented in Fig. 11-15, where hamstrings, cruciate ligament, and contact forces per unit load are plotted against flexion angle.

The hamstrings force rises from zero at 135° to a plateau of about 13 times the applied load before falling rapidly to zero again with the knee extended. Near extension, the tightening posterior capsule, this time acting agonistically, takes over the function of the muscle by providing a flexing moment to balance the ex-

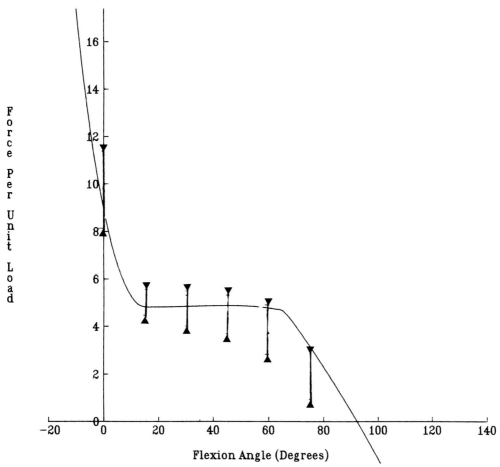

FIG. 11-13. Quadriceps force per unit load, plotted against flexion angle, for the configuration of Fig. 11-10 but with the femur held horizontal. The curve is the calculated result, and the bars indicate the range of Grood's data (16, fig. 3) from five specimens.

tending moment of the load. The maximum hamstrings force is larger than the maximum patellar tendon force in Fig. 11-11a because its lever-arm is smaller (Fig. 11-3).

The ligament forces shown in Fig. 11-15 are significantly different from those in Fig. 11-11b. The critical flexion angle for hamstrings-loaded cruciates is about 12°. The ACL forces are relatively small but the PCL forces are very large, with the maximum at 100° of flexion predicted to be larger than the maximum muscle force. These very large ligament forces arise because, at high flexion angles, the PCL is rotated at its

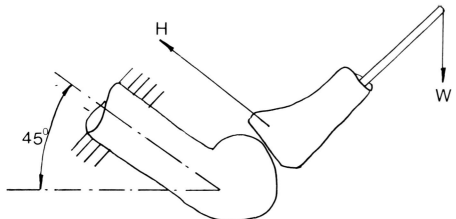

FIG. 11-14. Simulation of hamstrings-strengthening exercises. An extending load **W** is balanced by tension **H** in the hamstrings.

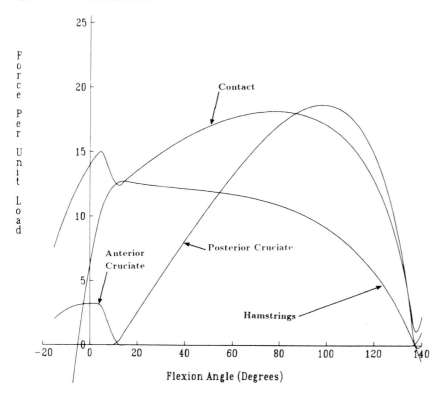

FIG. 11-15. Hamstrings, tibiofemoral contact, and cruciate ligament forces per unit applied load, plotted against flexion angle, for the configuration of Fig. 11-14.

maximum orientation from the tibial plateau (Figs. 10-8c and 10-16), where it can least efficiently provide the forward pull to the tibia needed to balance the backward pull of the hamstrings. These results are in reasonable agreement with measurements reported by O'Connor (27).

The tibiofemoral contact force reaches a maximum of about 18 times the applied load at 80° of flexion and remains large into high flexion. As flexion increases, the hamstrings force is directed more posteriorly (Fig. 10-31b and c), but the large PCL force is directed more proximally. A large distal push is required from the contact force over much of the flexion range to balance the combined proximal pull of hamstrings and the PCL.

Figure 11-15 also has a message for the ligament surgeon. Hamstrings exercises are not likely to be dangerous in remobilization after ACL injury, except near full extension. They should absolutely be avoided following PCL injury.

Discussion

Muscle Force Magnitudes

In proportion to the applied load, the very large muscle and ligament forces predicted by this analysis are a consequence of the system under study (Figs. 11-10 and 11-14), in which the external load has a large com-

ponent perpendicular to the leg so that its leverage about the knee is also large; indeed, in the experiment analyzed, the load acts entirely perpendicular to the leg at 45° of flexion, and the lever-arm of the load is then equal to the length of the tibia. The effect of load line of action on quadriceps force is seen by comparing Fig. 11-11a with Fig. 11-13. In normal activity, the line of the ground reaction passes much closer to the flexion axis of the knee, and the joint forces are then much smaller proportions of the load. However, in extreme activities such as weight-lifting, very large loads can be encountered. Zernicke (35) calculated a force of 14,500 N (17.5 times body weight) in the patellar tendon of a champion weight lifter at the instant of its avulsion from the tibia.

Ligament Forces

By considering a simple planar model of the knee, we have deduced the factors that determine which of the cruciate ligaments are subjected to tension by external loads in the sagittal plane.

Flexion angle is a factor because it controls the directions of the ligaments and muscle tendons. The direction and line of action of the load is the second factor, in part because it determines the value of the muscle force but also because the load generally has a component parallel to the tibial plateau. The balance between the components of the load and the muscle force parallel to the tibial plateau then requires either a backwards (anterior cruciate) or forwards (posterior cruciate) ligament contribution for equilibrium. The peculiar arrangement of the cruciate ligaments is such that one or the other is always available to provide the required ligamentous force.

The analysis clearly takes no account of the non-planar nature of the cruciates, the contributions of the collateral ligaments, the separate contributions of the medial and lateral tibiofemoral joints, the effects of axial rotation of the tibia, the extension of ligaments under load, the finite thicknesses of ligaments and tendons, the deformability of articular surfaces, or the presence of the menisci. Some of these factors will be discussed briefly in the following paragraphs. It is also necessary to distinguish the forces induced in the cruciates by external load and muscle action from those induced by passive flexion and extension. These latter are likely to be quite small in comparison.

The Collateral Ligaments

Figure 11-2 demonstrates that the lever-arms of the muscles are measured from the flexion axis at which the neutral fibers of the cruciate ligaments cross. Figure 10–20 suggests that there may also be a neutral fiber within the MCL which passes through the flexion axis in all positions of the joint and therefore remains isometric during passive flexion. If we take the line of the neutral MCL fiber to be the line of action of the resultant force transmitted by the entire ligament, then that force also passes through, and has no moment about, the flexion axis. Figure 10-19 supports the experimental observations that the lateral collateral ligament (LCL) goes slack during passive flexion and is unlikely to make a significant contribution to load transmission in the sagittal plane.

Since the force in the MCL may therefore be assumed to have no moment about the flexion axis, we can continue to argue that the value of the extensor or flexor muscle force is determined solely by the condition that it balances the flexing or extending effect of the external load. The relationship between the components of muscle force and load parallel to the tibial plateau determines whether a backwards or forwards ligament pull is required. If a backwards pull is required, Figure 10-20 suggests that the principal longitudinal fibers of the MCL could contribute, but only in association with the ACL. Our analysis of the drawer test above, taking account of the elasticity of the ligaments, concluded that the MCL may carry only 15–30% of an anterior drawer force. The longitudinal fibers of the MCL are unlikely to help the PCL in flexion, but the postero-oblique fibers could contribute and would reduce the forces demanded from the PCL. We

conclude that an analysis based on Fig. 11-9 is likely to overestimate the values of the forces transmitted by the cruciate ligaments.

Long Axis Rotation

From the point of view of load transmission in the sagittal plane, the main effects of rotation about the tibial axis would be to modify the directions of the ligaments and muscle tendons and therefore change the value of the critical flexion angle at which transfer of load from one cruciate to the other occurs. We showed above that stretching of the ligaments, allowing anterior or posterior displacement of the tibia, reduces the angle between the ligament and the tibial plateau (Fig. 11-7). The values of the forces in the elastic ligaments prove to be smaller than those calculated on the basis of inextensible ligaments.

ANTAGONISTIC MUSCLE ACTION

Athletes and others with proven ligament ruptures that are treated conservatively frequently return to their sports and achieve satisfactory function, at least for a time. This is particularly true of the isolated ACL injury, often leading to a questioning of its function when intact, since good function can sometimes be achieved without it. In this section, we shall demonstrate theoretically that antagonistic or agonistic muscle action can substitute for cruciate ligament action in the sagittal plane; moreover, we shall outline the price to be paid, in terms of increased muscle and contact forces, for such protection.

So far in this chapter, we have discussed (a) circumstances in which external loads passing through the flexion axis can be balanced by a combination of ligament and contact forces without muscle action (the drawer test) and (b) circumstances in which flexing or extending loads are balanced by the addition of a single muscle group, extensors or flexors (muscle-strengthening exercises). We now wish to discuss the possibility of two muscle groups acting simultaneously, either (a) the extensors with one of the flexors acting antagonistically or (b) the two flexors, hamstrings and gastrocnemius, acting agonistically.

Electromyographic (EMG) studies of level walking and other activities (Fig. 14-13) have demonstrated that antagonistic or agonistic action occurs frequently. During the walking cycle, hamstrings and quadriceps fire together before footstrike and in early stance phase. From the point of view of the mechanics of the lower leg, from the knee down to the ground, such antagonistic action is not necessary. A single muscle group together with one cruciate ligament force and the tibiofemoral contact force, as in Fig. 11-9, are mechanically sufficient for equilibrium for any arbitrary flexing or extending load applied in the sagittal plane. Why should antagonistic or agonistic action occur, and how can one calculate the values of the forces at the knee when it does?

Possible Combinations of Knee Joint Forces

In our analysis of Figs. 11-10 and 11-14, we used the laws of geometry to determine (a) the directions of the ligaments and tendons and (b) the line of action of the tibiofemoral contact force. We then used the laws of mechanics to calculate the forces at the joint. We said that the flexing or extending effect of the load about the flexion axis must be balanced by the extending or flexing effect of one muscle; the forward and backward pulls of load, muscle, and ligament must balance; the upward pulls of muscle and ligament must be balanced by the downward push of the tibiofemoral contact force. These are the only three conditions that mechanics can bring to bear in the sagittal plane, and they are sufficient to determine the absolute values of only three forces at the joint in that plane. Any combination of three (contact, ligament, and muscle forces) that satisfy those three conditions is sufficient for equilibrium and is sufficient to suppress the three degrees of freedom of the shank in the sagittal plane. (We are using the word *sufficient* here in the sense used in the field of mechanics. See also the discussion of degrees of freedom and equilibrium in Chapter 8.)

Although in our modeling we have simplified the picture by amalgamating the separate heads of quadriceps, of hamstrings and of gastrocnemius, by ignoring the contributions of the collateral ligaments and the separate contributions of the medial and lateral compartments, we have nonetheless recognized the possibility of forces transmitted by six elements: quadriceps **Q**, hamstrings **H**, gastrocnemius **G**, anterior cruciate ligament **A**, posterior cruciate ligament **P**, and the tibiofemoral contact **C**. There are, in fact, 20 possible combinations of three of these forces ($^6C_3$) which can be determined by the laws of geometry and mechanics. These combinations are listed in Table 11-1. It is always possible for one or two of the three forces

in any combination to be zero. In our analysis of the drawer test above, we showed that the combination **AC** (ACL force **A** with the tibiofemoral contact force **C**) could balance an anterior drawer force and that the combination **PC** (PCL force **P** with the tibiofemoral contact force **C**) could balance a posterior drawer force. The combination **AP** may be used when the tibia is hanging from the ligaments under its own weight. In our discussion of Fig. 11-9, we described how the combination **QAC** is sufficient for equilibrium near extension and how the combination **QPC** is sufficient for equilibrium in flexion (Fig. 11-11b). At the critical flexion angle, the ligament forces were zero; at that position alone, the combination **QC** (quadriceps force with the tibiofemoral contact force) was sufficient for equilibrium. The combinations **APC**, **QAC**, and **QPC** therefore each contain three possible subgroups of two forces, as do the other triads of Table 11-1.

It is also possible for the calculations to suggest that one or more of the forces in any combination could be negative, indicative of (a) a compressive muscle or ligament force or (b) a tensile contact force. By ruling out such possibilities, the number of geometrically and mechanically possible combinations that apply in a particular instance is much reduced. In the table, a distinction is drawn between distracting loads (as when the lower leg hangs under its own weight from the knee) and compressing loads (as when the knee has to transmit the ground reaction). Thus, if we were to evaluate the forces in the combination **QAC** in the presence of a purely distracting load, the contact force **C** would have a negative value and the possibility of that combination could be ruled out.

However, even though some of the 20 possible combinations of forces may not be physically realizable, we must face the fact that the results of calculations of joint forces from geometry and mechanics cannot be unique. We will show in chapter 14 that, over the gait cycle, more than one combination is frequently possible. Part of the problem is that until now we have regarded muscle forces, like ligament and contact forces, as passive reactions to load rather than active forces that the individual can choose consciously or subconsciously to apply.

TABLE 11-1. *Twenty combinations of three out of six possible forces at the knee[a]*

No muscle:	**APC**
One muscle—distracting load:	**QAP, HAP, GAP**
One muscle—compressing load:	**QAC, QPC, HAC, HPC, GAC, GPC**
Two muscles—distracting load:	**QHA, QHP, QGA, QGP, GHA, GHP**
Two muscles—compressing load:	**QHC, QGC, HGC**
Three muscles—distracting load:	**QHG**

[a] **Q**, quadriceps force; **H**, hamstrings force; **G**, gastrocnemius force; **A**, anterior cruciate ligament force; **P**, posterior cruciate ligament force; **C**, tibiofemoral contact force.

A full three-dimensional analysis of forces at the knee leads to even greater uncertainty. For example, we could attempt to evaluate five possible muscle forces (quadriceps and the medial and lateral heads of hamstrings and gastrocnemius), four ligament forces (the cruciates and the collaterals), and medial and lateral tibiofemoral contact forces. For their solution, we could apply the six conditions of mechanics for the equilibrium of the lower limb. There would then be 462 $^{11}C_6$ possible combinations of forces that could satisfy equilibrium. The advantages of seeking understanding through a two-dimensional analysis are obvious.

This is a complicated way of saying that the laws of geometry and mechanics can take us only so far. The individual, while remaining perfectly still, can decide to apply antagonistic muscle action and can decide to apply a little or a lot. The decision may be a conscious one or, as in walking and other activities, it may be quite unconscious. There has been considerable interest in proposing strategies that might be adopted during activity in choosing from the many geometrically and mechanically possible force combinations. These are reviewed in Chapter 14. In this section, we will demonstrate that it is geometrically and mechanically possible for antagonistic or agonistic action to be used to unload and therefore protect ligaments when they are present and functioning or to substitute for ligament forces when the ligaments are absent.

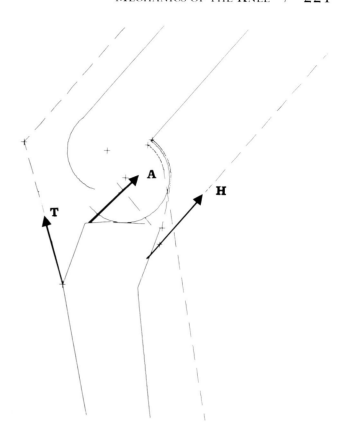

FIG. 11-16. The force in the ACL **(A)** or in the hamstrings **(H)** pull the tibia backward to balance the forward pull of the patellar tendon **(T)**.

Theory

The ACL of the knee prevents anterior displacement of the tibia by pulling the tibia backwards as well as upwards (Fig. 11-16.). Once the joint has been flexed beyond 20° or so, the hamstrings muscle also pulls the tibia backward. It is therefore geometrically and mechanically possible for the hamstrings to replace the action of the ACL in preventing anterior subluxation of the tibia when the limb is stabilized by the quadriceps, but only when the knee is sufficiently bent that the hamstrings force has a component backwards relative to the tibial plateau.

Similarly, the PCL prevents posterior displacement of the tibia by pulling it forwards as well as upwards. Between full extension and about 90° of flexion, so do both the patellar tendon or gastrocnemius. It is therefore possible that quadriceps or gastrocnemius action could be used to prevent posterior subluxation of the tibia—for instance, when the hamstrings are being used to terminate the swing phase of gait.

Theoretical Results—Quadriceps-Strengthening Exercises

Figure 11-17 shows the quadriceps, contact, hamstrings, and gastrocnemius forces required to balance the flexing load of Fig. 11-10, plotted in nondimensional form against flexion angle. Figure 11-17 should be compared with Fig. 11-12.

It will be seen that ligament-saving antagonistic solutions are geometrically and mechanically possible when the flexion angle of the knee is greater than about 25°. Below 25°, the line of action of the hamstrings force has a component along the tibial plateau directed *forward* (Fig. 10-31a). As shown in Fig. 11-10, near extension, equilibrium requires a *backward*-directed force, provided there by the ACL. Thus, below 20°, antagonistic action by the hamstrings cannot replace the action of the quadriceps-loaded ACL.

Above 25°, antagonistic action can replace the load-carrying functions of the cruciate ligaments in the sagittal plane completely. Between 25° and the critical flexion angle, 85°, hamstrings force can substitute for ACL force. Above 85°, gastrocnemius force can replace PCL force. At 85° (the critical flexion angle), neither antagonist is needed, just as in Fig. 11-11b, neither cruciate was needed; in both instances, the forward pull of quadriceps exactly balances the backward pull of the load. These conclusions are in general agreement with experimental measurements reported by Young (34).

Thus, antagonistic muscle action can entirely sub-

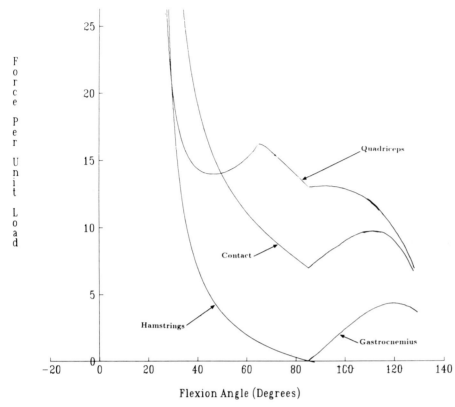

FIG. 11-17. Quadriceps, hamstrings, gastrocnemius, and tibiofemoral contact forces replacing ligament action in the configuration of Fig. 11-10.

stitute for ligament action, but only over a limited range of flexion. Unloading and protection of the ligaments is therefore a possible strategy for antagonistic action in normal activity. Replacement of load-bearing function of the ligaments in the injured knee is also possible.

The price to be paid for protection of the ligaments or replacement of their function can be deduced from Fig. 11-18. There the muscle ligament and contact forces of the single muscle solution of Figs. 11-11 and 11-12 are compared with the antagonistic solution of Fig. 11-17. The single muscle solution is shown by solid lines, and the antagonistic solution is shown by dashed lines. The two solutions are identical at the critical flexion angle, 85°. Elsewhere the quadriceps and contact forces of the antagonistic solution are larger than those of the single muscle solution. The hamstrings and gastrocnemius forces are larger than the corresponding ligament forces.

The larger forces in the antagonistic solution arise because the quadriceps, in addition to overcoming the flexing effect of the external load, has also to overcome the flexing effect of the flexor muscles and must be correspondingly larger than in the single muscle solution. The increased upward pulls of the muscles give rise to larger contact forces.

Thus, protection of the ligaments by antagonistic muscle action or replacement of their function requires significant increase in muscle and intraarticular con-

tact forces. Noting that McDevitt (23) uses division of the ACL in experimental animals as a model for promoting degenerative changes in the knee, we can speculate that the increased contact forces associated with antagonistic action may not be wholly benign.

Theoretical Results—Hamstrings-Strengthening Exercises

Antagonistic Hamstrings–Quadriceps Action

Next, consider the hamstrings-strengthening configuration (Fig. 11-14), but with simultaneous hamstrings and quadriceps action and no ligament forces. Figure 11-19 shows the values of hamstrings and quadriceps forces plotted against flexion angle. These somewhat bizarre results are best understood by reference to Fig. 11-15, which shows that, with hamstrings balancing the extending load, a forward pull on the tibia, provided by the PCL, is needed over the bulk of the flexion range but that a backward pull, provided by the ACL, is needed near extension. In Fig. 11-19, it will be seen that a physically realizable solution without ligament force can be obtained and quadriceps can act as an antagonist to hamstrings but only over a very narrow range of flexion, from 10° to 25°. Very large muscle and contact forces are required within that range.

Below 10°, the patellar tendon pulls the tibia forward

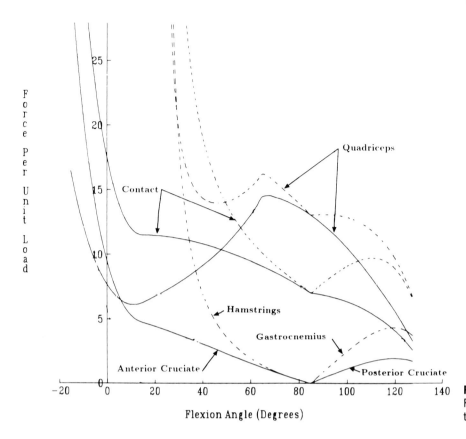

FIG. 11-18. Single muscle solution of Fig. 11-12 (——) compared with the antagonistic solutions of Fig. 11-17 (---).

and cannot provide the backward pull needed from ligament or antagonist.

Above 25°, the reason why the combination of hamstrings and quadriceps action, without ligament force, is not physically possible is more subtle. The antagonist must provide a forward pull to the tibia, and the patellar tendon is appropriately directed to do so. However, when quadriceps is applied to provide the necessary forward component, it tends, in addition, to extend the joint so that additional hamstrings force is needed to prevent extension. Beyond 25° of flexion, as the hamstrings force is increased above the level of Fig. 11-15, its backward component increases at a faster rate than the forward component of the patellar tendon force, and balance of forces parallel to the tibial plateau cannot be achieved.

Agonistic Hamstrings–Gastrocnemius Action

Now, consider the possibility of agonistic gastrocnemius action in the hamstrings-strengthening exercise, without ligament force. Figure 11-20 shows the calculated values of the hamstrings and gastrocnemius forces which are required to balance the extending load of Fig. 11-14. The agonistic solution is not possible near extension because gastrocnemius pulls the tibia forward when a backward pull is required. However, the ligament-free agonistic solution is possible over the large bulk of the flexion range.

When the single muscle solution of Fig. 11-15 is compared with the agonistic solution of Fig. 11-20, it will be seen that they are identical at the critical flexion angle of 12.5°, where the cruciate ligament forces in Fig. 11-15 and the gastrocnemius force of Fig. 11-20 are all zero. Above the critical flexion angle, all the forces of the agonistic solution are smaller than the corresponding forces of the single muscle solution.

Agonistic action can therefore be used to protect or replace the action of the PCL in the sagittal plane and can do so very efficiently.

Conclusion

When the ground reaction tends to flex the knee, the single muscle solutions such as those shown in Figs. 11-11 and 11-12 provide smaller muscle and contact forces than do the antagonistic solutions, but at the price of loading the cruciate ligaments. The cruciate forces can equal or even exceed the muscle forces in some circumstances. Antagonistic hamstrings action between about 25° and 85° (as well as antagonistic gastrocnemius action at higher flexion angles) can unload the cruciates, but at the price of increased quadriceps and contact forces.

When the ground reaction tends to extend the joint and is balanced by hamstrings, quadriceps action can unload the cruciates, but only over a very narrow range

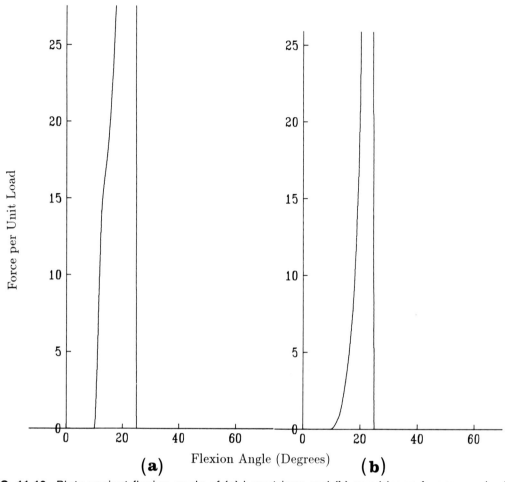

FIG. 11-19. Plots against flexion angle of **(a)** hamstrings and **(b)** quadriceps forces required to balance the load of Fig. 11-14 without ligament participation. This combination of forces is not possible outside the flexion range 12.5° to 25°.

of flexion and with very large forces. Agonistic hamstrings/gastrocnemius action can protect the PCL efficiently over the bulk of the flexion range in these circumstances and can reduce the values of the associated hamstrings and contact forces.

When only one muscle group, extensor or flexor, is used to balance an external load, the ligaments are inevitably loaded, except at the critical flexion angle.

ISOMETRIC MUSCLE CONTRACTION; SELF-EQUILIBRATING FORCES

In the previous sections, we have discussed forces set up at the knee by external load. There is also the possibility that the individual can contract extensor and flexor muscles simultaneously and build up muscle forces while keeping the limbs perfectly still and the external loads unchanged.

The contact, ligament, and muscle forces induced at the joint by such isometric contractions are in addition to those required to balance the external loads and may

be said to form self-equilibrating systems of forces, having no resultant. The proximal pull of the soft tissue forces applied to the tibia must balance the distal push applied by the femur. The backward and forward pulls of the soft tissue forces along the tibial plateau must balance. The moments of the muscle forces about the flexion axis must balance. Thus, as before, there are three conditions to be satisfied by the forces acting in the sagittal plane. How many forces can be involved in a typical self-equilibrating system?

If the extensor muscles are involved, then one or the other of the flexor muscles must also be. The requirement that they should neither extend or flex the joint determines the relative magnitudes of the extensor and flexor muscle forces, inversely proportional to their respective lever-arms (Fig. 11-3). The components of the two muscle forces parallel to the tibial plateau will pull the tibia either backward or forward and will require either a forward or backward ligament force for balance in this direction. Thus, either the ACL or PCL must also be involved. The three soft

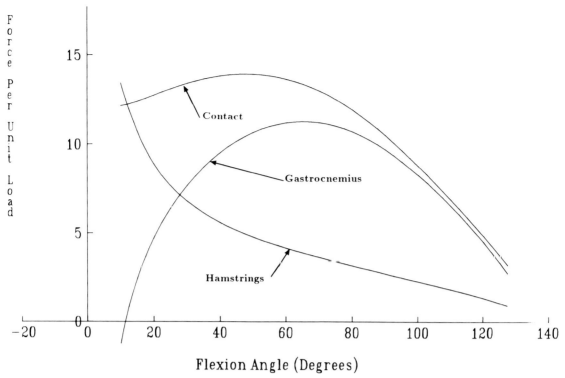

FIG. 11-20. Simultaneous hamstrings and gastrocnemius forces needed to balance the load of Fig. 11-14 without ligament participation. The associated contact force is also plotted against flexion angle.

tissue forces, pulling the tibia proximally, must be balanced by a tibiofemoral contact force, pushing the tibia distally. Hence, if muscle forces are involved in isometric contraction, a minimum of four forces—two muscle, one cruciate ligament, and one contact force—are required for equilibrium.

There is a further possibility—that the two flexor groups, hamstrings and gastrocnemius, should together balance not only the extending effect but also the anteroposterior displacing effect of the quadriceps. Ligament action would then not be required, and we would be left again with the possibility that appropriate simultaneous application of the extensors and flexors could unload and protect the ligaments during isometric contractions.

Possible systems of four self-equilibrating forces are listed in Table 11-2. The table indicates that there are five possibilities. We are then left with the problem of applying the three conditions of mechanics to evaluate four forces. Such a problem is said to be statically indeterminate. In structural mechanics, one would seek an additional condition to be applied, derived by studying the geometry of deformation. Such an approach was taken (Fig. 11-7) in our analysis of load-sharing between the ACL and the MCL in the drawer test. Here, the missing information derives from the will of the individual who decides the extent to which isometric contraction is applied and determines the absolute magnitudes of the forces. We can use mechanics only to determine their relative values, namely, the ratios of the values of three of the forces to the value of the fourth. Since our topic is ligament forces, it is convenient to evaluate the soft tissue forces (muscle and ligament) as nondimensional ratios of the tibiofemoral contact force.

Theoretical Results

We present in this section the values of the force ratios for each of the five systems in Table 11-2. The relative

TABLE 11-2. *Self-equilibrating muscle–ligament–contact force systems*

Two muscles, and one ligament—one contact:	**QHAC, QHPC, QGAC, QGPC**
Three muscles—one contact:	**QHGC**

[a] The notation is the same as that used for Table 11-1.

values of the forces vary with flexion angle because the directions of the soft tissue forces change, as shown in Fig. 10-31.

Quadriceps and Hamstrings

Figure 11-21 shows how the soft tissue forces per unit contact force vary with flexion angle when the quadriceps and hamstrings contract simultaneously. The hamstrings force is larger than the patellar tendon force over the entire flexion arc, reflecting the differences in their lever-arms (Fig. 11-3).

Near extension, the forward pull of the patellar tendon is larger than the backward pull of hamstrings, so a contribution from the ACL is required. When the knee is flexed beyond 22°, the backward pull of hamstrings dominates and a contribution from the PCL is required. There is a critical flexion angle at which the components of the two muscle forces parallel to the plateau exactly balance each other and no ligament forces are required.

Above 125°, a PCL force larger than the contact force is required, and the force ratio is greater than unity. This is because, in the highly flexed joint, the

hamstrings force pulls the tibia distally as well as posteriorly (Fig. 10-31c), and the sum of the upward components of the forces in the patellar tendon and the PCL now have to balance not only the downward push of the contact force but the downward pull of hamstrings as well.

Although the three conditions of mechanics are not sufficient to determine the absolute magnitudes of the forces, they are sufficient to determine the range of flexion over which each of the ligaments is loaded by isometric contractions. If simultaneous quadriceps and hamstrings contractions are used for rehabilitation following injury or surgery of the ACL, they should be applied only above the critical flexion angle—22° according to the calculations. They should be avoided if the PCL has been damaged.

Quadriceps and Gastrocnemius

Similar results are presented in Fig. 11-22 for simultaneous contraction of quadriceps and gastrocnemius. The gastrocnemius force required, with its relatively short lever-arm, is always about twice that in the patellar tendon. The combined pull of the two muscles

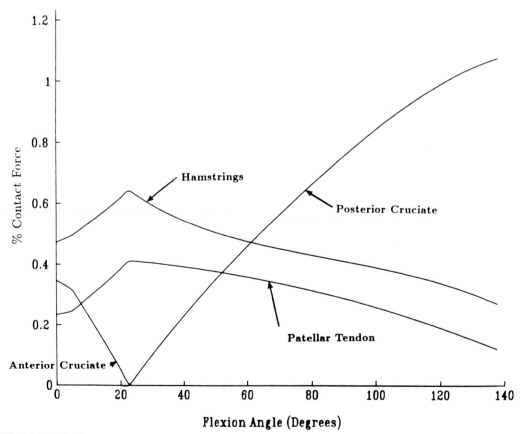

FIG. 11-21. Self-equilibrating forces. Isometric quadriceps and hamstrings contractions. Patellar tendon, hamstrings, ACL, and PCL forces per unit contact force, plotted against flexion angle.

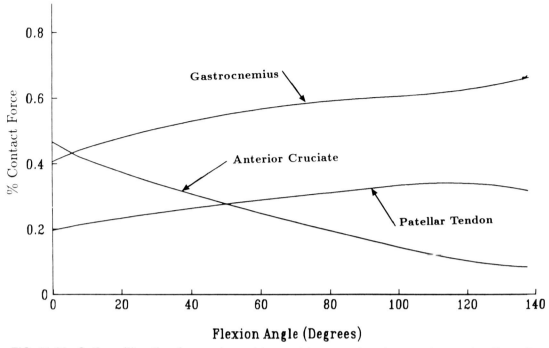

FIG. 11-22. Self-equilibrating forces. Isometric quadriceps and gastrocnemius contractions. Patellar tendon, gastrocnemius, and ACL forces per unit contact force, plotted against flexion angle. No PCL forces are involved.

parallel to the tibial plateau is always directed forward, requiring a contribution from the ACL, over the entire flexion range. The force required in the ACL decreases as the knee is flexed and the ligament comes to lie more closely along the plateau (Fig. 10-8c).

Whereas the combination of quadriceps and gastrocnemius would appear to be undesirable after damage to the ACL, it would appear to be ideal for rehabilitation of the PCL.

Quadriceps, Hamstrings, and Gastrocnemius

Figure 11-23 shows the calculated values of the forces when all three muscle groups act simultaneously, without ligament action. Since they all tend to pull the tibia forward when the knee is near extension, the combination is not physically realizable there, as indicated by the fact that the gastrocnemius force required would be negative and compressive. Above the critical flexion angle, the figure demonstrates that the combined action of the three muscle forces can be applied without loading either cruciate ligament.

Minimum Ligament Forces

Figure 11-24 is an amalgam of the above results, combined in such a way that the cruciate ligament forces required are minimized. Near extension, a contribu-

tion from the ACL is unavoidable. Hamstrings as the flexor requires a smaller force in the ACL than gastrocnemius, as may be seen by comparing Fig. 11-21 with Fig. 11-22. Near extension, Fig. 11-24 therefore includes the quadriceps–hamstrings–anterior cruciate solution. When flexed beyond the critical flexion angle, the three muscles can obviate the need for a contribution from either cruciate, and Fig. 11-25 therefore contains the three muscle solution in that region. The two solutions merge at the critical flexion angle, where quadriceps and hamstrings alone can satisfy the requirements of mechanics, with neither ligament nor gastrocnemius action.

Self-Equilibrating Ligament and Contact Forces

When attaching a ligament graft or prosthesis to bone, considerable attention has to be paid to the correct tensioning of the new structures. If the initial tension is too small, joint laxity may persist. If the tension is too large, stretching or rupture of the implant may occur. It is important to realize that tension applied to one of the cruciate ligaments induces tension in the other and that the ligament tensions so induced vary over the flexion range. Both ligament tensions, in turn, induce contact forces between the femur and the tibia.

Figure 11-1 illustrates a possible set of self-equilibrating ligament and contact forces. Since all three

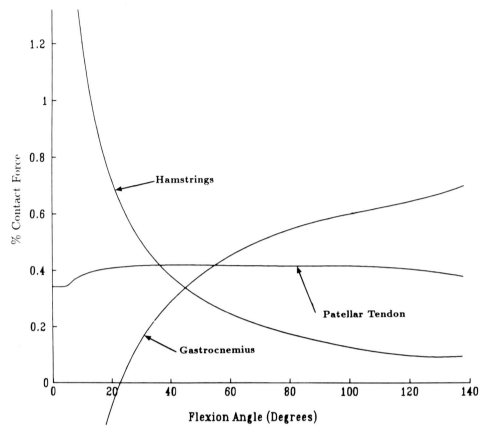

FIG. 11-23. Self-equilibrating muscles forces. Isometric quadriceps, hamstrings, and gastrocnemius contractions without ligamentous participation. Patellar tendon, hamstrings, and gastrocnemius forces per unit contact force, plotted against flexion angle. This system is not possible below 22.5° because compressive gastrocnemius forces would be required.

forces pass through the flexion axis, they have no moment about that axis, so that one of the three conditions of mechanics is always satisfied. Only two conditions are left to control the values of the three forces. The components of the ligament forces parallel to the tibial plateau must be equal and opposite. The sum of the components of the ligament forces perpendicular to the plateau is balanced by the contact force.

Since there are two conditions on three forces, only the relative values of the forces are controlled by mechanics. In the case of a graft or prosthesis, the absolute values of the forces would depend on the value of the tension that the surgeon chooses to apply when achieving fixation to the bone. Since we are concerned with ligament forces, we present the values of those forces expressed as proportions of the tibiofemoral contact force.

Figure 11-25 shows the calculated values of the cruciate ligament forces per unit contact force, plotted against flexion angle. It will be seen that the two ligament forces are equal at about 43° of flexion when they are equally inclined to the plateau, and their contributions to the contact force are also equal. The ACL

force decreases and the PCL force increases with increasing flexion as the former rotates towards, and the latter away from, the tibial plateau.

These results imply that an ACL graft tensioned near extension is likely to slacken with flexion. However, we have shown (Fig. 11-8b) that anterior laxity under a constant applied anterior load decreases with flexion as the ligament becomes more ideally aligned to resist anterior tibial displacement. Tensioning of an ACL graft fixed in extension may not therefore lead to undue anterior laxity in flexion. Conversely, if an ACL graft is tensioned in flexion, it is likely to tighten as the joint is extended, with the danger of stretching of the graft or limitation of extension. The opposite considerations would apply to the tensioning of a PCL graft.

Discussion

The study of self-equilibrating forces throws some light on the status of the single muscle and antagonistic/agonistic responses to load described in Figs. 11-11, 11-12, 11-15, 11-17, 11-19, and 11-20. It is clear that

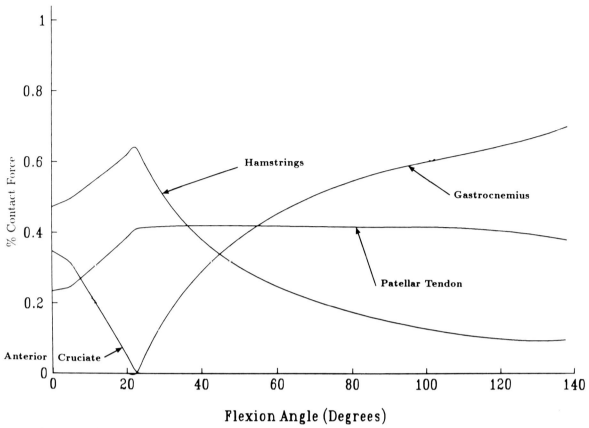

FIG. 11-24. Self-equilibrating forces. Isometric contractions with minimum ligament participation.

mechanics alone does not determine the forces transmitted by the structures of the knee and that there is not a unique solution for any loading situation.

Arbitrary values of either of (or both) the self-equilibrating solutions of Figs. 11-21 and 11-22 can be added to the single muscle solutions to give antagonistic solutions with ligament participation, valid over the entire range of flexion, with each superposition giving a system of joint forces in equilibrium with the loads. However, the key word is "added". Any addition of the self-equilibrating solutions to the single muscle load response solutions must increase the muscle and contact forces. The single muscle solutions therefore represent the minimal response of the joint to load, at least from the point of view of muscle and contact forces.

The ligament protecting antagonistic solutions of Figs. 11-17 and 11-19 represent particular combinations of single muscle and self-equilibrating forces which result in zero ligament forces and are not valid over the entire flexion range. Even when they are valid, there is not a unique ligament-protecting combination of muscle forces, since arbitrary values of the self-equilibrating ligament-protecting solution of Fig.

11-23 can be added to give a system of muscle and contact forces in equilibrium with the loads.

These results may have significance beyond the province of ligament injury and surgery. They show that simultaneous muscle action, agonistic or antagonistic, can dispose entirely of the need for ligament forces in stabilizing the limb or can minimize their contribution. Thus, there is not always an absolute need for ligaments to act as structural or mechanical elements. Barrack and Skinner, in Chapter 6, have provided powerful evidence of the sensory function of knee ligaments. Perhaps one of their functions is to act as sensory proprioceptive elements used in the control of limb position, providing the feedback signals needed in the choice of the correct balance of muscle forces required to position the bones upon each other precisely. The ligaments could be loaded when the bones occupy other than the desired positions, and muscle forces could then be adjusted until the desired position is attained. Minimum ligament strain would signal arrival at the desired position.

It is clear, however, that if EMG indicates that only one muscle group, extensor or flexor, is active, the ligaments must be loaded. If EMG indicates antago-

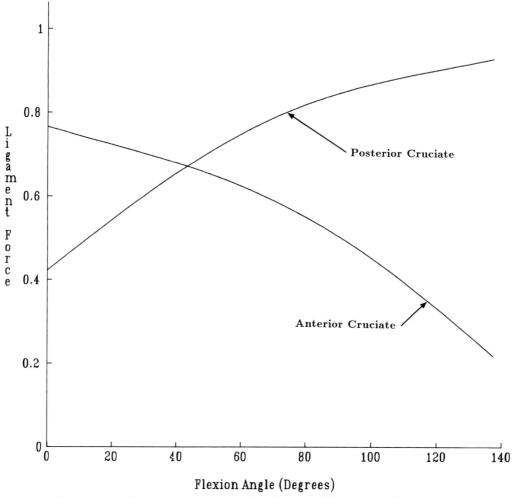

FIG. 11-25. Self-equilibrating ligament and contact forces. ACL and PCL forces per unit contact force, plotted against flexion angle.

nistic or agonistic action, the ligaments may or may not be loaded.

MECHANICS OF THE KNEE IN THE CORONAL PLANE

Coronal Plane Geometry

Next, we describe the outlines of a theory of knee mechanics in the coronal plane. Progress can be made with the mechanics of the joint in the coronal plane by making some simplifications in our descriptions of the geometry. We shall treat the two femoral condyles as circular, with centers at **C** laterally and **E** medially (Fig. 11-26) (21). The tibial plateaus are also considered circular, with centers at **B** laterally and **D** medially.

For reasons argued in the discussion of Fig. 10-7 above, the articular surfaces in each compartment of the joint must touch along the line joining their centers, which is the common normal to the articular surfaces at their point of contact.

The two common normals intersect at the point $\mathbf{I_T}$ (Fig. 11-26). This point has the same significance in the coronal plane as the intersection of the cruciates has in the sagittal. It is the instant center for movements of abduction or adduction, provided that contact is maintained in both compartments. Taking the femur to be fixed and the tibia to be moving into abduction or adduction, both points of contact move perpendicular to lines joining them to the instant center, a condition that can be satisfied only if the instant center is at $\mathbf{I_T}$. From a kinematical point of view, this result may be more of theoretical than practical interest, since movement of the bones about $\mathbf{I_T}$ would eventually result in separation of the articular surfaces in one or the other compartment. Once separation occurs, the instant center for subsequent movements is then located in the opposite compartment.

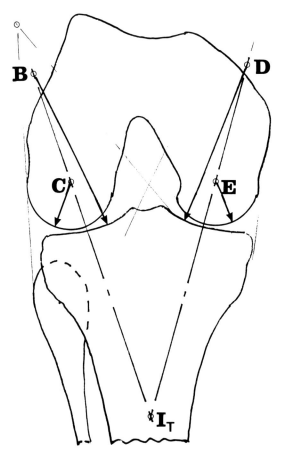

FIG. 11-26. Coronal plane geometry. Surfaces of the tibia and femur are taken to be circular, with centers at **B** and **C** laterally and **D** and **E** medially. The line of centers in each compartment passes through the point of contact of the bones. The two lines of centers intersect at I_T.

Lines of Action of the Compartmental Compressive Forces

If the articular surfaces are frictionless, then the two lines of centers are also the lines of action of the resultant compressive forces transmitted between the bones in the two compartments and they, too, intersect at I_T. The compressive forces have no moment about I_T.

Passive Stability in Abduction/Adduction

Response to an External Force

Loads applied to the limb purely in the coronal plane of the tibia can be balanced by some combination of (a) the contact forces in the two compartments and (b) forces in the collateral and cruciate ligaments. In this section, we describe the combinations of ligament and contact forces required to balance external loads pushing the tibia into varus or valgus, without muscle action.

Figure 11-27a is a diagram of a load **W**, applied to the tibia and passing through I_T but dividing the angle defined by the two center lines. The two contact forces F_M and F_L also pass through I_T and, in some combination, can balance the applied load, without ligament or muscle action. The values of the two contact forces can be calculated from the triangle of forces (Fig. 11-27b), where each of the forces is drawn parallel to its line of action in Fig. 11-27a. The contact forces are each proportional to and somewhat smaller than the load.

When the load lies precisely along the lateral center line, the compressive force F_L in the lateral compartment is exactly equal in magnitude to the load and the medial compartment is just unloaded and on the point of lift-off. Equally, a load applied along the medial line of centers just unloads the lateral compartment. The two lines of center therefore define the range in line of action of external loads which can be balanced by compressive forces in both compartments, without ligament force. If the line of action of the load is directed more medially or laterally, the soft tissues surrounding the lateral or medial compartments, respectively, have to provide tension forces to prevent lift-off.

Examples are shown in Figs. 11-28 and 11-29. In Fig. 11-28a, the load **W** is directed somewhat medially, pushing the tibia into varus. It compresses the surfaces of the medial compartment together, and they react by transmitting a compressive force F_M. The surfaces in the lateral compartment are no longer in contact. The ACL and the LCL provide the tensile forces necessary to prevent adduction. The resultant of the two ligament forces, **R** in Fig. 11-28a, must pass through the point I_L of their intersection. Since the tibia is loaded only by three forces, **W**, F_M, and **R**, their lines of action must be concurrent and the soft tissue force **R** must also pass through I_T where the other two forces meet. These considerations define the line of action of the soft tissue force **R** and make it possible to draw the triangle of force (Fig. 11-28b), which expresses the relationship between the load **W**, the contact force F_M, and the soft tissue force **R**. Once the value of **R** is known, its components **A** in the ACL and **L** in the LCL can also be determined from a secondary triangle of forces.

Essentially similar arguments make it possible to determine the lateral compartment compression F_L, as well as the forces **M** in the MCL and **P** in the PCL, when the line of action of the external load passes somewhat lateral to the lines of center, pushing the tibia into the valgus (Fig. 11-29). The relationships between load, compressive, and ligament forces vary with flexion because the shapes of the articular surfaces and the directions of the ligaments change.

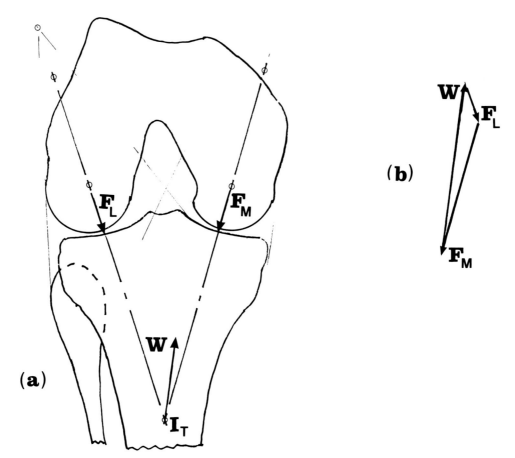

FIG. 11-27. Coronal plane mechanics. **a**: An external load **W** passing through I_T and dividing the angle defined by the lines of centers can be balanced by compressive forces in the two compartments, without ligament or muscle action. **b**: Triangle of forces giving the relationship between the load and the medial and lateral compressive forces F_M and F_L.

Response to a Pure Couple

Figure 11-30 is a diagram of a system of forces that could keep the tibia in equilibrium when subjected to a pure couple **C**, with zero resultant force. The sense of the couple rotates the tibia into abduction and is balanced by (a) a compressive force F_L in the lateral compartment and (b) tensile forces in the ACL and MCL. The resultant **R** of the ligament forces passes through their point of intersection **J** and is equal in magnitude and opposite in direction to the lateral contact force. The couple comprising the two forces **R** and F_L has a moment equal in magnitude and opposite in direction to the applied couple **C**.

Essentially similar arguments apply if the couple rotates the tibia into adduction. Figure 11-31 demonstrates that such a couple can be balanced by (a) a contact force in the medial compartment and (b) tension forces in the PCL and LCL.

General Loading of the Tibia

Our discussion of Fig. 11-4 above implied that any system of forces applied in a plane can be reduced to a single concentrated force acting through an arbitrary point and a pure couple. Thus, the passive response at the knee to any arbitrary forces applied to the tibia in the coronal plane must be some superposition of the systems of forces shown in Figs. 11-27 to 11-31 or combinations of three ligament forces balancing purely distractive loads. In general, therefore, any of the six possible forces—the two contact forces and the four ligament forces—could be involved in balancing any load applied to the tibia in the coronal plane.

Whereas in our discussion of possible combinations of contact, ligament, and muscle forces in the sagittal plane, three of the six possible forces are sufficient to balance any arbitrary load applied to the tibia in the coronal plane, most of the 20 possible combinations would be ruled out for a given loading by the fact that the contact forces should be compressive and the ligament forces tensile. What is clear is that the cruciate ligaments are as likely to be involved as the collaterals. The outcome of clinical tests that stress the limb into abduction and adduction is likely to be affected by deficiencies in the cruciates as well as by deficiencies in the collaterals.

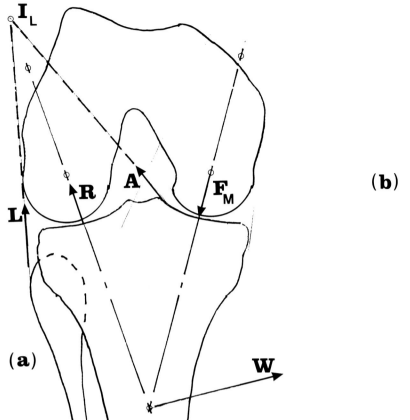
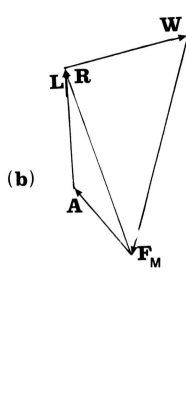

FIG. 11-28. Coronal plane mechanics. **a**: an external load **W**, passing through I$_T$ but outside the angle of the lines of centers, pushes the knee into varus and is resisted by a contact force **F**$_M$ in the medial compartment and by tension forces **L** and **A** in the LCL and ACL. The ligament forces have a resultant **R** which must pass through their point of intersection I$_L$ and through I$_T$. **b**: Values of **R** and **F**$_M$ in terms of **W** are determined by a triangle of forces. Values of the ligament forces are then determined from **R** by a triangle of forces.

DISCUSSION

This analysis shows how not only the collateral ligaments but the cruciates as well are needed to provide mediolateral stability of the knee and to control the alignment of the limb. Its conclusions verify the experimental results of Piziali (30), who showed that the ACL helps to resist medial displacement of the tibia and that the PCL helps to resist lateral displacement of the tibia. Seering (31), using the same apparatus, showed how the PCL cooperates with the MCL in resisting rotary movements in abduction. Admittedly, his evidence of the role of the ACL with LCL in resisting adduction was somewhat more equivocal.

The analysis suggests an important role for the cruciate ligaments in the control of leg alignment and may explain why alignment deformities rapidly increase when the ACL is damaged in arthritis and why release of the collateral ligaments is often necessary when the cruciate ligaments are sacrificed by the surgeon implanting a knee prosthesis.

It should be noted from the triangles of forces in Figs. 11-27 to 11-29 that when one compartment has lost contact, the contact force in the other is a much larger proportion of the load than when both compartments are compressed. This is because the compressive force has to balance not only the upward thrust of the load but also the upward pull of the soft tissues.

We have considered only loads applied purely in the coronal plane and have discussed only a very limited selection of the possible combinations of two contact forces and four ligament forces to such loads. Other combinations require further investigation.

Active intervention from the iliotibial tract and/or the separate lateral and medial heads of hamstrings or

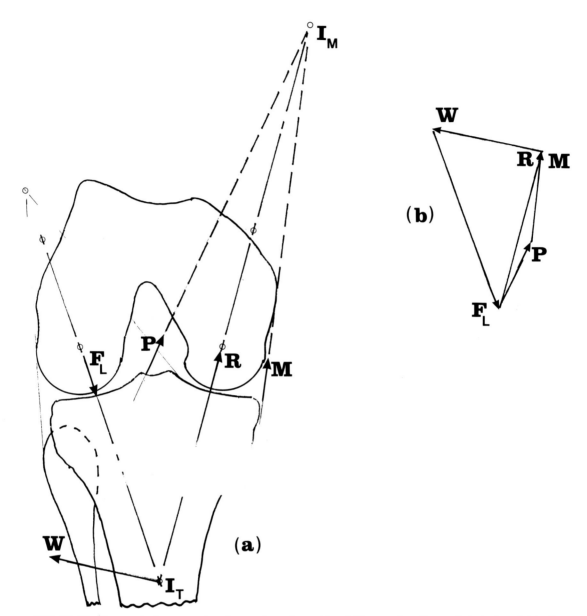

FIG. 11-29. Coronal plane mechanics. **a**:An external load **W**, passing through I_T but outside the angle of the lines of centers, pushes the knee into valgus and is resisted by a contact force **F**_L in the lateral compartment and by tension forces **M** and **P** in the MCL and PCL. The ligament forces have a resultant **R** which must pass through their point of intersection I_M and through I_T. **b**: Values of **R** and **F**_L in terms of **W** are determined by a triangle of forces. Values of the ligament forces are then determined from **R** by a triangle of forces.

gastrocnemius definitely contributes to the active control of abduction or adduction. These factors also require investigation.

Apart from clinical testing, loading purely in the coronal plane is rare. The values of the ligament forces are determined by the three-dimensional geometry and mechanics of the joint. Three-dimensional studies are now in hand but are guided by what has been learned from these studies in the sagittal and coronal planes.

The Menisci

In our discussions of the geometry and mechanics of the knee, we have not mentioned the menisci, although it is known (32) that they transmit the bulk of the compressive forces between the femur and the tibia. We have been concerned with methods to determine the resultant compressive force transmitted between the articular surfaces, not with the more complex problem of determining the distribution of contact stresses. It

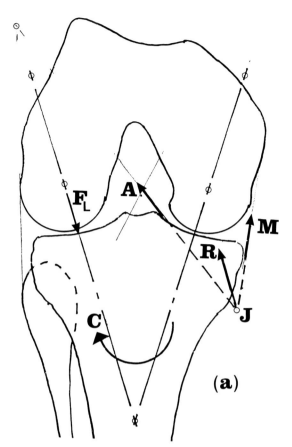

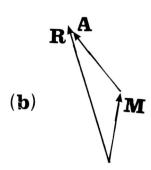

FIG. 11-30. Coronal plane mechanics. **a**: A pure couple **C**, stressing the limb into abduction, is balanced by an equal and opposite pure couple comprising the lateral contact force F_L and a ligamentous force **R**. The ligamentous force is provided by the ACL and the MCL and acts through the point **J** of their intersection. **b**: The relationship between the force **R** and its components **M** and **A** is given by the triangle of forces.

is therefore implied in the theory that the menisci do not restrain the movements of the bones upon each other or control the direction of the contact force. The menisci act as passive mobile conforming bearings that match the dissimilar shapes of the bones together and reduce the level of contact stresses.

CONCLUSION

The cruciate ligaments are directed anteroposteriorly, mediolaterally, and proximodistally. As such, they have roles to play in all three dimensions. The collateral ligaments are directed mainly proximodistally and, to some extent, anteroposteriorly. Their main roles are in controlling abduction/adduction and tibial rotation. Since we have concentrated on the sagittal plane, the collateral ligaments have played only a minor role in our discussion.

The simple two-dimensional methods of this chapter

have given some insight into (a) the forces transmitted by the structures of the knee in the drawer test, (b) the factors that govern loading of the ligaments by the muscles, and (c) the relationships between muscle and ligament forces during antagonistic, agonistic, and isometric muscle contractions. Clearly, a two-dimensional analysis cannot tell the whole story. The effect of coronal plane mechanics on the values of ligament and contact forces has been indicated and is currently being worked out in detail. Further study is required to include (a) transverse plane mechanics and (b) the effects of tibial rotation.

Apart from our analysis of the drawer test, the work presented here has been based on rigid-body geometry and mechanics, and the results are independent of the mechanical properties of the tissues. The elastic analysis of the drawer test suggests that rigid-body analysis can elucidate many features of the behavior of the joint but that the calculated values of the ligament forces may be somewhat overestimated. In the next chapter,

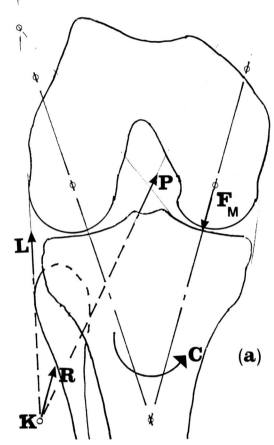

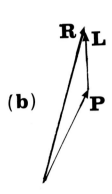

FIG. 11-31. Coronal plane mechanics. **a**: A pure couple **C**, stressing the limb into adduction, is balanced by an equal and opposite pure couple comprising the medial contact force F_M and a ligamentous force **R**. The ligamentous force is provided by the PCL and the LCL and acts through the point **K** of their intersection. **b**: The relationship between the force **R** and its components **L** and **P** is given by the triangle of forces.

we shall show surprising agreement between many of our calculated results and measurements on cadaver specimens.

The effects of soft tissue deformation, including that of articular cartilage, may be most important in the study of torsional laxity in the presence of muscle forces. Small changes in the directions of the muscle tendons could have significant influence on their contribution to torsional stability.

ACKNOWLEDGMENTS

The work described in this chapter was supported by a grant from the Arthritis and Rheumatism Council. Some of the ideas of this chapter were first developed while John O'Connor was a visitor at the Department of Orthopedics, University of California, San Diego.

REFERENCES

1. Bandi W. Chondromalacia patellae und femoro-patellare arthrose. Atiologie, klinik und therapie. *Helv Chir Acta* 1972 (Suppl II).
2. Baratta R, Solomonow M, Zhou BH, Letson D, Chuinard R, D'Ambrosia R. The role of the antagonistic musculature in maintaining knee stability. *Am J Sports Med* 1988;16:113–122.
3. Biden E. The mechanics of synovial joints. D. Phil. thesis, University of Oxford, 1981.
4. Bishop RED. On the mechanics of the human knee. *Eng Med* 1977;6:48–52.
5. Bishop RED, Denham RA. Mechanics of the knee and problems in reconstructive surgery. *J Bone Joint Surg* 1978;60B:345–351.
6. Butler DL, Noyes FR, Grood E. Ligamentous restraint to anterior–posterior drawer in the human knee. *J Bone Joint Surg* 1980;62A:259–270.
7. Crowninshield R, Pope MH, Johnson RJ. An analytical model of the knee. *J Biomech* 1976;9:397–405.
8. Dahlkvist NJ, Mayo P, Seedhom BB. Forces during squatting and rising from a deep squat. *Eng Med* 1982;11:7–15.
9. Dowson D, Atkinson JR, Brown K. The wear of high density polyethylene with particular reference to its use in artificial human joints. In: Lieng-Huang Lee, ed. *Advances in polymeric friction and wear*, vol 5B. New York: Plenum Press, 1975;533–547.
10. Draganich LF, Andriacchi TP, Andersson GBJ. Interaction between intrinsic knee mechanics and the knee extensor mechanism. *J Orthop Res* 1987;5:539–547.
11. Ellis MI, Seedhom BB, Amis AA, Dowson D, Wright V. Forces in the knee joint whilst rising from normal and motorized chairs. *Eng Med* 1979;8:33–40.
12. FitzPatrick DP, O'Connor JJ. Theoretical modelling of the knee applied to the anterior drawer test. *Proc Inst Mech Eng (London)* 1989;C384/033:79–83.

13. Frankel VH, Burstein AH. *Orthopaedic biomechanics*. Philadelphia: Lea & Febiger, 1970.
14. Goodfellow JW, O'Connor JJ. Clinical results of the Oxford knee. *Clin Orthop* 1986;205:21–42.
15. Grant PG. Biomechanical significance of the instantaneous center of rotation: the human temporomandibular joint. *J Biomech* 1973;6:109–113.
16. Grood ES, Suntay WJ, Noyes FR, Butler DL. Biomechanics of the knee-extension exercise. *J Bone Joint Surg* 1984;66A:725–733.
17. Hanley P, Lew WD, Lewis JL, Hunter RE, Kirstukas S, Kowalczyk C. Load sharing and graft forces in anterior cruciate ligament reconstructions with the ligament augmentation device. *Am J Sports Med* 1989;17:414–422.
18. Haxton H. The function of the patella and the effects of its incision. *Surg Gynecol Obstet* 1945;80:389–396.
19. Hungerford DS, Barry M. Biomechanics of the patellofemoral joint. *Clin Orthop* 1979;144:9–15.
20. Kaufer H. Mechanical function of the patella. *J Bone Joint Surg* 1971;53A:1551–1560.
21. Kurosawa H, Walker PS, Abe S, Garg A, Hunter T. Geometry and motion of the knee for implant and orthotic design. *J Biomech* 1985,18.487–499.
22. Malcolm L, Daniel D. A mechanical substitution technique for cruciate ligament force determinations. *Trans Orthop Res Soc* 1980;26:303.
23. McDevitt CA, Muir, H. Biochemical changes in the cartilage of the knee in experimental and natural osteoarthritis of the dog. *J Bone Joint Surg* 1976;58B:94–101.
24. Nissell R. Mechanics of the knee. *Acta Orthop Scand* 1985;56 (Suppl 216).
25. Noyes FR, Grood E. The strength of the anterior cruciate ligament in humans and rhesus monkeys. *J Bone Joint Surg* 1976;58A:1074–1082.
26. O'Connor J, Goodfellow J, Biden E. Designing the human knee. In: Stokes IAF, ed. *Mechanical factors and the skeleton*, London: John Libbey, 1981.
27. O'Connor JJ, Goodfellow JW, Young SK, Biden E, Daniel D. Mechanical interactions between the muscles and the cruciate ligaments in the knee. *Trans Orthop Res Soc* 1985;31:140.
28. O'Connor J, Shercliff T, Goodfellow J. Mechanics of the knee in the sagittal plane—mechanical interactions between muscles, ligaments and articular surfaces. In: Muller W, Hackenbruch W, eds. *Surgery and arthroscopy of the knee*. Berlin: Springer-Verlag, 1988;12–30.
29. Piziali RL, Rastegar C, Nagel DA. Measurement of the coupled non-linear stiffness characteristics of the human knee. *J Biomech* 1977;10:45–51.
30. Piziali RL, Rastager J, Nagel DA, Schurman DJ. The contribution of the cruciate ligaments to the load–displacement characteristics of the human knee joint. *Trans ASME, J Biomed Eng* 1980;102:277–283.
31. Seering WP, Piziali RL, Nagel DA, Schurman DJ. The function of the primary ligaments of the knee in varus–valgus and axial rotation. *J Biomech* 1980;13:785–794.
32. Shrive NG, O'Connor JJ, Goodfellow JW. Load-bearing in the knee joint. *Clin Orthop* 1978;131:279–287.
33. Smidt GL. Biomechanical analysis of knee flexion and extension. *J Biomech* 1973;6:79–82.
34. Young SK, Rigby H, Shercliff TL, O'Connor JJ. Antagonistic quadriceps–hamstrings action. *Trans Orthop Res Soc* 1988;34:197.
35. Zernicke RF, Garhammer J, Jobe FW, Human patellar tendon rupture. *J Bone Joint Surg* 1979;59A:179–183.

Knee Ligaments: Structure, Function, Injury, and Repair, edited by D. Daniel, et al.

CHAPTER 12

The Muscle-Stabilized Knee

John O'Connor, Edmund Biden, John Bradley, David FitzPatrick, Stephen Young, Christopher Kershaw, Dale M. Daniel, and John Goodfellow

In contrast to Chapters 10 and 11, this chapter presents mainly experimental evidence. In the first section, we report experiments designed to test the sagittal plane theories of Chapters 10 and 11. The remainder of this chapter deals with the effects of muscle forces on the stability of the knee in torsion and abduction/adduction.

SAGITTAL PLANE MECHANICS

Muscle Lever-Arms

Direct experimental verification of the lengths of the muscle lever-arms is rendered difficult by the translu-

J. O'Connor and D. FitzPatrick: Department of Engineering Science, University of Oxford, Oxford OX1 3PJ, England.

E. Biden: Department of Mechanical Engineering, University of New Brunswick, Fredericton, New Brunswick, Canada E3B 5A3.

J. Bradley: Department of Orthopaedic Surgery, Colchester General Hospital, Colchester, Essex CO4 5JL, England.

S. Young: Department of Orthopaedic Surgery, South Warwickshire Hospital, Warwick CV34 5BW, England.

C. Kershaw: Department of Orthopaedics, Leicester Royal Infirmary, Leicester LE1 5WW, England.

D. Daniel: Department of Orthopedic Surgery, University of California, San Diego, School of Medicine, La Jolla, California 92037; and Kaiser Permanente Medical Center, San Diego, California 92120.

J. Goodfellow: Department of Orthopaedic Surgery, Nuffield Orthopaedic Centre, Oxford OX3 7LD, England.

cency of soft tissues, ligament, and tendon to x-ray. Also, Duke (6) has discussed possible errors in the application of the method of Rouleaux to the determination of the instant center, the focus of the lever-arms (Fig. 11-2). We have preferred an indirect method, namely, comparison of calculations and *in vitro* measurements of muscle tendon forces.

Apparatus

For measurement of quadriceps forces, two rigs were used. One rig was a simulation of the quadriceps-strengthening exercise (Fig. 11-10), with (a) the femur held at 45° to the horizontal, (b) the patellar facet pointing upwards, and (c) the weight suspended distally on the tibia; this arrangement allowed 135° of flexion. The other rig was a simulation of flexed knee stance (Fig. 8-13), with (a) the knee flexing or extending to allow the hip to move vertically above the ankle and (b) a vertical load applied on the hip/ankle axis by means of dead weight. In both arrangements, tension force **Q** applied through the quadriceps tendon and measured with a proving ring was used to balance the flexing effect of the applied load. Different positions of flexion were obtained by lengthening the quadriceps tendon wire.

For measurement of hamstrings forces, the specimens were held as in Fig. 11-14, with the femur at 45° to the horizontal and the patellar facet pointing down-

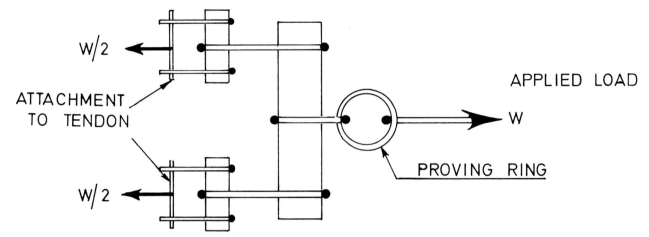

FIG. 12-1. The yoke used to give attachment to the medial and lateral heads of the hamstrings and gastrocnemius muscles. The circular proving ring was used to measure the total applied force, shared equally between the two limbs of the yoke which are equidistant from the axis of the proving ring. The medial and lateral heads of the muscles were attached to the two limbs of the yoke.

wards. A load applied distally on the tibia was balanced by a single force, **H**, shared between the hamstrings tendons. A yoke (Fig. 12-1) was used to gain attachment to the tendons of biceps laterally and semimembranosis medially. A tension force applied centrally through a proving ring balanced the extending effect of the applied load, shared equally between the medial and lateral tendons.

For measurement of gastrocnemius forces, the arrangement shown in Fig. 12-2 was used. The tibia was fixed at 45° to the horizontal, with the tibial tubercle pointing downwards. Weight hung distally from the femur was balanced by a force **G** in the tendons of the gastrocnemii. The yoke arrangement shown in Fig. 12-1 was used to share the load equally between the medial and lateral heads.

The design of each of these fixtures allowed the two

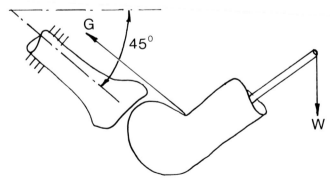

FIG. 12-2. Loading of the gastrocnemius muscles. The tibia was fixed at 45° to the horizontal. A force **G** was applied to the muscle tendons through the yoke of Fig. 12-1 to balance the load **W** hung from the free end of the femur.

bones to move freely relative to each other, subject only to the restraints applied by the ligaments and articular surfaces of the knee. When external load was applied, simulated muscle action was necessary for equilibrium.

Materials

Fresh cadaveric knees were frozen at autopsy and stored until required. They were then thawed, prepared, and used for a single experiment. Firstly, the skin and muscles were removed. The muscle tendons were identified, and a small loop of canvas strapping was sutured to each to allow the attachment of a wire; 15 cm each of femur and tibia were left on each specimen. A 3-mm-diameter hole was drilled across through each bone. The intramedullary canals were reamed; and a 10-mm bolt, with a 3-mm-diameter transverse hole 20 mm from its end, was fixed into each of the cut bone ends with methylmethacrylate cement. While the cement was setting, a pin was passed through the transverse holes in bone and bolt for increased rotational stability. Locking nuts were screwed onto the bolts and were tightened against the bone ends to provide a secure bone–bolt connection. The studs protruding from each bone could then be used to attach the specimen to either one or other of the rigs used in the tests.

Method

For each specimen, the quadriceps, hamstrings, and gastrocnemius forces necessary to balance a range of external loads were measured at different points in the flexion arc, from full extension to 135° of flexion. The wire attached to the muscle tendon was successively lengthened to stabilize the joint at different positions.

Calculation of Muscle Forces

The computer model of Chapters 10 and 11 was used to calculate the values of the muscle forces for each of the experimental configurations. Graphs similar to those in Fig. 11-11 were obtained—that is, plots of muscle force per unit load versus flexion angle. Two sets of calculations were performed: One set was based on the parameters given in the appendix to Chapter 10, derived from anthropometrical measurements on four specimens. The second set was based on the values of the parameters deduced from similar measurements on a single specimen, specimen A, these measurements being made after the specimen had been subject to the range of muscle force measurements.

Results

Quadriceps Forces in Leg-Lift

Figure 12-3A is a plot of the measured quadriceps tendon force versus flexion angle for specimen A at six values of the applied load. It will be seen that the quadriceps force varies with flexion angle and with applied load. In Fig. 12-3B, the same data are presented in nondimensional form: Measured quadriceps force divided by the value of the applied load is plotted against flexion angle, in the manner of Fig. 11-11.

Expressing measured forces in the form of a nondimensional ratio allows direct comparisons to be made between the results of tests carried out at different applied loads. In this form, the experimental results coalesce onto a single curve with only slight scatter. The coalescence indicates that, within the range of the loads used in these experiments, the quadriceps force at any flexion angle is proportional to the applied load; the quadriceps force per unit load is therefore independent of the absolute value of the applied load, as suggested by the theory of Chapter 11.

Figure 12-3B also includes a solid line, the theo-

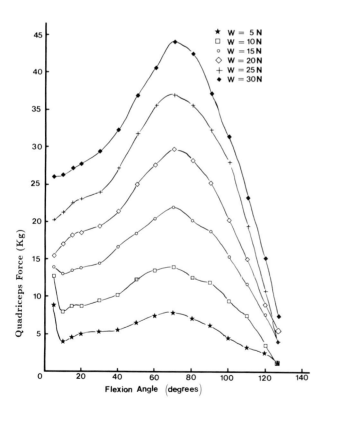

A

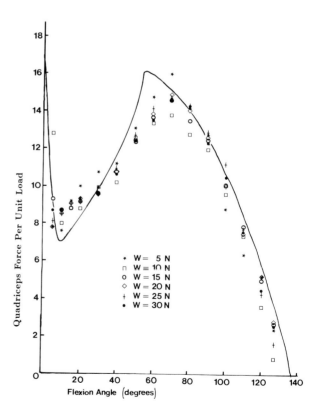

B

FIG. 12-3. Specimen A. **A:** Forces in the quadriceps tendon during leg-lift, plotted against flexion angle, for six values of the applied load. **B:** quadriceps force per unit load, plotted against flexion angle. The solid line was calculated from the computer model using specimen A parameters.

retical quadriceps force per unit load based on the parameters for the same specimen. There is quite close agreement between theory and experiment.

Figure 12-4A is a similar nondimensional plot for six separate specimens, indicating some specimen-to-specimen variation. The solid curve was calculated from the computer model using the averaged parameters of Chapter 10. The differences between theory and experiment are barely more pronounced than the specimen-to-specimen differences.

The increasing resistance of the posterior capsule to hyperextension is indicated by the sharp increase in both experimental and theoretical quadriceps force values as extension is approached. To emphasize the effect of the posterior capsule in resisting extension,

the dashed curve in Fig. 12-4A shows how the quadriceps force would diminish as extension is approached in the absence of capsular forces. The difference between the solid and dashed curves is a quantitative demonstration of the effect of the posterior capsule in preventing hyperextension of the knee. This effect could be further demonstrated because, fortuitously, one of the specimens tested was osteoarthrotic with a flexion deformity of about 25°. The experimental results for this specimen at five different loads are shown in Fig. 12-4B. In order to match the computer calculation to the measurements in this case, it was necessary to assume that the posterior capsule began to tighten at 45° of flexion as opposed to 15° in Fig. 12-4A.

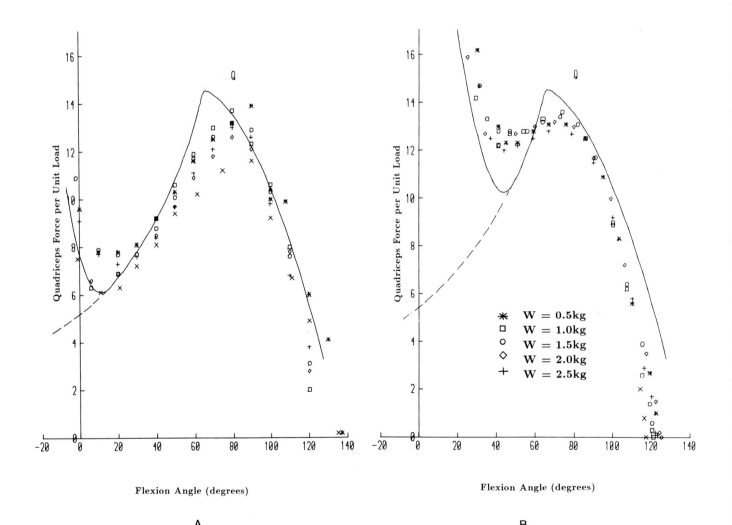

FIG. 12-4. A: Quadriceps force per unit applied load, plotted against flexion angle, for six specimens under a load of 20 N (2 kg). The solid line was calculated from the computer model for the parameters of Chapter 10. The dashed line excludes the contribution of the posterior capsule. **B:** Quadriceps force per unit load, plotted against flexion angle, at five values of the load for an osteoarthritic specimen with a flexion deformity. Solid and dashed lines were obtained from the computer model with and without the contribution of posterior capsule.

Quadriceps Forces in Flexed Knee Stance

Figure 12-5 shows the measured values of the quadriceps force per unit vertical load from 11 specimens, plotted against flexion angle. The results for a single specimen at different loads again coalesced onto a single curve, but the examples of such curves in Fig. 12-5 showed some scatter from specimen to specimen. The figure also contains data calculated from the results of Perry (26), which are quite consistent with ours.

The solid line, calculated from the computer model, gives an upper bound to the measurements. From about 10°, the quadriceps force increases steadily with flexion in this experiment, in contrast to what is shown

in Figs. 12-3 and 12-4. In the flexed knee stance rig, the specimen had to be pushed backwards to achieve hyperextension against the resistance of the posterior capsule. In the absence of such a push but in the presence of vertical load, full extension could only rarely be achieved; the appropriate theoretical curve is probably the dashed curve of Fig. 12-5, calculated without the contribution of the posterior capsule.

Hamstrings Forces

Figure 12-6A shows the measured values of the hamstrings force needed in specimen A at five values of the applied load. Dividing the measured value of the

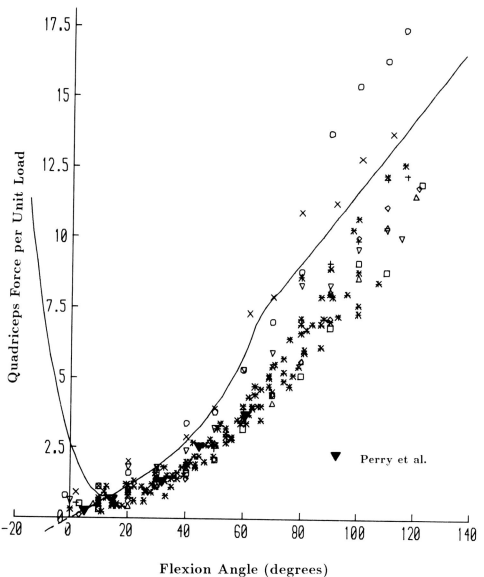

FIG. 12-5. Quadriceps force per unit applied load, plotted against flexion angle, for 11 specimens in the flexed knee stance rig. Solid and dashed lines were obtained from computer model with and without the contribution of the posterior capsule for the parameters of Chapter 10.

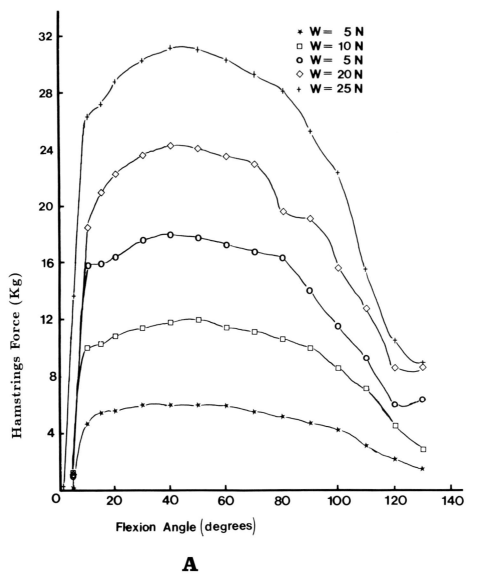

A

FIG. 12-6. A: Specimen A. Hamstrings force plotted against flexion angle for five applied loads. **B:** Specimen A. Hamstrings force per unit applied load in leg-lift, plotted against flexion angle, for five applied loads. The solid line was obtained from the computer model using specimen A parameters. **C:** Hamstrings force per unit applied load in leg-lift, plotted against flexion angle, for five specimens under a load of 2 kg. Solid and dashed lines were obtained from the computer model using the parameters of Chapter 10 with and without the contribution of the posterior capsule, respectively.

hamstrings force by the value of the applied load, the same data are plotted in nondimensional form in Fig. 12-6B, where they will be seen to coalesce onto a single curve. For this specimen, the maximum hamstrings force per unit load was found near 45° of flexion, where the lever-arm available to the external load was maximum.

The solid line in Fig. 12-6B was calculated from the computer model using the parameters of specimen A.

Similar results for six specimens are plotted in Fig. 12-6C. There is rather more scatter from specimen to specimen than was found with the quadriceps force

measurements. In particular, the flexion angle at which the maximum hamstrings tension occurred varied from about 60° in some specimens down to 20° in others. In all specimens, near full extension the tension fell very rapidly as the posterior capsule tightened, and its fibers worked agonistically with the hamstrings to balance the extending effect of the load. Eventually, in hyperextension, the extending effect of the load was entirely balanced by the posterior capsule and no hamstrings action was required. Larger loads produced more hyperextension.

Most of the behavior just described was reproduced

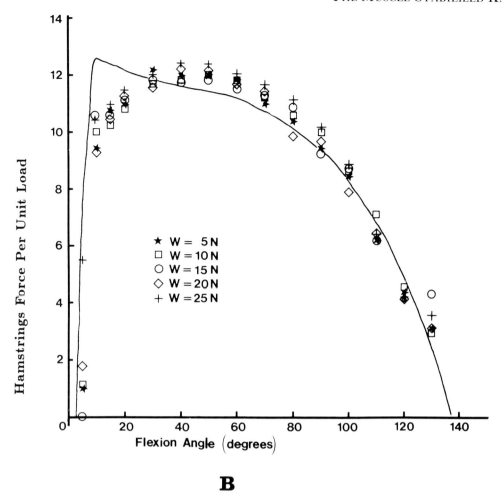

B

FIG. 12-6. (*Continued*)

by the solid line calculated from the computer model. The calculation predicts muscle forces nearer the lower level of the observations from different specimens. The calculated hamstrings force increases slowly as extension is approached and falls rapidly as the posterior capsule tightens. The differences between solid and dashed lines near extension demonstrate the agonistic action of the posterior capsule when acting with the hamstrings to limit extension.

Gastrocnemius Forces

Figure 12-7A shows the measured gastrocnemius force in the loading configuration of Fig. 12-2 for specimen A under five values of the external load. The same data, nondimensionalized, are presented in Fig. 12-7B. The coalescence onto a single curve to be expected in Fig. 12-7B is perhaps not quite as convincing as in Figs. 12-3B and 12-6B. The trend towards increasing values of the gastrocnemius force per unit load at high flexion may be an artifact of the experiment for this specimen where the canvas straps sutured to the muscle tendons were being squeezed in the decreasing gap between the backs of the bones. The solid line, calculated from the computer model with specimen A parameters, underestimates the measured forces at high flexion, predicts quite closely the maximum gastrocnemius force per unit load at about 60° of flexion, and somewhat overestimates the forces as extension is approached.

Figure 12-7C shows the gastrocnemius force per unit applied load for five specimens. There was some scatter from specimen to specimen, with the maximum gastrocnemius force varying from about 18 to 23 times the applied load between 45° and 60° of flexion. Near full extension, as with the hamstrings, the tightening posterior capsule acted agonistically with the gastrocnemius muscles until, at about 10° of hyperextension, no muscle action was needed in any specimen. The solid line from the computer model with the parameters of Chapter 10 gives values on the lower side of the observations. The differences between the solid and dashed lines near extension show how the posterior capsule progressively takes over from the muscle complete responsibility for limiting extension.

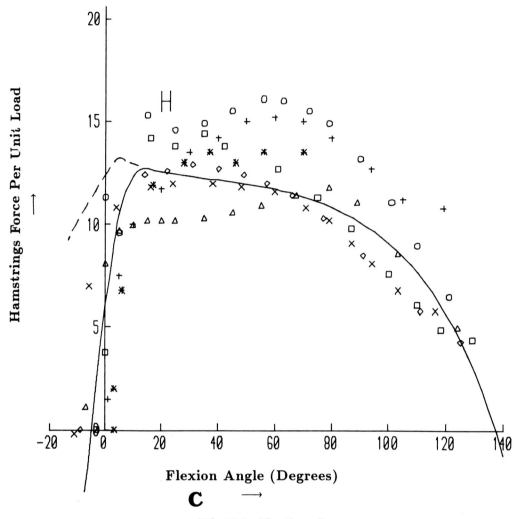

FIG. 12-6. *(Continued)*

Discussion

Comparison of Figs. 12-3 and 12-5 shows that muscle force depends on flexion angle, on the value of the applied load, and on the lever-arm available to the applied load. In the configuration of Fig. 11-10, from which Figs. 12-3 and 12-4 were obtained, the lever-arm of the applied load was longest at 45° of flexion and smallest at 135°. In the flexed knee stance rig, the lever-arm of the external load was zero at full extension and increased steadily with flexion. These differences in external leverage explain entirely the different patterns of variation of quadriceps force per unit load in the two experiments.

In general, the results of the measurements have provided some confirmation of the predictions of the calculations. The comparison between theory and measurement for specimen A shows particularly good agreement. The relative scatter of results from different specimens suggests that, for precise prediction, parameters appropriate to each particular specimen are

required. The average parameters of Chapter 10 were chosen to give a reasonable fit to the whole range of data from several specimens. Nonetheless, the theoretical calculations give the general trend and order of magnitude of the muscle force data.

The measurements and calculations showed that the muscle forces acting through small lever-arms (Fig. 11-2) can be much larger than the applied loads acting through lever-arms whose length is equal to that of the tibia. Looking at the measurements from all specimens, the maximum gastrocnemius forces (18–23 times the applied load) were larger than the maximum hamstrings forces (11–16 times the applied load) or the maximum quadriceps forces (11–14 times the applied load). This follows inversely the general trend of the calculated lever-arm lengths (Fig. 11-3), where gastrocnemius has the shortest lever-arms and quadriceps the longest. In the case of specimen A, the lever-arm of hamstrings was calculated to be longer than that of quadriceps over most of the flexion range, and the measured forces of the hamstrings were slightly

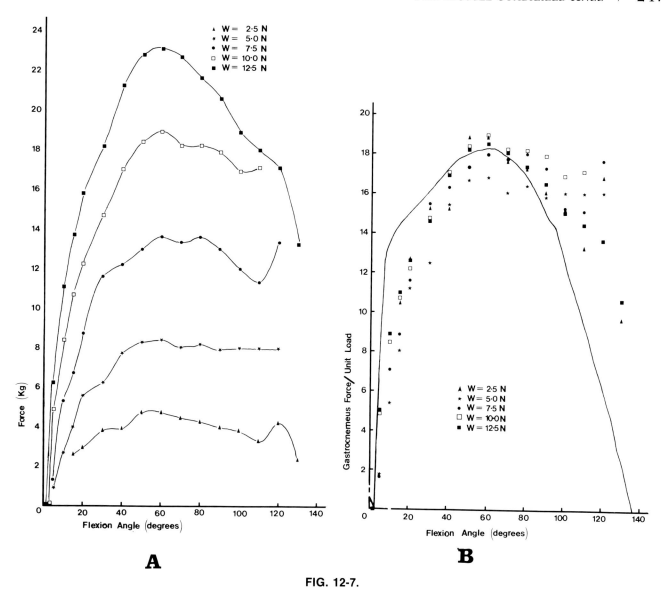

FIG. 12-7.

smaller than those of the quadriceps. Equality of hamstrings and quadriceps lever-arms would appear to be the hallmark of good design.

The values of the muscle forces per unit load reported here should not be taken to be typical of normal activity. Our experiments were designed to maximize the external leverage by applying loads perpendicular to the limb. In normal activities such as walking, the line of action of the ground reaction (Chapter 14) always passes much closer to the joints so that forces in excess of five times body weight are rarely encountered.

The calculations suggested that the forces induced in muscles in the presence of external load and in the absence of antagonistic or agonistic muscle action should be proportional to the value of the external load. This prediction is clearly confirmed by the results of Figs. 12-3B and 12-6B, where the values of muscle

force per unit load are shown to be independent of the load. This simple observation appears to have been overlooked in previous investigations from other laboratories.

When the results from different specimens are compared, there is considerably more scatter, particularly for hamstrings and gastrocnemius forces. This may have arisen because the lever-arms available to the external loads in these experiments were kept the same from test to test whereas the specimens, which were not selected for size, presumably varied. It would seem likely that the intrinsic lever-arms available to the muscle tendons would be larger in large specimens than in small ones. More careful control of the choice of external lever-arm in relation to the size of the specimen may have reduced the specimen-to-specimen scatter.

The experiments demonstrated the effects of the posterior capsule in preventing hyperextension, a sud-

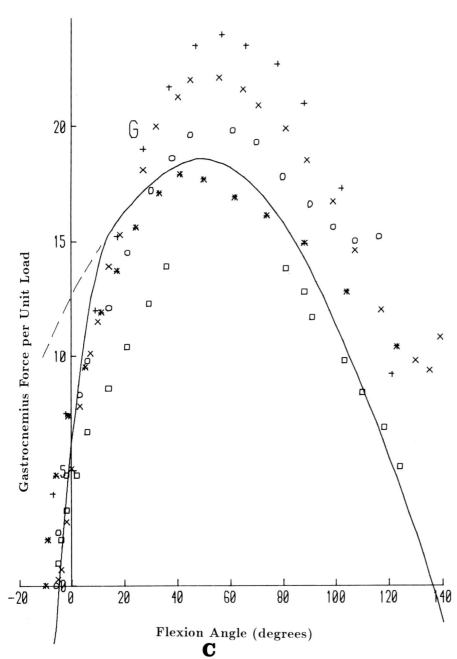

FIG. 12-7. A: Specimen A. Gastrocnemius force plotted against flexion angle for five applied loads. **B:** Specimen A. Gastrocnemius force per unit applied load in leg-lift, plotted against flexion angle, for five applied loads. The solid line was obtained from the computer model using specimen A parameters. **C:** Gastrocnemius force per unit applied load in leg-lift, plotted against flexion angle, for five specimens under a load of 1 kg. Solid and dashed lines were obtained from the computer model using the parameters of Chapter 10 with and without the contribution of the posterior capsule, respectively.

den rise in the quadriceps force and reduction in hamstrings and gastrocnemius forces as extension was approached. Grood (11) attempted to determine the length of the quadriceps lever-arm by dividing the measured flexing moment (taken to be the product of measured external load times its lever-arm about the tibiofemoral contact point) by the measured quadriceps force (Fig. 11-13), which we have already shown to be consistent with our calculations. While our calculations of lever-arm length (Fig. 11-3) are in reasonable agreement with Grood's for the flexed joint, he showed a dramatic decrease in the lever-arm below 20° by not accounting for the antagonistic effect of the posterior capsule.

One of the main deficiencies of the theory is that it does not account for the contributions of the collateral ligaments, medial or lateral. In Chapter 10, we suggested that the flexion axis of the knee penetrates not only the two cruciate ligaments but the medial collateral ligament (MCL) as well. It follows that any force in the MCL would have no moment about the flexion axis and would make no contribution to resisting the flexing or extending effect of external load. The lateral collateral ligament (LCL) lies entirely behind the flexion axis and therefore slackens during passive flexion. It may be expected to make relatively little contribution to the transmission of loads applied in the sagittal plane. Agreement between theory and experiment for specimen A therefore supports the notion that the focus of the muscle lever-arms at the knee is an axis through the intersection of the cruciate ligaments, the instant center of the joint in the sagittal plane.

Cruciate Ligament Forces in Flexion and Extension

Our analysis in Chapter 11 suggested that one or the other of the cruciate ligaments must be loaded when a single muscle group is acting to extend or flex the knee. We postulated the existence of a critical flexion angle. Between extension and the critical angle, the anterior cruciate ligament (ACL) would be loaded by all muscle groups. Above the critical angle, the posterior cruciate ligament (PCL) would be loaded. The value of the critical angle would depend on the muscle group active and on the line of action of the applied load. In this section, we report experiments designed to test these propositions.

Direct measurement of ligament force in an intact joint under a variety of loads in a variety of positions is difficult. Chapters Eight and Nine described how sequential dissection of ligaments has been used as a method of determining which ligaments resist different modes of relative movement of the bones; such methods can given quantitative information only about the increase in movement or reduction in resistance to movement consequent to ligament dissection.

In Chapter 8, we described a number of transducers used to measure ligament fiber strain or extension. These give only an indirect measure of ligament force. Having measured fiber strain under load in various positions with the transducer fixed to the ligament, it would be necessary to calibrate the strain transducer so as to relate measured strain to ligament force. The specimen would have to be disarticulated and loaded in tension, with the bones connected only by the ligament under tests and with the transducer still *in situ*. Since, as we described in Chapter 10, the shape and configuration of the ligament changes with flexion angle, the calibration would have to be performed at a number of flexion angles, with the bones and the ligament attachment areas in precisely the same relative positions as in the intact joint to reproduce the distribution of strain throughout the ligament. Account would also have to be taken of the strain induced by passive flexion from one position to another. Because of these difficulties, the literature contains only a few reports of experimental measurements of ligament forces (22,27). We have preferred an alternative method, also indirect but with the advantage of giving a more direct read-out of force.

Materials and Methods

The specimens used for the measurements of muscle forces above were also used in the present experiments. The specimens were held in one or the other of the configurations of (a) Fig. 11-10 or 8-13 for testing of the cruciate–quadriceps interaction, (b) Fig. 11-14 for the testing of the cruciate–hamstrings interaction, and (c) Fig. 12-2 for the testing of the cruciate–gastrocnemius interaction. A specimen could be used to test only one combination of a muscle with a cruciate, since the method involved division and replacement of the relevant cruciate with a substitute wire, as first described by Malcolm (22).

A series of three tests was carried out on each specimen. Firstly, the specimen was loaded and taken over the range of flexion from full extension to 135°. Measurements were made of the appropriate tendon force (Figs. 12-3 to 12-7), and the track of one bone on the other was recorded by using an optical method. One or the other of the cruciate ligaments was then divided, and the first test was repeated. The new track of one bone upon the other was recorded. Where the new track diverged from that of the intact joint, it was inferred that the divided cruciate ligament had been loaded in the intact specimen. Where the tracks coincided, the ligament had not been loaded. The flexion angle at which divergence occurred was the critical flexion angle for the particular muscle in the configuration of the experiment.

The last phase of the experiment involved replacing the cut ligament with a wire and measuring the tension needed in the wire to restore the track of the bones upon each other to that of the previously intact joint (Fig. 12-8). A 5-mm drill hole was made from the attachment of the ligament through each of the bones to the outer cortex. A section of bicycle-brake cable sheath was placed in each bone tunnel. The wire was passed through the cable sheath and along the line of the divided ligament. A reaction plate on one end of the wire was held against the outer cortex of one of the bones. To reduce friction, a teflon (PTFE) sheath was placed around the wire where it passed through the cable sheath. The wire was passed through a proving ring and attached to the moving jaw of a screw-thread vice. Between the fixed jaw of the vice and the proving ring, the wire was surrounded by a bicycle-brake cable sheath. By moving the jaws of the vice apart, tension force was applied to the wire and, by reaction, equal compression force was applied to the sheath and measured by the proving ring.

In the final phase of the experiment, the specimen was again taken over the full arc of flexion under load. The force in the ligament replacement wire required to bring the bones back to the track of the previously intact joint was measured. The measured value of the

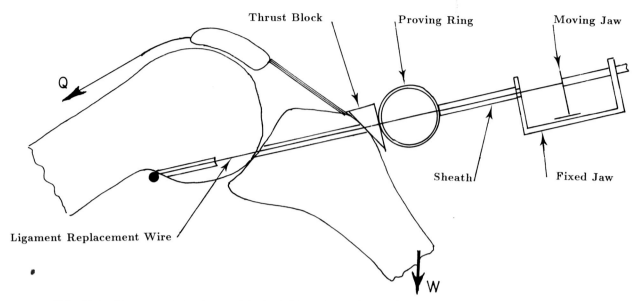

FIG. 12-8. Diagram of the knee with the ACL replaced by a wire. The wire is shown fixed to the femur and passing through tunnels in both bones and then passing through a thrust block, a proving ring, and a sprung metal sheath to the moving jaw of a screw-thread vice. The screw thread was used to apply tension to the wire. The resulting compressive reaction in the sheath was measured with the proving ring.

force was deemed to be equal to that transmitted by the ligament in the intact joint.

Optical Method

A simple optical method was used to record the track of one bone upon the other during the excursion from full extension to 135°. A perspex (plexiglass) plate (Fig. 12-9) containing a line of 0.5-mm-diameter holes, at 1-cm spacing, was attached through a ball-and-socket joint to the fixed bone. A cardboard sheet was attached through a similar joint to the movable bone. The positions of the plate and cardboard were adjusted relative to each other until the cardboard sheet moved in a plane parallel to that of the perspex plate over the flexion arc. At every 10 degrees of that arc, pins were passed through two holes in the perspex plate about 10 cm apart to puncture the cardboard sheet. The two curves created by the successions of holes gave an accurate record of the position of one bone upon the other. The method was found to be reproducible; when the specimen was taken over the flexion arc again, the pins could be passed through the holes previously created, without strain.

The recorded track reflected changes in all six possible degrees of freedom (cf. Chapter 8). The track could be altered manually by rotating the movable bone about each of three axes or translating it parallel to such axes. Thus, when a ligament was divided, the change in track reflected not only anteroposterior sub-

luxation but other possible movements as well. All these movements were reversed when force was applied through the ligament replacement wire to return the specimen to its intact track.

The force in the ligament replacement wire could be adjusted until the two bones were returned to positions where the pins could again be passed through the holes created when the joint was intact. Figure 12-10 shows the tracks that were made on a cardboard sheet before and after the PCL was divided in the presence of tension in the hamstrings tendons. The images of the holes have been enlarged for clarity.

Results

In the following graphs, the x-axis represents the angle of flexion of the knee. The y-axis represents the value of the measured tension in the ligament replacement wire, divided by the value of the applied load. The theoretical analysis of the experimental configurations of Chapter 11 suggested that the ligament forces, like the muscle forces, should be proportional to applied load, and it also suggested that the ligament forces per unit load should be independent of the load. In each of the graphs, we present not only the points representing the measurements but also lines representing the values of the ligament forces calculated from the computer model, using the parameters of Chapter 10.

The method described above for the measurement of ligament forces worked reasonably well in the pres-

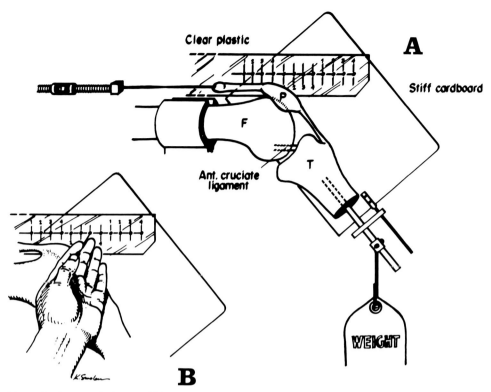

FIG. 12-9. Optical technique of Malcolm (22) used to record the track of the moving tibia on the fixed femur. **A:** A perspex sheet was fixed to the femur, with the line of holes lying parallel to the long axis of the bone. A cardboard sheet was fixed to the tibia. **B:** Pins through two holes in the perspex sheet were used to punch holes in the cardboard.

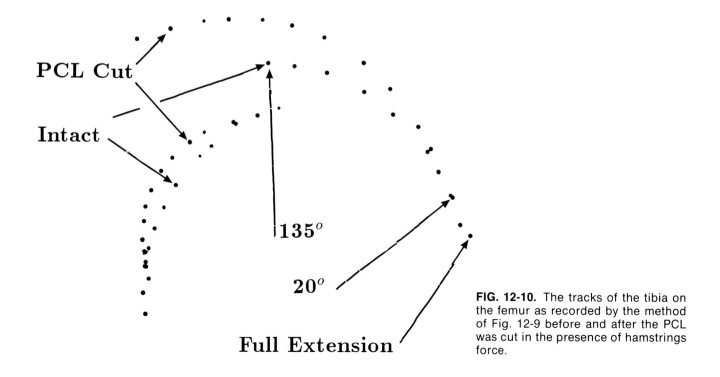

FIG. 12-10. The tracks of the tibia on the femur as recorded by the method of Fig. 12-9 before and after the PCL was cut in the presence of hamstrings force.

ence of quadriceps and hamstrings action but not with gastrocnemius. Possible reasons are discussed below. We can therefore compare measurement and calculation of ligament forces with quadriceps and hamstrings action in the muscle-strengthening simulation and with quadriceps in flexed knee stance.

ACL Forces with Quadriceps in Leg-Lift

Values of the force in the ACL replacement wire per unit external load are plotted against flexion angle in Fig. 12-11A, which contains measurements made by Malcolm (22) on four specimens at four different loads and by the present authors on two specimens. The Malcolm experiment was the same as ours except that he held the femur horizontal, rather than at 45° to the horizontal. Although the measurements exhibit considerable scatter, they demonstrate that the critical flexion angle beyond which the quadriceps does not load the ACL is slightly greater than 60°. They further demonstrate how the ACL force increases as extension is approached. In all these tests, the track followed by the bones after the sectioning of the ACL was the same as that of the intact joint above 60° of flexion, implying that the ACL in the intact joint was not loaded by quadriceps action above 60°.

The two lines drawn in Fig. 12-11A are the calculated values of the ACL force for the configuration of Fig. 11-10 with the femur inclined at 45° to the horizontal and for that of Malcolm (22) with the femur horizontal. The calculations provide an upper bound for the bulk of the experimental data. They suggest that the results obtained from the two slightly different configurations should be quite similar.

PCL Forces with Quadriceps in Leg-Lift

Measured values of the force in the PCL replacement wire with quadriceps action in the configuration of Fig. 11-10 are shown for four specimens in Fig. 12-11B. In each of the specimens, PCL force was required above a critical flexion angle which was more than 80° in three specimens and 70° in the fourth. Below the critical angle, the track of the intact specimen was reproduced in each case after the PCL had been divided. The solid line in Fig. 12-11B is the calculated value of the PCL force. The calculation suggests a slightly higher critical angle than given by the measurements, and it also suggests slightly higher maximum PCL forces.

ACL Forces with Quadriceps in Flexed Knee Stance

Values of the ACL force per unit vertical load measured in the flexed knee stance rig (Fig. 8-13) are plot-

ted against flexion angle in Fig. 12-12 for four specimens. As in Fig. 12-11, there is considerable scatter in the results but the value of the critical flexion angle is less clearly defined. For three specimens, it lay in the region 50–70°, for a fourth it lay at about 110°, and for the fifth specimen no critical angle was apparent and the value of the ACL force appeared to continue to grow with increasing flexion. The calculation, the solid line, suggested a critical flexion angle of 87.5° for this configuration and provided an upper bound for most of the data obtained below that angle. The large ACL forces near extension in some of the specimens could only be reproduced by the model with the inclusion of the effect of the posterior capsule. The dashed curve near extension is the predicted ACL force in the absence of the posterior capsule.

Whitmer (37) described the use of a Hall Effect transducer (1) (Chapter 8) to measure strain in the ACL when supported and loaded in a manner similar to our experiment. His graph of ACL strain plotted against flexion angle is very similar in form to our theoretical curve without the posterior capsule contribution. We have explained the difficulties in transforming such strain data to give values of ligament force.

PCL Forces with Quadriceps in Flexed Knee Stance

Although this experiment was performed on five specimens at various positions up to 120° of flexion, the results were difficult to interpret. In three of the specimens, the original track of the intact joint was recovered over the entire range of flexion after sectioning of the PCL without the application of additional forces. In two others, the track of the intact joint was not recovered at any point in the range of movement after sectioning of the PCL. In these two specimens, the track could subsequently be recovered by the application of force in the PCL replacement wire, with quite substantial force being applied in one of these specimens. These sets of results were therefore contradictory: One set implied that the PCL is inactive in flexed knee stance over the flexion range up to 120°, whereas the second set implied the reverse. The calculation, the dotted line in Fig. 12-12, suggested that very large PCL forces are required above the critical angle of 87.5°.

ACL Forces with Hamstrings in Leg-Lift

The ACL replacement experiment was performed in four specimens with hamstrings forces in the configuration of Fig. 11-14. In two of them, the track of the intact joint was reproduced over the entire range of movement after sectioning the ACL, implying that the ACL was not loaded by hamstrings action in these

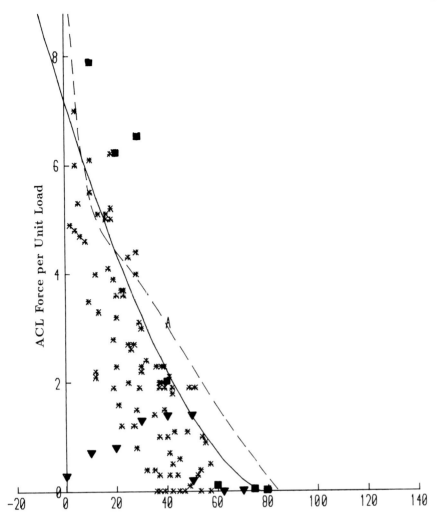

Flexion Angle (degrees)

A

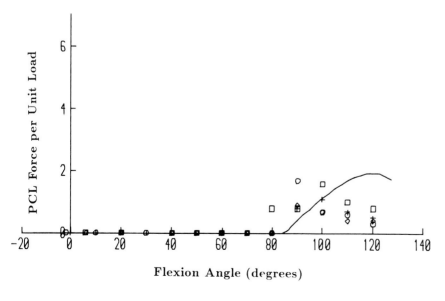

Flexion Angle (degrees)

B

FIG. 12-11. Values of the ACL **(A)** and PCL **(B)** forces per unit applied load, plotted against flexion angle for the leg-lift experiment with quadriceps action. In part A, square and triangular points are from two specimens under 2 kg load, with the femur fixed at 45°. The remaining points were obtained by Malcolm (22) from four specimens at four loads with the femur held horizontal. The solid line plots the theoretical ACL force per unit load versus flexion angle for a horizontal femur, and the dashed line is for a femur at 45° to the horizontal; both were calculated from the computer model for the parameters of Chapter 10.

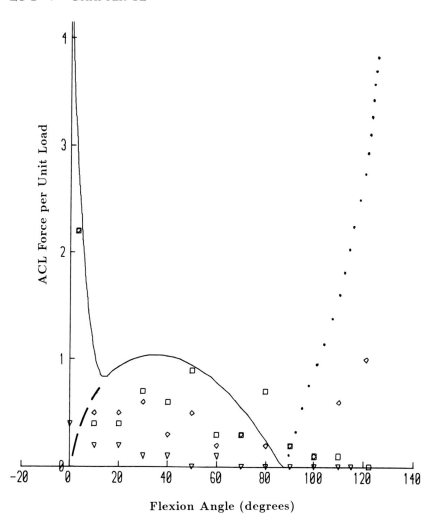

FIG. 12-12. ACL force per unit load, plotted against flexion angle, for five specimens in the flexed knee stance rig. The solid line, calculated from the computer model, includes the effect of the posterior capsule near extension. The dashed line near extension shows the modification to the calculation when the contribution of the posterior capsule is not included. The dotted line gives the calculated PCL force per unit load.

specimens. In two further specimens, there was a distinct deviation from the track of the intact joint below 25° requiring the values of the ACL forces shown in Fig. 12-13A to recover the intact track. The calculated value of the ACL force, the solid line in the figure, gave a reasonable estimate for these two specimens but suggested a critical flexion angle of 12.5°.

PCL Forces with Hamstrings in Leg-Lift

Values of the forces in the PCL replacement wire for the configuration of Fig. 11-14 are plotted against flexion angle in Fig. 12-13B for five specimens. Although there is considerable scatter in the values of the measured forces, all specimens exhibited a critical flexion angle below which the track of the intact joint was recovered after PCL sectioning. The critical angle varied from above 40° in one specimen to below 10° in another, with the remaining three specimens falling within this range. Very large forces had to be applied by the PCL replacement wire in the range 60–100°, reaching values of 18 times the applied load in one

specimen and certainly reaching values of the same order of magnitude as the maximum hamstrings forces in all specimens. These values are nonetheless smaller than those suggested by the calculation, the solid line in Fig. 12-13B.

Ligament Forces with Gastrocnemius Action

Attempts to use the same techniques with gastrocnemius action were not successful. Repeated runs with intact specimens did not reproduce the same track of the femur on the tibia. In the presence of quadriceps or hamstrings forces, tibial rotation was completely stable and there was a preferred position to which the bones would return when disturbed. Gastrocnemius forces conferred no such stability; within a limited range of tibial rotation, the bones lay in positions of neutral equilibrium and could be moved from one position of rotation to another without resistance. Thus there was no preferred track of one bone on the other, the basis of the method of ligament force measurement.

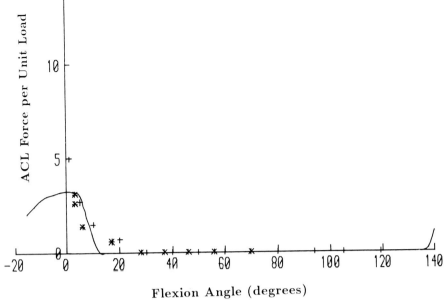

Flexion Angle (degrees)

A

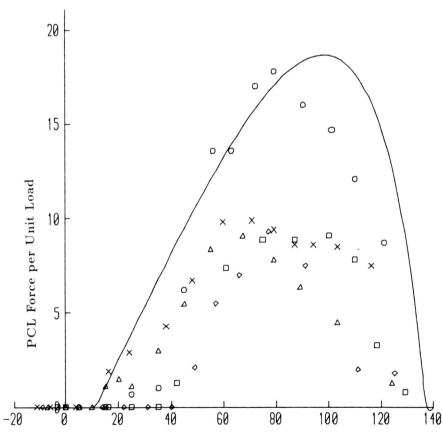

Flexion Angle (degrees)

B

FIG. 12-13. ACL **(A)** and PCL **(B)** forces per unit load, plotted against flexion angle, in the hamstrings leg-lift experiment. The solid lines were calculated from the computer model.

Discussion

Critical Flexion Angle

In general, the results of the ligament force measurements have confirmed the existence of a critical flexion angle separating the range of ACL action from that of PCL action. The fact that each ligament was under load over only part of the flexion range was confirmed by the observation that, when outside that range, the track of the intact joint could be accurately reproduced after the ligament had been divided. In association with the quadriceps, the critical angle appears to be between 60° and 80°. With hamstrings action, it appears to be much nearer full extension, around 20°. On the basis of theoretical argument alone, the critical angle with gastrocnemius action would be expected to be in the highly flexed region.

Further investigation is needed to establish the values of the critical angle more precisely, especially when the separate heads of the flexors are under load. Knowledge of the critical angles associated with different activities enables the clinician to suggest muscle exercise regimes in the early postoperative period which avoid loading a ligament graft or prosthesis.

Ligament Forces

The values of the forces measured in the ligament replacement wire showed much more scatter than did the corresponding measurements of muscle force. The method of the replacement wire can only be precise if the wire is placed exactly along the line of action of the resultant force transmitted by the intact ligament and if there is no friction between the wire and the cable through which it passes. Both of these conditions are clearly difficult to meet.

In the experiments with the leg-lift apparatus, the form of the ligament force variation with flexion was generally similar from specimen to specimen, though there were some very significant variations in the magnitudes of the measured forces and some scatter in the value of the critical flexion angle. The same was true of the measurements of the ACL forces in the flexed knee stance rig, with an even bigger scatter in the value of the critical flexion angle (from 50° in one specimen to beyond 120° in another).

The scatter was most marked in the case of PCL forces with hamstrings action; in one specimen, forces of up to 18 times the applied load were measured. In our discussion of the calculation of PCL forces as reported in Fig. 11-15, we showed that, in high flexion, the PCL lies close to perpendicular to the tibial plateau so that the ligament force has only a small component parallel to the plateau. Small errors in the placing of

the ligament wire would then give disproportionately large errors in the measured ligament force. This may also be the reason why PCL forces were difficult to detect in the flexed knee stance rig. A slight anterior subluxation of the tibia resulting from the dead weight of the tibial and femoral arms of the rig could make small but very significant changes in the orientation of the PCL.

Comparison Theory and Experiment

The calculations of the ligament forces generally provided upper bounds to the measurements, as was suggested in the discussion in Chapter 11. There are two possible reasons for this overestimate. The calculations were based on the assumption that the cruciate ligaments alone provided the components of force parallel to the tibial plateau necessary for equilibrium and ignored possible contributions from the collateral ligaments and capsular structures. Elastic stretching of the ligaments and indentation of the articular surfaces were also ignored. We showed in our elastic analysis of the drawer test in Chapter 11 that such assumptions would lead to overestimates of the angles between the ligaments and the tibial plateau and, therefore, to overestimates of the ligament forces.

Choice of Parameters

The parameters used for these calculations were those of Chapter 10. The adjustments that had to be made to the average values from measurements on specimens were mainly concerned with attempts to reduce estimates of the PCL forces required with hamstrings action. Parameter changes that reduced the angle between the PCL and the tibial plateau increased the angle of the ACL and therefore increased the value of the critical flexion angle. In Figs. 12-11A and 12-12, the calculated critical flexion angle is clearly about 20° too high. It proved perfectly possible to choose parameters that fitted the quadriceps–cruciate interaction very much better, but at the price of a worse fit between theory and measurement of the cruciate–hamstrings interaction. Extensive parametric studies to study these effects are required and have obvious application to ligament surgery. The ligament surgeon, when attaching grafts or prostheses to the bones, determines the parameters of the living cruciate linkage.

Ligament Surgery

From the point of view of ligament surgery, the relationship between ligament angle and ligament force is important. Placement of a graft or prosthesis at steeper than natural angles to the tibial plateau could lead to unnaturally high ligament forces. This would be particularly important in the case of the PCL in flexion. Using grafts or prostheses that are too rigid would not lead to the reduction in ligament angle and reduction in ligament force seen as the natural ligaments stretch. We have alluded to the significance of the critical flexion angle in devising programs of rehabilitation following ligament surgery.

TIBIAL ROTATION

Introduction

Passive flexion and extension of the knee are accompanied by an involuntary rotation of the bones about the long axis of the tibia. The tibia rotates internally on the femur during flexion and rotates externally during extension. Because this movement is easiest to observe near extension, it is often termed the "screw-home" mechanism and is said to be the mechanism by which the knee "locks" at extension. However, the rotation can be much increased by the application of torque about the tibial axis. Lindahl (21) observed that the screw-home motion was easily changed by passive restraint of the knee.

Many authors have commented on tibial rotation. Interest has concentrated more on the mechanisms which limit or resist tibial rotation than on those which cause and control it. Brantigan (3) noted that while the LCL and the joint capsule contributed to rotational stability, it was the MCL which resisted the largest portion of any applied tibial torque. This view was reinforced by Kennedy (16) when he tested knees to failure in tibial rotation and found that the MCL and the medial capsule were the first structures to fail. In 1977, Kennedy (17) showed that the strain in the MCL was largest when torsional load was applied. Morrison (25) observed that the MCL always resists rotation, as did Robichon (28). Shoemaker and Daniel (Chapter 9) have concluded from their survey of the recent literature that the medial structures provide the primary restraint to internal rotation but the ACL provides the major secondary restraint. Conversely, the lateral structures provide the primary restraint to external rotation but the PCL provides the major secondary restraint.

Both Wang (36) and Markolf (23) tested cadaver joints in an attempt to quantify tibial rotation. Wang (36) held specimens in a two-degree-of-freedom testing machine that allowed (a) axial rotation about a fixed axis and (b) axial displacement along that axis. He applied transverse loads at a distance from the axis to rotate the tibia relative to the femur. Their torque–rotation curves showed a region of relative laxity about a neutral position, with low resistance to rotation, sur-

rounded by a stiff region with increased resistance to rotation. When compressive forces were applied along the axis of the testing machine, the region of laxity was diminished. In our view, the reduction in laxity may not have been entirely physiological, since the large compressive forces were not accompanied by simulated muscle action and since the axis of tibial rotation was imposed by the test device. However, Markolf (23), using an unconstrained testing device, observed similar effects.

In this section, we present results from cadaver experiments designed to clarify some of the above-mentioned points. A simple mathematical model of the knee is also described in which we attempted to quantify the contribution of the soft tissues, muscles, and ligaments to the transmission of torque across the knee. We describe and explain tests of passive and forced tibial rotation with flexion. Tests and model results are presented for both loaded and unloaded joints.

Relations Between Flexion, Torque, Load, and Rotation

Materials and Methods

Experiments were performed using the flexed knee stance rig described in Chapter 8. The specimens were prepared as described in the first section of this chapter. They were mounted in the rig, configured as in Fig. 8-13A. Tests were performed at a number of flexion angles, both with vertical load applied along the hip/ankle axis and the corresponding quadriceps force (Fig. 12-5) and without vertical load and quadriceps force.

A pure couple was applied about an axis parallel to the long axis of the tibia by means of a pair of equal and opposite forces (Fig. 8-13A). Since a pure couple has the same moment about any point in space, this method of loading did not presuppose any particular axis of tibial rotation. Furthermore, it does not induce either flexion/extension or abduction/adduction. Movements relative to the six degrees of freedom were measured, and the relative rotation of the bones about the long axis of the tibia was calculated. In the following graphs, tibial rotation is expressed relative to the positions adopted by the bones in full extension.

Results and Discussion

Natural Tibial Rotation

Consider first the natural tibial rotation that accompanies flexion and extension. Figure 12-14 shows the mean tibial rotation for eight knees while they were flexed in the absence of applied tibial torque. All knees

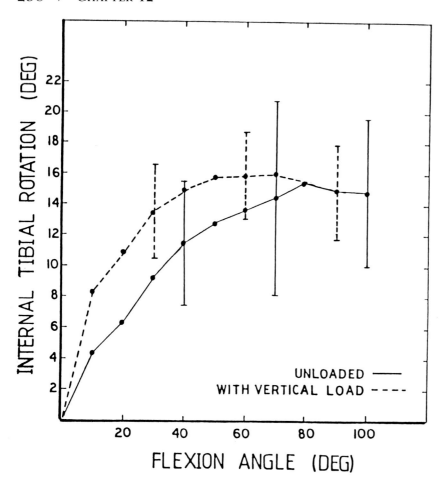

FIG. 12-14. Internal tibial rotation as a function of flexion angle for eight knees with and without vertical load and associated quadriceps force. Note that rotation and flexion are coupled motions observed when no tibial torque was applied.

underwent internal tibial rotation as the knee flexed. This rotation for the unloaded case is shown as the solid line in Fig. 12-14.

Internal rotation varied nearly linearly during the first 50–60° of flexion and then achieved an approximately constant value. For the unloaded joint, the "screw-home" mechanism was much more gradual than that described by Shaw (30). He stated that there is a large tibial rotation between full extension and 20–30° of flexion. Markolf (23) found that tibial rotation changed almost linearly with flexion, reaching a maximum of about 8° of internal rotation at 120°, consistent with our findings. However, his values of both the range of rotation and the flexion angle at which the maximum occurs differ from ours, perhaps because he tested complete legs with the muscles, skin, etc. in place.

When vertical load was applied at the hip and balanced by quadriceps tension, the knee usually underwent some additional tibial rotation. The dashed line in Fig. 12-14 shows the mean rotation for the loaded knee. In general, even a small load (in the region of 20 N applied through the hip in the Oxford rig) was sufficient to cause this additional tibial rotation. Fur-

ther increases in load had little effect. With load and quadriceps action, there was a much more marked final tibial rotation as extension was approached than in the unloaded case. The rotation occurred mainly within 30° of full extension.

The bones appear to have preferred or null positions of tibial rotation which vary from high flexion to full extension, positions that differ. These preferred positions must represent a balance of the forces transmitted by the structures of the knee. This balance would appear to be dominated by quadriceps action, when it is present. It is possible that quadriceps pull lines up the tibial tubercle under the trochlear groove. In this experiment, the quadriceps force increases rapidly with flexion (Fig. 12-5), as would its consequent effect on rotational alignment. Near extension, the null position is dominated by the soft tissue structures that tighten to prevent hyperextension, notably the posterior capsule. At both full extension and high flexion angles, the null positions are the same in the loaded and unloaded states.

Figure 12-15 shows results for three knees tested before and after meniscectomy. The changes in natural rotation characteristics induced by meniscectomy are

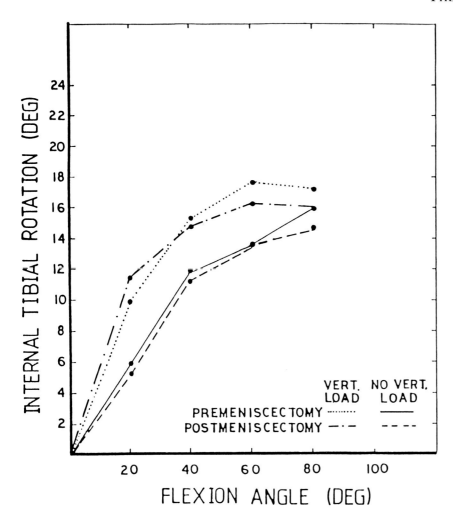

FIG. 12-15. Internal tibial rotation pre- and post-meniscectomy.

insignificant both for the loaded and unloaded knee, suggesting that the detailed geometry of the articular surfaces does not control these movements. An interesting feature of these three particular knees is that tibial rotation increased with application of load at both high and low flexion angles.

Tibial Rotation and Applied Torque

Seven knees were tested for their response to tibial torque. Average results are shown in Fig. 12-16, with separate families of curves at different values of the vertical load and different flexion angles. The null position for the curves corresponds to that shown in Fig. 12-14 for the appropriate flexion angle. For all the knees tested, the pattern shown was observed. However, there was considerable variation from knee to knee with regard to the magnitude of the rotation for a given torque. Standard deviations for selected points are shown in Fig. 12-16C. These were typical of those observed and illustrate the variation from knee to

knee. They have been omitted in the other plots to show more clearly the effects of increasing vertical load.

For the response with no vertical load applied and hence no quadriceps force, several features may be observed. At all positions except full extension, there was a region of laxity about the null position, with only small torque being required in order to achieve about 20–25° of rotation. Further rotation met with increased resistance and required much larger torques. These effects were similar to those described by Wang (36) and Markolf (23). The amount of external rotation of the tibia was considerably larger than the corresponding internal rotation at each tested flexion angle and torque amplitude. This has been observed by others (3,16,30). The ratio of the external to internal rotation ranged from about 1.5 to 1 at 20° to about 1.8 to 1 at 80°. The range of rotation, from the maximum external limit to the maximum internal limit, gradually increased with flexion so that, at 80°, it was about 30% larger than at 20°. When knees were tested near full extension, laxity decreased and the range of rotation

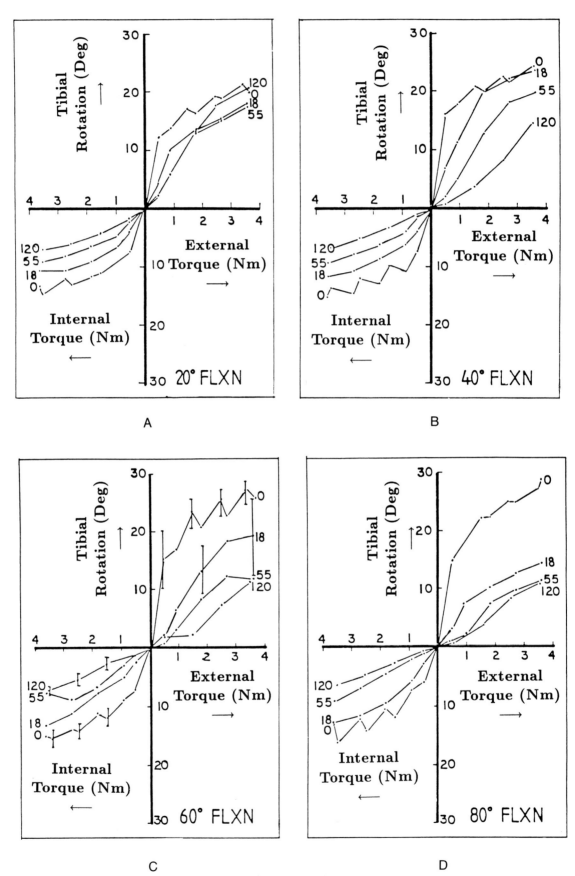

FIG. 12-16. Tibial rotation plotted against torque at 20° **(A)**, 40° **(B)**, 60° **(C)**, and 80° **(D)** of flexion for seven specimens. Results are presented for vertical loads of 0, 40, 80, and 120 N with associated quadriceps forces as in Fig. 12-5. Part C contains bars to indicate one standard deviation from the mean of seven measurements.

was much diminished because of the effects of the tightening posterior capsule. It was not possible to perform tests precisely at full extension because, in the flexed knee stance rig, this is a position of unstable equilibrium.

When vertical load was applied along with the appropriate quadriceps force, the laxity of the knee decreased. At low flexion angles (Fig. 12-16A), increasing the load to 120 N decreased the range of rotation by only 19% at 20° of flexion. As the flexion angle increased, the effect of applied load became more and more marked, with a 120-N load decreasing the range by up to 60% at 80°. The principal change was a reduction in the lax regions of the curves, and thus the external rotation was reduced more than internal rotation for a given vertical load and torque amplitude. This effect became more pronounced with increasing flexion and hence higher forces in the quadriceps mechanism and in the passive structures of the knee. The slope of the torque–rotation curve under load was similar to that of the unloaded curve in the stiff region.

Effect of Meniscectomy

Figure 12-17 shows average tibial rotation in three knees before and after bilateral meniscectomy. The laxity in the unloaded case was increased by meniscectomy by approximately 18% at 20° flexion and by 14% at 80°. This is consistent with the findings of Wang (36), who found a 14% increase in laxity for the knee flexed to 25° and under no compressive load. When the menisci are removed, the soft tissues become more slack as the bones move closer together (31), and hence the laxity of the joint is increased. However, Markolf (23) found a minimal increase in rotational laxity following meniscectomy.

Figure 12-17 suggests that the effects of meniscectomy on the torsional characteristics of the joint become less noticeable as load is applied, with an increased laxity of only 4% or less under a 120-N load. This is consistent with the view that the dominant restraint of tibial rotation under load is the quadriceps tendon force.

Axes of Tibial Rotation

The position of the axis about which the rotations just described occur has been a matter of some conjecture. Shaw (30) found that, up to 30° flexion, the axis of rotation passed through the medial intercondylar eminence. Steindler (33) and Kapandji (15) stated that the axis lay toward the medial side of the knee, with Kapandji arguing that the lateral condyle moves much more than the medial condyle in rotation. There do not appear to have been subsequent investigations of the

"impression" formed by Slocum (32) that the rotational axis "moves posteriorly progressively as flexion takes place", as does the axis of flexion (see Chapter 10). In this section we have studied movement of the axis of rotation by two separate methods.

The Screw Axis Method

The relative motion between any two bodies may be defined as a set of translations along and rotations about a so-called "screw axis" (19). The screw axis is the three-dimensional analog of the two-dimensional instant center described in Chapter 10. Just like the instant center, the screw axis may move relative to both bodies.

For pure tibial rotation relative to the femur, the screw axis corresponds to the physical axis of rotation. In this case, the translation along the screw axis is zero since such translation would involve either distraction or interpenetration of the bones. From knowledge of the five rotations and one translation measured by the transducers of the Oxford rig (Chapter 8), programs were written based on Kinzel's method (19) for locating the screw axis. The method was applied to the experiments of Fig. 12-16.

Shear Center Method

Theory

In the theory of beams in structural mechanics, the shear center is defined as the point about which the distributed shear stresses on the cross-section of the beam have zero twisting moment about the beam axis. It coincides with the axis of twist of the beam. If the line of action of a shear force applied in the plane of the cross-section passes through the shear center, no rotation occurs.

In the laboratory, the position of the shear center is found by applying a shear force along various lines of action and measuring the consequent rotation. The shear center lies on the particular line of action at which the rotation changes sign (i.e., from clockwise to anti-clockwise), this being the line of action that produces no twist.

The concept of the shear center can be applied to the knee, with certain reservations. In discussing the rotation of the tibia induced by anteroposterior forces as an example of coupled motions in Chapter 8 (Fig. 8-3b, c, and d), we implicitly used the concept. An anterior force applied to the tibia produces (a) internal rotation when applied lateral to the axis of rotation and (b) external rotation when applied medial to the axis. Posteriorly directed forces produce rotations of the opposite signs. Similarly, medially directed forces pro-

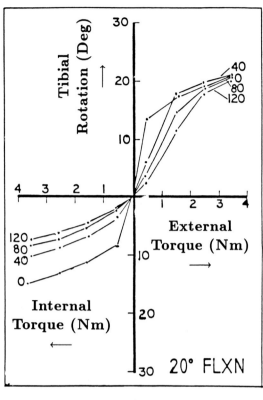 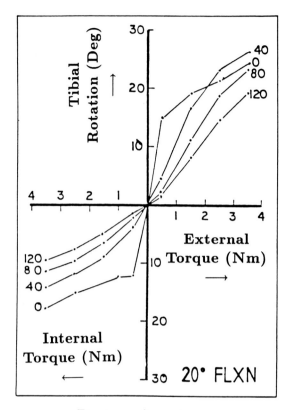

Premeniscectomy   Postmeniscectomy

A

FIG. 12-17. Torque–rotation characteristics for three knees before and after meniscectomy at 20° **(A)** and 60° **(B)** of flexion.

duce (a) internal rotation when applied anterior to the axis of rotation and (b) external rotation when applied posterior to the axis of rotation. Laterally directed forces produce opposite rotations.

These arguments gave rise to a method for locating the axis of twist of the human knee directly. The reservation in the application of the method to synovial joints is that, unlike a steel beam, the structures which transmit medially and laterally directed loads are not necessarily the same (see Figs. 11-28 and 11-29), so that the position of the axis of tibial rotation may depend on the direction of the applied load.

Experiment

Figure 8-13B shows a plate that was attached to the tibial arm of the Oxford rig, replacing the pulley used to apply torque to the tibia in Fig. 8-13A. Two sides of the plate contained dove-tailed grooves in which a pair of slider elements could be moved from one position to another. Hooks attached to the sliders could

be used for the application of transverse forces to the specimen. Scales attached to the plate were used to define the positions of the sliders relative to the position of the tibial intramedullary stud.

With specimens prepared and mounted in the rig as previously described, a series of tests were performed at 30°, 60°, and 90° of flexion. Either an abducting or an adducting load was applied parallel to the plane of the tibial plateau by hanging weight in the mediolateral direction to a string attached to one of the slider hooks. The slider was moved posteriorly in 5-mm steps; at each position, the positions of the bones were recorded by the transducers and the rotation of the tibia was calculated. Figure 12-18 shows the outcome of such a series of tests, with results from the three positions of flexion. For each position, the reference point of zero induced rotation was taken to be the null rotary position of the tibia at the corresponding flexion angle, as in Fig. 12-14. The position of the slider at the reference point was taken to lie on a line through the axis of tibial rotation.

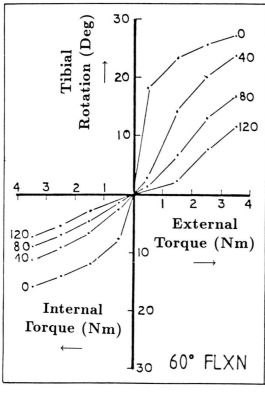

Premeniscectomy

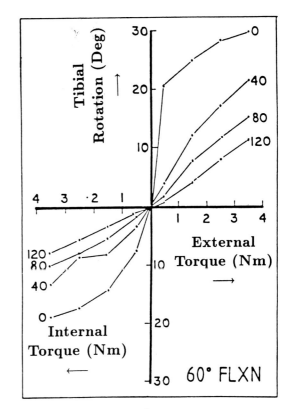

Postmeniscectomy

B

FIG. 12-17. (Continued)

Similar tests were performed with the line of action of the load in the plane of the tibia plateau at 45° anteriorly and posteriorly to the mediolateral direction. In theory, the three lines through the axis of tibial rotation should intersect at a point on that axis. In practice, because of experimental error, the intersections of each of the three pairs of lines formed a triangle (a "cocked hat" in the language of navigation) within which the true axis probably lay.

Tests were performed on each specimen under both abducting and adducting loads. The tests were repeated with the addition of (a) a vertical load on the hip/ankle axis and (b) the corresponding quadriceps force (Fig. 12-5).

The method just described located the axis of tibial rotation relative to the intramedullary stud used to fix the tibia on the rig, as described in the first section of this chapter. The final step, therefore, was to disarticulate the specimen and to locate the intramedullary stud relative to the tibial plateau by taking x-ray pictures of the tibia with its plateau lying on the photographic plate.

Results

Screw Axis

Figure 12-19 shows a plan view of the tibial plateau, with the location of the screw axis between the tibia and femur marked. Results are shown for four knees without vertical load and for three further knees unloaded and with 80-N vertical load. A circle indicating the estimated error in the calculation of the position of the axis is included. Taking account of possible error, the results suggest that, in all specimens, the axis of rotation lay on the medial side of the tibial plateau, as suggested by Shaw (30), Kapandji (15), and Steindler (33).

It should also be observed that the axis moved anteroposteriorly, but its track for external rotation is not necessarily the same as that for internal rotation. In four of the six assessments, the axis moved progressively backwards with increasing flexion; in the fifth (internal rotation in knees 1–4, unloaded) the track moved initially forward and then backward, and in the

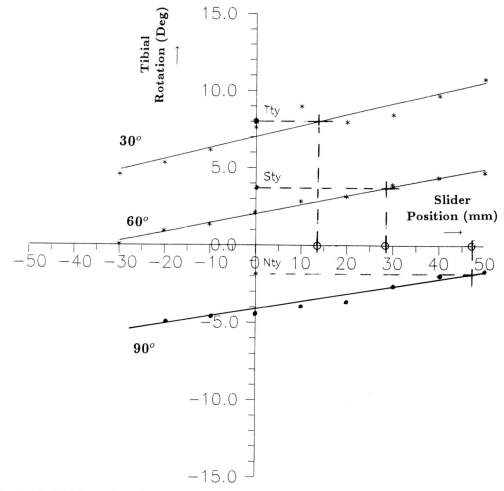

FIG. 12-18. Tibial rotation plotted against slider position at 30°, 60°, and 90° of flexion. The points marked Tty, Sty, and Nty indicate the values of tibial rotation at the null positions at each of those flexion angles. The dashed lines show the construction used to find the slider position corresponding to zero induced rotation.

sixth (external rotation in knees 5–7, 80-N load) the track moved initially backward and then forward. In two of the assessments (unloaded external rotation, knees 1–4, loaded internal rotation, knees 5–7), the backwards movement of the axis of tibial rotation appeared to follow the instant center of flexion/extension (Chapter 10) at the sagittal plane intersection of the cruciates.

Shear Center

Figure 12-20 shows a set of estimates of the position of the axis of tibial rotation by the shear center method, for both a loaded and an unloaded specimen. The error triangles were, in general, much smaller for the unloaded specimens, and the axis of rotation was further forward. In the presence of vertical load, the tibial rotations were generally smaller than in the unloaded state (Fig. 12-16), and thus the method less sensitive.

A summary of such results for five unloaded specimens and four loaded specimens is shown in Fig. 12-21.

To show the positions of the axis, averaged from a number of specimens, the tibial plateau is represented as a square; the distances within that square imply proportions of the dimensions anteroposteriorly and mediolaterally within the plateau. Crossed arrows represent the position of the axis within the plateau, with the arrow lengths representing the error bands. Thus, in Fig. 12-21B, all tests at 60° and 90° of flexion gave axis positions behind the plateau, near the center of the medial condyle under abducting loads and about halfway between the condyles under adducting loads.

In the unloaded state (Fig. 12-21A), the rotation axis lay near the center of the plateau at 30° of flexion; moreover, there was a slight drift medially and a pronounced drift posteriorly with increasing flexion, from the center of the plateau at 30° to the back of the plateau or beyond at 90°. Using Student's *t*-test, the differences between the anteroposterior positions of the

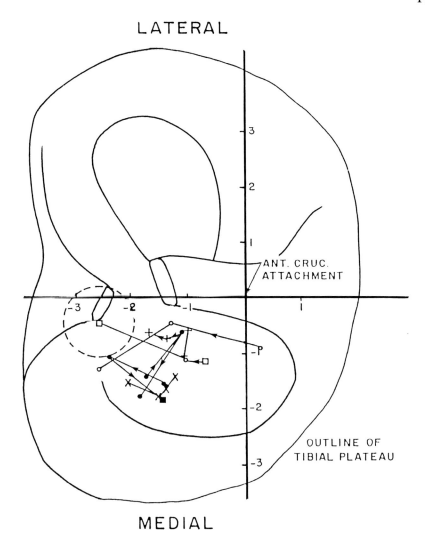

LATERAL

ANT. CRUC. ATTACHMENT

OUTLINE OF TIBIAL PLATEAU

MEDIAL

FIG. 12-19. Plan view of the tibial plateau showing position of the screw axis in four unloaded specimens and three specimens with and without 80-N vertical load and associated quadriceps force. Tracks of the screw axis from 30° to 60° to 90° under internal and external torques are shown. The dashed circle indicates the possible error in each estimate of position. (●) Internal rotation, knees 1–4, no load; (○) external rotation, knees 1–4, no load; (+) internal rotation, knees 5–7, no load; (×) external rotation, knees 5–7, no load; (□) internal rotation, knees 5–7, 80-N load; (■) external rotation, knees 5–7, 80-N load.

axis at 30° and 90° were highly significant (p < 0.001). The application of a 50-N vertical load with associated quadriceps force moved the axis under abducting loads medially and, under both loads, posteriorly.

Discussion

Both methods of assessment strongly suggest a backward progression of the rotation axis with increasing flexion. In the unloaded knee, it might serve as a first approximation to say that the axis of rotation follows the axis of flexion backwards and forwards on the tibial plateau. In Chapter 10, we showed that the position of the flexion axis is defined by the geometry of the ligaments. The movement of the flexion axis was associated with changes in that geometry. A precise theory to locate the rotation axis and explain its movement in terms of ligament geometry is not yet available, but the evidence points to such an explanation.

The shear center method involved applying either abducting or adducting loads. In the absence of vertical

load and quadriceps force, either the lateral or medial condyles were out of contact and yet, with only little error, the paths of the rotation axis within the tibial plateau were much the same, suggesting that the geometry of the articular surfaces cannot be the main determining factor. The importance of the ligaments, and of the cruciate ligaments in particular, may be deduced from the phenomenon of pivot shift after disruption of the ACL. The relationship between flexion and tibial rotation implied by the screw-home mechanism and quantified by graphs such as Fig. 12-14 cannot fully be explained by models such as the four-bar planar linkage of Chapter 10 but requires a three-dimensional analysis of a space linkage comprising the two bones and the collateral as well as the cruciate ligaments.

The anteroposterior movement of the rotation axis has previously been described by Slocum (32), and the rotation axis' position in the center of the plateau or towards the medial side has been described by several authors (3,32,34). The posterior movement may be important in prosthesis design. In several current de-

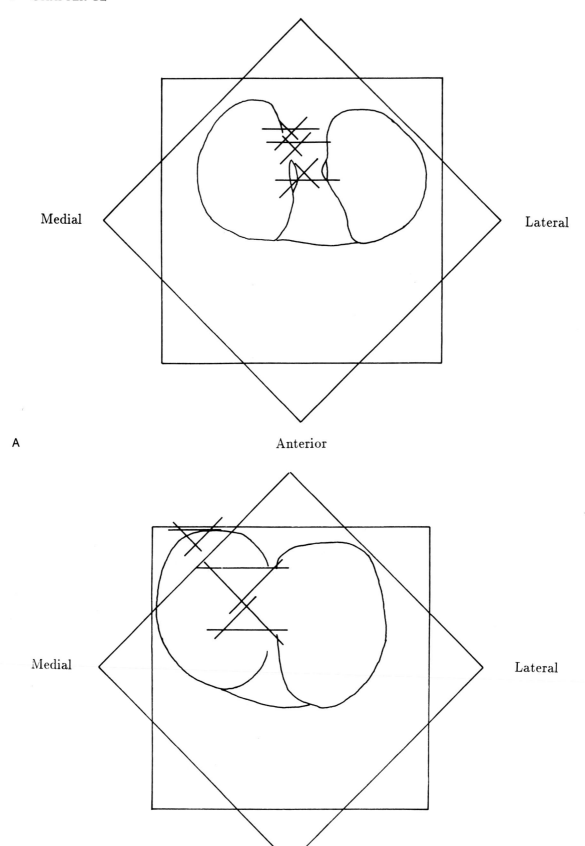

FIG. 12-20. Error triangles for loads applied medially and at 45° anteromedially and postero-medially parallel to the plane of the tibial plateau without **(A)** and with **(B)** vertical load and associated quadriceps force.

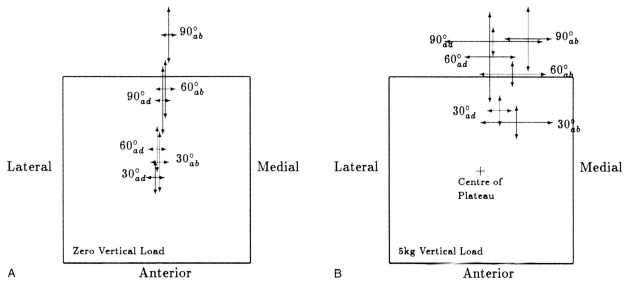

FIG. 12-21. Diagrammatic plan view of the tibial plateau. Horizontal distances represent proportional distances mediolaterally on the plateau. Vertical distances represent proportional distances anteroposteriorly on the plateau. Intersections of arrowed lines represent the position on the plateau of the rotation axis under abducting (*ab*) and adducting (*ad*) loads; the lengths of the arrowed lines indicate the error bands, without **(A)** and with **(B)** vertical load and associated quadriceps force.

signs, attempts are made to minimize the loosening effects of torsional loads on hinge or other constrained prostheses by including a facility for long axis rotation as well but about a fixed axis.

The posterior position of the rotation axis under even small axial loads implies that adducting loads applied within the span of the tibial plateau would virtually always be accompanied by internal rotation, abducting loads by external rotation. This would explain the remarks of Haynes (12) that "varus/valgus and rotational movements are inexorably linked". We have shown that the nature of the coupling between these movements depends critically on the line of action of the mediolateral loads. It does not occur when the mediolateral load passes through the rotation axis or when rotation is produced by a pure torque, as in the tests of Fig. 12-16. Similarly, the nature of the coupling reported by Fukubayashi (8) between anteroposterior force and rotation depends on the mediolateral location of the line of action of the force in relation to the axis of rotation. Coupling between the various degrees of freedom at the knee will finally be understood only when the factors that determine the axes of such movements are themselves fully understood.

Effect of Load on Torsional Characteristics—A Calculation

Wang (36) explained the reduction in laxity under axial load by arguing that the femoral condyles climb the tibial eminence, with the horizontal forces thus produced serving to resist the applied torque. Goodfellow (9) suggested that this could be only a minor part of the explanation, since it does not account for the contributions of the soft tissues. Those contributions may have been minimal in the constrained rig used by Wang (36). The fact that the resistance to rotation is reduced by soft tissue sectioning (Chapter 9) indicates that the soft tissues play an important role.

The reduction of rotational laxity with load and quadriceps force was found also (10) in knees in which both compartments had been replaced with meniscal prostheses which allowed retention of all the ligaments and which reproduced the rolling action of the femur on the tibia during flexion/extension (Fig. 10-10). The tibial articular surfaces of the prosthesis were entirely flat and offered no resistance to anteroposterior movement. Apart from friction, there could be no resistance to rotation due to surface shapes until the meniscal bearings contacted the tibial eminence. In the experiments, considerable tibial torque was resisted by the replaced joint with no apparent contact between the meniscal bearings and the tibial eminence. This resistance can only have come from the soft tissues. Of course, the articular surfaces play an important role in the sense that the soft tissues can develop the tension forces necessary to hold the bones together only if the articular surfaces develop the compressive forces necessary to hold the bones apart.

In this section, we estimate the torque/tibial-rotation characteristics of the knee on the assumption that all torsional resistance comes from the ligaments, the muscles (when active), and the menisci.

Method of Calculation

Calculation of the relative contributions of different elements within the knee to resisting tibial rotation requires, like our study of the drawer test in Chapter 11, a statically indeterminate analysis. The forces in the various soft tissue elements were calculated on the assumption that they are all compatible with a specified rotation of the femur on the tibia about the screw axis appropriate to the flexion angle (Fig. 12-19). Since they pass close to the screw axis, the contributions of the cruciates to transmitting the torque were not included in the calculation.

The null positions of the collateral ligaments in the sagittal plane were taken to be those defined by the sagittal plane theory (Fig. 10-18). Their mediolateral coordinates on the tibia and femur were measured from specimens. Under a specified tibial rotation, the directions of the collateral ligaments and the patellar tendon change in a calculable way (Fig. 12-22).

For the collateral ligaments, the analysis of Fig. 12-22A was used to calculate the extension of each ligament corresponding to a specified angle of tibial rotation. Various authors [e.g., Decraemer (4) and Vidik (35)] have described the stress–strain relationship for connective tissue such as ligaments. Figure 12-23 shows a typical load–extension curve from a human MCL strained in an INSTRON testing machine. The essential characteristics are that there is (a) a soft "toe in" region where large displacements occur with small forces and (b) a stiff, approximately linear, region where additional displacement requires a higher force. Such force–extension relations for the collateral ligaments were used to estimate from the calculated extension the values of the forces that these ligaments transmitted. The moment about the screw axis of the circumferential components of the collateral ligament forces for a chosen angle of tibial rotation was then calculated.

For the patellar tendon, the geometric analysis of

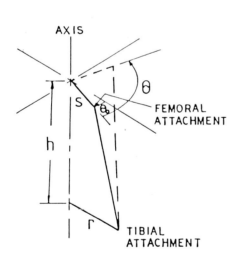

A

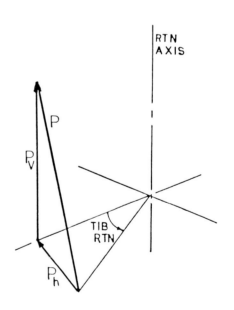

B

FIG. 12-22. Movements of a collateral ligament **(A)** and the patellar tendon **(B)** during tibial rotation about the screw axis. In A, the tibial and femoral attachments lie at radii r and s from the screw axis and are separated axially by a distance h. Initially, the ligament is inclined at an angle θ_0 to the vertical but it is rotated through an angle θ by the action of tibial rotation. The relative movement of the bony attachments in part A determines the extension of the ligament. In this illustration, the circumferential direction of the ligament has to be reversed before it is appropriately directed to resist rotation. In B, the component of the patellar tendon force in the sagittal plane, P_v, is determined from the sagittal plane theory (Chapter 11). The rotation of the tendon out of the sagittal plane is used to determine its circumferential component P_h and its resultant P.

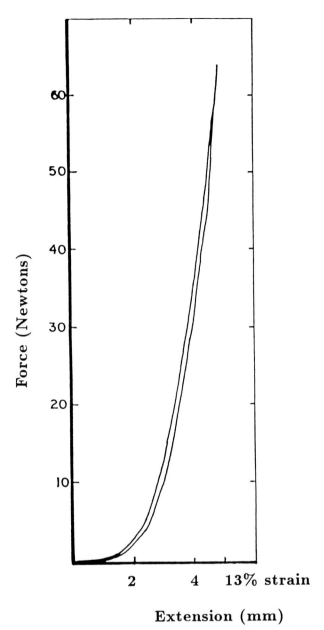

FIG. 12-23. Typical load–extension curve for an MCL. The preparation included a bone block at each end, gripped by the testing instrument.

Fig. 12-22B was used to calculate the direction of the tendon for a specified tibial rotation. The sagittal plane theory (Chapter 11) was used to calculate the component P_v of the tendon force in the sagittal plane during flexed knee stance and, from this and the calculated inclination of the tendon, to deduce the circumferential component.

An estimate of the contributions of the menisci were also included in the calculation on the argument that meniscectomy was found to lead to an increase in rotational laxity (Fig. 12-17). Figure 12-24 shows the geometry of a femur climbing a curved meniscus. A pair of anteroposterior forces are thereby developed, in-

creasing with rotation of the tibia. Assuming the contact force to be equally shared between the two compartments, their anteroposterior components were taken to be equal in magnitude and opposite in direction, separated by a distance equal to half the width of the tibial plateau. The value of the anteroposterior force was estimated from the geometry of Fig. 12-24, assuming the menisci to be rigid. The torsional moment for a specified tibial rotation could then be estimated. The assumption of rigid menisci doubtlessly leads to an overestimate of their contribution; to make allowance for their deformability would greatly complicate the calculation.

Results and Discussion

Figure 12-25 shows predicted torque–rotation curves based on the values given in Table 12-1 for the parameters and variables. The curves are of similar form to the experimental results of Fig. 12-16. The calculated range of rotation at any specified torque amplitude rises with increasing flexion and decreases with increasing compressive load.

From the method of calculation, the resistance to rotation offered by the collateral ligaments was independent of load. The contributions of the patellar tendon and the menisci came into effect only with vertical load present. The curves at zero vertical load therefore define the contributions of the collateral ligaments, with the differences between the zero and nonzero load curves at a specified rotation representing the combined contributions of patellar tendon and menisci.

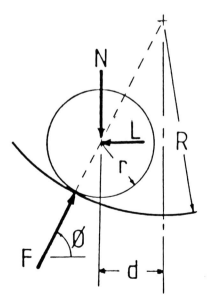

FIG. 12-24. A circular femoral condyle climbing the circular surface of a meniscus, giving rise to an anteroposterior component, *L*, of the contact force.

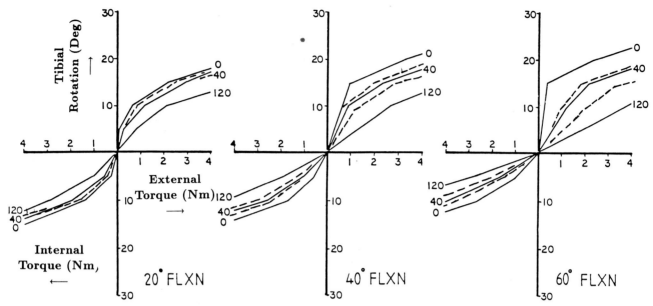

FIG. 12-25. Calculated torque/angle-of-twist characteristics at 20°, 40°, and 60° of flexion. The solid lines include the contributions of the collateral ligaments, patellar tendon, and menisci to the transmission of the torque. The dashed lines omit the meniscal contribution.

The dashed curves are the outcome of the calculation when the contribution of the menisci was omitted, allowing the assessment of their relative contribution. While the bulk of the loss of rotational laxity would appear to be due to the contribution of the patellar tendon, a significant contribution would appear to come from the menisci. As we observed above, the present calculation probably overestimates that contribution.

Of course, the quantitative results given in Fig. 12-25 depend entirely on the chosen values of the parameters, and a further parametric study is necessary be-fore the exact porportions of different contributions to resistance to rotation can be calculated with confidence. Such a calculation would also require a theory to explain the position of the rotation axis relative to the cruciate ligaments so their contribution could also be assessed. The important contributions of the flexor muscles and of popliteus also need to be studied.

What is clear from the fact that the simple theory presented here is in general agreement with observation is that the peripheral ligamentous structures provide much of the unloaded resistance but allow significant rotational laxity. When load is applied, the forces in the muscle tendons greatly reduce the rotational laxity of the knee. The menisci may also transmit a proportion of the torque.

ABDUCTION/ADDUCTION

Introduction

In addition to flexion/extension and long-axis tibial rotation, the knee allows a small amount of abduction/adduction—that is, rotation about an anteroposterior axis in the plane of the tibial plateau. In the previous section, we described experiments conducted in the flexed knee stance rig in which the position of the axis of tibial rotation was determined by finding the line of action of abducting or adducting loads at which no rotation occurred. From one such experiment, Fig. 12-26 shows the range of abduction/adduction plotted against the magnitude of the abducting/adducting

TABLE 12-1. *Data for calculating torque–rotation characteristic*

Width of tibia:	9.0 cm
Stiffness of MCL:	100 N/mm
Stiffness of LCL:	60 N/mm
Patellar tendon force per unit load (Fig. 12-22B)	
At 20° of flexion:	0.6
At 40° of flexion:	1.8
At 60° of flexion:	2.8
Normal compressive force per unit load (Fig. 12-24)	
At 20° of flexion:	1.6
At 40° of flexion:	2.7
At 60° of flexion:	3.8
Difference between condyle and meniscal radii (Fig. 12-24)	
At 20° of flexion:	1.7 cm
At 40° of flexion:	2.0 cm
At 60° of flexion:	2.3 cm

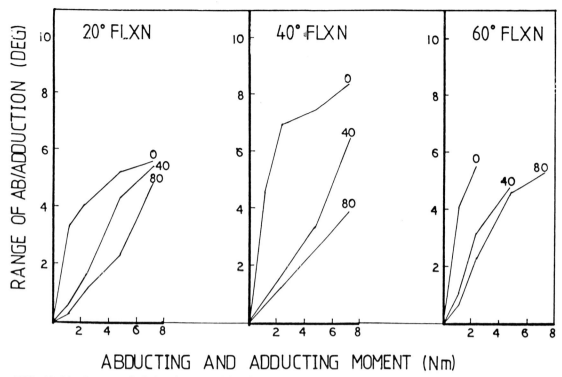

FIG. 12-26. Range of abduction to adduction, plotted against amplitude of abducting/adducting torque, at 20°, 40°, and 60° flexion under 0-, 40-, and 80-N vertical load with corresponding quadriceps force.

torque applied. The range of movement was that which occurred between the application of first an abducting moment and then an adducting moment of the same magnitude. Results are shown for three angles of flexion and for three values of the applied vertical load.

At zero vertical load, the graphs show a typical lax region, where about 5° of varus/valgus rock occurs at very low applied moments, followed by a stiffer region where increased resistance to movement was found. The laxity diminished as full extension was approached. When vertical load was applied and balanced by quadriceps tension, the region of laxity was eliminated and the specimens showed increased resistance to varus/valgus rock over the range of moments applied. This pattern was very similar to that for tibial rotation (see Fig. 12-16).

Bond Sharing Between the Compartments

We showed in Chapter 11 that the distribution of compressive force between the two compartments of the joint depends on the direction of the line of action of the applied load. Figures 11-28 and 11-29 showed how abducting or adducting loads could result in lift-off of the medial or lateral compartments, respectively. Even if lift-off does not occur, Fig. 11-27 showed how the total compressive force could be shared unequally be-

tween the two compartments. Abducting or adducting loads would reduce the compressive force transmitted by one compartment at the expense of an increase in the other. After lift-off, the contact force in the contacting compartment is much increased to balance the ligament forces restraining lift-off. The much reduced abduction/adduction shown in Fig. 12-26 in the presence of vertical load and quadriceps force is interpreted as an indication that such loads prevent lift-off and result in a more equable sharing of compressive force between the two compartments. However, many authors assert that the larger condyle on the medial side of the tibial plateau implies that it habitually carries the larger compressive force.

In the modern practice of knee arthroplasty, great emphasis is placed on restoring the alignment of the limb to normal. Correction of varus/valgus malalignment is seen as crucial in preventing excessive loading in either the medial or lateral compartments, with the consequent risk of early failure of the prosthesis.

The natural knee has a tibiofemoral angle of 6–8° such that, with the limb straight, a line drawn from the center of the femoral head vertically down to the center of the ankle joint passes through the medial side of the intercondylar eminence when viewed in the coronal plane. This line is often referred to as the "mechanical axis" of the leg. In the two-legged stance and with the leg straight, the line of the ground reaction coincides with the mechanical axis; in the one-legged stance, however, the line of the ground reaction passes medial to the knee, and consequently a greater proportion of the load would be expected to be borne medially.

The distribution of load between the medial and lateral compartments of the knee has been estimated by various means: hypothesis based on anatomical studies (33); gait and force-plate data analyzed by a mathematical model (25,14); x-ray data applied to a mathematical model (18,13); experiments using cadaveric knees on force plates (20) and strain-gauged bones (7). All these methods are indirect and entail simplifications and approximations in the analysis.

Direct measurement of loads acting across the hip joint have been made (a) *in vitro* (24) using strain gauges beneath the articular cartilage and (b) *in vivo* by the use of an instrumented implant (29). Such studies quantitatively corroborate the forces estimated to act across the hip by mathematical modeling from measurements of ground reaction forces and limb position. At the knee, mechanisms of load-sharing between the compartments are not fully understood and a direct means of measurement is desirable. We have undertaken a series of tests in the flexed knee stance rig (see Chapter 8).

Measurement of Compartmental Loads

Methods and Materials

Six specimens were prepared, as described above, for testing in the flexed knee stance rig. A unicompartmental meniscal knee prosthesis (2,10) was inserted into the medial and lateral compartments of the specimens. This prosthesis was a totally unconstrained surface arthroplasty, excising the minimum of bone and preserving all the ligaments. By measuring the gaps remaining between the fixed metal components after implantation, the appropriate thickness of meniscal bearing was chosen for each compartment to restabilize the joint, thus restoring ligament tension. The femur then resumed its rolling/sliding movement relative to the tibia (Fig. 10-10). Figure 12-27 shows that when quadriceps force in the replaced joint was compared with that in the previously intact joint, no significant differences could be detected. Thus, some degree of normal knee kinematics and mechanics was reproduced by the arthroplasty.

The meniscal bearings were instrumented with a flat-line load cell (Entran) to measure the compressive force transmitted by each compartment.

The specimens were mounted in the flexed knee stance rig in the configuration shown in Fig. 8-13B. As shown in Fig. 8-14, the slider on the hip assembly could be set such that the sagittal plane containing the flexed

TABLE 12-2. *The mean angular adjustment at the ankle for the six specimens required to alter the line of the vertical load through the four loading conditions*

Change in orientation[a]	Mean angular adjustment
CLC → CTE	3.2
CTA → CMC	3.1
CMC → MMC	1.8

[a] CLC, center of lateral compartment; CTE, center of the tibial eminence; CMC, center of the medial compartment; and MMC, medial to the medial compartment.

limb could be fixed in any desired plane through the ankle assembly of the rig. The plane of flexion could therefore be set in any desired relation to the line of action of the vertical load over 100° of flexion.

Method

The specimens were mounted such that the ratio of the femoral arm (distance from center of the hip to the center of the knee) to the tibial arm (center of the knee to the center of the ankle) was 1.1:1, corresponding to anthropometric data (5). The vertical load was applied, acting (a) through the center of the lateral compartment (CLC), (b) through the center of the tibial eminence (CTE), (c) through the center of the medial compartment (CMC), and (d) on a line just medial to the medial compartment (MMC).

The last position was chosen to correspond approximately to the line of the vertical load in single-leg stance. Shown in Table 12-2 is the mean angular adjustment of the plane of flexion required to alter the specimens from one configuration to the next.

Vertical loads of 50 N and 80 N, tending to flex the knee, were applied. Static measurements of the tension force in the quadriceps tendon and of the compressive forces in each of the two compartments of the specimen were taken at 10° increments over the flexion range.

In three of the six specimens, tension was also applied via a second proving ring to the iliotibial tract (ITT) to examine how a 40-N force in this structure redistributed the total compressive load in the medial and lateral compartments.

Results

Figure 12-27 shows measured values of the quadriceps force per unit applied vertical load, plotted against flexion angle, for the specimens when intact and after replacement by the prosthetic components. There is no significant difference between the two sets of results.

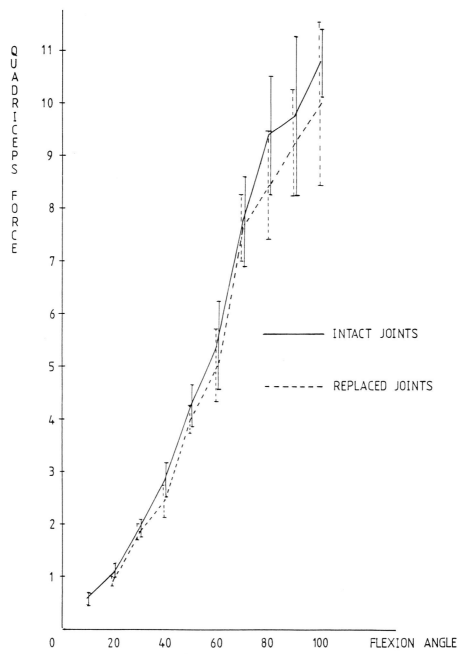

FIG. 12-27. Quadriceps force per unit load in the flexed knee stance rig, plotted against flexion angle, for six specimens when intact and after bicompartmental meniscal arthroplasty.

Figure 12-28 shows the total contact force per unit vertical load, plotted against flexion angle, for each of the four loading configurations. There was no significant difference between the four sets of results.

The proportion of the total compressive force borne by the medial compartment for each of the four loading configurations is plotted against flexion angle in Fig. 12-29. The values plotted are the mean values of the measurements. These results demonstrate the predictable increase in the proportion of the total load borne by the medial compartment as the line of the load passes from laterally to medially. However, the range of the data for each load configuration was much smaller at extension than it was in flexion; thus, while the differences between the values for different load configurations were significant near extension, there was much overlap in the data in flexion, and the differences between load configurations were not significant. The line of vertical load therefore had the greatest effect on the distribution of the force between the medial and lateral compartments near extension, where the total compressive load and the muscle forces acting across the joint were least (Figs. 12-27 and 12-28).

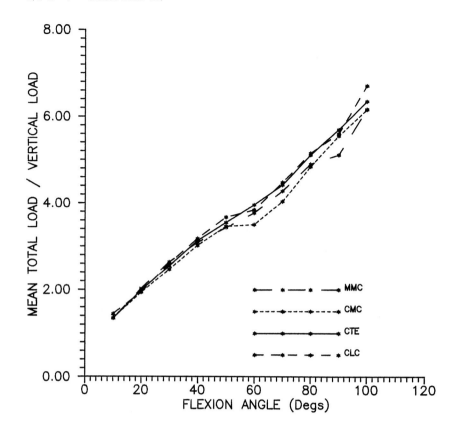

FIG. 12-28. Total contact force per unit load, plotted against flexion angle, for each of four loading configurations.

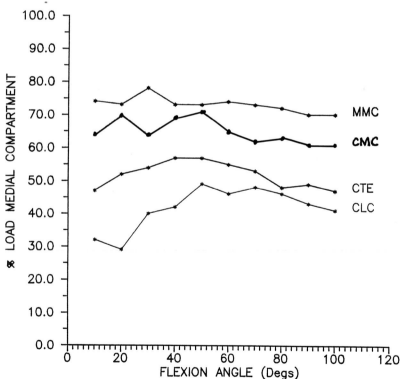

FIG. 12-29. Mean values of the percentage of the total contact force carried by the medial compartment, plotted against flexion angle, for each of four loading configurations.

TABLE 12-3. *Percentage reduction in the medial compartment load over the flexion range when 40-N tension was applied to the iliotibial tract*

Flexion angle	Mean percentage reduction in medial compartment load
10	22
20	20
30	13
40	11
50	13
60	15
70	15
80	13
90	9
100	4

Tension in the ITT, at the expense of some increase in the total compressive force, significantly unloaded the medial compartment at low angles of flexion, but not at high angles (Table 12-3).

Discussion

Direct measurement of compartmental loads in a complex joint such as the knee is difficult. Previous attempts at estimation have been theoretical or indirectly derived from ground reaction forces, requiring simplifications and approximations in the model. The method described measures the compartmental loads after an unconstrained meniscal arthroplasty directly and therefore is of value in itself. However, it is contended that by correct retensioning of the ligaments with appropriately sized bearings, near-normal joint kinematics and mechanics are restored. The similarity between the measured quadriceps forces before and after arthroplasty adds support to this contention. The measurements of compartmental forces may therefore be of relevance to the natural knee.

Previous reports have differed widely in estimating the distribution of load between the medial and lateral compartments of the knee (Table 12-4). This study shows that when the line of vertical load passes through the tibial eminence, along the so-called "mechanical axis" of the limb and clinically a situation occurring in the two-legged stance, the total compressive force is evenly distributed between the two compartments (Fig. 12-29, curve CTE). When the line of vertical load is altered to pass just medial to the knee joint curve (MMC), corresponding to the single-leg stance, the medial compartment bears about 75% of the total compressive load. This quantifies, in a manner more direct than ever before, the effects of external load direction and changes in compartmental loads achieved by altering limb alignment by joint replacement or osteotomy.

From these results and knowing the anthropometric measurements, it is possible to calculate the load redistribution in the compartments per degree of angular deviation of the load from the mechanical axis or angular correction achieved either by replacement or by osteotomy. This works out at (a) 2% unloading of the total compressive load in one compartment and (b) a corresponding increase in the other per degree of deviation or correction.

The effects of external load direction on load-sharing proved not to be statistically significant at high flexion angles. This can hardly be the effect of flexion in and of itself but is, instead, the effects of the large muscle and contact forces set up in high flexion in this experiment. In contrast, large muscle and contact forces are set up during the single-leg stance in gait (Chapter

TABLE 12-4. *Literature review of previous studies examining load distribution in the medial and lateral compartments of the knee*

Author (ref.)	Year	Study	Method	Load distribution
Steindler (33)	1955	Walking	Hypothesis based on anatomical study	Lateral > medial compartment
Morrison (25)	1970	Walking	Gait analysis/force-plate date → a mathematical model	Medial > lateral compartment during stance phase
Kettlekamp (18)	1972	Two-legged stance	Mathematical model and x-ray data	90% Medial compartment
Engin (7)	1974	Extension	Strain-gauged cadaveric bones in loading device	25% Medial compartment
Kostuik (20)	1975	Extension	Cadaveric knees on force platform	Medial = lateral compartment
Johnson (14)	1980	Walking	Gait analysis/force-plate + x-ray data	Medial > lateral compartment even in valgus knees
Hsu (13)	1988	Two-legged stance	X-ray data input to mathematical model	76% Medial compartment

14), although the knee is then only slightly flexed. Load-sharing between the compartments is the result of a balance between (a) the forces applied externally to the limb and (b) the soft tissue forces generated at the knee in response. As the patellar tendon force, acting in the midline of the knee as seen from the front, increases in relation to the loads and the other soft tissue forces, the line of action of the resultant contact force must also approach the midline of the joint, and its distribution between the two compartments should tend to equalize.

There is therefore a significant contribution to load-bearing on the outer side of the knee even when the line of the vertical load passes medial to the medial compartment. Johnson (14) has argued that the medial compartment load will in fact be greater in the dynamic than in the static situation in their model based on gait analysis measurements. However, probably underestimated to date is the lateral stabilizing effect of the ITT, especially in the dynamic situation, where tension will tend to off-load the medial compartment in favor of the lateral. In our experiments (Table 12-3), the effect of a 40-N force in the ITT had a clear equalizing effect near extension, where the effect of load direction was greatest. In flexion, the ITT comes to lie more nearly parallel to the joint line, and ITT tension would then act more as an external rotator of the tibia than as a lateral stabilizer.

It would be surprising if the lateral compartment, endowed as it is with thick articular cartilage for weight-bearing, is functionally little more than an outrigger for the medial compartment. This study would suggest that it plays a more important role in the overall normal kinematics and mechanics of the knee.

CONCLUSION

The work described in this chapter had two objectives: to present experimental descriptions of the behavior of the knee and to compare, where possible, these descriptions with the predictions of the theory of Chapters 10 and 11. Good agreement between theory and experiment gives confidence not only that the mechanisms which underlie the theory are correct but also that the theory can be applied to situations not studied experimentally. Good agreement therefore widens the applicability of experimental results.

When viewed in this context, we have found excellent agreement between our measurements and calculations of muscle forces, implying that our estimates of the lengths of the muscle lever-arms are correct. However, we noted the need to use subject-specific parameters if quantitative precision is required. More important, agreement establishes the view that the length of the lever-arm of a muscle tendon is its distance from the flexion axis of the joint. Since the location of the flexion axis is controlled by the geometry of the ligaments, repair of ligament injury is necessary, not only to restore the passive stability of the joint but also to restore physiological muscle function.

Comparison between theory and our attempts at measurement of ligament force was less satisfactory. The existence of a critical flexion angle at which the changeover of loading from ACL to PCL occurs was vindicated by the measurements, but the values of the critical angles were less precisely predicted. That part of the experimental method should not be too inaccurate, so the errors may lie with the theory. The predictions of the values of the ligament forces were, in general, too high; however, not all the blame should lie with the theory. The experimental method of estimating ligament forces in situ was obviously crude and needs refinement.

The shortcomings of the theory are clear. It is two-dimensional and based, in the main, on the assumption that the ligaments are single, inextensible line elements. A three-dimensional theory based on elastic linkage systems is the ultimate objective. We have reported in Chapters 10 and 11, as well as in this chapter, some work aimed at that objective. The elastic analysis of the drawer test should be regarded as an exercise to establish possible methods of analysis. The experiments that we reported on tibial rotation and abduction/adduction, while possibly of some interest in themselves, are aimed at collecting the experimental evidence upon which a three-dimensional elastic theory should be based.

Despite its shortcomings, it is remarkable that a two-dimensional theory based upon inextensible ligaments can give such reliable insights into the kinematics and mechanics of the knee, vindicating such a simple-minded approach. It is hoped that further theoretical work can be kept as simple as possible.

ACKNOWLEDGMENTS

The work reported in this chapter was supported by the Arthritis and Rheumatism Council, 41 Eagle Street, London. John Bradley was supported by a one year fellowship from the Leverhulme Trust. Mr. Chris Dodd, FRCS, helped with the experiments reported in Fig. 12–21B.

REFERENCES

1. Arms SW, Renstrom P, Stanwyck TS, Hogan M, Johnson RJ, Pope MH. Strain within the anterior cruciate during hamstrings and quadriceps activity. *Trans Orthop Res Soc* 1985;31:139.
2. Bradley J, Goodfellow J, O'Connor J. A radiographic study of bearing movement in unicompartmental Oxford knee replacement. *J Bone Joint Surg [Br]* 1987;69B:598–601.

3. Brantigan OC, Voshell AF. The mechanics of the ligaments and menisci of the knee joint. *J Bone Joint Surg [Am]* 1941;23A:44–66.

4. Decraemer W, Maes M, Vanhuyse V. An elastic stress–strain relation for soft biological tissue based on a structural model. *J Biomech* 1980;13:463–468.

5. Dempster W. *Space requirements of the seated operator.* Ohio: Wright–Patterson Air Force Base, Report No WADCTR 55-159, 1955.

6. Duke RP, Somerset JH, Blacharski P. Some investigations of the accuracy of knee joint kinematics. *J Biomech* 1977;10:659–673.

7. Engin A, Korde M. Biomechanics of the normal and abnormal knee joint. *J Biomech* 1974;7:325–334.

8. Fukubayashi T, Torzilli PA, Sherman MF, Warren RF. An in vitro biomechanical evaluation of antero-posterior motion of the knee. Tibial displacement, rotation and torque. *J Bone Joint Surg [Am]* 1982;64A:258–264.

9. Goodfellow J, O'Connor J. The mechanics of the knee and prosthesis design. *J Bone Joint Surg [Br]* 1978;58B:291–299.

10. Goodfellow J, O'Connor J. Clinical results of the Oxford knee. *Clin Orthop* 1986;205:21–42.

11. Grood ES, Suntay WT, Noyes FR, Butler DL. The biomechanics of the knee-extension exercise. *J Bone Joint Surg [Am]* 1984;66A:725–733.

12. Haynes DW, Hungerford DS, McLeod PC, Connor, KM. Sectioning the anterior cruciate creates a valgus laxity which automatically increases rotational laxity. *Trans Orthop Res Soc* 1986;32;309.

13. Hsu R, Himeno S, Coventry M, Chao E. Normal axial alignment of the lower extremity and load bearing capacity at the knee. *Trans Orthop Res Soc* 1988;34:282.

14. Johnson F, Leidl S, Waugh W. The distribution of load across the knee; a comparison of static and dynamic forces. *J Bone Joint Surg [Br]* 1980;62B:346–349.

15. Kapandji I. *The physiology of the joints*, vol II. London: Churchill Livingstone, 1970.

16. Kennedy J, Fowler PJ. Medial and anterior instability of the knee. *J Bone Joint Surg [Am]* 1971;53A:1257–1270.

17. Kennedy J, Hawkins R, Willis R. Strain gauge analysis of knee ligaments. *Clin Orthop* 1977;129:225–229.

18. Kettlekamp D, Chao E. A method for quantitative analysis of medial and lateral compressive forces at the knee during standing. *Clin Orthop* 1972;83:202–213.

19. Kinzel G, Hall A, Hillberry B. Measurement of the total motion between two body segments. *J Biomech* 1972;5:93–105.

20. Kostuik J, Schmidt O, Harris W, Wooldridge C. A study of weight transmission through the knee joint with applied varus and valgus loads. *Clin Orthop* 1975;108:95–98.

21. Lindahl O, Movin A. The mechanics of extension of the knee joint. *Acta Orthop Scand* 1967;38:226–243.

22. Malcolm L, Daniel D. A mechanical substitution technique for cruciate ligament force determinations. *Trans Orthop Res Soc* 1980;26:303.

23. Markolf K, Mensch J, Amstutz H. Stiffness and laxity of the knee. The contributions of the supporting structures. *J Bone Joint Surg [Am]* 1976;58A:583–594.

24. Mizrahi J, Solomon L, Kaufman B, Duggan T. An experimental method for investigating load distribution in the cadaveric human hip. *J Bone Joint Surg [Br]* 1981;63B:610–613.

25. Morrison J. The mechanics of the knee joint in relation to normal walking. *J Biomech* 1970;3:51–61.

26. Perry J, Antonelli D, Ford W. Analysis of knee joint forces during flexed knee stance. *J Bone Joint Surg [Am]* 1975;57A:961–967.

27. O'Connor JJ, Goodfellow JW, Young SK, Biden E, Daniel D. Mechanical interactions between the muscles and the cruciate ligaments in the knee. *Trans Orthop Res Soc* 1985;31:140.

28. Robichon J, Romero C. The functional anatomy of the knee joint with special reference to the medial collateral and anterior cruciate ligaments. *Can J Surg* 1968;11:36–40.

29. Rydell N. Forces acting on the femoral head prosthesis. *Acta Orthop Scand [Suppl]* 88;1966.

30. Shaw J, Murray D. The longitudinal axis of the knee and the role of the cruciate ligaments in controlling transverse rotation. *J Bone Joint Surg [Am]* 1974;56A:1603–1609.

31. Shrive N, O'Connor J, Goodfellow J. Load bearing in the human knee. *Clin Orthop* 1977;131:279–287.

32. Slocum D, Larson R. Rotary instability of the knee. *J Bone Joint Surg [Am]* 1968;50A:211–226.

33. Steindler A. *Kinesiology of the human body under normal and pathological conditions.* Springfield, IL: Charles C Thomas, 1955.

34. Trent PS, Walker PS, Wolf B. Ligament length patterns, strength and rotational axes of the knee joint. *Clin Orthop* 1976;117:263–270.

35. Vidik A. Functional properties of collagenous tissues. *Int Rev Connect Tissue Res* 1973;6.

36. Wang C, Walker P. Rotary laxity of the human knee joint. *J Bone Joint Surg [Am]* 1974;56A:161–170.

37. Whitmer GG, Haynes DW, Hungerford DS. The effect of different axial loads upon the anterior cruciate ligament. *Trans Orthop Res Soc* 1988;34:60.

Knee Ligaments: Structure, Function, Injury, and Repair, edited by D. Daniel, et al.
© 1990 by Raven Press, Ltd. All rights reserved.

CHAPTER 13

The Tensile Properties of Human Anterior Cruciate Ligament (ACL) and ACL Graft Tissues

Savio L-Y. Woo and Douglas J. Adams

Knowledge of the tensile properties of the human ACL is a prerequisite for the selection, design, and evaluation of ACL replacements such as autografts, allografts, and synthetic substitutes. Moreover, these data are needed for kinematic analyses of the human knee in order to understand the role the ACL plays in joint function. The literature contains a large number of studies of human knee kinematics, with the majority designed to evaluate the contribution of the ACL to guide or to restrain joint motion. A detailed literature review of knee kinematic studies can be found in Chapters 7 and 8. The establishment of a tensile load–deformation relationship for the human ACL will aid in the estimation of the forces in the ligament if the deformation is measured. Likewise, the motion between the femur and tibia can be predicted if the loads in the ACL are known.

The tensile properties of the femur–ACL–tibia complex (FATC) have been evaluated by many authors, but the majority of the work has been related to animal models such as rabbit (2,17,39,41), swine (26), dog (1,5,8,12,13,19,30,43), goat (23), and monkey (8,10,28), as well as others. Some studies addressed

the tensile properties of various autografts, including those of the patellar tendon (2,5,11), iliotibial tract (5,22,29,38), and semitendinosus (25). Surprisingly little work has been done on the tensile properties of the human ACL. Kennedy (24) measured the strength of the isolated ACL and found the ultimate loads to be in the range of 480 ± 30 N and 640 ± 20 N. Trent (37) studied the bone–ACL–bone complex from human donors of various age and reported ultimate loads no higher than 1750 N. The fact that these two reports have provided limited biomechanical data on the human FATC and, particularly, lower-than-expected ultimate load values stimulated Noyes (28) to perform a landmark study on the tensile properties of the human ACL as a function of age. Using a strain rate of approximately 100%/sec (based on a calculation of elongation with respect to distance between the femoral and tibial insertion sites), the load–deformation relationship was obtained for six ACLs from young donors (16–26 years) and for 20 ACLs from older donors (48–86 years). Significantly higher values of linear stiffness, ultimate load, and energy absorbed at failure were found for the younger group. The ultimate load for the young ACL was 1725 ± 269 N (mean ± SEM). Since that study, the guidelines and criteria for the strength of autograft, allograft, and synthetic substitutes have been based on 1730 N, since this value has become the gold standard in the field.

S. L.-Y. Woo and D. J. Adams: Orthopedic Bioengineering Laboratory, Division of Orthopedic Surgery, University of California, San Diego, School of Medicine, La Jolla, California 92093.

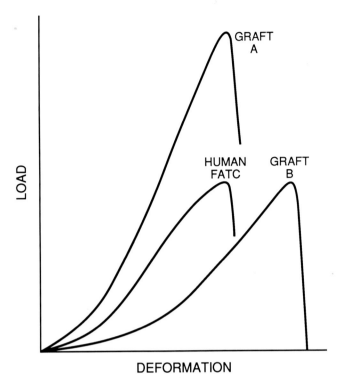

FIG. 13-1. The structural properties (load–deformation curves) of the FATC and two ACL replacement grafts.

As described in Chapter 7, a number of biomechanical properties of the ligament may be described in addition to the ultimate load that the bone–ligament–bone structure can sustain prior to failure. Structural properties of the FATC involve the examination of the entire load–deformation curve as well as other parameters, including linear stiffness, ultimate deformation, and energy absorbed at failure. The need to look at the entire load–deformation curve must be emphasized. To illustrate, Fig. 13-1 is a schematic diagram of the structural properties of two ACL replacement grafts (A and B) plotted together with that for the native FATC. Both grafts are strong enough; however, the question regarding whether these grafts are ideal replacements for the ACL remains. The answer is no! In spite of the equal or high ultimate load values, the load–deformation curve in tension of both grafts does not mimic that of the normal ACL. During normal function, the tensile forces in the ACL have been estimated (not measured) by Chen (9) to range from 67 N (for ascending stairs) to 630 N (for jogging). Note also that an ACL replacement graft must be subjected to these load levels for millions of cycles. It seems clear that graft A would be too stiff while graft B would be too compliant for these purposes, and neither would have appropriate elasticity in order to provide the knee with appropriate motion during physiological function. As such, the selection of the medial patellar tendon–bone units as an autograft replacement should also be questioned (Fig. 13-2). Although its ultimate load is almost double that of the native FATC, its linear stiffness (650 ± 68 N/mm) is significantly higher than that of the native FATC (182 ± 33 N/mm). Therefore, when implanted, it could not have satisfactorily served as an ACL replacement based on its biomechanical behavior. Likewise, the polytetrafluoroethylene (PTFE) Gore-Tex synthetic ligament graft, in spite of its reported ultimate load being as high as 4830 ± 280 N, is questionable in its effectiveness to serve as an ACL replacement. This is because the stiffness (322 N/mm) is very high and the load–deformation curve does not

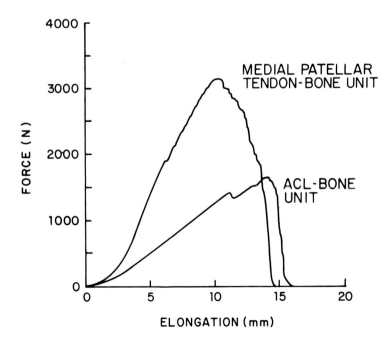

FIG. 13-2. The structural properties (load–deformation curves) of the FATC and of the patellar tendon–bone unit. (Redrawn from ref. 27.)

match that of the normal FATC (4). Matching the tensile load–deformation curve for the grafts with that for the native FATC should be a goal of graft design and selection. In the least, linear stiffness should be added to the design criteria in addition to the ultimate load.

This chapter will describe the tensile properties of the human FATC available in the literature based on the fundamentals. We will also discuss some of the state-of-the-art techniques that are used to measure these properties and the methods used to deal with the complex geometry and anatomy of the ACL. The effects of direction of the applied load with respect to the anatomical axis of the ACL will be emphasized. The data obtained will be used as a basis to evaluate the properties of autografts as well as to assess synthetic replacement grafts that are described in the literature.

TENSILE PROPERTIES OF HUMAN FEMUR–ACL–TIBIA COMPLEX (FATC)

Data from the Literature

Trent (37) tested human ACL from autopsy specimens between 29 and 55 years old. The ACL was removed from the knee as a bone–ligament–bone complex and maintained in a "physiologic" position for tensile testing. The author reported an averaged ultimate load of 633 N, with a maximum of 1750 N and a stiffness of 141 N/mm for these specimens. Although most of his ACL failures occurred at midsubstance, frequent insertion site failures occurred which resulted in lower failure loads. Noyes (28) was the first to emphasize the importance of specimen age on the structural properties of FATC. He reported values of 1725 ± 269 N and 182 ± 33 N/mm for the ultimate load and stiffness of the younger specimens (16–26 years of age), respectively, while the older specimens had an averaged ultimate load of 734 N and averaged stiffness of 129 N/mm.

In a recent workshop on the Biomechanics of Human Ligaments sponsored by the University of Ulm and the European Society of Biomechanics, Rauch (32) presented tensile properties of human FATC tested at 30° of knee flexion. The age of the donors ranged from 17 to 84 years, and the ultimate loads ranged from 250 N to 2500 N. There was a significant correlation between age of specimen and ultimate load. The linear stiffness and ultimate load for the five specimens from the younger group (17–28 years) were 203 ± 34 N/mm and 1716 ± 538 N, respectively. For the 44 older specimens (34–84 years of age) the values were lower (124 ± 39 N/mm and 814 ± 356 N, respectively).

Tensile testing of FATC from younger (22–49 years) and older (60–97 years) human donors in our laboratory indicate that the linear stiffness and ultimate load are significantly affected by age and angle of knee flexion, as well as by the direction of tensile loading with respect to the anatomy of the ACL. The details will be given in the following section.

Data from our Laboratory (UCSD)

Consideration of the Effects of Knee Flexion and Direction of Applied Load

The ACL has a very complex anatomy and an equally complex function. As the knee undergoes flexion–extension as well as internal–external and varus–valgus rotation, the length and orientation of the ACL change significantly. The broad attachments of the ACL to both the femur and the tibia allow various portions of the ligament to be relatively taut while others are lax, depending on the knee motion. Given a particular orientation of the knee, some collagen bundles of the ACL experience tension while other bundles are unloaded. In addition, the orientation of the ACL changes with different knee positions (16). Therefore, the tensile behavior of the ACL will depend on knee orientation as well as on the direction of applied load.

Previous studies of tensile properties of the FATC were performed at various positions with respect to the ligament orientation relative to the direction of applied load. An early study by Viidik (39) on the structural properties of the FATC in rabbits was performed with the knee in a fully extended position and with the femur, tibia, and ACL all aligned along the axis of the applied tensile load. Gupta (20) used a similar experimental setup to test the FATC of canines, but with the tibia externally rotated 90° relative to the femur to eliminate the natural twist in the ACL. Noyes (28) tested the FATC of rhesus monkeys as well as of young and old humans. In his study, the knee was placed in approximately 45° flexion and the loading axis was aligned with the axis of the ACL in the sagittal plane but not in the coronal plane. Dorlot (12) tested the canine FATC with a knee flexion angle of 90°, without detailing direction of applied load.

Several authors have used a simulated anterior drawer loading to assess the failure properties of canine FATC (5,30,33). Other investigators examined the structural properties of the FATC using various knee flexion angles and axes of tensile loading. Clancy (10) tested the FATC of rhesus monkeys at 30° flexion. Yoshiya (43) tested canine FATC with the femur aligned along the loading axis and the knee flexed to 30°. Jackson (23) also used a knee flexion angle of 30°, but he aligned the ACL (or ACL graft) vertically along the direction of loading. Figgie (13) demonstrated that the angle of knee flexion had a significant effect on the structural properties of the canine FATC. When the FATC was stretched along the axis of the tibia, the ultimate load decreased significantly with increasing angles of flexion. Our laboratory confirmed these findings using a rabbit model (41). Furthermore, we have found the tensile stiffness and strength of the FATC to be dependent upon the direction of the applied tensile force. A special clamp was designed to accomplish this goal (Fig. 13-3). A comparative study of paired rabbit legs was performed, in which loading was applied either along the ACL axis or along the tibial axis. Cyclic hysteresis, linear stiffness, ultimate load, and energy absorbed at failure were determined (41).

The ultimate load values for the rabbit FATC decreased with increased knee flexion for those loaded along the tibial axis, whereas no such change was detected for FATC tested along the ligament axis (Fig. 20-3). Other tensile properties also followed similar

trends. It is concluded that the structural properties of the rabbit FATC change minimally with knee flexion (from 0° to 90°) when loaded along the ligament axis, but they decrease significantly with knee flexion when loaded along the axis of the tibia. Therefore, the method of evaluating the structural properties of the FATC needs to be taken into account before the data obtained for a specific animal model, particularly with respect to the direction of loading, can be properly evaluated (18,26,42).

Design of New Experimental Apparatus for Human Knee

As a result of knowing the effects of knee flexion and direction of applied tension on the properties of the rabbit FATC, our laboratory designed and fabricated an apparatus for testing human knee specimens. The apparatus can measure the tensile behavior of the FATC at any desired loading direction and knee flexion angle (Fig. 13-4A and B). In order to compare the direction of the applied load on the tensile properties of the FATC, the clamps are adjusted to accommodate two chosen directions, namely, the ACL (or ligament) axis and the tibial axis. Paired human knees are tested, with one knee of each pair randomly assigned to a tensile test to failure with the load applied along the ligament axis. The other knee is tested along the tibial axis (Fig. 13-5).

Experimental Procedure

Using the apparatus and methodology described in Figs. 13-4 and 13-5, pairs of human cadaveric knees were evaluated in our laboratory. Seven pairs were obtained from younger donors (age 22–49 years, with a mean age of 34). Five died following acute trauma, one died from hepatic failure, and one died from pneumonia. An additional seven pairs were from older donors (age 60–97, years with a mean age of 74). All knees were tested at a flexion angle of 30°. The protocol used for tensile testing of the human FATC was as follows: A 2.5-N tensile preload was applied, and the specimen was preconditioned cyclically between 0 and 2 mm of deformation at an extension rate of 20 mm/min for 10 cycles. Subsequently, the specimen was loaded to failure at a rate of 200 mm/min. The displacement and loads were recorded on a strip chart recorder. Linear stiffness, ultimate deformation, ultimate load, energy absorbed at failure, and failure mode of each specimen were determined. Linear stiffness was defined as the slope of the load–deformation curve between 3 and 7 mm of displacement. It is also important to consider the stiffness of the experimental apparatus. The linear stiffness for each FATC was cor-

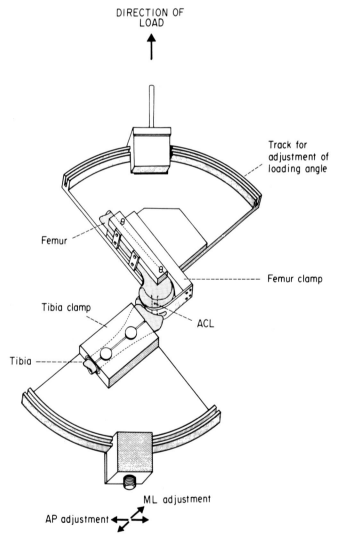

FIG. 13-3. Schematic diagram of the testing device used to evaluate the tensile structural properties of the rabbit FATC.

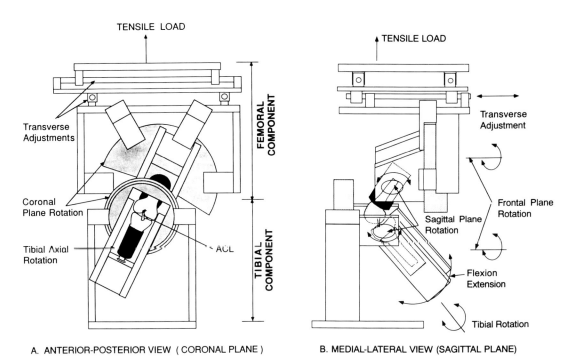

A. ANTERIOR-POSTERIOR VIEW (CORONAL PLANE)   B. MEDIAL-LATERAL VIEW (SAGITTAL PLANE)

FIG. 13-4. Schematic diagram of the testing device used to evaluate the tensile structural properties of the human FATC. Adjustments are possible in all six degrees of freedom for tensile testing, permitting precise alignment of the direction of loading with respect to the knee ligament. Knees are dissected free of muscle tissue, leaving the ligaments and capsule intact. The femur and tibia are cut to a length of 15 cm from the joint line, and they are fixed within aluminum mounting cylinders using three transfixing bolts for each bone. The knee is then placed in the femoral and tibial components of the device, and necessary adjustments are made. **A:** Coronal view. **B:** Sagittal view.

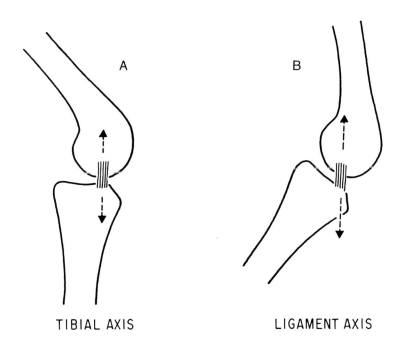

TIBIAL AXIS   LIGAMENT AXIS

FIG. 13-5. Schematic diagram of FATCs at 30° knee flexion, demonstrating the difference in alignment for the tibial axis **(A)** and for the ligament axis **(B)** during tensile testing. For testing along the tibial axis, the tibia is secured vertically along the loading axis in the coronal and sagittal planes. The soft tissues around the knee are removed, leaving only the ACL. The femur is moved anteriorly and medially on the tibia, positioning the femoral origin of the ACL directly over its tibial insertion. The FATC is secured in this position, permitting joint motion along the loading axis only. For testing along the ligament axis, the knee is rotated in the sagittal and coronal planes to align the long axis of the ACL visually along the vertical loading axis using a plumb line.

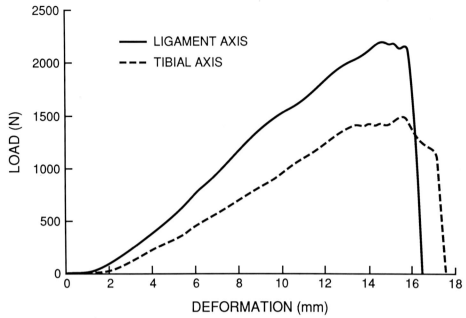

FIG. 13-6. Typical load–displacement curves for FATC tested along the ligament and tibial axes.

rected for the stiffness of the experimental apparatus, which was measured by bolting a stainless steel plate between the femoral and tibial cylinders. The device stiffness is constant at 508 N/mm throughout a range of tensile load of up to 2500 N.

Experimental Results

Typical load–displacement curves obtained during tensile testing of the FATC along the tibial and liga-ment axes are shown in Fig. 13-6. It can be seen that the structural properties are significantly affected by the direction of the applied load. The ligament axis specimens demonstrate a significantly steeper linear stiffness, higher ultimate load, and slightly less ulti-mate deformation than for the tibial axis specimens. The modes of failure were also different. The speci-mens tested along the ligament axis mostly failed by midsubstance tear, whereas the specimen tested along the tibial axis mostly failed by sequentially "tearing off" at the tibial insertion.

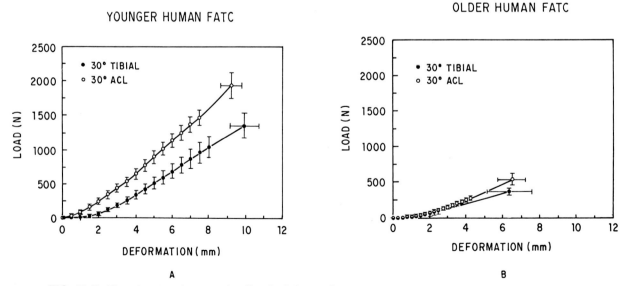

FIG. 13-7. The structural properties (load–deformation curves) of the FATC tested at 30° of flexion along the tibial and ACL axes for **(A)** younger donors and **(B)** older donors.

TABLE 13-1. *Structural properties of the FATC for younger and older donors along the ACL and tibial axes*[a]

Property	Younger donors		Older donors		Significance level	
	ACL	Tibia	ACL	Tibia	Age	Axis
Linear stiffness (N/mm)	292 ± 28	226 ± 41	179 ± 29	129 ± 19	$p < .05$	$p > .05$
Ultimate load (N)	1954 ± 187	1373 ± 180	642 ± 164	470 ± 108	$p < .001$	$p < .05$
Ultimate deformation (mm)	9.0 ± 0.3	9.8 ± 0.6	5.8 ± 0.9	6.4 ± 1.0	$p < .001$	$p > .1$
Energy absorbed (N-m)	8470 ± 950	5880 ± 900	1690 ± 596	1270 ± 380	$p < .001$	$p < .05$

[a] Values are expressed as mean ± SEM. Levels of significance are given for both age and axis of loading.

The load–deformation curves for all the FATC specimens tested are plotted in Fig. 13-7. It can be seen that both the direction of applied load and age of donors have a significant effect on the outcome (Table 13-1). Statistical analysis using two-way analysis of variance showed a significant effect of age on linear stiffness ($p < 0.05$), with the younger specimens having a higher linear stiffness than the older specimens (Fig. 13-8). For specimens tested along the ligament axis, the values were 292 ± 28 N/mm for the younger specimens and 179 ± 29 N/mm for the older specimens, whereas those tested along the tibial axis were 226 ± 41 N/mm and 129 ± 19 N/mm, respectively. There was no statistically significant effect of loading direction ($p > 0.05$). On average, however, FATCs tested along the ligament axis had a 33% higher linear stiffness than did those tested along the tibial axis.

Both specimen age and loading axis had a significant effect on the ultimate load values ($p < 0.05$). The mean ultimate load of the younger specimens was three times higher than that of the older specimens, whereas the

mean ultimate load for the FATC tested along the ligament axis was 41% higher than that for the tibial axis. A decrease in ultimate load was seen with increasing age, regardless of loading axis, and the difference in FATC ultimate load between the ligament and tibial loading axes also diminished with increasing age (Fig. 13-9).

The ultimate deformation was significantly affected by age, but not by the axis of loading (p < .001, p > 0.1, respectively; Table 13-1). The younger FATCs had higher ultimate deformation than the older ones. This was probably due to the higher linear stiffness and ultimate load. For specimens from the same age group, there were relatively small differences in the ultimate deformation with respect to axis of loading.

The energy absorbed at failure values for the FATCs followed those for the ultimate load (i.e., were affected significantly by both age and loading axis) (Table 13-1). The younger specimens absorbed more energy at failure than did the older specimens, whereas the specimens tested along the ligament axis absorbed more

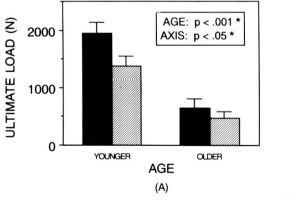

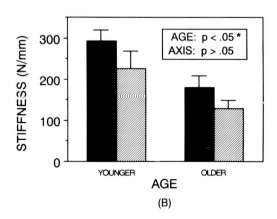

■ LIGAMENT AXIS

▨ TIBIAL AXIS

* STATISTICALLY SIGNIFICANT TWO WAY ANOVA

FIG. 13-8. The effect of axis of loading and specimen age on average values of **(A)** linear stiffness and **(B)** ultimate load.

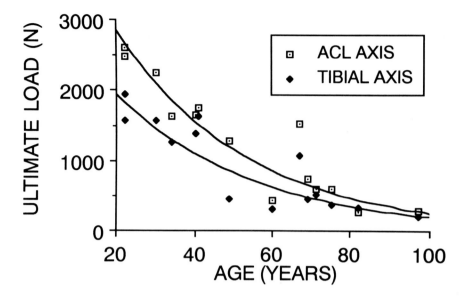

FIG. 13-9. The effect of specimen age on FATC tensile ultimate load.

energy at failure than did those tested along the tibial axis.

The failure modes changed with both specimen age and loading axis. The older specimens had a higher incidence of substance failure than did the younger specimens, regardless of the axis of applied load. Presumably, the higher incidence of substance failures in the older specimens was due to a deterioration of the ligament substance with increasing age, since the insertion site appears to be relatively stronger than the ligament substance. However, the ultimate load of the insertion site and ligament substance in the younger specimens are comparable, since the failure modes included a variety of substance, avulsion, and insertion failures, or a combination thereof.

The specimens tested along the ligament axis had a higher percentage incidence of substance failures than did those tested along the tibial axis, regardless of specimen age (50% of the younger age group and 86% of the older age group). The contrast in the failure modes of the two loading axes is quite important. The higher percentage of ligament substance failures for the FATCs tested along the ligament axis resulted in higher ultimate load values, since the data are more representative of the ACL substance strength than of the ligament insertion-site failures. Specimens tested along the tibial axis had a higher incidence of insertion-site failures, probably due to the ACL being out of its normal anatomical alignment during tensile loading. Presumably, a smaller number of its fiber bundles were loaded simultaneously, and, as a result, the fiber bundles under load (presumably the shorter ones) would fail first before other (longer), initially unloaded fiber bundles began to take load. This process would continue until the entire ligament is "peeled off" at the insertion site or avulsed with some bony fragments from around the insertion site.

FATC alignment relative to the loading axis is crit-

ical in tensile testing. The complex arrangement of ACL fiber bundles with different lengths makes uniform loading of the entire ACL an impossibility. Presumably, testing the FATC along the long axis of the ACL, while maintaining anatomical knee alignment, allows a greater proportion of fiber bundles to be loaded simultaneously during tensile testing. This premise is substantiated by the higher values of FATC stiffness, ultimate load, energy, and deformation to ultimate load for specimens tested along the ligament axis, compared with those tested along the tibial axis. Furthermore, we have documented a higher ultimate load for the human FATC tested along the anatomical axis of the ACL than has previously been reported for younger specimens. The mean ± SEM values for the samples under 35 years of age were 2246 ± 216 N. In the study by Noyes (28), the specimens were tested with a flexion angle of 45°. However, the orientation of the ACL with respect to the axis of loading in his study and in the study by Rauch (32) is not specified. Therefore, it is difficult to compare the published data, even though similar angles of knee flexion were used in all three studies.

Although the axis of the ACL is difficult to define uniquely because of the complexity of its anatomical structure of the ACL, we feel that an attempt to align the direction of applied load along the ACL axis would be a significant improvement over an arbitrarily selected direction of loading. Repeatable data as well as a consistently higher ultimate load for the FATC obtained in this study substantiate this approach.

TENSILE PROPERTIES OF BIOLOGICAL GRAFTS

There exist only limited data on the tensile properties of tissue grafts used for ACL replacement (6,27). In

1984, Noyes (27) performed a comprehensive study on the biomechanical properties of nine different autograft tissues. A total of 90 specimens of autograft tissues, obtained from 14 male and 4 female young donors (mean age 26 years) were tested. The major cause of death for the donors was trauma. The autograft tissues included central and medial portions (14 mm wide) of the bone–patellar tendon–bone complex, semitendinosus tendons, gracilis tendons, distal iliotibial tract, and fascia lata, as well as the medial, central, and lateral aspects of the quadriceps–patellar retinaculum–patellar tendon complexes. The width of the tissue grafts ranged from 14 to 18 mm. The grafts were subjected to tensile tests, with an extension rate of 100% of the initial length of the specimen per second. This investigator found that the bone–patellar tendon–bone complex was the strongest among all grafts; for example, a 14-mm-wide graft was approximately 1.6 times that of the human FATC. The weakest was the quadriceps–patellar retinaculum–patellar tendon complex, which was only 14–21% that of the human FATC (Table 13-2). The mean ultimate load value for the semitendinosus tendon was 70% that of the FATC, whereas those for the gracilis and the distal iliotibial tract were approximately 50% that of the FATC.

Noyes (27) also reported other important structural properties such as the linear stiffness and energy absorbed at failure (Table 13-2). Again, the central and medial third of the bone–patellar tendon–bone complex had the highest linear stiffness (approximately four times that of the FATC). Other grafts such as the semitendinosus tendon, gracilis tendon, and fascia lata (16 mm in width) were within the same order of magnitude as the FATC. The energy-absorbing capability of the bone–patellar tendon–bone complex was identical to that of the FATC, whereas those of the others were significantly lower (Table 13-2). Our laboratory

has long advocated that the ultimate load is only one of the many biomechanical parameters to be considered in order to describe the structural characteristics of a bone–ligament–bone complex. Noyes (27) also emphasized that linear stiffness and other biomechanical parameters must be considered when selecting an appropriate graft for ligament reconstruction. In spite of these cautions, many investigators continue to limit their concerns to the ultimate load value as the only parameter for matching the grafts for ACL replacement.

There are also a few animal studies relating to the effects of storage and sterilization on the biomechanical properties of allografts for ACL replacement. The results are generally preliminary as well as contradictory. Barad (3) showed that deep-freezing of allografts from the Rhesus monkey at −80°C has no effect on the properties of the FATC. Thomas (36) showed no effect of freeze-drying on the biomechanical properties, whereas Webster (40) demonstrated a significant decrease in strength of the flexor tendon as a result of freeze-drying.

Recently, gas and cobalt irradiation sterilization techniques as well as freeze-drying have been proposed as a means to increase the supply of allograft tissues. Butler (7), Paulos (31), France (14), and Gibbons (15) have carefully evaluated the mechanical properties (stress–strain relationship) of the allografts before and after sterilization and preservation. These studies are a significant improvement over previous work where only the ultimate load (one of the structural properties) was compared. Although the data are preliminary, the general conclusion is that cold ethylene oxide gas sterilization and low-dosage irradiation do not appear to change the mechanical properties of allografts, whereas high-dosage cobalt irradiation may

TABLE 13-2. *A comparison of structural properties of various autograft tissues commonly used for ACL reconstruction*[a]

Tissue	Number of specimens	Width (mm)	Ultimate load (N)	Ultimate load as % of ACL	Stiffness (N/mm)	Energy absorbed to failure (N-m)
Anterior cruciate ligament	6	—	1725 ± 269	100	182 ± 33	12.8 ± 2.2
Bone–patellar tendon–bone						
Central third	7	13.8 ± 1.4	2900 ± 260	168	685 ± 86	12.8 ± 2.4
Medial third	7	14.9 ± 1.1	2734 ± 298	159	651 ± 85	12.8 ± 2.2
Semitendinosus	11	—	1216 ± 50	70	186 ± 9	8.9 ± 0.5
Fascia lata	18	15.6 ± 0.8	628 ± 35	36	118 ± 5	3.0 ± 0.4
Gracilis	17	—	838 ± 30	49	171 ± 11	3.5 ± 0.4
Distal iliotibial tract	10	18.0 ± 1.6	769 ± 99	44	—	—
Quadriceps–patellar retinaculum–patellar tendon						
Medial	7	14.4 ± 1.9	371 ± 46	21	—	—
Central	6	16.3 ± 3.5	266 ± 74	15		
Lateral	7	13.7 ± 1.8	249 ± 54	14	—	—

[a] Adapted from ref. 27.

cause the mechanical properties of the tissue to become compromised.

Haut (21) recently examined the effect of order of irradiating and freeze-drying on the biomechanical properties of young (29 ± 3 years) human bone–patellar tendon–bone preparations, finding significant decreases in strength (75%) and modulus (40%) if the specimens were lyophilized prior to irradiation. No significant effect was found for specimens lyophilized after irradiation. Further work is warranted to investigate sterilization techniques that provide allografts without compromised mechanical properties.

FUTURE DIRECTIONS

Biomechanical Criteria for Appropriate Graft Selection

All too frequently, criteria for ACL replacement have focused on reproducing or surpassing the natural strength of the ACL. Much attention has been placed on the strength of the ACL and autografts adopted from the work of Noyes (27,28) as "gold standards" for ACL replacement. Although strength is an important consideration, the stiffness, as well as other parameters such as deformation and energy absorbed at failure, must also be considered. In other words, the entire load–deformation behavior of the FATC should be reproduced by the graft in order to achieve normal joint kinematics. Most autografts, allografts, and synthetic grafts do not come close to reproducing the load–deformation behavior of the FATC. Furthermore, our current data show that the tensile characteristics of the human FATC are not unique. When the FATC from young donors is tested along the ligament axis, the stiffness and strength values substantially exceed the previously published data. It is evident that more data are needed pertaining to the load–deformation properties of the ACL, tissue grafts, and synthetic replacements. It is also important to point out that stronger grafts may not necessarily be better grafts. Should a synthetic graft be designed with a failure strength several times greater than that of the native ACL, a fully incorporated graft could conceivably present a serious problem. A very large applied external load that would normally cause failure of the ACL may now instead cause catastrophic damage to the entire knee.

Utility of Present Knowledge

Various animal models have been used to gain objective information on ACL replacement, but these studies have limitations in applicability to patient management. Firstly, the joint anatomy and kinematics are different between animals and humans, creating a problem in the evaluation of the stress demands on the grafts. Moreover, the physiological response of an animal joint to surgical procedures may not match that of a human. In most cases, these models represent an accelerated case of healing. In addition, synthetic grafts designed for humans are often implanted in animals, and, as such, the graft size is not appropriate for the size of the joint. The lack of appropriate rehabilitation in animal studies further clouds the picture. Since it is impossible to impose a fully controlled rehabilitation program, data obtained from animal models must be evaluated accordingly.

Presently, clinical follow-up in evaluating ACL reconstruction is only a few years at best. Problems may develop as a result of changes in the joint or in the long-term integrity of the graft. Therefore, optimistic short-term follow-up may yield misleading results. Indeed, at least 5 years or more are necessary in order to fully evaluate the use of ACL grafts.

Much progress has been made and knowledge gained in the last decade on the treatment of ACL injury using grafts. However, it is expected that replacement of the ACL with grafts will remain an important and widely discussed topic for many years. In order to adequately evaluate innovative treatments, a further understanding of the structural behavior of the human ACL itself is warranted. Significantly high numbers of knee specimens of all ages must be tested in order to provide a sufficient data base for the purpose of graft design and selection. A graft should have characteristics that match the entire tensile load–deformation curve of the ACL that it is designed to replace. As discussed elsewhere in this book, graft fixation remains foremost of the problems to overcome, since this is the weakest link of the bone–graft system.

ACKNOWLEDGMENTS

The authors wish to thank the many students and laboratory staff at the Orthopedic Bioengineering Laboratory. We also gratefully acknowledge the financial support of the following: the RR&D Grant A188-3RA of the Veterans Administration; NIH Grants AR34264 and AR39683; and the Malcolm and Dorothy Coutts Institute for Joint Reconstruction and Research.

REFERENCES

1. Alm A, Ekstrom H, Stromberg B. Tensile strength of the anterior cruciate ligament in the dog. *Acta Chir Scand* 1974; 445:15–23.
2. Ballock RT, Woo SL-Y, Lyon RM, Hollis JM, Akeson WH. Use of patellar tendon autograft for anterior cruciate ligament reconstruction in the rabbit—a long term histological and biomechanical study. *J Orthop Res* 1989;7:474–475.

3. Barad S, Cabaud HE, Rodrigo JJ. Effects of storage at −80°C as compared to 4°C on the strength of rhesus monkey anterior cruciate ligaments. *Trans Orthop Res Soc* 1982;7:378.
4. Bolton CW, Bruchman WC. The GORE-TEX™ expanded polytetrafluoro-ethylene prosthetic ligament: an *in vitro* and *in vivo* evaluation. *Clin Orthop Rel Res* 1985;196:202–213.
5. Butler DL, Hulse DA, Kay MD, Grood ES, Shires PK, D'Ambrosia R, Shoji H. Biomechanics of cranial cruciate ligament reconstruction in the dog. II. Mechanical properties. *Vet Surg* 1983;12:113–118.
6. Butler DL, Kay MD, Stouffer DC. Comparison of material properties in fascicle–bone units from human patellar tendon and knee ligaments. *J Biomech* 1986;19:425–432.
7. Butler DL, Noyes FR, Walz KA, Gibbons MJ. Biomechanics of human knee ligament allograft treatment. *Trans Orthop Res Soc* 1987;12:128.
8. Cabaud HE, Rodkey WG, Feagin JA. Experimental studies of acute anterior cruciate ligament injury and repair. *Am J Sports Med* 1979;7:18–21.
9. Chen EH, Black J. Materials design analysis of the prosthetic anterior cruciate ligament. *J Biomed Mater Res* 1980;14:567–586.
10. Clancy WG, Narechania RG, Rosenberg TD, Gmeiner JG, Wisnefske DD, Lange TA. Anterior and posterior cruciate ligament reconstruction in rhesus monkeys. *J Bone Joint Surg* 1981;63A:1270–1284.
11. Clancy WG, Nelson DA, Reider B, Narechania RG. Anterior cruciate ligament reconstruction using one-third of the patellar ligament augmented by extra-articular tendon transfers. *J Bone Joint Surg* 1982;64:352–359.
12. Dorlot JM, Ait Ba Sidi M, Tremblay GM, Drouin G. Load elongation behavior of the canine anterior cruciate ligament. *J Biomech Eng* 1980;102:190–193.
13. Figgie HE, Bahniuk EH, Heiple KG, Davy DT. The effects of tibial–femoral angle on the failure mechanics of the canine anterior cruciate ligament. *J Biomech* 1986;19:89–99.
14. France PE, Paulos LE, Rosenberg TD, Harner CD. The biomechanics of anterior cruciate allografts. In: Friedman MJ, Ferkel RD, eds. *Prosthetic ligament reconstruction of the knee.* Philadelphia: WB Saunders, 1988;180–185.
15. Gibbons MJ, Butler DL, Grood ES, Chun KJ, Noyes FR, Bukovec DB. Dose-dependent effects of gamma irradiation on the material properties of frozen bone–patellar tendon–bone allografts. *Trans Orthop Res Soc* 1989;35:513.
16. Girgis FG, Marshal JL, Al Monajem ARS. the cruciate ligament of the knee joint. *Clin Orthop* 1975;106:216–231.
17. Goldberg VM, Burstein AH, Dawson M. The influence of an experimental immune synovitis on the failure mode and strength of the rabbit anterior cruciate ligament. *J Bone Joint Surg* 1982;64A:900–906.
18. Grood ES, Butler DL, Noyes FR. Comment on 'Effects of knee flexion angle on the structural properties of the rabbit femur–anterior cruciate ligament–tibia complex'. *J Biomech* 1988;21:688–689.
19. Gupta BN, Brinker WO, Subramanian KN. Breaking strength of cruciate ligaments in the dog. *J Am Vet Med Assoc* 1969;155:1586–1588.
20. Gupta BN, Subramanian KN, Brinker WO, Gupta AN. Tensile strength of canine cranial cruciate ligaments. *Am J Vet Res* 1971;32:183–190.
21. Haut RC, Powlison AC. Order of irradiation and lyophilization on the strength of patellar tendon allografts. *Trans Orthop Res Soc* 1989;14:514.
22. Holden JP, Grood ES, Butler DL, Noyes FR, Mendenhall HV, VanKampen CL, Neidich RL. Biomechanics of fascia lata ligament replacements: early postoperative changes in the goat. *J Orthop Res* 1988;6:639–647.
23. Jackson DW, Groof ES, Arnoczky SP, Butler DL, Simon TM. Freeze dried anterior cruciate ligament allografts: preliminary studies in a goat model. *Am J Sports Med* 1987;15:295–303.
24. Kennedy JC, Hawkins RJ, Willis RB, Danylchuk KD. Tension studies of human knee ligaments, yield point, ultimate failure and disruption of the cruciate and tibial collateral ligaments. *J Bone Joint Surg* 1976;58A:350–355.
25. Kennedy JC, Roth JH, Mendenhall HV. Presidential Address: Intraarticular replacement in the anterior cruciate ligament-deficient knee. *Am J Sports Med* 1980;8(1):1–8.
26. Lyon RM, Woo SL-Y, Hollis JM, Marcin JP, Lee EB. A new device to measure the structural properties of the femur–anterior cruciate ligament–tibia complex. *J Biomech Eng* 1989;submitted for publication.
27. Noyes FR, Butler DL, Grood ES, Zernicke RF, Hefzy MS. Biomechanical analysis of human ligament grafts used in knee-ligament repairs and reconstructions. *J Bone Joint Surg* 1984;66A:344–352.
28. Noyes FR, Grood ES. The strength of the anterior cruciate ligament in humans and rhesus monkeys. Age-related and species-related changes. *J Bone Joint Surg* 1976;58A:1074–1082.
29. O'Donoghue DH, Frank GR, Jeter GL, Johnson W, Zeiders JW, Kenyon R. Repair and reconstruction of the anterior cruciate ligament in dogs: factors influencing long term results. *J Bone Joint Surg* 1971;53A:710–718.
30. O'Donoghue DH, Rockwood CA, Frank GR, Jack SC, Kenyon R. Repair of the anterior cruciate ligament in dogs. *J Bone Joint Surg* 1966;48A:503–519.
31. Paulos LE, France EP, Rosenberg TD, Drez DJ, Abbott PJ, Straight CB, Hammon DJ, Oden RR. Comparative material properties of allograft tissues for ligament replacement: effects of type, age, sterilization and preservation. *Trans Orthop Res Soc* 1987;33:129.
32. Rauch G, Allzeit B, Gotzen L. Tensile strength of the anterior cruciate ligament in dependence on age. In: *Biomechanics of human knee ligaments.* Proceedings of the European Society of Biomechanics. Ulm, West Germany: University of Ulm, 1987;24.
33. Ryan JR, Drompp BW. Evaluation of tensile strength of reconstructions of the anterior cruciate ligament using the patellar tendon in dogs: a preliminary report. *South Med J* 1966;59:129–134.
34. Shino K, Kawasaki T, Hirose H, Gotoh I, Inoue M, Ono K. Reconstruction of the anterior cruciate ligament by allogenic tendon graft: an operation for chronic ligamentous insufficiency. *J Bone Joint Surg* 1986;68B:739–746.
35. Simon TM, Jackson DW. Anterior cruciate ligament allografts. In: Jackson DW, Drez D, eds. *The anterior cruciate deficient knee.* St. Louis: CV Mosby, 1987;211–225.
36. Thomas ED, Gresham RB. Comparative tensile strength study of fresh-frozen and freeze-dried human fascia lata. *Surg Forum* 1963;14:442–443.
37. Trent PS, Walker PS, Wolf B. Ligament length patterns, strength and rotational axes of the knee joint. *Clin Orthop* 1976;117:263–270.
38. vanRens TJG, van den Berg AF, Huiskes R, Kaypers W. Substitution of the anterior cruciate ligament: a long-term histologic and biomechanical study with autogenous pedicled grafts of the iliotibial band in dogs. *Arthroscopy* 1986;2:139–154.
39. Viidik A. Elasticity and tensile strength of the anterior cruciate ligament in rabbits as influenced by training. *Acta Orthop Scand* 1968;74:372–380.
40. Webster DA, Werner FW. Mechanical and functional properties of implanted freeze-dried flexor tendons. *Clin Orthop Rel Res* 1983;180:301–309.
41. Woo SL-Y, Hollis JM, Roux RD, Gomez MA, Inoue M, Kleiner JB, Akeson WH. Effects of knee flexion on the structural properties of the rabbit femur–anterior cruciate ligament–tibia complex (FATC). *J Biomech* 1987;20:557–563.
42. Woo SL-Y, Hollis JM, Lyon RM. Authors' response. *J Biomech* 1988;21:689–691.
43. Yoshiya S, Andrish JT, Manley MT, Kurosaka M. Augmentation of anterior cruciate ligament reconstruction in dogs with prostheses of different stiffnesses. *J Orthop Res* 1987;4:475–485.

Knee Ligaments: Structure, Function, Injury, and Repair, edited by D. Daniel, et al.
© 1990 by Raven Press, Ltd. All rights reserved.

CHAPTER 14

Gait Analysis

Edmund Biden, John O'Connor, and J. J. Collins

Walking is perhaps the most fundamental of all human movements. It is learned when one is an infant and taken for granted by the time one is 2 or 3 years old. The complexity of the control mechanisms and biomechanics underlying human gait is often not appreciated until one's walking is disrupted by injury, pathology, or fatigue.

According to legend, modern gait analysis originated with a bet on a horse (34). In the 1870s, Leland Stanford, former governor of the state of California, became involved in an argument with Frederick Mac-Crellish over the placement of the feet of a trotting horse. Stanford put $25,000 behind his belief that at times during the trot, the horse had all of its feet off the ground. To settle the wager, a local photographer, Eadweard Muybridge, was asked to photograph the different phases of the gait of a horse. Though this tale may be apocryphal, Stanford eventually commissioned Muybridge to photograph the movement of other animals, including humans, engaged in various activities. Later in his career, Muybridge applied his novel photographic technique to clinical assessment: He collaborated with Dr. Francis Dercum of the University of Pennsylvania Medical School to study the abnormal movements of patients suffering from various disorders.

Until the recent advent of electronic equipment that links computers with video cameras, gait analysis was used mainly to analyze patients with relatively static disorders, such as cerebral palsy and stroke. With the development of improved and cost-effective equipment, gait analysis has emerged as a valuable tool for clinicians and is seeing increasing use in many areas. Quantitative measurement of walking, running, and other activities gives the clinician the opportunity to analyze and document the changes and compensations in gait patterns due to the progress of pathological conditions and to evaluate the effects of surgical procedures and rehabilitative techniques.

In this chapter we will discuss the use of gait analysis to study knee function. We will describe the fundamental aspects of walking, present an overview of the methods of experimental measurement, and discuss the relatively small number of studies that have utilized gait analysis to examine dynamic compensatory responses and alterations secondary to ligament disruption. This chapter will conclude with a section describing the use of a two-dimensional mathematical model of the knee to calculate the values of muscle,

E. Biden: Department of Mechanical Engineering, University of New Brunswick, Fredericton, New Brunswick, Canada E3B 5A3.
J. O'Connor: Department of Engineering Science, University of Oxford, Oxford OX1 3PJ, England.
J. J. Collins: Orthopaedic Engineering Centre, University of Oxford, Oxford OX3 7DL, England.

ligament, and tibiofemoral contact forces developed at the knee during walking.

FUNDAMENTAL ASPECTS OF HUMAN WALKING

Human walking can be represented as a symmetrical, cyclic pattern of movements. With the assumption that successive cycles are very similar, a single cycle is usually taken as representative of the locomotion pattern.

Figure 14-1 contains sketches (31) of an individual going through one gait cycle. The walking cycle for each leg is made up of two phases—stance and swing. Stance phase, which begins when the foot strikes the ground, applies to the period when any part of the foot is in contact with the walking surface. Swing phase, which begins with toeing-off of the foot, involves the period when the foot is not in contact with the floor. By convention, one gait cycle spans the interval from the onset of stance phase until the onset of the next stance period (i.e., footstrike to consecutive footstrike). The word "footstrike" is used instead of "heelstrike" because it is quite possible for the forefoot to be the first part of the foot to contact the floor, as in the case of the slow walking gait of some cerebral palsy patients or the running gait of some individuals.

The stance phase of each foot takes up about 60% of the gait cycle. During the interval just after footstrike and just prior to opposite footstrike, both feet are simultaneously in contact with the walking surface. This period is called "double-stance" or "double-support." During double-stance, the support of the weight of the body is transferred from one foot to the other.

KINEMATICS OF THE GAIT CYCLE

Kinematics is the study of movement. Kinematics does not consider the forces that cause the movement but, instead, is concerned with the details that describe the actual motion. Kinematic measures of gait include stride length, step length, walking speed, cadence and linear and angular displacements. In order to give some sense of the complexity of the coordinated movements of the hip, knee, and ankle during walking, we shall describe the changes in the respective sagittal plane joint angles over one gait cycle (Figs. 14-1 and 14-2).

Sagittal Plane Joint Angles

Throughout the gait cycle, the pelvis is tilted slightly anteriorly. At footstrike, the hip is flexed to about 40°, the knee is flexed to about 10°, and the ankle is near the anatomical neutral. In a normal pattern where the

NORMAL WALK CYCLE

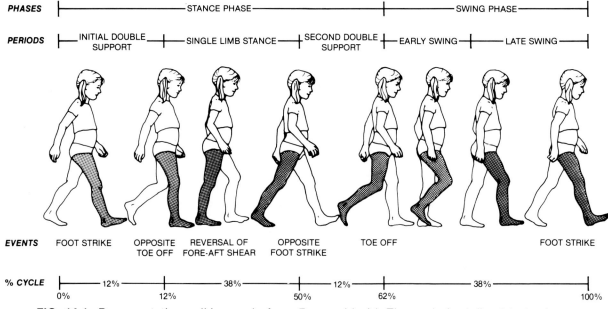

FIG. 14-1. Representative walking cycle for a 7-year-old girl. The cycle is defined to be from footstrike through opposite footstrike until footstrike again on the same side. The basic divisions are (a) stance phase when the foot being considered is in contact with the floor and (b) swing phase when the foot is off the floor and moving forward, preparing for the next step. (From ref. 31.)

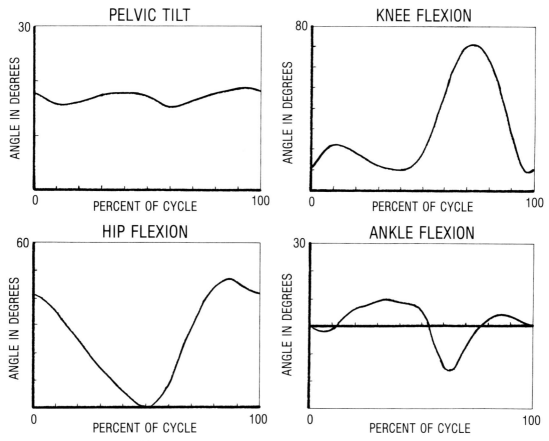

FIG. 14-2. Typical sagittal angles for walking gait.

heel is the first part of the foot to make contact with the ground, the ankle immediately begins to move into plantarflexion, the knee flexes, and the hip begins to extend. This ankle plantarflexion brings the bottom of the foot into overall contact with the floor to provide a stable base. The combined motions of the three joints serve to keep the trunk moving forward in a smooth and controlled way.

After footstrike, the subject is in double limb support. As one leg is beginning to support the weight of the body, the other leg is unloading, in preparation to swinging ahead for the next step. Once the support of weight has been transferred, the opposite limb leaves the floor (opposite toe-off) and begins to swing ahead. At opposite toe-off, the loaded knee and hip are flexed and the ankle is returning to neutral from its plantarflexed position. As the opposite leg is swung ahead, the body continues to move forward over the loaded foot. At mid-stance, the loaded hip is still flexed, the knee is extended, and the ankle is in dorsiflexion. This has the effect of lifting the body so that the swinging leg has sufficient ground clearance. The knee begins to flex at about 45% of the cycle, but the hip does not begin to flex until after opposite footstrike. Between opposite footstrike and toe-off, weight is transferred

to the opposite leg. As the subject comes to the end of stance, the ankle goes progressively into more plantarflexion as the tibia moves ahead and the heel begins to rise. At toe-off, the hip is flexed about 20°, the knee is flexed nearly 40°, and the ankle is plantarflexed. After toe-off, the knee continues to flex and the ankle to dorsiflex in order to shorten the leg. Knee flexion peaks at about 70° in mid-swing and then declines; the hip continues to flex throughout late stance in preparation for the next step.

Looking at the pelvic orientation, it is clear that it changes little during normal level walking. Hip flexion is more or less a sinusoidal function, whereas knee and ankle flexion include higher harmonics. It is generally the case that motions get simpler as one moves proximally (22), and a deviation from this pattern is likely pathological.

Running Versus Walking

Most sports activities are more complicated than walking. One of the most basic athletic activities is jogging or running. The fundamental difference between walking and running is that running involves some time dur-

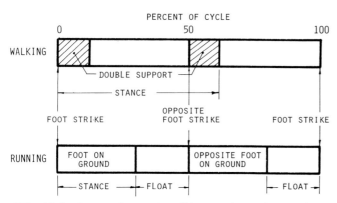

PERCENT OF CYCLE

FIG. 14-3. Comparison of walking and running cycles. The major difference between walking and running is that in walking a person is always in contact with the ground, whereas in running there are times when a person "floats" with neither foot in contact. Also, during running there is no "double support" period with both feet in contact.

ing each cycle when the runner is not in contact with the ground. Figure 14-3 shows the phases of running gait. Whereas in walking the stance phase averages about 60% of the cycle and swing about 40%, in running the phase porportions are reversed. At a jogging pace of 8 min/mile, stance phase is reported by Mann (17) to be about 35% of the cycle. This decreases further as one shifts into a run or a sprint. After footstrike, the foot is on the ground and the opposite leg is in the midst of swinging forward for the next step. When toe-off occurs, the opposite leg is still in swing and the runner loses contact with the ground. This period is often referred to as the "float phase." Opposite foot-strike occurs at about 50% of the cycle. (It is worth remembering that for symmetrical gait, be it walking or running, the two legs function 180° or 50% out of phase so that opposite footstrike always occurs very near 50% of the cycle.) The opposite foot is then in contact as the limb being considered swings ahead. There is a second float phase just prior to the footstrike which concludes the cycle and begins the next.

The timing of the running cycle is also different from the timing of walking. Running cycle times tend to be shorter; Mann (17) reported that a jogging pace has a period that is about two-thirds the period for walking. The resulting higher cadence in concert with longer strides in running yield much higher speeds than in walking gait.

Joint motions in running are generally similar to those seen in walking gait, but the range of motion is exaggerated. For example, the range of hip flexion in walking is about 40–45° (32). Mann (17) reported a similar range for jogging but found that in running and sprinting, the ranges increased to about 60° and 75°, respectively. Motions at the other lower limb joints are similarly affected.

METHODS OF MEASUREMENT

Motion Analysis Systems

Goniometers Versus Video-Based Systems

Limb segment orientations and joint angles are usually measured with cine-film, by video-based systems, or by goniometry (which measures limb orientations directly). Cine and video techniques allow detailed analysis and permanent records of gait patterns. The majority of systems rely on the attachment of markers to anatomical landmarks on the subject's legs. In the past, the use of cine-film was laborious and time consuming; the spatial coordinates of each marker for each frame of film had to be determined and analyzed by hand. The introduction of video-based systems and the integration of computers and automated digitizing systems has reduced the processing time, making it reasonable to perform kinematic studies on a routine clinical basis.

Goniometers are electrical potentiometers producing an output voltage proportional to angle. The uncertainties of measurement of joint angles are comparable for both goniometer and video systems, with typical errors of ± 3°. There are disadvantages associated with both types of system. Goniometers are heavier and more bulky than reflective markers used for cine-film or video. Goniometers can weigh up to about 10 N (1 kg mass), whereas reflective markers usually have a mass of only a few grams. The attachment of the goniometers may cause subjects to alter their gait. Moreover, goniometers are sensitive to positioning errors and have difficulty in measuring axial rotations. Cine-film and video suffer from similar problems but can compensate by attaching wands to the limb segments to amplify the movements caused by the axial rotation.

Definition and Measurement of Joint Angles

In gait analysis, the most common measure of segment motion is the joint angle—for example, the sagittal plane angles that we have used in the earlier descriptions. The question is: What do we really mean when we say knee flexion or hip flexion? Figure 14-4 shows how knee flexion is usually measured. If the measurement is made from a sagittal view only, then internal or external rotation of the leg as a whole will decrease the apparent knee flexion. If knee flexion is defined as the angle between vectors aligned with the tibial and femoral axes, then the problem of angles changing with rotation disappears, but it is difficult to separate knee flexion from knee abduction/adduction. For example, a knee with a slight flexion deformity might be thought

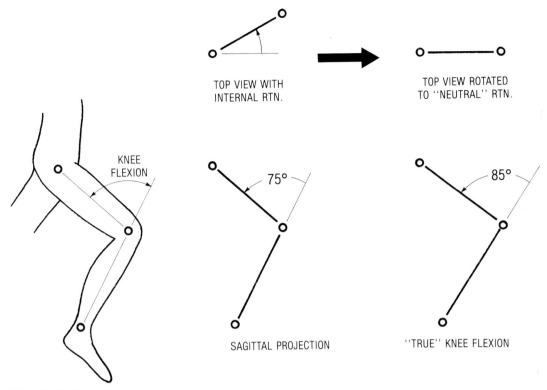

FIG. 14-4. Errors in assessing knee flexion from a strictly sagittal view. A subject observed from the side has apparent flexion of 75° but also is internally rotated. If the effect of internal rotation were removed, the "true" angle of flexion would be measured as 85°. The internal rotation moves the apparent position of the knee closer to a line joining the hip and ankle, thereby reducing the apparent flexion of the observed ankle. RTN, rotation.

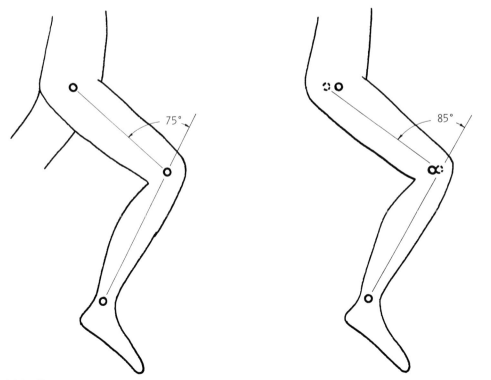

FIG. 14-5. Example of marker malpositioning. In this case, the "hip center" is displaced posteriorly and the "knee center" is displaced anteriorly. As can be seen, this has a significant effect on the measured angle. Poor positioning of goniometers can lead to similar problems.

to be in varus when the leg is externally rotated. If the measurement is based on markers attached to the body or is from a goniometer attached to the limb, then the location of the markers or the orientation of the goniometer influences the absolute value of the angles measured. Figure 14-5 shows the effect of misplacing the markers or misorienting the goniometer. Great care must be taken in the approach to this problem. If one simply has the patient stand in the anatomically neutral position, then one will miss any tendency for the knee to be either hyperextended or slightly flexed in neutral. It is often useful to consider the pattern of motion independent of the absolute values—that is, to observe the changes in the joint angle rather than the actual angles. This removes the effects of marker malpositioning at the expense of not knowing the absolute angles. Figure 14-6 shows an example of this technique.

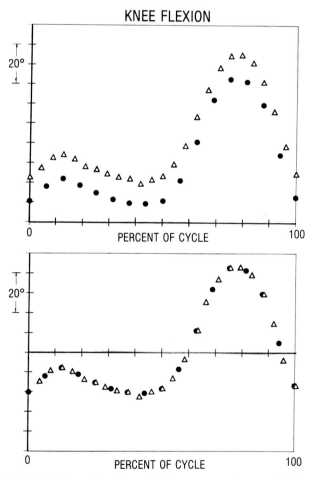

FIG. 14-6. Top: Two knee flexion curves that are similar in "shape" but have different numbers of data points and different minimum and maximum values. **Bottom:** The same data but with the average value subtracted from each data point. The curves now appear even more similar. This method allows more direct comparison of the "pattern" of the curve.

Sampling Rates

The rate at which kinematic data are sampled is an important variable in gait investigations. Yang (39) reported that the natural cadence for an adult population has a mean of about 120 steps/min. Thus, a typical adult completes one walking cycle in about a second. The minimum number of data points needed to describe a walking cycle is between 16 and 20 (6,31). Therefore, one of the following is required: (a) a frame rate for cine or video of about 25 frames/sec or (b) recording goniometric measurements with a bandwidth of at least 10 cycles/sec. Usually there is some noise or error associated with the data collection process. In order to be able to average out some of the noise, one needs more than the minimum number of data points. Typical television cameras operate at either 30 frames/sec (Canada and the United States) or 25 frames/sec (Europe and most of the rest of the world), making them useful in analyzing walking (13,35). Although this is adequate for analytical measures, a rate nearer 50 frames/sec is commonly used to allow for smooth slow-motion observation. Analysis of running, cutting, and other sports activities requires higher sampling rates, on the order of 200–500 frames/sec.

Site-to-Site Variability

Different measurement systems are likely to lead to somewhat incompatible results, making comparison of data from different research centers difficult. Biden (3) described tests to compare the gait of a number of normal subjects walking in four different laboratories. The labs chosen all used video-based gait systems but were different in the data collection hardware, the positioning of markers on the subjects, and the algorithms used to reconstruct angles from the point position data. Biden's findings were that for angles which are unambiguous, such as hip, knee, and ankle flexion; the pattern of motion was the same for all laboratories. Even then, the absolute values of the angles were variable, and a subject could apparently have the knee (a) in extension at mid-stance in one center and (b) in 10 degrees of flexion at the same point in the cycle when measured in another lab. For angles in the frontal and transverse planes, the agreement between sites was poor (Fig. 14-7), reflecting the difficulty in accounting for axial rotation. This illustrates the need to follow a well-recognized protocol or to do the tests to establish "normal" for the measurement system being used.

Normal Database

If the clinician is to compare normal and abnormal gait quantitatively and qualitatively, he or she needs either

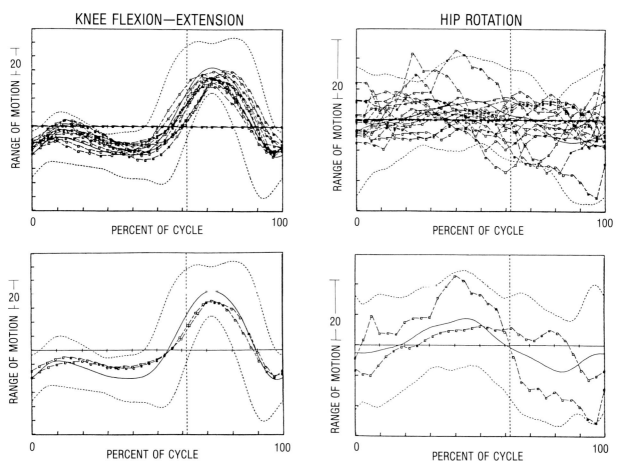

FIG. 14-7. Top: Knee flexion and hip rotation (transverse of plane) for eight subjects studied in various combinations of four different gait labs. **Bottom:** Data for one subject in two different labs. Note that mean values have been removed from each curve, as illustrated in Fig. 14-6. Knee flexion is quite consistent across subjects and laboratories, but hip rotation is almost chaotic.

to establish a database describing normal walking or to duplicate the measurement system used by someone who has already established "normal" for the desired motion. It is possible to determine means values and to make estimates of the variability in the population as a whole if one considers data for normal subjects using consistent data collection and analysis techniques. Evaluation of the range of data for a continuous variable, such as knee flexion, is a complex process. It is often the case than an individual's data will be near the mean at one point during the gait cycle and well away from the mean at another. Statistical techniques can be used to create boundaries that account for these variations (22,32,33). The width of the boundary needed to define "normal" is surprisingly wide (Fig. 14-8). These data represent normal, mature gait; the scatter is well defined by the bands. In this case, the bands are positioned 3.2 standard deviations away from the mean. Data are often presented in the form of the mean ± 1 standard deviation. Even for a normal

distribution, the mean ± 1 standard deviation encloses only 68% of the data. Such a boundary will misclassify about one in three measures in the best of situations and, in this case, would classify only one in three subjects as normal.

Symmetry and Coordination of Gait

Smooth gait, whether for running or walking, requires a high degree of coordination. Nearly everyone has had the experience of tripping over a bump on a sidewalk which was barely high enough to see. The usual ground clearance of the swinging leg in gait is on the order of 1 or 2 cm. The maintenance of such control requires a high degree of coordination in the motions of the joints. Thus, despite the fact that there are considerable differences in hip, knee and ankle angles from person to person, the movements of the lower limb in normal walking or running gait are controlled

KNEE FLEXION—EXTENSION

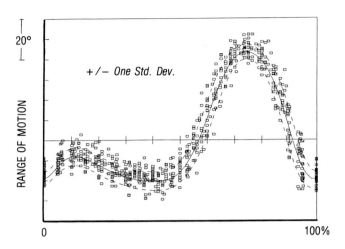

+/− One Std. Dev.

RANGE OF MOTION

20°

0   100%

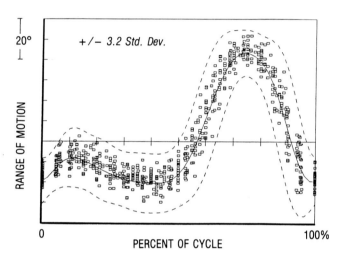

+/− 3.2 Std. Dev.

RANGE OF MOTION

20°

0   PERCENT OF CYCLE   100%

FIG. 14-8. The data points plotted on both curves are for a group of normal children. The solid line through the middle of the data points are, in each case, the mean for the data. **Top:** Dashed lines are drawn at ±1 standard deviation from the curve. Clearly, only a few subjects' data would be completely enclosed. **Bottom:** Curves are drawn at ±3.2 standard deviations as suggested by "bootstrap" processing. This level should enclose about 95° of subjects' data completely. In this case it somewhat overestimates the width of the boundary, since all subjects' data are enclosed fully. (Data were supplied by the Motion Analysis Lab, Children's Hospital, San Diego, and were collected under NIH Grant HD08520.)

for minimal ground clearance, symmetrical steps, and so forth. The key to looking at movement data to assess function is to observe this coordination and symmetry.

As we saw in Fig. 14-8, the range of normal is considerable and may mask many gait deviations. Figure 14-9 shows the measures of change in what we call "effective leg length" and "leg angle." When compared to knee flexion, the measure of leg angle, which reflects movements of the pelvis, hip, knee, and ankle,

is much more tightly bounded. Similarly, it can be seen that the distance from the hip to the fifth metatarsal (effective leg length) is closely controlled by subjects as they walk—the only area of large variation occurs around the time of toe-off (60–65% into the walking cycle).

Figure 14-10 shows the pattern of transverse plane knee rotation, measured in this case as the difference between the orientation of the tibia and the orientation of a plane defined by the hip, knee, and ankle. The average difference from side to side for this measure when comparing left and right gait cycles can be over 10°. This being the case, minor differences in this variable for a single individual are likely to fall well within the normal range. Thus, it is important to look for patterns as well as absolute values in order to detect abnormality. For example, a combination of knee flexion differences, knee rotation differences, and differences in actions at the ankle is much more likely to reflect some disorder than is a single gait measure.

Time–Distance Parameters

Measures of time–distance parameters offer yet another way to analyze gait. In the face of an injury or unstable limb, the usual response is to slow down and to favor the affected side. Measures of walking speed, cycle time, cadence, and step or stride length can be used to detect the slowing process. Measures of the relative percentage of single stance for each side and the timing of toe-off and opposite footstrike can be used to determine the degree of gait symmetry for the subject. For example, normal individuals are very symmetrical in measures such as the timing of opposite footstrike despite the variation from side to side in joint angles. Sutherland (32) reported that by the age of 7 years, the range of values for the timing of opposite footstrike expressed as a percent of the gait cycle is only about ±2% around the 50% mark expected for a perfectly symmetrical cycle. Thus, assessment of symmetry is one of the most powerful techniques in gait analysis.

Force Platforms

Ground Reaction Forces

The study of forces involved in human walking is known as *kinetics*. Force platforms can be used to define the magnitude and direction of the resultant ground reaction force (GRF) applied by the ground to the foot. The measured GRF is the superposition of two components: (i) the support of the weight of the body and (ii) the forces required for the horizontal, vertical, and lateral accelerations of the body. Thus,

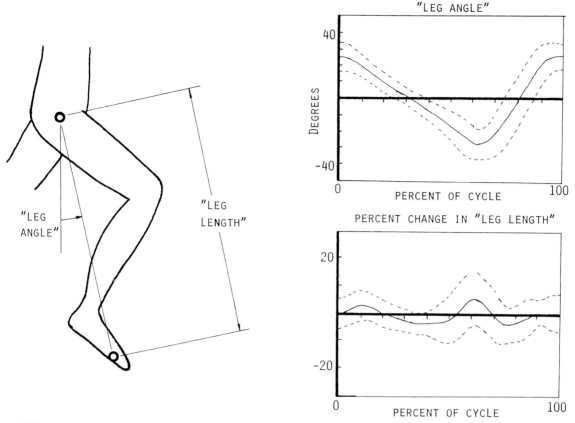

FIG. 14-9. "Effective leg length" and "leg angle." The way these are defined is shown at left, and data with 95% boundaries are shown on the right. These measures, which combine motions of the hip, knee, and ankle, have very narrow bands around them. They are narrower, in fact, than the corresponding bands for hip, knee, or ankle flexion. This suggests that normal individuals coordinate the movements of all joints functioning together rather than trying to control each joint individually.

the force platform acts as a weighing machine and as a whole-body accelerometer. By convention in gait analysis, many investigators describe the forces applied by the foot to the ground. However, from the standpoint of joint mechanics, where one is interested in the response of joint structures (such as muscles and ligaments) to external loads, it is more appropriate to refer to the forces applied by the ground to the foot.

Force platforms can resolve the GRF into three mutually perpendicular directions (Fig. 14-11): vertical, mediolateral, and anteroposterior. These latter two are called *shear forces* because they are applied parallel to the ground and require friction. Walking on ice is difficult because of the lack of friction.

If the GRF reflected only the support of weight (neglecting the dynamic effects of the body), the plot of the vertical force would resemble that of Fig. 14-12A During early stance, the vertical force would rise smoothly to a value equal to body weight; it would remain at a constant value of body weight throughout mid-stance, and then decline at the end of stance as the support of weight is transferred. Typical patterns

of the forces seen in normal gait differ from the static ideal and are shown in Fig. 14-12B.

As the foot contacts the floor, there is often a foot-strike transient produced by the impact between the foot and the floor. Following this brief spike, the vertical force rises steadily as the support of weight is transferred from one limb to another. The first peak of vertical force usually occurs at the same time the opposite leg is about to toe-off. As the trunk shifts forward over the foot, the center of mass is moving upward. As the person goes through mid-stance, the load on the planted limb falls to below body weight. As the trunk continues forward, the vertical force rises again to a second peak above body weight, occurring when the opposite foot contacts the floor. Vertical force then declines rapidly as the support of weight is transferred to the opposite limb. Differences between the static ideal (Fig. 14-12A) and the observed vertical component of the GRF (Fig. 14-12B) are attributable mainly to dynamic effects, to provide the external forces necessary to accelerate the center of mass of the body upwards and downwards.

KNEE ROTATION

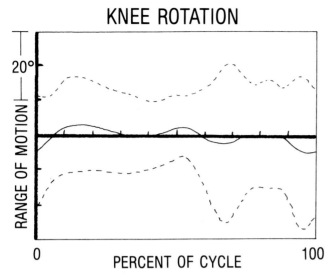

FIG. 14-10. Transverse knee rotation showing the range of normal data. These data have been processed to remove the mean value so that the curves are centered on zero. Absolute knee rotation would show the knee to be normally somewhat externally rotated.

After the initial high-speed events of footstrike, the walker pushes the floor forward and, in reaction, the floor pushes the foot backward. This push backward reaches its maximum at about opposite toe-off and then decreases to zero at mid-stance as the weight of the body moves directly over the loaded foot. Once past mid-stance, the direction of the force changes and the floor pushes the foot forward. Vertical forces peak at about 110% of body weight, whereas maximum fore/aft shear is usually closer to 15% of body weight.

The usual pattern of medial/lateral shear is to have a brief lateral "blip" (ground/foot force) just after footstrike with the subsequent ground/foot force being directed medially. From a purely static point of view, a medially directed component is necessary during single leg stance to ensure that the resultant ground reaction passes through or close to the center of gravity of the body. These forces are quite small, of the order of 5% of body weight. The presence of larger medial or lateral forces is often indicative of some pathological condition that is altering the gait.

Torque, the twisting moment applied by the floor to the subject during walking, has a generally sinusoidal pattern of internal torque until mid-stance, followed by external torque until toe-off. Torque values are quite small, and large values are again often indicative of some alteration to normal gait.

Running Versus Walking

The forces observed in running are somewhat different from those of walking. The vertical force shows no mid-stance valley and is characterized by a single "hill," with its maximum value often in excess of twice that seen in walking. Fore/aft shear has much the same shape as seen in walking, but the magnitudes of the forces are increased.

Center of Pressure

Force platforms measure the resultant force applied by the ground to the foot, but they do not describe how that force is distributed across the base of the foot. The center of pressure, the point about which the distributed forces applied to the foot have zero moment, is found by determining the line of action of the forces measured by the platform and calculating where that

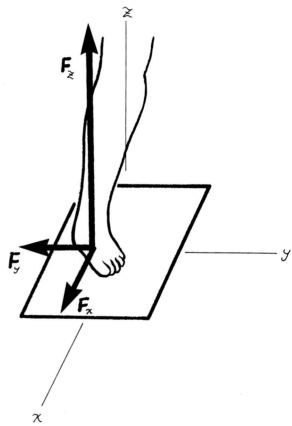

FIG. 14-11. Force plate showing three principal forces. $\mathbf{F}_z$ is the vertical force, $\mathbf{F}_x$ is fore–aft shear, and $\mathbf{F}_y$ is mediolateral shear. Just as a body has 6 degrees of freedom, a load applied has six components: three forces and three moments. Note that the origin of the three forces is in the xy plane (plane of the floor) but that it is not coincident with the origin of our xyz coordinate system. The force $\mathbf{F}_z$ gives a moment about both x and y, and the two forces $\mathbf{F}_x$ and $\mathbf{F}_y$ produce a moment about the z axis. More commonly, the data used for gait studies are the three forces, their location (which defines where the ground reaction force passes through the foot), and the moment about z.

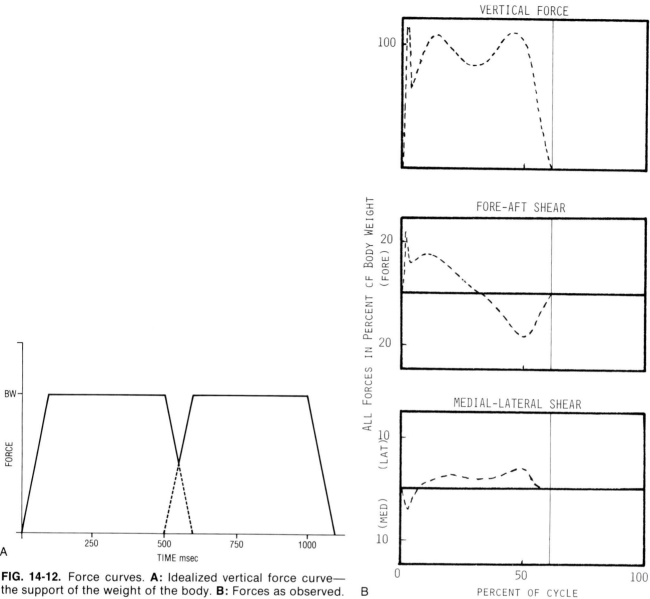

FIG. 14-12. Force curves. **A:** Idealized vertical force curve—the support of the weight of the body. **B:** Forces as observed.

line intersects the surface of the force platform. Normally, there is an initial loading under the heel, followed by a rapid progression forward along a curving track that is somewhat lateral to the midline of the foot. During the last portions of stance, the line of action of the resultant force is applied through the forefoot. In normal gait, this smooth progression from heel to forefoot is clearly evident on center-of-pressure plots.

Sampling Rates

Kinetic measurements require relatively high sampling rates, often 10 times faster than those used for kinematic analysis. Footstrike transients have durations on the order of 10–20 ms, which is less than the 33 ms

between frames in a standard television setup. A rate of 500 frames/sec (i.e., one frame every 2 msec) would give several data points during the transient, allowing it to be observed reliably, although higher sampling rates are often desirable.

Accuracy of Measurement

Force platform accuracy is usually quoted at a fraction of the full-scale load. If, for example, the maximum load the platform will accept is a vertical force of 2000 N and the error is quoted at ±1%, then the uncertainty of measurement is approximately 20 N. Such errors tend to be small when compared to the maximum values of the large vertical forces observed in gait, but they can be substantial if the sensitivity of the fore/aft shear or medial/lateral shear measurements is not adjusted to take account of their lower magnitudes. For example, if the uncertainty is 20 N for all channels and the maximum fore/aft shear is 150 N, then the uncertainty is over 13% for that measure. Because medial/lateral and fore/aft forces have such large lever-arms along the lower limbs, such errors can have very significant effects on calculations of resultant moments at the joints.

Site-to-Site Variability

Force platforms, because they do not rely on the placement of markers as do motion measurements, are generally reproducible from site to site. The principal force platform technologies use either piezoelectric or strain gauge force transducers. From a practical standpoint, there is little difference between the two when applied to gait analysis.

Clinical Assessment

Force data have been shown to be indicative of pathologies and injuries, including ligament problems. As mentioned earlier, slowing down is a common response to conditions that affect gait. Force patterns are sensitive to walking speed; the faster one walks, the more exaggerated are the peaks and valleys of the curves. Similarly, conditions that slow gait will tend to smooth out these changes. It is also observed that the rate at which the limb is loaded (measured from the slope of the force–time plots) is often lower in subjects with unstable limbs. Thus, a combination of lower loading rates and relatively flat force curves probably indicates some pathology. Tibone (36), in his study of anterior cruciate ligament (ACL)-deficient subjects during walking, running, cutting, and stair climbing, found that the peaks and valleys in the force measures were altered relative to normals. He also noted that some of the differences disappeared in later trials when the subjects were asked to repeat a maneuver several times. Although the subjects were not a particularly homogeneous group, his findings suggest that there are differences in ligament-deficient patients but that, with practice and familiarity, a patient may be able to compensate for the ligament deficiency.

Electromyography

ON/OFF Patterns

Walking is the direct result of the actions of different muscles across the joints of the lower limbs. Electro-

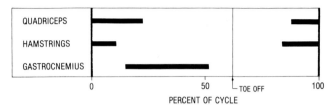

FIG. 14-13. EMG patterns for three muscle groups as reported by Sutherland (32).

myography (EMG), the process of recording the electrical signals associated with muscle activity, is a useful investigative technique in gait analysis. There are many difficulties in correlating the EMG signal amplitude with muscle force magnitude (24,30). Both linear and nonlinear relationships between the force level in skeletal muscle and the EMG signal have been reported. Consequently, EMG is most commonly used in clinical practice and gait analysis to determine phasic patterns for individual muscles or muscle groups. One can examine simple ON/OFF patterns (32,36), or one can process the EMG to find an envelope that encloses the signal and then examine EMG patterns as defined by the shape of the envelope over the gait cycle (14,28). In the latter process, it is common to normalize the signal as a percentage of voluntary maximum muscle contraction. The process of detecting when a muscle is turned ON or OFF is usually one of testing whether the average level of the singal is above some set limit. This can be done by recording the EMG signal on a chart recorder and visually identifying the ON and OFF times. For facilities with access to more sophisticated data acquisition and processing systems, the determination of ON/OFF times is often done by calculating the shape of the EMG envelope and then testing for occasions when the envelope exceeds some threshold value. EMG ON/OFF times are generally more variable from step to step than either kinematic or kinetic gait measurements. Our experience is that variation from the average ON or OFF time is approximately ±3% of the gait cycle. Typical EMG patterns for quadriceps, hamstrings, and gastrocnemius activity during gait as reported by Sutherland (32) are shown in Fig. 14-13.

Surface Electrodes Versus Needle Electrodes

The two main types of electrodes used in EMG studies are surface electrodes and intramuscular needle electrodes. Surface electrodes usually consist of pairs of metal pads. These are attached to the skin over the muscle to be studied. In many cases, the pads are built into a holder which ensures consistent spacing between pads and which frequently contains an amplifier to increase the signal strength. Needle electrodes are made of pairs of fine wire (usually 0.002-mm-diameter stainless steel). The wires are insulated except for the tips, which are bared and bent into a hook (2). Needle electrodes are loaded into the barrel of a fine-gauge hypodermic needle that is inserted into the muscle to be studied. When the needle is withdrawn, the electrodes remain hooked in the muscle tissue. The free ends of the fine wires are then connected to the EMG recording devices.

Each type of electrode has its advantages and disadvantages. Surface electrodes are convenient, easy to apply to the skin, and cause little (if any) pain, irritation, or discomfort to the subject. They pick up signals from active muscles in the general area of application. This feature makes surface electrodes the ideal choice for analysis of global activity in superficial muscles or muscle groups. On the other hand, surface electrodes are sensitive to movement of the skin under the electrodes and have poor specificity. They are influenced by significant muscle crosstalk, where the electrical signals of one muscle interfere with the signals from another. Thus, the activity of neighboring muscles (adjacent or deeper) can falsify results.

The major advantage of needle electrodes is selectivity. Needle electrodes can be used to measure the activity of specific deeper muscles in isolation. The influence of the electrical activity of nearby muscles is greatly reduced. Nonetheless, there are a number of disadvantages to needle electrodes. Pain on insertion, the difficulty of accurate placement, and wire movement with muscle contraction are some of the associated drawbacks. Because they are to be inserted in the subject's body, needle electrodes must be sterile and sufficiently strong to resist breakage.

Sampling Rates

Recorded EMG signals can span frequencies from 50 to 3000 cycles/sec (15). If these signals are to be recorded accurately, very high sampling rates (considerably higher than those used in kinematic and kinetic gait measurements) must be employed.

Clinical Assessment

Evaluation of EMG ON/OFF data is usually restricted to determination of whether or not the phasic pattern is altered significantly from normal. It has been observed that faster movement produces more consistent patterns of muscle activity (20,27). Thus, muscles tend to be active more during running than during walking. It is our observation that if a joint is unstable, the patient will use more muscle activity than normal. Consistent with these general observations, Tibone (36) studied EMG in 18 subjects with unilateral ACL de-

ficiency and found that during running, the vastus medialis obliquus of the ACL-deficient leg had earlier onset of activity and that the medial hamstrings of the same leg fired longer than the respective muscles on the sound side. Limbird (14), in a similar study of 12 unilateral ACL-deficient subjects, reported significant EMG pattern differences between normal and ACL-deficient subject populations. For example, at foot-strike, the ACL-deficient subjects demonstrated less quadriceps and gastrocnemius and more biceps femoris activity than the normal subjects. These findings are consistent with our observations (Chapter 11) that hamstrings action can compensate for ACL action.

Summary of Gait Analysis

Gait analysis can provide measures of the motions, GRFs, and EMG activity during walking and other activities. In its simplest form, as a collection of video or film images, it enables direct visual comparison of the patient at different times during treatment. Although measurement limitations exist, the degree of refinement in gait measures is such that it is becoming practical to incorporate gait results into patient assessment. While kinematic and kinetic measures are valuable in isolation, the most useful information related to these measures can be derived when the relationship between the position of the joint and the external forces is incorporated into the joint force calculations. In the following section, such an analysis for the sagittal plane is developed.

KNEE LIGAMENT FORCES DURING WALKING

Literature Review

Although there have been numerous studies of the forces transmitted by the human knee during gait, very few of them have attempted to analyze ligament forces. The reason is simple. The problems of analysis are difficult.

If we attempt to simplify the problem by considering only the resultant tensile forces transmitted by the patellar tendon, by the medial and lateral heads of hamstrings and gastrocnemius, by the iliotibial tract, by the two cruciate and the two collateral ligaments and the resultant compressive forces transmitted by the medial and lateral compartments of the knee, we are concerned with the values of 12 separate forces. However, it is clear from EMG that not all the muscles are active all the time during gait. The flexors are often quiet when the extensors are active, and vice versa; the hamstrings are quiet when the gastrocnemii are active, and vice versa. It would seem reasonable to suppose, similarly, that not all the ligaments are loaded all the time. What governs the choice of loaded structures?

Mechanical analysis can help only up to a point. If we consider the three-dimensional mechanics of the lower leg, from the joint cleft of the knee down to the ground, we have available only six equations of mechanics from which to determine the knee forces required to accelerate the lower limb and balance the applied external loads. There are then 924 combinations of six forces out of a possible 12 which could satisfy those equations. As we shall see, the number of combinations is much reduced by applying the simple criterion that muscle and ligament forces must be tensile and that intraarticular contact forces must be compressive.

Many authors (9,38) circumvent these difficulties by calculating only the resultant force and moment transmitted at the knee, without attempting to determine the values of the forces transmitted by the individual structures. By using linked segment models with the flexion axis of the knee fixed in relation to the bones and thus not allowing for the rolling movement of the femur on the tibia, errors not only in the magnitude but even in the sign (flexing or extending) of the moment at the knee can be made.

The problem of evaluating the forces transmitted by the structures of the knee can be much simplified by ignoring the ligaments and their control of the movements of the bones upon each other, applying the full sophistication of gait analysis to a rather primitive model of the joint. This still leaves the intriguing question of the criteria used during walking in selecting which muscles should fire at any instant. MacConaill (16) had postulated the Principle of Minimum Total Muscular Force, which stated that "no more total muscular force is used than is both necessary or sufficient for the task to be performed" (16). Rohrle (25), without reference to MacConaill, analyzed a model of the leg in which the hip allowed rotation about each of three axes, the knee about one fixed axis, and the ankle about two. He considered 42 muscles and found the combination of six active and 36 passive ones which minimized the sum of the muscle forces at the three joints. Seireg (26) minimized the sum of all muscle forces plus a weighted sum of their moments at the knee. Hardt (10) minimized a linear objective function based on a thermodynamic model of the energy requirements of the muscles. Crowninshield (7), Patriarcho (23), and Calderdale (5) used various inequality constraints that limited muscle stress. These studies, too, considered the flexion axis of the knee to be fixed in relation to the bones.

Implicit account of the functions of the ligaments in transmitting load across the knee can be taken by recording (e.g., by x-ray analysis) the positions of the bones upon each other as they move under the control of the ligaments. The lines of action of the muscle tendons can then be deduced. This was the approach of Smidt (29), giving a more accurate view of the lever-arms of the muscle tendons about the moving instant center of the joint and their variation with knee flexion. Bishop (4) also performed a mechanical analysis based upon x-ray analysis of position. Ligament forces were not calculated explicitly in either study, merely the component of force parallel to the tibial plateau. Draganich (8) used pressure-sensitive film to detect the center of pressure of each femoral condyle on the tibial plateau at various positions of flexion; with this information and x-ray pictures, he deduced the changing lever-arm available to the quadriceps mechanism with respect to the tibial center of pressure. Mikosz (18) used this model in gait analysis, but he assumed that the directions of the flexor muscles were fixed in relation to the tibia and did not attempt to evaluate ligament forces explicitly.

The only gait analysis known to us which takes explicit account of knee ligament function is that of Morrison (19). He assumed that the joint flexes and extends about an axis fixed in the bones. He could then calculate the directions of the ligaments and muscle tendons at a series of instants in the gait cycle from a knowledge of their flexion angles and their points of insertion into the bones. He calculated the resultant force and moment at the knee from measured force plate and kinematic data. From EMG, he chose the principal muscle group active at each instant, but he did not attempt to account for antagonistic muscle action. His analysis of forces was three-dimensional and dynamic, albeit based on two-dimensional knee motion, leading to calculations of the forces in all the ligaments of the knee at each instant of the gait cycle. We shall discuss his results below in the context of our own. Harrington (11) used Morrison's methods, with some simplification, to compare the gait of normal and pathological subjects. Nissan (21) suggested that the assumption of a fixed axis of flexion could lead to substantial errors in the calculated values of the forces.

In summary, there is not available in the literature an analysis of knee ligament forces in gait which takes account of the movements of the flexion axis relative to the bones and which, in that context, considers the possibility of antagonistic or agonistic muscle action. Part of our current research is aimed at filling this void, and we will now give a preliminary report.

In this section, the two-dimensional mathematical model of the knee presented in Chapters 10 and 11 will be used to calculate the values of muscle, ligament, and tibiofemoral contact forces developed at the knee during normal level walking. By considering the two-dimensional problem, we need deal only with the 20 possible sets of joint forces described in Chapter 11 (Table 11-1) rather than the 924 mechanically possible solutions discussed above. We can nonetheless gain some understanding of possible muscle–ligament interactions in walking without having to confront their full complexities.

Analysis of Forces at the Knee

Calculations are presented for a single representative subject studied in the gait laboratory of the Oxford Orthopaedic Engineering Centre. A description of the Vicon gait analysis system and Kistler force plate, similar in all respects to equipment described above, was given by Whittle (37). A further nine normal subjects (four female and five male) were studied, and variations from the behavior of the representative subject will be discussed. The parameters of the knee and lower leg model used were the average parameters of the model listed in the Appendix to Chapter 10.

We considered the equilibrium of the lower leg (from the joint cleft of the knee down to the ground) when loaded by the foot/ground reaction and its own weight. From gait analysis, the position of the lower leg in space was known at each of the data sampling points. Data from the force platform defined the magnitude and direction of the resultant force applied by the ground to the foot and its relation in space to the lower leg. Lower leg weights were determined for each subject from Winter's data (38), according to height and body weight. The accelerations of the lower leg were not measured in this preliminary study. Since the measured GRF involves inertial as well as gravitational effects for the whole body, the errors involved in neglecting the accelerations of the lower leg in stance phase are small. Inertial effects of the lower leg are likely to be more significant in swing phase, although, then, the joint forces themselves are relatively small.

Firstly, calculations were made of the values of the resultant force through the instant center of the knee (at the intersection of the cruciate ligaments) and the associated couple needed to balance the external forces (the ground reaction and lower leg weight). Calculation of the values of muscle, ligament, and contact forces at the knee needed to transmit that resultant force and moment is possible only if the position and direction of the line of action of each of these forces is known. We used the computer model of the knee (Chapter 10) to deduce (a) the lines of action of the quadriceps, hamstrings, and gastrocnemius tendons and the two cruciates and (b) the tibio femoral contact force at each sampling point of the walking cycle, taking account of the movement of the contact point on the tibial plateau.

The values of the 20 possible sets of three joint forces at each sampling point were obtained (Table 11-1). A combination was rejected if any of the forces were neg-ative—a physically impossible condition corresponding to compressive muscle or ligament forces or to a tensile contact force. There remained at least one set of valid solutions at each sampling point.

It will be recalled that the 20 possible solutions involve (a) single muscle solutions with a ligament and a contact force and (b) antagonistic or agonistic muscle solutions with a contact but no ligament force. These solutions would be expected during stance phase when the knee joint forces are dominated by the ground reaction. The antagonistic or agonistic solutions, with no ligament action, could be thought of as instances where the muscles act to protect the ligaments. When the knee supports the lower leg hanging vertically during swing phase, the distracting solutions of Table 11-1 would be expected to come into play.

In the single muscle solutions, the muscle force is determined solely by the condition that its moment about the instant center of the knee must balance the flexing or extending effect of the external load (ground reaction plus lower leg weight). The ligament force is then determined by the condition that its component parallel to the plateau must balance the vector sum of the corresponding components of muscle force and external load. Finally, the combined upwards pull of the soft tissue forces plus the upward push of the external load determines the value of the tibiofemoral contact force. Since the anterior cruciate ligament (ACL) pulls the tibia backward and the posterior cruciate ligament (PCL) pulls it forward, a single muscle solution is always possible. Agonistic or antagonistic solutions are possible only when the direction of the antagonistic/agonistic force is appropriate to provide force balance parallel to the plateau.

Results

Figure 14-14A shows the pattern of knee flexion angle during the gait cycle for the representative subject, and Fig. 14-14B shows the value of the resultant flexion/extension moment of the loads about the instant center of the knee during the gait cycle for the same subject. Figure 14-15 shows the corresponding EMG data. The temporal patterns of the predicted solutions for that subject and the number of solutions available at each data point are presented in Fig. 14-16. Sample force calculations over one complete gait cycle for the representative subject are shown in Figs. 14-17, 14-18, and 14-19, where we have selected combinations that most closely agree with EMG findings, both published (32) and our own (Fig. 14-15).

During early stance (which corresponds to the first 25% of the walking cycle for our representative subject), the line of action of the external load passed behind the instant center of the knee, tending to flex the

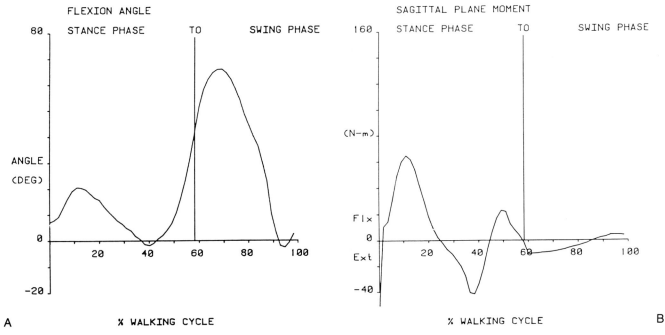

FIG. 14-14. A: Knee flexion angle plotted aginst time during the gait cycle for the representative subject. **B:** Knee flexion/extension moment of the external loads about the instant center of the knee during the gait cycle for the representative subject.

joint, and an extending moment was required (Fig. 14-14). Only one solution, QAC (quadriceps, ACL, and tibiofemoral contact force), was found to be physically realizable (Fig. 14-16). For the bulk of mid-stance, two single muscle solutions, HAC and GAC, were obtained. In this interval, the line of action of the load passed in front of the instant center to produce an extending moment, and flexor action was needed. Throughout most of late stance, only the single muscle solution QAC was obtained. However, for two frames preceding toe-off, the antagonistic solution QHC was also calculated.

Immediately following toe-off, there was no longer a GRF acting on the system. The weight of the lower leg was the only external force acting on the lower limb. The external moment was an extending one (Fig. 14-14B), and, consequently, flexor muscle activity was required. Three solutions were calculated for the initial 60% of the swing phase: two single muscle solutions (HPC and GAC) and one agonistic solution (HGC). Contact forces were involved because the extending effect of lower leg weight dominates the distracting effect. Mid-swing phase was characterized by distracting solutions (i.e., solutions not involving the joint contact force). During late swing, there was only one solution calculated—QAC.

The estimated quadriceps force patterns are in excellent agreement with the EMG patterns, both during stance and during late swing phase. Predicted gastrocnemius activity in mid-stance phase was found

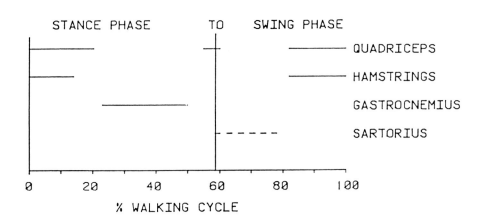

FIG. 14-15. Periods of muscle activity for the representative subject, as indicated by EMG.

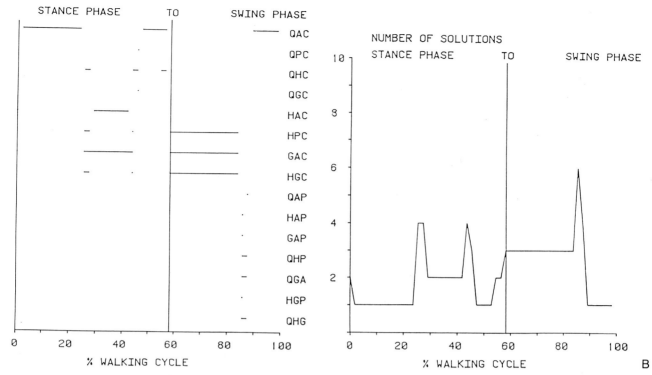

FIG. 14-16. A: Temporal patterns of mechanically possible solutions for the representative subject. Q, quadriceps; H, hamstrings; G, gastrocnemius; A, anterior cruciate ligament; P, posterior cruciate ligament; C, tibiofemoral contact. Thus, QAC is the solution involving forces in the quadriceps and the anterior cruciate with the tibiofemoral contact force. **B:** The number of such solutions calculated at each data point of the gait cycle.

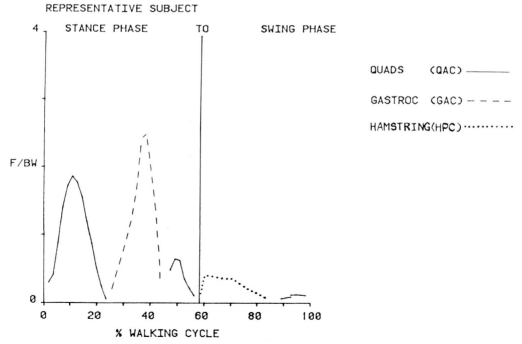

FIG. 14-17. Muscle forces for the EMG-consistent solutions for the representative subject during the gait cycle.

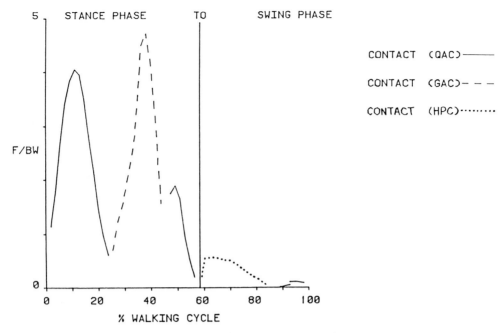

FIG. 14-18. Tibiofemoral contact force.

with EMG, but swing-phase activity was not. The predicted hamstrings solution HPC in early swing matches EMG observation of sartorius activity at this stage. Elsewhere, EMG patterns for the hamstrings activity are not consistent with the force calculations. Firstly, EMG indicated hamstrings activity in late swing and early stance, but such solutions were not found in the force calculations. Secondly, hamstrings EMG activity was not found during mid-stance, although the force calculations show such activity to be geometrically and mechanically possible.

The pattern of possible solutions at different phases of the walking cycle for all 10 subjects are summarized in Table 14-1. There was remarkable unanimity in the

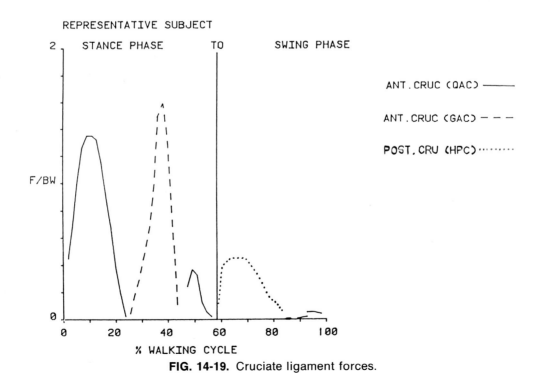

FIG. 14-19. Cruciate ligament forces.

TABLE 14-1. *Subject-to-subject variability: temporal force patterns*

Period of gait cycle	Calculated combination(s)[a]	Number of subjects (10 total)
Early stance	QAC	9
Mid-stance	Flexor muscle activity	8
Late stance	QAC	8
Early swing	HPC, GAC, HGC	10
Mid-swing	Distracting solutions	10
Late swing	QAC	9

[a] Q, quadriceps; A, anterior cruciate ligament; C, tibiofemoral contact; H, hamstrings; P, posterior cruciate ligament; G, gastrocnemius.

patterns for eight of the subjects during stance phase and for nine of them during swing. The tenth walked so as to eliminate the need for flexor activity during stance. In nearly all subjects, the single muscle combination of QAC, involving ACL forces, proved to be the only theoretical possibility in 35–60% of the walking cycle, corresponding to early stance, late stance, and late swing. Of the 20 possible, the maximum number of simultaneous physically realizable solutions for any subject at any instant was six, occurring only for an instant in swing phase. Multiple solutions were found mainly near the instants when the external moment was changing from flexing to extending (or vice versa), when the associated forces would be expected to be small.

Discussion

Numbers of Calculated Solutions

Although 20 possible solutions could arise at each point of the walking cycle, the condition that ligament and muscle forces should be tensile and the contact force compressive ruled out a large majority of them.

When the resultant force transmitted across the joint had a compressive component, the distractive combinations of Table 14-1 were inappropriate, and vice versa. Flexing loads ruled out the single muscle flexor solutions. Similarly, extending loads ruled out the single muscle extensor solutions. Since the ACL pulls the tibia backward and the PCL pulls it forward, one or other can provide a shear force in the appropriate direction so that a single muscle solution involving cruciate ligament force was found at every instant. The same is not true of the muscle forces; near extension, all muscle groups pull the tibia forward and some antagonistic and agonistic solutions were ruled out because the direction of pull was inappropriate. For instance, in mid-stance with the knee nearly straight, the solutions found involved each of the flexors with the

ACL, indicating that a backwards pull on the tibia was required to balance the combined effect of either flexor with the external load. Antagonistic action of either flexor with the quadriceps did not occur because, near extension, the patellar tendon pulls the tibia forward when a backwards pull was required. Agonistic hamstrings/gastrocnemius action was not found because, near extension, both muscles pull the tibia forward and neither can provide the necessary backwards component to counteract the other. Thus, the laws of geometry and mechanics, rather than some more abstruse criterion, determined which muscle combinations were active at most instants.

Muscle Selection Criteria

These studies, taking account of possible ligamentous contribution to load-bearing, appear to rule out many of the criteria previously considered as possible bases for the selection of muscle activity. The preferred gastrocnemius solution in mid-stance involves higher peak total muscle force than the hamstrings solution, suggesting that lowest total muscle force is unlikely to be the criterion. By the same token, since the cross-sectional area of gastrocnemius is smaller than that of hamstrings, a minimum muscle stress criterion is even less likely. The domination of single muscle activity throughout the gait cycle implies that the muscles do not always act to protect the ligaments.

EMG/Theory Discrepancies

The anomalies between EMG and the absence of hamstrings solutions can be attributed to several factors. Firstly, in its present form, the model will always predict separate hamstrings and gastrocnemius single muscle solutions to provide flexor action at the knee joint. Thus, during mid-stance, the model calculates independent hamstrings and gastrocnemius activity (as single muscle solutions), whereas EMG demonstrates only gastrocnemius action. Secondly, these calculations were only applicable to the lower leg, from the knee down to ground level. However, the hamstrings are biarticular in nature, acting as flexors of the knee and extensors of the hip. Thus, hamstrings EMG patterns detected during late swing and early stance could be the result of the hamstrings' role as a hip extensor, assisting gravity in terminating forward swing of the leg. During this time, the knee requires mainly extensor action, provided by quadriceps with an associated requirement for anterior cruciate force. A similar backwards pull on the tibia cannot be provided by hamstrings because the knee flexion angle is too low.

The discrepancy between the calculation and the EMG signal can be overcome by adding to the QAC solution in late swing and early stance an appropriate contribution from the self-equilibrating QHAC solution of Fig. 11-9. The appropriate level of the hamstrings force could be determined by considering the dynamics of the leg as seen from the hip. The addition of this self-equilibrating solution to the forces at the knee would increase the quadriceps, anterior cruciate, and contact forces from the levels shown in Figs. 14-17 to 14-19. Our current research is aimed at evaluating this contribution.

Force Magnitudes

Throughout the stance phase, there are periods when calculated muscle forces are considerably greater than body weight (Fig. 14-17). These calculations reflect the differences in leverage of the external loads and the respective muscles. The lever-arms of the muscle tendons in the knee joint can be much shorter than the lever-arms of the external loads acting along the limb. Thus, large muscle forces acting along small lever-arms are required to be in equilibrium with smaller external loads acting with longer lever-arms. The mechanical disadvantage of the muscles relative to the external loads has consequences for the tibiofemoral contact force (Fig. 14-18). Large contact forces are required to balance the upwards pull of the muscles; that is, the tibiofemoral contact force for our representative subject reaches a peak value of 4.7 times body weight.

The Role of the Ligaments in Force Transmission During Gait

Figure 14-19 shows the calculated cruciate ligament forces required for the representative subject. These results are consistent with the EMG data for that subject, except in late swing and early stance where, as we have explained above, the addition of the hamstrings forces detected by EMG would be expected to increase the ACL forces given by Fig. 14-19. The correspondence between EMG and theoretical predictions of single muscle activity suggests that single muscle activity detected by EMG implies significant ligament participation in load transmission in 65% of the gait cycle in the representative subject. The absence of antagonistic or agonistic solutions for the bulk of the gait cycle implies that, for this subject, compensation for injury to or disruption of the ACL can only be achieved by altering the gait pattern. More flexion would be required at the knee during stance to allow the hamstrings pull the tibia backwards in the manner of an intact ACL.

The results for the 10 subjects tested were similar: The ACL was shown to have a possible role in 65–100% of the cycle (Table 14-1). Moreover, the maximum ACL forces, ranging from 0.7 to 1.7 times body weight, were significantly larger than the maximum PCL forces, ranging from 0.3 to 0.4 times body weight.

It is interesting to compare these calculations with those of Morrison (19) (Fig. 14-8). Both sets of solutions show three waves of ACL activity during stance, but our calculations yielded much higher force values, up to 1.6 times body weight. In two of the three subjects on whom he reported in detail, Morrison found PCL activity during stance, not found in his third subject or in any of our 10 subjects. Both solutions found PCL action during swing, persisting in Morrison's results into early stance. The discrepancy in phasing is not accounted for by the absence from our results of the self-equilibrating effect described above since Morrison did not consider antagonistic action. In our solutions, possible PCL participation was confined mainly to swing phase, where neglect of lower leg accelerations most significantly affect accuracy.

Morrison's three-dimensional analysis could estimate forces in the collateral ligaments. The medial collateral ligament (MCL) was found to be loaded only during swing phase, but significant forces were required in the lateral structures, resisting a lapse into adduction when the line of action of the foot/ground reaction passes medial to the joint in single-leg stance. Although in his calculations these forces were attributed to the lateral collateral ligament (LCL), Morrison points out that the iliotibial tract is likely to participate.

Subject-Specific Parameters

The patterns of muscle and ligament activity suggested by Fig. 14-16 have been found to be quite sensitive to the choice of parameters, not only those of the knee model (Chapter 10, Appendix) but also those describing the leg down to the floor. Figures 14-16 to 14-19 should therefore be regarded as preliminary results that demonstrate the arguments of this section. The variation in the patterns of predicted solutions probably vary from subject to subject, a matter currently under investigation.

CONCLUSIONS AND FURTHER WORK

The results of our analysis emphasize the importance of intact ligaments for proper load transmission during walking, apart from their possible roles in position control and proprioception. Whole-leg models are required to take account of the interaction at the different joints of diarthrodial muscle groups. Subject-specific parameters must be investigated to establish the variation in the role ligaments play during gait. Computer modeling could then be used to study possible variations to the gait pattern which could compensate for injured or ruptured ligaments.

The significant role played by the ligaments in gait could justify the development of surgical procedures to repair or replace injured ligaments in order to restore the normal muscle–ligament interactions that guide knee motion and transmit load.

ACKNOWLEDGMENTS

The work described in the section entitled "Methods of Measurement" was carried out in the Oxford Orthopaedic Engineering Centre with the help and encouragement of Dr. M. W. Whittle and Dr. R. J. Jefferson.

REFERENCES

1. Adelaar RS. The practical biomechanics of running. *Am J Sports Med* 1986;14(6):497–500.
2. Basmajian JV, DeLuca C. *Muscles alive*, 5th edition. Baltimore: Williams & Wilkins, 1985.
3. Biden E, Olshen R, Simon S, Sutherland D, Gage J, Kadaba M. Comparison of gait data from multiple labs. *Trans 33rd Mtg Orthop Res Soc.* 1987;504.
4. Bishop RED. On the mechanics of the human knee. *Eng Med* 1977;6:48–52.
5. Calderdale PM, Scelfo G. A mathematical model of the locomotor apparatus. *Eng Med* 1987;16:141–161.
6. Capozzo A, Leo T, Pedotti A. A general computing method for the analysis of human locomotion. *J Biomech* 1975;8:307–320.
7. Crowninshield RD, Brand RA. A physiologically based criterion of muscle force prediction in locomotion. *J Biomech* 1981;14:793–801.
8. Draganich LF, Andriacchi TP, Andersson GBJ. Interaction between intrinsic knee mechanics and the knee extensor mechanism. *J Orthop Res* 1987;5:539–547.
9. Gilbert JA, Maxwell GM, McElhaney JH, Clippinger FW. A system to measure the forces and moments at the knee and hip during level walking. *J Orthop Res* 1984;2:281–288.
10. Hardt DE. Determining muscle forces in the leg during normal human walking—an application and evaluation of optimisation methods. *J Biomech Eng* 1978;100:72–78.
11. Harrington IJ. A bioengineering analysis of force actions at the knee in normal and pathological gait. *Biomed Eng* 1976; May:167–172.
12. Inman VT, Ralston HJ, Todd F. *Human walking*. Baltimore: Williams & Wilkins, 1981.
13. Jarrett MO. A television/computer system for human locomotion analysis. Ph.D. thesis, University of Strathclyde, Glasgow, 1976.
14. Limbird TJ, Shiavi R, Fracer M, Borra H. EMG profiles of knee joint musculature during walking: changes induced by anterior cruciate ligament deficiency. *J Orthop Res* 1988;6:630–638.
15. Loeb GE, Gans C. *Electromyography for experimentalists*. Chicago: University of Chicago Press, 1986.
16. MacConaill MA. The ergonomic aspects of articular mechanics. In: Evans FG, ed. *Studies on the anatomy and function of bones and joints*. Berlin: Springer-Verlag, 1967;69–80.
17. Mann RA, Moran GT, Dougherty SE. Comparative electromyography of the lower extremity in jogging, running and sprinting. *Am J Sports Med* 1986;14(6):501–510.
18. Mikosz RP, Andriacchi TP, Andersson GBJ. Model analysis of factors influencing the prediction of muscle forces at the knee. *J Orthop Res* 1988;6:205–214.
19. Morrison JB. The mechanics of the knee joint in relation to normal walking. *J Biomech* 1970;3:51–61.
20. Murray M, Mollinger L, Gardner G, Sipic S. Kinematic and EMG patterns during slow, free and fast walking. *J Orthop Res* 1984;2:272–280.
21. Nissan M. Review of some basic assumptions in knee biomechanics. *J Biomech* 1979;14:513–525.
22. Olshen R, Biden E, Wyatt M, Sutherland D. Gait analysis and the bootstrap. *Ann Stat* 1989;17:4, 1419–1441.
23. Patriarco AG, Mann RW, Simon SR, Mansour JM. An evaluation of the approaches of optimization models in the prediction of muscle forces during human gait. *J Biomech* 1981;14:513–525.
24. Perry J, Bekey GA. EMG-force relationships in skeletal muscle. *CRC Crit Rev Biol Eng* 1981;7(1):1–22.
25. Rohrle H, Scholten R, Sigolotto C, Solbach W, Kellner H. Joint forces in the human pelvis-leg skeleton during walking. *J Biomech* 1984;17:409–424.
26. Seireg A, Arvikar RJ. The prediction of muscular load sharing and joint forces in the lower extremities during walking. *J Biomech* 1975;8:89–102.
27. Shiavi R, Bugle H, Limbird T. Electromyographic gait assessment, part 1: adult EMG profiles and walking speed. *J Rehab Res Dev* 1987;24:13–23.
28. Shiavi R, Green N. Ensemble averaging of locomotor electromyographic patterns using interpolation. *Med Biol Eng Comput* 1983;21:573–578.
29. Smidt GL. Biomechanical analysis of knee flexion and extension. *J Biomech* 1973;6:79–92.
30. Solomonow M, Baratta R, Binghe HZ, Shoji H, D'Amrosia R. Historical update and new developments on the EMG–force relationships of skeletal muscles. *Orthopedics* 1986;9:1541–1543.
31. Sutherland D. The events of gait. *Bull Prosthet Res* 1981; 10(35):281–282.
32. Sutherland D, Olshen R, Biden E, Wyatt M. *Development of mature walking*. London: MacKeith Press, 1988.
33. Sutherland D, Olshen R, Cooper L, Woo S. Development of mature gait. *J Bone Joint Surg* 1980;62A:354–363.
34. Taft, R. An introduction: Eadweard Muybridge and his work. In: Muybridge E. *The human figure in motion*. New York: Dover Publications, 1955;vii–xiv.
35. Taylor KD, Mottier FM, Simmons DW. An automated motion measurement system for clinical gait analysis. *J Biomech* 1982;15:505–516.
36. Tibone J, Antich T, Fanton G, Moynes D, Perry J. Functional analysis of anterior cruciate ligament instability. *Am J Sports Med* 1986;14(4):276–284.
37. Whittle MW. Calibration and performance of a three dimensional television system for kinematic analysis. *J Biomechanics* 1982;15:185–196.
38. Winter DA. *Biomechanics of human movement*. New York: John Wiley & Sons, 1979.
39. Yang J, Winter DA. Surface EMG profiles during different walking cadences in humans. *Electroenceph Clin Neurophys* 1985;60:485–491.

PART IV

Repair

Knee Ligaments: Structure, Function, Injury,
and Repair, edited by D. Daniel, et al.
© 1990 by Raven Press, Ltd. All rights reserved.

CHAPTER 15

The Response of Ligaments to Stress Modulation and Overview of the Ligament Healing Response

Wayne H. Akeson

The purpose of this chapter is to summarize and place in perspective several of the more detailed basic research observations described in Chapters 16 through 22. In addition, a few of the most pressing questions of contemporary research on knee biology, pathophysiology, and repair will be highlighted. In particular, emphasis will be placed on some of the specific issues where the application of animal experimentation results to human surgical questions is problematic. Naturally, this is a tall order and cannot be comprehensive. Nevertheless, it should be of value to clarify and place into focus some of the more important observations and controversies from the large amount of research data on knee injuries accumulated during the past decade.

The importance of daily musculoskeletal activity for maintenance of connective tissue homeostasis and general well-being of synovial joints has become so universally accepted as to presently stand as therapeutic catechism. Yet, the basis for this general understanding is relatively recent in the history of orthopedic surgery. Generally, and to our good fortune (for patients and surgeons alike), the underlying understanding of the favorable interactions of biological

processes with the physical environment has been in concert with modern therapeutic goals and with the constraints of health-care economics. Examples abound, but they are characterized by the needs of successful trauma management. In the modern trauma center, patients with multiple system injuries, including major long bone and/or pelvic fractures, seldom leave the operating suite on the day of admission before achievement of internal fixation or external skeletal fixation of the principal fracture instabilities. The improved survival rates resulting from better cardiopulmonary nursing, as well as the improved musculoskeletal rehabilitation made possible by prompt mobilization of the patient, have been extensively documented (10,22,23). These benefits have been extended in recent years to stabilization of the injured spine as well (18,19). These advances have been made possible by the triumphs of bioengineering and biomaterials research in collaboration with dedicated and resourceful orthopedic surgeons. The resulting array of spinal internal fixation devices and supportive instrumentation permits early mobilization of all but the most devastated spinal injury patients. In present days of mounting medical costs, the dividends of economies achieved through shortened hospital stays are hardly inconsequential. No longer are rounds through orthopedic wards a jungle of patients in traction waiting desperately day after day for an x-ray verdict of "early

W. H. Akeson: Department of Surgery, Division of Orthopedics and Rehabilitation, University of California, San Diego, School of Medicine, La Jolla, California 92093.

union'' so they might leave the hospital, only to be sentenced to weeks of imprisonment in the skin-tight walls of the spica cast, the equivalent of the medieval iron maiden. Shortened hospitalizations are accompanied in such cases by an accelerated rehabilitation course and earlier return to work. Such rewards are, fortunately, not contrary to favorable healing and sound physiological principles; rather, they provide mutual reinforcement.

The understanding of the rationale for aggressive and early rehabilitation requires familiarity with the effects of stresses on specialized connective tissues of the locomotor system. These effects and the derivative therapeutic principles will be outlined below.

STRESS DEPRIVATION EFFECTS ON SYNOVIAL JOINTS

For some time there has been a general understanding of the fact that orthopedic surgery is commonly defeated by contractures, failure of ligament repair, and articular cartilage damage. But while every orthopedist has known for decades of Wolff's law of bone (47), until recent years few knew of the dependence of connective tissue well-being on regular exposure to physical forces. In support of Rasch (36), we have proposed that Wolff's law be expanded to include connective tissue and be restated to say that the *musculoskeletal system* adapts to stresses applied (6,19). With this enlargement in conception, all connective tissues (cartilage, tendon, and ligament, as well as bone) are enveloped by the argument, and we have come a long way toward understanding what is probably the key concept in musculoskeletal rehabilitation.

It was important that data be accumulated to document the effects of stress enhancement and stress deprivation on the musculoskeletal system. However, the central question, What are the effects of stress modulation on the musculoskeletal system?, was not given rigorous attention until after the mid-1950s. In part, the subject was ignored simply out of low ranking on the ladder of research priorities. The feeling of many surgeons was that the subject lacked excitement and, furthermore, that the implications were few, since most therapeutic choices of cast immobilization were dictated by the presenting condition. Eventually, detailed studies unfolded and the extensive ramifications of stress effects on the broad range of musculoskeletal tissues became apparent. Along with heightened awareness of the stress dependence of the musculoskeletal system came new developments in internal fixation which permitted a revolution in orthopedic therapeutic strategies. This combination of advances in knowledge and technology was associated with a heightened awareness of the costs of long-term hospitalization which were approaching almost crisis proportions. A widespread acceptance of early internal fixation of most long bone fractures and rapid institution of the rehabilitation process quickly followed in the decades of the 1970s and 1980s (25,27,37).

There are protean effects of stress deprivation on synovial joints. Some of the effects can be observed by gross and histological techniques. Animal and human studies have shown consistent and complementary results supporting the view that a large price is paid for immobility when it is imposed as a therapeutic measure. The historical dichotomy of ''resters'' versus ''movers'' has decisively been resolved in favor of advocates of early functional activity. Whether dealing with injury or disease, there are few exceptions to this conclusion.

MORPHOLOGICAL OBSERVATIONS FOLLOWING STRESS DEPRIVATION

Morphological effects of stress modulation are seen in all the synovial joint structures, including articular cartilage, bone, synovium, ligament, and ligament insertion sites. And, strikingly, the troublesome deprivation changes occur in a few short weeks.

Numerous studies have demonstrated the proliferation of fibrofatty connective tissue within the joint as a consequence of immobility (15,16). Fibrofatty structures within the mammalian joints presumably serve a lubricating function by facilitating the coating of articular surfaces with synovial fluid during normal articular motion. In the stress-deprived condition, the fibrofatty connective tissue proliferates gradually into the joint space and becomes adherent to exposed synovial and cartilage surfaces, eventually obliterating the joint space.

Articular cartilage deteriorates when overgrown by the fibrofatty connective tissue described above. The tissue overgrowth of articular cartilage is reminiscent of the pannus of rheumatoid arthritis and has a similarly deleterious effect (15,16). The morphological deterioration includes loss of metachromatic staining characteristics of the matrix, as well as an erosion of the surface cartilage layers. Matrix alterations besides surface erosion include (a) deep fibrillation and (b) intracartilaginous cyst formation. Later, cells from the subchondral layer penetrate the subchondral plate into the deeper layers of articular cartilage. Contact from opposing cartilage surfaces may lead to full-thickness cartilage ulceration, depending upon the load applied and the duration of the compression (38,44). The limited repair potential of articular cartilage does not allow effective recovery from such deep structural damage.

The synovial lining does not contribute significantly

to joint stability. However, synovial tissue provides the cells that proliferate as the fibrofatty connective tissue layer that grows over the joint surfaces after a period of immobility. The confluence of such tissue between the accordion fold pleats of relaxed synovium, such as found in the inferior aspect of the shoulder or the posterior aspect of the flexed knee, mature with time and may markedly restrict joint motion. Such adhesions must be stretched by prolonged physical therapy. If such treatment fails, the joint may require manipulation or surgical release before joint motion can be restored.

The process of connective tissue homeostasis at the ultrastructural level is also seriously disrupted by stress deprivation, and these effects are seen prominently in ligaments. Morphologically, the effect is observed as a pattern of increased fiber randomness as compared to control tissue. Loss of parallelism of collagen fibrils in cruciate ligaments has been observed in experimental animal models, and even changes in cell characteristics have been described (3,29). These findings are consistent with the conclusions of mechanical studies, showing reduced ligament stiffness and lower ultimate tensile strength of the affected ligaments (30,51). The details of the biomechanical and biochemical effects of stress deprivation on ligaments are described at length in Chapters 16 and 17.

LIGAMENT INSERTION SITES

The attachment of ligaments to bone requires a continuity of collagen fibers from the ligament into bone at the attachment site. The attachment of ligament and tendon are conceptually similar in this respect. In the most complex arrangement, the fibers enter bone through a fibrocartilage layer and then travel through a calcified fibrocartilage layer before proceeding into the osseous tissue (14). The fibrocartilage and ossified fibrocartilage layers are separated by a blue stained line in hematoxylin and eosin (H&E)-processed sections. Transmission electron-microscopic (TEM) sections show individual collagen fibers passing across the mineralization front (28). The stress deprivation process has a deleterious effect on bone at these ligament attachment sites. Laros (28) has shown dramatic mechanical and morphological changes in bone at these sites in immobilized limbs. In animal studies the process is seen most prominently at the tibial and fibular insertion sites of collateral ligaments. In a few weeks, osteoclasts produce cortical resorption, weakening the ligament insertion sites by interrupting the collagen fiber continuity between the two structures. At the conclusion of the process, the only remaining major attachment of the ligament may be to the periosteal portion of its attachment. Regional variations in this

process seem to be dependent upon the extent of local osteoclastic resorption that occurs as a part of the osteoporosis of disuse. Mechanical testing of the bone–ligament–bone preparations of such joints predictably shows weakening of the ligament attachment sites, and failure commonly occurs at this point (42,43). Laros speculated that the approximation of the periosteum at the distal ligament insertions of the collaterals might provide the anatomical explanation for the difference in response to stress deprivation at those sites, compared to the proximal attachment and to cruciate attachments. The periosteal layer is lacking at the proximal collateral ligament junctions and at both ends of cruciate insertion sites (41).

These studies indicate that comparison of results between different ligaments is invalid and point out the importance of monitoring activity of so-called control animals. Caged animals cannot serve as controls, and animals recently acquired must be placed on standardized activity programs for several weeks before acceptance as controls in studies where biomechanical testing of ligaments is performed.

BIOMECHANICAL OVERVIEW OF STRESS DEPRIVATION ON SYNOVIAL JOINTS

It should also be no surprise that the profound biological response to stress deprivation is reflected in changes in cell metabolism and, ultimately, in matrix characteristics.

Chapter 13 details the biochemical changes that occur in periarticular connective tissue of stress-deprived joints. Both the fibrous component of the connective tissue and the "ground substance" that lubricates the fiber–fiber interfaces are involved in this process. In brief, the ground substance undergoes atrophy along with the fibrous component (4). The ground substance changes consist of loss of water and loss of the proteoglycans (4). The component of proteoglycan most drastically changed is hyaluronic acid, which is reduced by about 40% after an 8- to 9-week period of immobility (1). Hyaluronic acid is the component of connective tissue responsible for lubrication of the fiber–fiber interface (40). The fibrous component also atrophies about 10% in this time period. More dramatically, an increased turnover of the fibrous component occurs with evidence of increased collagenase activity, increased reducible collagen crosslinks, and increased collagen turnover (2). Implications of these changes are several. Ground substance atrophy permits a centripetal collapse of the matrix so that fiber–fiber distances are decreased. Enhanced collagen turnover without the guiding influence of normal mechanics results in a random disposition of fibers. The random configuration is less able to respond to stress application in the tensile loading configuration than the usual parallel-type structured ligament. The net effect is an apparent paradoxical one in which the joint as a whole becomes more stiff while at the same time the individual ligaments themselves exhibit a ''softer'' profile on stress strain diagrams and exhibit a lowered ultimate failure load (51).

RECOVERY FROM STRESS DEPRIVATION

During the recovery from immobilization, it is the ligament insertion site which is the slowest to return to normal strength (31,49). In the sense of a chain failing at its weakest link, the failure condition in the studies performed following remobilization is usually at the insertion site. The reversal of the processes described above is very slow. Twenty-four weeks after immobilization was discontinued, the insertion site properties had not returned to normal in the studies cited above (28). The histological changes had not reverted completely by 30 weeks after immobilization was discontinued. The implications with respect to rehabilitation are as follows: (a) The recovery process is not a mirror image of the development of the stress-deprived state, and (b) greater time is required for recovery than for the development of these changes. Experimental studies in animals indicate that a year is the minimum time requirement for full recovery of insertion-site strength (31,49). This pattern of rapid development of structural weakness from stress deprivation and the importance of recognition of slow recovery from this process is of crucial importance in designing clinical treatment protocols and in prescribing rational rehabilitation programs (Fig. 17-6).

STRESS ENHANCEMENT EFFECTS ON SYNOVIAL JOINTS

Periarticular connective tissue is capable of hypertrophy. But in the studies that follow, it is clear that the time course of its hypertrophy is much slower than is seen in its response to stress deprivation. In studies of pigs exercised five times a week, 3 months of exercise increased flexor tendon maximum load to failure 6%, and with 12 months of exercise the maximum load to failure was 19% (versus controls $p < 0.005$) (52). These studies indicate that a great deal of time and effort is required to achieve even small stress enhancement effects in the fibrous connective tissue of the musculoskeletal system.

In answer to the question posed earlier in this chapter, What are the effects of stress modulation on the musculoskeletal system?, we can see that the effects are wide-ranging and are central to rational therapeutic decision-making. The fundamental studies correspond closely to clinical observations. The themes are consistent and pervasive.

The extension of Wolff's law of bone to include the entire musculoskeletal system, including synovial joints and supporting fibrous periarticular structures, is now widely accepted. The implications of the stress dependence of connective tissue in the clinical arena has been dramatic. As will be seen in the following chapters, not only is this axiom applicable to normal musculoskeletal homeostasis, but it is also necessary for the enhancement of the rate and quality of healing. Furthermore, the axiom is key to the design of rational rehabilitation programs and must be considered as one of the common pillars to successful orthopedic treatment in all its aspects.

PROBLEMS OF LIGAMENT HEALING

One of the questions confounding clinicians is, Why do certain ligaments fail to heal while others heal readily? In the focus on the knee, the obvious target of the question is the anterior cruciate ligament (ACL), which consistently fails to heal (26,32,33). Part of the answer to the failure of ACL healing may rest with an important concept that has received increasing emphasis in the past decade—namely, that fibrous connective tissues are not uniform structurally, biomechanically, biochemically, or biologically. In Chapters 5 and 7, biochemical and biomechanical differences between tendon and ligament, as well as between certain ligaments, are detailed.

An example of the differences between tendon and ligament is as follows: Ligaments contain elastin, whereas tendons do not (8). The existence of elastin fibers in ligaments is not surprising. Their absence from tendon at first glance was unexpected, but on reflection one recognizes that a tendon has muscle to serve as an energy damper and hardly requires elastic fibers for that purpose.

Nowhere is the variability of ligaments more striking than between the ACL and medial collateral ligament (MCL). The unique gross structural features of these ligaments are well known, but the variability in crimp pattern, biochemical composition, and biomechanical characteristics have only recently been elucidated (5,48,49). The cellular patterns of ACL and MCL are also distinctively different. ACL cells are arranged in columns, similar to pearls on a string (Fig. 15-1A). The cells are rounded, resembling the cells of fibrocartilage, resting in an amorphous matrix several microns wide (29). These cells lack any of the elongated processes characteristic of the usual fibroblast. The MCL, by contrast, is populated by spindle-shaped cells with processes extending many times the length of the cell in several directions (Figs. 15-1 to 15-5). These pro-

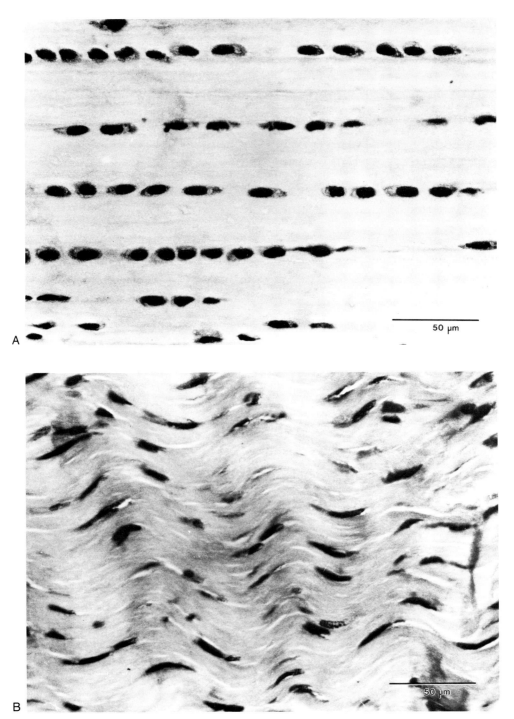

FIG. 15-1. A: Longitudinal H&E section from the midportion of rabbit ACL. The cells are strung out like pearls on a string and lack long cellular processes. **B:** Photomicrograph of longitudinal H&E section from the midportion of rabbit MCL. The cells are spindle-shaped with long cytoplasmic processes extending distances many times the length of the cell body.

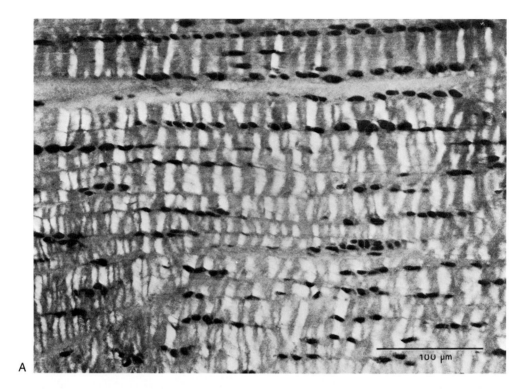

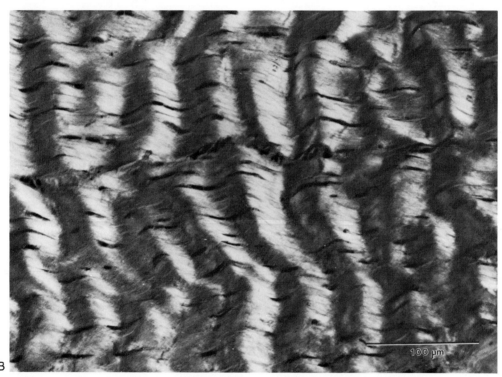

FIG. 15-2. A: Polarized light appearance of rabbit ACL showing lack of register of wave forms of adjacent bundles. Cells are not tightly adherent to matrix, and they do not deform in register with the wave forms of the matrix. **B:** Polarized light photomicrograph of midportion of the MCL showing the sharp wave forms in register across the section. The cell bodies and processes closely follow the wave-form configuration.

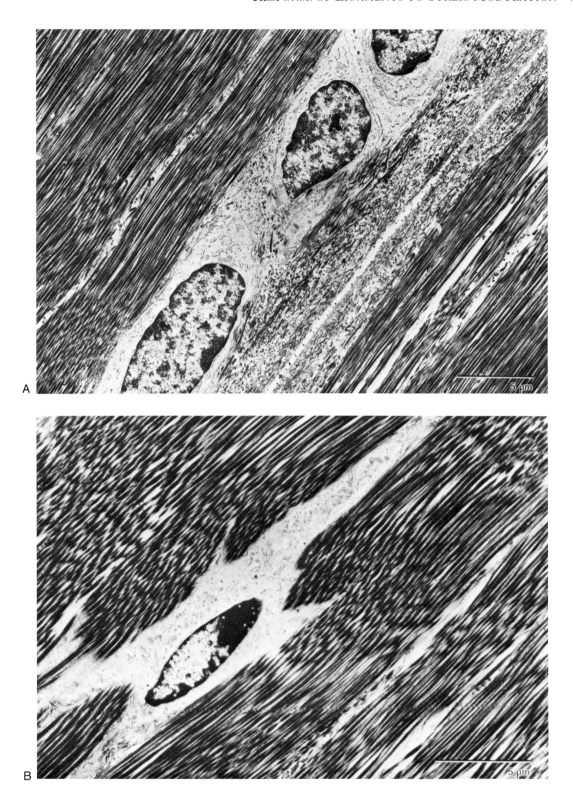

FIG. 15-3. A: Low-power TEM of rabbit ACL showing an amorphous matrix separating the cytoplasmic membrane and the adjacent collagen fibrils. The cells lack long cytoplasmic processes. The rounded nature of the cells is obvious. **B:** Low-power TEM of rabbit MCL showing a fibroblast with long cytoplasmic processes extending outward into the surrounding matrix. Close proximity of the cytoplasmic membrane to the mature collagen fibrils is evident. Ray-like processes from adjacent cells are seen extending between fibrils of the matrix.

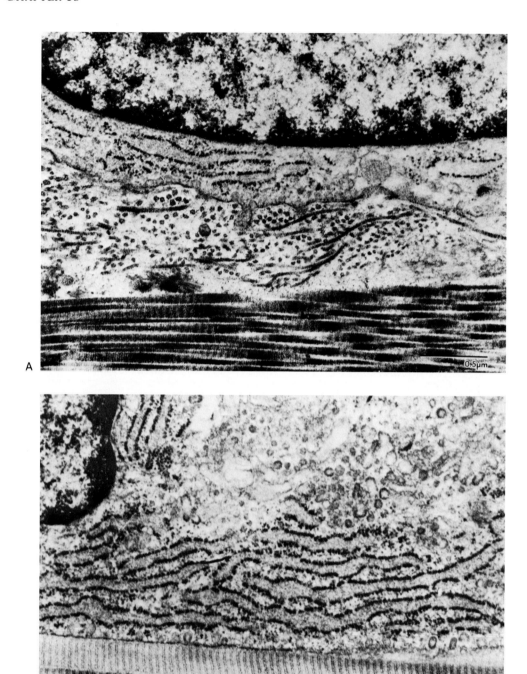

FIG. 15-4. A: Higher-power TEM of rabbit ACL showing separation of the cytoplasmic membrane from the adjacent collagen fibrils by a zone of amorphous material containing fine fibrils, some of which lack clear periodicity. **B:** High-power TEM of longitudinal section through rabbit MCL. The precise apposition of the cytoplasmic membrane to the adjacent mature collagen fibrils is clearly evident. CM, cytoplasmic membrane.

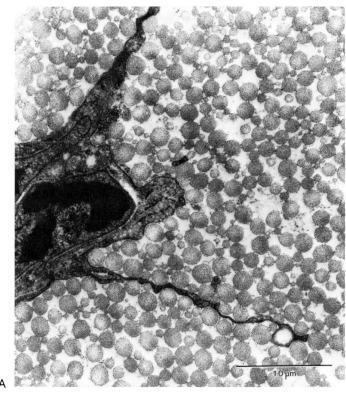

A

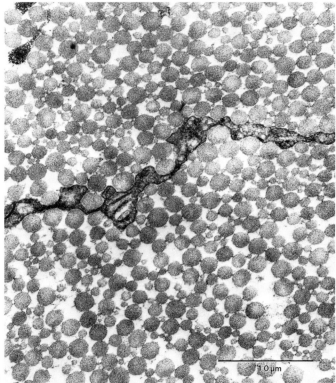

B

FIG. 15-5. A&B: High-power TEM cross-section through rabbit MCL showing the intimate relationship between the cytoplasmic membrane and the collagen fibrils. In some cases the long processes of the MCL partially enfold the adjacent fibrils in a lacunar-like fashion.

cesses are in intimate contact with adjacent matrix and the processes of adjacent cells. Unlike the ACL, cells of the MCL have no amorphous matrix separating the cell membrane from matrix collagen fibers; rather, the cell membrane rests directly on the collagen fibers (29). The ACL cells more resemble the cells of meniscus (Fig. 15-6) than they do the cells of the MCL. The full functional implications of these cellular differences is as yet unclear. However, one striking biological difference between the two ligaments, their differing response to injury, raises at once the question of relevance of the difference of cell form to the difference in healing response. The MCL readily heals, whereas the ACL invariably does not (except for avulsion injuries in which the healing response is one of bone, not of ACL substance). It is tempting to speculate that the failure of healing of the ACL is related to its fibrocartilage-like cellular features (29). Failure of cartilage and fibrocartilage healing is well known.

We have proposed that in ligaments there exists a continuum of cells between the fibroblast and the chondroblast, and that cellular features of one phenotype can be transformed to another under altered environmental conditions (29). Known examples of this type of transformation include (a) the transformation of cartilage cells to fibroblasts under conditions of cell culture (11,39) and (b) the transformation of fibroblasts of tendon to fibrocartilage cells at points of tendon compression (21,34,45). It seems likely that the cellular characteristics of the ACL are modulated by the unique features of its environment. These features include (a) its proximity to the joint space and (b) its complex fiber orientation, which is twisted to adapt to the cam-like configuration of the femoral condyle. Proximity to the joint space due to its location within the intercondylar notch exposes the ligament to the so-called "hostile environment" of that space. Hostile factors include synovial fluid, which in injury and disease states contains hemorrhagic breakdown products and/or a variety of catalytic enzymes. This location also dictates that a significant portion of the nutritional supply of the ACL derives from synovial fluid (7,46). The bathing action of the joint fluid also inhibits the formation of a fibrin clot after injury, thereby undoubtedly removing growth factors that normally aid the healing response.

When immobilized, the cells of the ACL assume an appearance more typical of fibroblasts, suggesting that mechanical factors may be a paramount modulating factor (29). The twisted fiber configuration of the ACL creates unusual forces within the ligament. In particular, compressive as well as tensile forces are inevitable because of the intermittent wringing action that occurs during flexion and extension. Such compressive forces might favor a fibroblast-to-fibrocartilage

transition, such as occurs in tendon at locations of compressive load (21,34,45).

The relative importance of the environmental factors influencing the ACL biological, morphological, and biochemical signatures in inhibiting the ACL's healing response remains to be elucidated. New opportunities for modifying the healing response with growth factors should be explored. Additional opportunities to study the response of ACL to injury using techniques of modern molecular biology are also intriguing.

The enhancement of healing of tendon and ligament by controlled motion has been recently reported (20,50). In the case of flexor tendon lacerations in "no man's land," the healing can be accelerated by controlled passive motion. Until recently, it was thought that flexor tendons could heal only by the extrinsic healing mechanisms. In this type of healing, primitive neovascular tissue grows into the defect from overlying tissue. In fact, the confluence of scar from the skin through tendon sheath into the laceration led to the term "one wound concept" (35). For this type of healing to be operative, motion of the tendon must be restricted during healing. Healing by this mechanism is usually successful; however, restricted tendon gliding is a common complication because tendon becomes locked by scar.

We have been able to demonstrate clearly that intrinsic healing of a tendon laceration can occur if the tendon is passively moved after repair (20). Motion inhibits ingrowth of tissue from the overlying tendon sheath. Intrinsic healing is less apt to compromise tendon mobility as compared to extrinsic healing, so the benefits of passive motion are multiplied. Similarly, our laboratory showed benefits of improved healing in the MCL in animals by allowing early motion (17,24,50). Thus, the knowledge of the interaction of physical forces with biological response to injury can be usefully exploited in postinjury or postsurgery rehabilitation programs involving the knee. Recent widespread clinical employment of these concepts with respect to Grade I and II injuries of the MCL have confirmed the utility of this approach.

RECONSTRUCTION OF THE ACL

What is the fate of biological tissue used for ACL reconstruction? Studies using animal models indicate that cells of autograft tissue do not survive in the synovial environment. The outcome has not been shown to be improved by transferring the graft along with an intact blood supply (13). Apparently the intrasynovial environment will not support cells transplanted to this site. The graft quickly loses its cellular population: By 2 weeks, only ghosts of cells remain (9). However, the matrix quickly becomes repopulated with new cells,

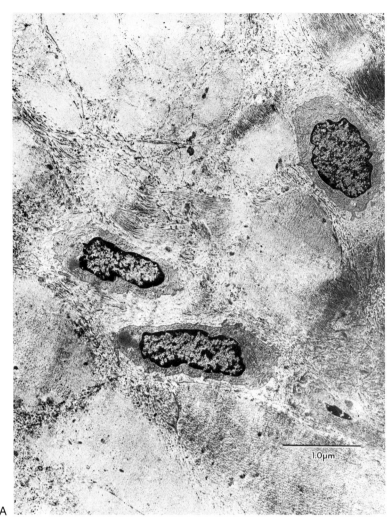

A

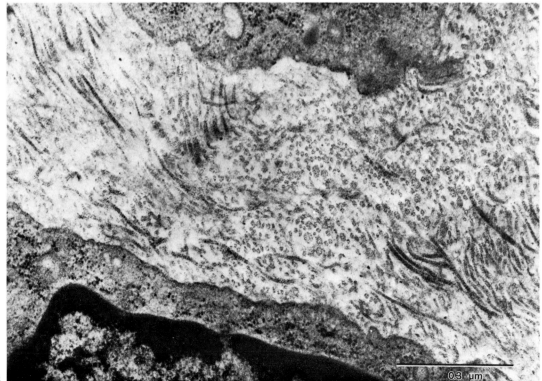

B

FIG. 15-6. A&B: Low- and high-power TEM section through rabbit knee meniscus. The rounded cytoplasmic configuration with very short projecting processes is similar to the ultramicroscopic morphology of the cells of the ACL. An apparently random configuration of the fine collagen fibrils in the immediate cellular environment is evident.

even prior to revascularization. The phenomenon of "ligamentization"—the change in biochemical characteristics of tendon matrix into ACL-type matrix—is described in Chapter 20.

RELEVANCE OF ANIMAL RESEARCH

What is the relevance of studies of animal ligament healing to the biology of ligament healing and clinical management of ligament injuries in humans? A perplexing problem persists in the majority of reports on mechanical properties of the reconstructed ACL in animals. Although the grafts become repopulated with cells and actively metabolize matrix components, they do not achieve the structural characteristics of the normal ACL. As described in Chapters 20 and 21, most animal studies show the ultimate failure load to be well below 50% of the normal ACL even up to 1 year past reconstruction (12,49). Several studies show the ultimate failure load to be only 20% of normal. Yet, in human ACL reconstructions the functional improvement is obvious and usually of lasting benefit, although precise mechanical data are lacking. Many differences between the animal models and the human knee can be cited (Chapter 22). For the present, the animal models have great utility in searching for mechanisms and insights into human knee ligament healing, but these results obviously cannot be transferred to the clinical arena directly. Rather, they require careful interpretation and integration with the empirical clinical evidence.

Despite their shortcomings, animal studies will continue to be required for studies of mechanisms of healing and for development of new, improved therapeutic strategies in treatment of knee injuries. Many challenging new possibilities for improved treatment of ligament injuries must be explored. These range from (a) molecular biology and growth factors on one extreme to (b) synthetic substitutes and allografts on the other. The ability to take advantage of these opportunities will depend on the viability of the collaboration between basic and clinical scientists focusing on these problem areas.

REFERENCES

1. Akeson WH, Amiel D, LaViolette D. The connective tissue response to immobility. *J Bone Joint Surg* 1966;48(A):808.
2. Akeson WH, Amiel D, Mechanic GL, Woo SL-Y, Harwood FL, Hamer M. Collagen cross-linking alterations in joint contractures: changes in the reducible cross-links in periarticular connective tissue collagen after nine weeks of immobilization. *Connect Tissue Res* 1977;5:15–19.
3. Akeson WH, Amiel D, Woo SL-Y. Immobility effects joints: the pathomechanics of joint contracture. *Biorheology* 1980; 17:95–110.
4. Akeson WH. An experimental study of joint stiffness. *J Bone Joint Surg* 1961;43(A):1022–1034.
5. Akeson WH, Frank C, Amiel D, Woo SL-Y. Ligament biology and biomechanics. In: Finerman G, ed. *AAOS: Symposium on sports medicine—The knee*. St. Louis: CV Mosby, 1984; 111–151.
6. Akeson WH, Woo SL-Y, Amiel D, Frank CB. The biology of ligaments. In: Hunter LY, Funk FJ, eds. *Rehabilitation of the injured knee*. St. Louis: CV Mosby, 1984;93–148.
7. Amiel D, Abel MF, Kleiner, JB, Akeson, WH. Synovial fluid nutrient delivery in the diathrial joint: an analysis of rabbit knee ligament. *J Orthop Res* 1986;4:90–95.
8. Amiel D, Frank CB, Harwood, FL, Fronek J, Akeson WH. Tendons and ligaments: a morphological and biochemical comparison. *J Orthop Res* 1984;1:257–265.
9. Amiel D, Kleiner JB, Akeson WH. The natural history of the anterior cruciate ligament autograft of patellar tendon origin. Sports Injury Research Award, American Orthopedic Society. *Am J Sports Med* 1986;14:445–462.
10. Baker C, Oppenheimer L, Stephens B, et al. Epidemiology of trauma deaths. *Am J Surg* 1980;140:144–150.
11. Benya PD, Shaffer, JD. Dedifferentiated chondrocytes reexpress the differentiated collagen phenotype when cultured in agarose gels. *Cell* 1982;30:215–224.
12. Butler DL, Hulse DA, Kay MD, Grood ES, Shires PK, D'Ambrosia R, Shoji H. Biomechanics of cranial cruciate ligament reconstruction in the dog. II. Mechanical properties. *Vet Surg* 1983;12:113–118.
13. Clancy WG, Thomsen E, Dueland RT, Wilson JM, Vanderby R, Graft BK. Anterior cruciate and posterior cruciate ligament reconstruction with patellar tendon using a medial vascularized graft, lateral vascularized graft and free patellar tendon graft. *Am J Sports Med* 1987;15:399–400.
14. Cooper RR, Misol S. Tendon and ligament insertion. *J Bone Joint Surg* 1970;52A:1–20.
15. Enneking WF, Horowitz M. The intra-articular effects of immobilization on the human knee. *J Bone Joint Surg* 1972; 654(A):973–985.
16. Evans EB, Eggers GWN, Butler JK, et al. Experimental immobilization and remobilization of rat knee joints. *J Bone Joint Surg* 1960;42(A):737–758.
17. Frank C, Woo SL-Y, Amiel D, Harwood F, Gomez M, Akeson WH. Medial collateral ligament healing—a multidisciplinary assessment in rabbits. *Am J Sports Med* 1983;11:379–389.
18. Garfin SR, Shackford SR, Marshall LF, Drummond JC. Care of multiply injured patient with cervical spine injury. *Clin Orthop* 1989;239:19–29.
19. Garfin SR. Thoracolumbar injuries. In: Poss R, ed. *Orthopaedic Knowledge Update III*. Chicago: AAOS, 1990.
20. Gelberman RH, Woo SL-Y, Lothringer K, Akeson WH, Amiel D. Effects of early intermittent passive mobilization on healing canine flexor tendons. *J Hand Surg* 1982;7(2):170–175.
21. Gillard GC, Reilly HC, Bell-Booth PG, Flint MH. The influence of mechanical forces on the glycosaminoglycan content of the rabbit flexor digitorum profundus tendon. *Connect Tissue Res* 1979;7:37–46.
22. Goris R, Draaisma J. Causes of death after blunt trauma. *J Trauma* 1982;22:141–146.
23. Hansen S. Concomitant fractures of the long bones. In: Meyers M, ed. *The multiply injured patient with complex fractures*. Philadelphia: Lea & Febiger, 1984;401–411.
24. Inoue M, McGurk-Burleson E, Hollis JM. Treatment of the medial collateral ligament injury. 1. The importance of anterior cruciate ligament on the varus–valgus knee laxity. *Am J Sports Med* 1987;15:15–21.
25. Johnson KD, Cadambi A, Seibert GB. Incidence of adult respiratory distress syndrome in patients with multiple musculoskeletal injuries: effect of early operative stabilization of fractures. *J Trauma* 1985;25:375–383.
26. Kleiner JB, Amiel D, Harwood FL, Akeson WH. Early histologic, metabolic and vascular assessment of anterior cruciate ligament autografts. *J Orthop Res* 1989;7:235–242.
27. LaDuca J, Bone L, Seibel R, et al. Primary open reduction and internal fixation of open fractures. *J Trauma* 1980;20:580–586.

28. Laros GS, Tipton CM, Cooper RM. Influence of physical activity on ligament insertions in the knees of dogs. *J Bone Joint Surg* 1971;53A:275–286.

29. Lyon RM, Billings E Jr, Woo SL-Y, Ishizue KK, Kitabayashi L, Amiel D, Akeson WH. The ACL: a fibrocartilaginous structure. *Trans 35th Mtg Orthop Res Soc.* Las Vegas, February 6–9, 1989; 189.

30. Noyes FR. Functional properties of knee ligaments and alterations induced by immobilization. *Clin Orthop* 123:210–242.

31. Noyes FR, Torvik PJ, Hyde WB, DeLucas JL. Biomechanics of ligament failure. II. An analysis of immobilization, exercise and reconditioning effects in primates. *J Bone Joint Surg* 1974;56A:1406–1418.

32. O'Donoghue DH, Frank CG, Jeter GL, Johnson W, Zeiders JW, Kenyon R. Repair and reconstruction of the anterior cruciate ligament in dogs. Factors influencing long-term results. *J Bone Joint Surg* 1971;53A:710–718.

33. O'Donoghue DH, Rockwood CC Jr. Repair of the anterior cruciate ligament in dogs. *J Bone Joint Surg* 1966;48A:503–519.

34. Okuda Y, Gorski JP, An KN, Amadio PC. Biochemical, histological and biomechanical analyses of canine tendon. *J Orthop Res* 1987;5:60–68.

35. Peacock EE. Comparison of collagenous tissue surrounding normal and immobilized joints. *Surg Forum* 1963;14:440–444.

36. Rasch PJ, Maniscalco R, Pierson WR, Logan GA. Effect of exercise, immobilization and intermittent stretching on strength of knee ligaments of albino rats. *J Appl Physiol* 1960;15:289–290.

37. Riska E, von Bonsdorff H, Hakkinen S, et al. Primary operative fixation of long bone fractures in patients with multiple injuries. *J Trauma* 1977;17:111–121.

38. Salter RB, Field P. The effects of continuous compression on living articular cartilage: an experimental investigation. *J Bone Joint Surg* 1960;42A:31–49.

39. Schiltz JR, Mayne R, Holtzer H. The synthesis of collagen and glycosaminoglycans by dedifferentiated chondroblast in culture. *Cell Differ* 1973;1:97–108.

40. Swann DA, Radin EL, Nazimiec M. Role of hyaluronic acid in joint lubrication. *Ann Rheum Dis* 1974;33:318–326.

41. Tipton CM, Matthes RD, Maynard JA, Carey RA. The influence of physical activity on ligaments and tendons. *Med Sci Sports Exerc* 1975;7:165–175.

42. Tipton CM, Schild RJ, Flatt, AE. Measurements of ligamentous strength in rat knees. *J Bone Joint Surg* 1967;49A:63–72.

43. Tipton CM, Schild RJ, Tomanek RJ. Influence of physical activity on the strength of knee ligaments in rats. *Am J Physiol* 1967;212:783–787.

44. Trias A. Effect of persistent pressure on the articular cartilage: an experimental study. *J Bone Joint Surg* 1961;43B:376–386.

45. Vogel KG, Heinegard D. Characterization of proteoglycans from adult bovine tendon. *J Biol Chem* 1985;260:9298–9306.

46. Whiteside LA, Sweeney RE. Nutrient pathways of the cruciate ligament. *J Bone Joint Surg* 1980;62:1179.

47. Wolff J. *Das Gesetz der Transformation der Knochen.* Berlin: August Hirschwald, 1892.

48. Woo SL-Y, Akeson WH. Response of tendons and ligaments to joint loading and movements. In: Helminen HJ, et al., eds. *Joint loading: biology and health of articular structures.* Bristol: Wright, 1987;287–315.

49. Woo SL-Y, Gomez MA, Sites T, Newton PO, Orlando CA, Akeson WH. The biomechanical and morphological changes of the MCL following immobilization and remobilization. *J Bone Joint Surg* 1987;69A:1200–1211.

50. Woo SL-Y, Inoue M, McGurk-Burleson E. Treatment of the medial collateral ligament injury. 2. Structure and function of canine knees in response to differing treatment regimens. *Am J Sports Med* 1987;15:22–29.

51. Woo SL-Y, Kuei SC, Gomez MA, Winters JM, Amiel D, Akeson WH. The effect of immobilization and exercise on the strength characteristics of bone–medial collateral ligament–bone complex. *Am Soc Mech Eng Symp* 1979;32:67.

52. Woo SL-Y, Ritter MA, Gomez MA, Kuei SC, Akeson WH. The biomechanical and structural properties of swine digital flexor tendons secondary to running exercise. *Orthop Trans* 1980;4:165–166.

Knee Ligaments: Structure, Function, Injury, and Repair, edited by D. Daniel, et al.
© 1990 by Raven Press, Ltd. All rights reserved.

CHAPTER 16

The Response of Ligaments to Stress Deprivation and Stress Enhancement

Biochemical Studies

David Amiel, H. von Schroeder, and Wayne H. Akeson

BIOCHEMICAL SEQUELAE OF STRESS DEPRIVATION

Collagen

In the stress-deprived knee there are a number of changes in metabolism and in matrix composition which occur in the periarticular connective tissue as well as in the ligaments. Within the tissues there is an increase in collagen turnover (4,8,15,38) and in certain types of collagen crosslinking (4,10).

In ligaments per se there is a small reduction in the total collagen content but no change in the ratio of collagen types present (10,29,48). As with the periarticular tissues, stress deprivation also causes an increase in collagen turnover in the ligaments (9,13,29), with increases in both collagen synthesis and degradation as is evident from labeling studies (10). The rate of degradation exceeds the rate of synthesis, and the resulting 5–10% net decrease in collagen contributes to an overall reduction in the mass of the ligaments

(13,48,52). The cruciate ligaments are particularly susceptible to these changes (30). Since the ligament size and collagen mass change minimally, observed structural weakening of the ligaments must be due to changes of the ligament substance itself and not solely to atrophy. This physical change derives from an increase in immature collagen content. The less mature collagen fiber is more pliable and has reduced stiffness. The newly synthesized collagen is randomly dispersed and may be poorly disposed to resisting tensile forces. It also interferes with the functional gliding between fibers, and therefore it contributes to the alteration in the mechanical properties of the ligaments.

Substantial changes in collagen crosslinking are observed with immobilization of joints. Increases of the dihydroxylysinonorleucine (DHLNL), hydroxylysinonorleucine (HLNL) and histidinohydroxymerodesmosine (HHMD) crosslinks are observed (4) (Fig. 16-1 and Table 16-1) which correlate with the decrease in mechanical stiffness of the tissues. The crosslinks are associated with new collagen synthesis, and the increase of crosslinks indicates an increase of immature collagen in the ligament and may play a role in the contracture process that occurs with immobilization (2,5).

D. Amiel, H. von Schroeder, and W.H. Akeson: Department of Surgery, Division of Orthopedics and Rehabilitation, University of California, San Diego, School of Medicine, La Jolla, California 92093.

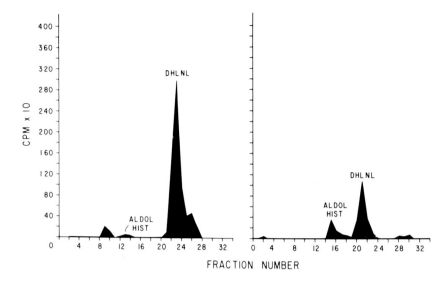

FIG. 16-1. Elution profiles of aldol-histidine–DHLNL peak from immobilized (**left**) and control (**right**) periarticular connective tissue collagen rechromatographed on an extended basic column. (From ref. 4.)

Ground Substance and Water

The components of ground substance have a relatively fast turnover rate compared to those of collagen, and changes in these components are more apparent. Loss of water (50,51) and glycosaminoglycans (3,6,43) in immobilized ligaments, together with the small decreases in collagen content, decrease the mass of the ligaments (13,48). The water loss (up to 6%) and the decrease in hyaluronic acid (40%), dermatan sulfate (8%), and chondroitin-4-SO$_4$ and chondroitin-6-SO$_4$ (20%) result in decreased spacing between fibers and reduced lubrication ability of the matrix. The net effect is decreased independent gliding of microfibrils past one another, which appears to have a considerable effect on the soft tissue mechanics (2). Glycosaminoglycans (GAGs) may also play a role in the stabilization of the collagen fibril and fiber (27). They are also presumed to be important in the alignment of collagen fibers and in the formation of larger fibers during collagen synthesis (33). These roles of the matrix indicate its importance in maintaining normal functional integrity of the ligament and suggest that alterations in the matrix in the absence of controlling factors such as stress may have profound effects of the function of the ligament.

Contrary to the above observations that GAG concentrations decrease with stress deprivation, Vindeman (54) has shown an increase in the synthesis and content of the GAGs uronic acid and hexosamine. In his model, rabbit knees were immobilized in extension for up to 87 days, and increases were noted as early as 2 days. Observations using the same techniques have shown that GAG synthesis increases in ligaments of non-weight-bearing joints but decreases in ligaments of weight-bearing joints (55). Increases versus decreases in GAGs may also be due to the position of immobilization. Knees fixed in flexion infrequently develop osteoarthritis, whereas fixation in extension has been used as a model to produce arthritic changes. GAG content has also been observed to decrease in degenerative areas of human menisci (21). Increases in GAGs seen with osteoarthritis and immobilization may be secondary to an increased inflammatory and hence metabolic response or may be secondary to the stresses on the joint in a given fixed position.

Metabolic and Enzymatic Changes

Several investigators have shown that ligaments are not inert but, instead, are metabolically active structures (20,22,25). Repaired medial collateral ligament (MCL) lacerations from knees subsequently immobilized have been shown to have decreased DNA concentrations (52) as compared to their contralateral control. This change is apparently related to the observed decrease in collagen synthesis. This study indicates that stress deprivation is deleterious not only to normal ligaments but also to damaged or healing ligaments (see Chapter 15).

After 4 weeks of immobilization, anterior cruciate ligaments (ACLs) and MCLs have been shown to ex-

TABLE 16-1. *Mean values in the changes in the reducible crosslinks in normal and immobilized periarticular connective tissue from rabbit knees (eight animals)*

Reduced crosslinks	$(E - C/C) \times 100$[a]	Paired t-test
HLNL	+49%	$p < .005$
DHLNL	+116%	$p < .005$
HHMD	+29%	$p < .05$

[a] E: experimental, C: contralateral control

press lowered levels of collagenase (23). Although increased catabolism is noted with stress deprivation, this result would indicate that there is less catabolic activity. Decreased collagenase may be due to more rapid degradation of the enzyme itself during immobilization, or it may reflect decreased production of the enzyme or of the collagen. Since collagen is produced on demand, and there is less demand in the stress-deprived state resulting in less collagen production, it is hypothesized that less collagenase is required (23). Alternatively, immobilization for longer periods may be required before changes are apparent. During immobilization, fibroblasts undergo other enzymatic adaptations to a state of catabolism. Lysomal hydrolase activity (β-glucuronidase, β-xylosidase, and β-N-acetylgalactosaminidase), which is responsible for GAG degradation, is increased (19) and is consistent with the observed decreases in GAGs outlined above. Vailas (53) has shown that immobility can cause a 36% reduction in cytochrome oxidase activity of fibroblasts in MCLs. The activities of both lactic dehydrogenase (a cytoplasmic glycolytic enzyme) and malic dehydrogenase (an oxidative mitochondrial enzyme) were also decreased with immobility (19). All of these changes illustrate the change in function of the fibroblasts (i.e., from an anabolic synthetic state to a catabolic state) during stress deprivation.

Duration of Stress Deprivation

The magnitude of the biochemical changes that occur with stress deprivation are dependent on the duration of deprivation. Differences in the animal species, limb position, and rigidity of fixation must always be considered; however, immobility for 12 weeks is likely to be necessary before there is a noticeable reduction in ligament mass (13). The hypermetabolic response induced by immobility causes both increased synthesis and increased degradation of collagen. Up to 9 weeks of stress deprivation of the MCL, these processes balance each other with no significant change in total collagen (Fig. 16-2A). A decrease in total collagen is observed in the ACL beyond 9 weeks of immobilization, resulting from a relative increase in collagen degradation over new collagen synthesis (Fig. 16-2A). After 12 weeks there is a further decrease in the rate of synthesis, whereas collagen degradation has been observed to double in some studies (9). Figure 16-2 illustrates the changes in amounts of MCL collagen after 9 and 12 weeks of immobilization. At 12 weeks there is less collagen added to the ligament than at 9 weeks, indicating a reduction of collagen synthesis during the 3 additional weeks of immobilization. During these 3 weeks there is also an increase in collagen degradation, with a collagen mass loss of 14% at 9 weeks and 28%

for the MCL at 12 weeks. There is an insignificant net change (2%) in the amount of collagen after 9 weeks of MCL immobilization, but there is a large decrease (27%) after 12 weeks of immobilization (Fig. 16-2B). The changes for the ACL are more marked, and for both the ACL and the MCL these changes represent a relatively exponential degradative process; the duration of stress deprivation is illustrated in the descending portion of the graph in Fig. 16-4. The recovery process of the ligament substance after immobilization almost mirrors the changes of stress deprivation. This is illustrated by the normalization of the total collagen mass of the rabbit ACL and MCL after a 9 week and 12 week recovery period following 9 weeks of immobilization (Fig. 16-3A and B). After a 9-week recovery period, collagen synthesis and degradation balance each other, but both are still higher than normal, indicating increased metabolic activity (Fig. 16-3A). By comparison, after a 12-week recovery period, slower rates of both synthesis and degradation are observed; however, both are still higher than normal, and both processes balance each other, resulting in normal collagen mass. The return to normal collagen mass of the ligament substance after immobilization is represented in Fig. 16-4. This process occurs within a time frame similar to the duration of immobilization. In contrast to the ligament substance, the recovery of the insertion site is extremely slow (24,37,59); longer periods of stress deprivation require even longer periods of recovery, and chances of complete recovery are less likely to occur with increases in the period of immobility, represented by the gradual ascending portion of the graph in Fig. 16-4.

Degradative lysosomal hydrolase enzymes increase (whereas oxidative and glycolytic anabolic enzymes decrease) with the duration of immobility of MCLs (19). These changes reflect the transition within the ligament from an anabolic to a catabolic state which increases with time. Theoretically, if these data are extrapolated, continued stress deprivation could conceivably lead to complete dissolution of the ligament; however, such studies have not been conducted.

Joint Contracture Etiology

A variety of pathological mechanisms result in joint contracture. Whether the contracture is caused by immobility, pain, paralysis, joint destruction, or incongruity, the result is a loss of range of motion. The resistance to motion is due to structural changes secondary to a common underlying biochemical process. The fibrous capsular structures of the knee, like the ligaments, are predominantly collagen by mass; but instead of being oriented in a parallel array, their pattern is a criss-crossed weave. A variety of models of

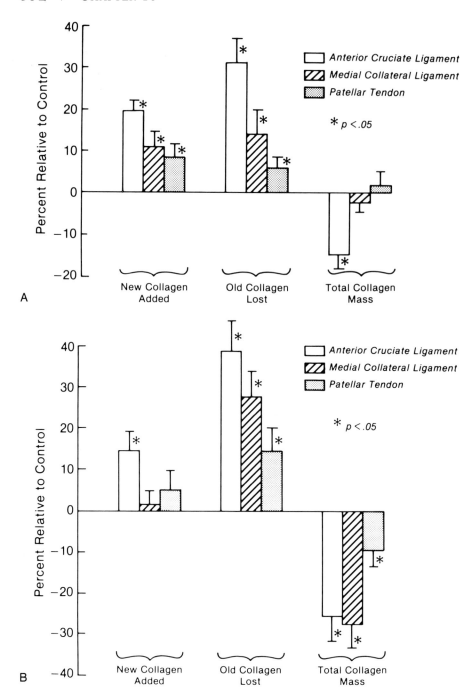

FIG. 16-2. A: The effect of 9 weeks of immobilization of the rabbit knee illustrates an increase in production of new collagen and an increase in the degradation of old collagen, resulting in a net decrease of total collagen in the ACL but no change in total collagen of the MCL or patellar tendon. **B:** Twelve weeks of immobilization results in minimal new collagen formation, a marked increase of collagen degradation, and a significant decrease in total collagen mass of the ligaments and tendon.

immobilization of joints have been used to study stress-dependent changes not only of the ligaments but also of the remainder of the joint. Changes in the fibrous connective tissue of the periarticular structures reflect changes in the ligaments described above, with decreased collagen mass, increased collagen turnover and degradation, increased reducible collagen crosslinks, and reduced GAGs and water (2). Disordered deposition of collagen fibrils appears to impede the normal flexibility of the joint capsule by impeding the fiber–fiber gliding at nodal points. One of the differences between the joint capsule and the ligaments of the knee is that changes in the capsule contribute to contractures, whereas the ligaments decrease in stiffness (14) with immobilization and therefore are less likely to contribute to the contracture. Intraarticular adhesions and muscle shortening also contribute to contractures, but the relative importance of each of these factors needs to be determined.

Treatment of contractures should focus on prevention, and joint mobility becomes a key consideration when choosing a treatment modality. Treatment of established contracture deformities include collagen synthesis inhibitors, collagen crosslink inhibitors (D-pen-

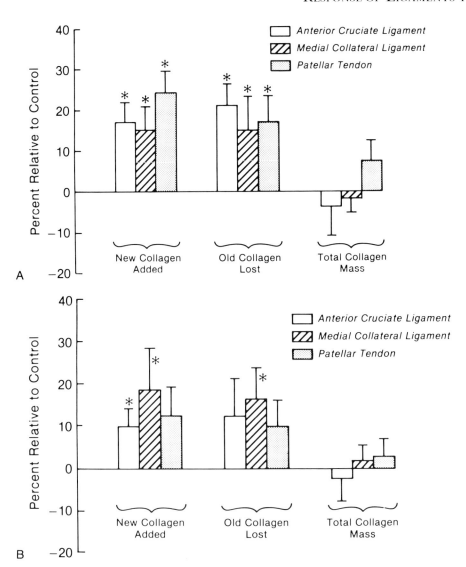

FIG. 16-3. A: Nine weeks of re-mobilization of the rabbit knee following 9 weeks of immobilization shows increased collagen turn-over with normalization of the total collagen mass. B: Twelve weeks of remobilization following 9 weeks of immobilization shows a decreasing collagen turnover with normal collagen mass, indicating a return to the baseline metabolic rate of control tissue. Note that the time frame for recovery is similar to the duration of immobilization.

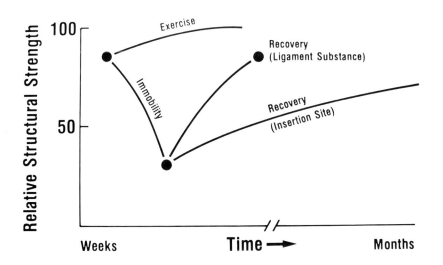

FIG. 16-4. Schematic representation of the effects of exercise, immobilization, and recovery on ligament complex properties. The effects of immobility occur rapidly, and recovery of the ligament substance with remobilization occurs within a similar time-frame. In contrast, the recovery curve for the ligament insertion site and the exercise curve illustrate slow change over a prolonged period of time. (From ref. 18.)

icillamine), hormones (estrogen), and hyaluronic acid. Corticosteroids, most notably cortisone, inhibit collagen synthesis and decrease contracture strength. However, corticosteroids also inhibit useful collagen synthesis during healing responses, and the practical applications of steroids are therefore limited. Crosslink inhibitors, such as lathyrogenic agents (β-aminoprorionitrile) (39) and proline analogues (cis-hydroxyproline) (32), prevent the crosslinking of immature collagen necessary for its maturation into collagen fibrils. As with corticosteroids, crosslink inhibitors decrease both undesirable and useful collagen synthesis and are therefore of limited practical application. Penicillamine acts as a competitive collagen crosslink inhibitor (36) and has been used experimentally to inhibit contracture development and block the increase of DHLNL, HLNL, and HHMD in the rabbit immobilized knee (11). D-Penicillamine and cysteamine form thiozolidine complexes with lysine-derived aldehydes, which prevent Schiff base formation and hence collagen crosslinks. At higher doses, D-penicillamine blocks the enzyme lysyl oxidase, which plays a role in aldehyde formation and therefore in the development of collagen crosslinks. Nevertheless, D-penicillamine is not a practical agent for the same reasons that apply to the corticosteroids and lathyrogenic agents. Estrogen (17β-estradiol) has been observed to reduce joint contractures by approximately 50% and to partially prevent the loss of hexosamine and water which occurs with immobilization (7). The mechanism of these changes, as well as the observed reduction in soluble collagen following estrogen administration, is poorly understood, and more work to pursue the potential of such hormones for orthopedic purposes is required. Hyaluronic acid has also been observed to decrease contractures in an experimental model (12). A single intraarticular injection has been shown to reduce contractures by approximately 50% after 9 weeks of immobilization (12). GAG concentrations increased and collagen mass remained unchanged in the periarticular connective tissue. Although hyaluronic acid is a prime lubricant at soft tissue interfaces (46), it is unlikely that a single injection could provide such a lasting effect without some cellular stimulus, and it has been postulated that hyaluronic acid increases the production of more hyaluronic acid through positive feedback, although the exact mechanism of action remains to be elucidated.

Stress Enhancement

The effects of exercise do not appear to cause significant morphological changes in ligaments, although several investigations have led to confusing and contradictory results (1,16,40,48,52,58,62,63). However, acutely after exercise there is a suggestion of decreased water content, with a duller appearance and a slight loss of fiber waviness (56). Increases in ligament mass may occur with certain long-term exercise programs and are associated with increases in cross-sectional area, weight, and strength of the ligament (31,34,48). The increase in mass may be due to the fiber bundle hypertrophy and increase of collagen between cell bodies seen microscopically (47–49). Collagen turnover in exercised ligaments may also be increased (26); however, other studies have noted no changes in collagen, water, or GAG content as a result of exercise (60). Additional studies will be necessary in order to further examine the changes of ligaments in the stress-enhanced state and to review the observation that exercise induces a laxity within ligaments (42,44,56). The type and duration of exercise create a matrix of variables and must also be considered in these studies. An increase in prolyl hydroxylase activity (35,45), the enzyme which hydroxylates proline into hydroxyproline in procollagen (28), has been noted in exercise-induced enlargements of cardiac and skeletal muscle, and it is interesting to postulate that a similar potential may exist within ligaments. Likewise, the biochemical changes resulting from exercise remain to be elucidated. Vailas (53) has shown a minimal increase of cytochrome oxidase of approximately 10% in the exercised MCL. This change is small when compared to the large changes that occur in muscle and tendons with chronic exercise.

Ligament complex strength has been shown to be increased not only by exercise but also by exogenous testosterone and thyroxine (16,48). For this reason, systemic hormonal mediation of changes in ligament properties has been suggested. Hypophysectomy causes a significant 60% reduction in the cytochrome oxidase activity of ligaments, much greater than the 43% observed with immobilization (53). Although this finding is confounded by a contradictory increase in oxygen consumption, these results may imply a synergistic action of hormones and exercise on the structural and material properties of the ligaments (51) and may suggest that exercise effects on ligaments may vary, depending not only on hormones but also on age, sex, species, nutrition, type of ligament, and the specific ligament involved.

The role of continuous passive motion (CPM) to favorably influence rehabilitation after stress deprivation or to inhibit stress deprivation remains to be established. CPM has been shown to increase range of motion in the early postoperative period after total knee replacement and has also been shown to decrease the requirements for pain medication (17). Since the cruciate ligaments and articular cartilage rely heavily on synovial fluid for nutrition (41), and the joint motion influences intrasynovial nutrition (61), CPM may play a significant role in the process of synovial fluid circulation and thereby increase the nutrition to the intraarticular ligaments. The motion itself has obvious clinical benefits to the postoperative and healing knee by decreasing knee effusions and pain and by increasing range of motion; however, the link between motion and response of the fibroblasts and connective tissue remains unclear.

CONCLUSIONS

This chapter summarizes the present knowledge of the histological and biochemical properties of ligaments of the knee and the changes that occur under conditions of stress enhancement and of stress deprivation. Ligaments are influenced both quantitatively and qualitatively under these conditions, with changes being more pronounced with stress deprivation than with stress enhancement. Stress deprivation illustrates the relationship between form and function of the ligament and implies that the stimulation of physical activity is required for homeostasis of the connective tissue, which includes (a) regulation of metabolic rate of both synthesis and degradation and (b) control of orientation of extracellular matrix proteins. The manner in which cells interpret physical signals, or lack of them, is unknown. Postulated are (a) mechanical sensors for tension or compression and (b) electrical sensors that sense the piezoelectrical signals generated by the physical forces on the collagen fibers. Regardless of the mechanism, the fibroblasts respond by changing the extracellular matrix to meet the functional need or lack of it. In the latter case (i.e., with stress deprivation), the morphological and biochemical aspects of the catabolic process within the ligament is readily apparent. The clinical implications of this information is that joint immobilization is not an innocuous therapeutic modality. The benefits of joint rest in terms of pain relief, decreasing inflammation, or increasing potential healing must be weighed against the adverse effects of stress deprivation. Following a period of immobilization, the weakened mechanical state of the ligaments must be taken into account when considering rehabilitation and the return to regular activities and exercise.

With reversal of the stress-deprived state, the recovery process is slow, and full recovery may not be reached. Data available indicate that ligament complexes from joints immobilized for a few weeks require more than a year to recover. The slow process of ligament recovery is also reflected in the minimal improvements that occur in the ligament under exercise conditions. Hypertrophy of ligaments with exercise does occur, but the process requires a large expenditure of effort over a long period of time to achieve a small increment of change. Appreciation of the re-

sponse of ligaments to stress deprivation and stress enhancement represents an important step in understanding the changes of these tissues under various conditions and illustrates that Wolff's law (57) not only applies to bone but also applies broadly to highly specialized connective tissues.

ACKNOWLEDGMENTS

This work was supported by the Easter Seal Research Foundation and NIH Grants AR15918 and AR39159.

REFERENCES

1. Adams A. Effect of exercise upon ligament strength. *Res Q Exerc Sport* 1966;37:163–167.
2. Akeson WH, Amiel D, Abel MF, Garfin SR, Woo SL-Y. Effects of immobilization on joints. *Clin Orthop* 1987;219:28–37.
3. Akeson WH, Amiel D, LaViolette D. The connective tissue response to immobility: a study of chondroitin-4 and -6 sulphate and dermatan sulphate changes in periarticular connective tissue of control and immobilized knees of dogs. *Clin Orthop* 1967;51:183–197.
4. Akeson WH, Amiel D, Mechanic GL, Woo SL-Y, Harwood FL, Hamer ML. Collagen cross-linking alterations in joint contractures: changes in the reducible cross-links in periarticular connective tissue collagen after nine weeks of immobilization. *Connect Tissue Res* 1977;5:15–19.
5. Akeson WH, Amiel D, Woo SL-Y. Immobility effects on synovial joints: the pathmechanics of joint contracture. *Biorheology* 1980;17:95–110.
6. Akeson WH, Woo SL-Y, Amiel D, Coutts RD, Daniel D. The connective tissue response to immobility: biochemical changes in periarticular connective tissue of the immobilized rabbit knee. *Clin Orthop* 1973;93:356–362.
7. Akeson WH, Woo SL-Y, Amiel D, Doty DH, Rutherford L. Value of 17 β-oestradiol in prevention of contracture formation. *Ann Rheum Dis* 1976;35:429–436.
8. Deleted in proofs.
9. Amiel D, Akeson WH, Harwood FL, Frank CB. Stress deprivation effect on metabolic turnover of the medial collateral ligament collagen. *Clin Orthop* 1983;172:265–270.
10. Amiel D, Akeson WH, Harwood FL, Mechanic GL. The effect of immobilization on the types of collagen synthesized in periarticular connective tissue. *Connect Tissue Res* 1980;8:27–32.
11. Amiel D, Akeson WH, Harwood FL, Schmidt DA. Effects of low dosage schedule of D-penicillamine in collagen cross-linking in a nine-week immobilized rabbit knee. *Connect Tissue Res* 1977;5:179–183.
12. Amiel D, Frey C, Woo SL-Y, Harwood F, Akeson WH. Value of hyaluronic acid in the prevention of contracture formation. *Clin Orthop* 1985;196:306–311.
13. Amiel D, Woo SL-Y, Harwood FL, Akeson WH. The effect of immobilization on collagen turnover in connective tissue: a biochemical–biomechanical correlation. *Acta Orthop Scand* 1982;53:325–332.
14. Blinkley JM, Peat M. The effects of immobilization on the ultra structure and mechanical properties of the medial collateral ligament of rats. *Clin Orthop* 1986;203:301–308.
15. Brooke JW, Slack HGB. Metabolism of connective tissue in limb atrophy in the rabbit. *Ann Rheum Dis* 1959;18:129–136.
16. Cabaud HE, Chatty A, Gildengorin V, Feltman RJ. Exercise effects on the strength of the rat anterior cruciate ligament. *Am J Sports Med* 1980;8:79–86.
17. Coutts RD, Kaita J, Barr R, Mason R, Dube R, Amiel D, Woo SL-Y, Nickel V. The role of continuous passive motion in the postoperative rehabilitation of the total knee. *Trans Orthop Res Soc* 1982;7:195.
18. Frank CB, Amiel D, Woo SL-Y, Akeson WH. Joints: clinical

and experimental aspects. In: Nahum AM, Melvin J, eds. *The biomechanics of trauma*. New York: Appleton-Century-Crofts, 1985;369–397.

19. Gamble JG, Edwards CC, Max SR. Enzymatic adaptation in ligaments during immobilization. *Am J Sports Med* 1984;12:221–228.

20. Gerber G, Gerber G, Altman KI. Studies on the metabolism of tissue proteins. I. Turnover of collagen labelled with proline-U-C^{14} in young rats. *J Biol Chem* 1960;235:2653–2656.

21. Gosh P, Ingam AM, Taylor TFK. Variations in collagen, non-collagenous proteins and hexosamine in menisci derived from osteoarthritic and rheumatoid arthritic knee joints. *J Rheumatol* 1975;2:100–107.

22. Harper J, Amiel D, Harper E. Collagenase production by rabbit ligaments and tendons. *Connect Tissue Res* 1988;17:253–259.

23. Harper J, Amiel D, Harper E. Collagenases from periarticular ligaments and tendon: enzyme levels during the development of joint contracture. *Matrix* 1989;9(3):200–205.

24. Heerkens YF, Woittiez RD, Huijing PA, Husan A, Schenau, van Ingen GJ, Rozendal RH. Passive resistance of the human knee: the effect of remobilization. *J Biomed Eng* 1986;9:69–76.

25. Heikkinen E, Souminen H, Vihersaari M, Vouri I, Kiiskinen A. Effect of physical training on enzyme activities of bones, tendons, and skeletal muscle in mice. In: *Proceedings of the 2nd International Symposium on Biochemical Exercise, Magglingen,* 1975;448–450.

26. Heikkinen E, Vuori I. Effect of physical activity on the metabolism of collagen in aged mice. *Acta Physiol Scand* 1972;84:543–549.

27. Jackson DS, Bentley JP. Collagen–glycosaminoglycan interactions. In: Gould BS, ed. *Treatise on collagen*. New York: Academic Press, 1968.

28. Kivirikko KI, Prockop DJ. Purification and partial characterization of the enzyme for the hydroxylation of proline in protocollagen. *Arch Biochem Biophys* 1967;118:611–618.

29. Klein L, Dawson MH, Heiple K. Turnover of collagen in the adult rat after denervation. *J Bone Joint Surg* 1977;59A:1065–1067.

30. Klein L, Player JS, Heiple KG, Bahniuk E, Goldberg VJ. Ligament–bone failure mechanics correlated with radioassay of collagen and calcium loss during immobilization atrophy. Presented at the 26th Annual Orthopaedic Research Society Meeting, 1980.

31. Kuei SC, Woo SL-Y, Gomez MA, Amiel D, Akeson WH. The study of strength characteristics of bone–ligament complex—a new methodology. *Trans Orthop Res Soc* 1980;5:355.

32. Lane JM, Bora FW, Block J. *Cis*-hydroxyproline limits work necessary to flex a digit after tendon surgery. *Clin Orthop* 1975;109:193–200.

33. Laros GS, Cooper RR. Electron microscopic visualization of protein polysaccharides. *Clin Orthop* 1972;84:179–192.

34. Laros GS, Tipton CM, Cooper RM. Influence of physical activity on ligament insertions in the knees of dogs. *J Bone Joint Surg* 1971;53A:275–286.

35. Lindy S, Turto H, Uitto J. Protocollagen proline hydroxylase activity in rat heart during experimental cardiac hypertrophy. *Circulation Res* 1972;30:205–209.

36. Nimni ME. Collagen: structure, function and metabolism in normal and fibrotic tissues. *Sem Arthritis Rheum* 1983;13:1–85.

37. Noyes FR, Torvik PJ, Hyde WB, DeLucas JL. Biomechanics of ligament failure. II. An analysis of immobilization, exercise and reconditioning effects in primates. *J Bone Joint Surg* 1974;56A:1406–1418.

38. Peacock EE. Comparison of collagenous tissue surrounding normal and immobilized joints. *Surg Forum* 1963;14:440–441.

39. Peacock EE. Biology of tendon repair. *N Engl J Med* 1967;276:680–683.

40. Rasch PJ, Maniscalco R, Pierson WR, Logan GA. Effect of exercise, immobilization and intermittent stretching on strength of knee ligaments of albino rats. *J Appl Physiol* 1960;15:289–290.

41. Renzoni SA, Amiel D, Harwood F, Akeson WH. Synovial nutrition of knee ligaments. *Trans Orthop Res Soc* 1984;9:277.

42. Skinner HB, Wyatt MP, Stone ML, Hodgdon JA, Barrack RL. Exercise-related knee joint laxity. *Am J Sports Med* 1986;14:30–34.

43. Slack HGB. The metabolism of sulphated polysaccharides in limb atrophy in the rat. *Biochem J* 1955;60:112–118.

44. Stoller DW, Markolf KL, Zager SA, Shoemaker SC. The effects of exercise, ice, and ultrasonography on torsional laxity of the knee. *Clin Orthop* 1983;174:172–180.

45. Suominen H, Heikkinen E. Enzyme activities in muscle and connective tissue of M. vastus lateralis in habitually training and sedentary 33- to 70-year old men. *Eur J Appl Physiol* 1975;34:249–254.

46. Swann DA, Radin EL, Nazimiec M. Role of hyaluronic acid in joint lubrication. *Ann Rheum Dis* 1974;33:318–326.

47. Tipton CM, James SL, Mergner W, et al. Influence of exercise on strength of medial collateral knee ligaments of dogs. *Am J Physiol* 1970;218:894–902.

48. Tipton CM, Matthes RD, Maynard JA, Carey RA. The influence of physical activity on ligaments and tendons. *Med Sci Sports Exerc* 1975;7:165–175.

49. Tipton CM, Schild RJ, Flatt AE. Measurements of ligamentous strength in rat knees. *J Bone Joint Surg* 1967;49A:63–72.

50. Tipton CM, Schild RJ, Tomanek RJ. Influence of physical activity on the strength of knee ligaments in rats. *Am J Physiol* 1967;212:783–787.

51. Tipton CM, Tcheng T-K, Mergner W. Ligamentous strength measurements from hypophysectomized rats. *Am J Physiol* 1971;221:1144–1150.

52. Vailas AC, Tipton CM, Matthes RD, Gart M. Physical activity and its influence on the repair process of medial collateral ligaments. *Connect Tissue Res* 1981;9:25–31.

53. Vailas AC, Tipton CM, Laughlin HL, Tcheng TK, Matthes RD. Physical activity and hypophysectomy on the aerobic capacity of ligaments and tendons. *J Appl Physiol* 1978;44:542–546.

54. Vindeman T, Eronen I, Friman C, Langenskiold A. Glycosaminoglycan metabolism of the medial meniscus, the medial collateral ligament and the hip joint capsule in experimental osteoarthritis caused by immobilization of the rabbit knee. *Acta Orthop Scand* 1979;50:465–470.

55. Vindeman T, Nichelsson J-E, Langenskiold A. The development of radiographic changes in experimental osteoarthritis provoked by immobilization of the knee in rabbits. *Int Res Comm Syst Med Sci* 1977;5:62–68.

56. Weisman G, Pope MH, Johnson RJ. The effect of cyclic loading on knee ligaments. *Trans Orthop Res Soc* 1979;4:24.

57. Wolff J. *Das Gesetz der Transformation der Knochen*. Berlin, 1892.

58. Woo SL-Y. Mechanical properties of tendons and ligaments II. The relationship of immobilization and exercise on tissue remodeling. *Biorheology* 1982;19:397–408.

59. Woo SL-Y, Gomez MA, Sites TJ, Newton PO, Orlando C, Akeson WH. The biomechanical and morphological changes in the medial collateral ligament of the rabbit after immobilization and remobilization. *J Bone Joint Surg* 1987;69A:1200–1211.

60. Woo SL-Y, Kuei SC, Gomez MA, Winters JM, Amiel D, Akeson WH. The effect of immobilization and exercise on the strength characteristics of bone–medial collateral ligament–bone complex. *Am Soc Mech Eng Symp* 1979;32:67–70.

61. Yaru NC, Danzig LA, Hargens AR, Gershuni DH, Simpkins A, Gorball MA, Johnson MA, Amiel D, Akeson WH. Facilitation of meniscal nutrition by continuous passive motin. *Trans Orthop Res Soc* 1984;9:279.

62. Zuckerman J, Stull GA. Effects of exercise on knee ligament separation force in rats. *J Appl Physiol* 1969;26:716–719.

63. Zuckerman J, Stull GA. Ligamentous separation force in rats as influenced by training, detraining, and cage restriction. *Med Sci Sports Exerc* 1973;5:44–49.

CHAPTER 17

The Response of Ligaments to Stress Deprivation and Stress Enhancement

Biomechanical Studies

Savio L-Y. Woo, Caroline W. Wang, Peter O. Newton, and Roger M. Lyon

Ligaments, like other tissues of the body, have the ability to respond to environmental demands. This homeostatic response appears to be stress-dependent, with the ligament adapting positively to increased stress and negatively to decreased stress. The biomechanical properties of ligaments have been studied extensively in situations of both stress deprivation and stress enhancement. Tensile testing of the bone–ligament–bone complex allows determination of the structural properties of this composite, which is made up of bone, ligament insertion site, and ligament substance. The structural properties that characterize the bone–ligament–bone complex include: linear stiffness, ultimate load, ultimate deformation, and energy absorbed at failure. (For a definition of these terms and the detailed experimental methodology, see Chapter 7). It is also possible to determine the mechanical (material) properties of the ligament substance from the same tensile test (28). With measurements of the cross-sectional area and tensile strain of the ligament, a stress–strain relationship for the ligament can be generated. From this relationship, tensile strength, ulti-

mate strain, and the tangent modulus can be obtained. Technological advances have permitted accurate determination of the biomechanical behavior of a bone–ligament–bone complex and its changes relating to applied motion and forces. The following section will discuss the experimental findings regarding changes in the biomechanical properties of various knee ligaments through a wide spectrum of treatment modalities (i.e., from the conditions of joint immobilization, followed by subsequent remobilization, to increased ligament tension and exercise training).

EFFECTS OF IMMOBILIZATION

Treatment of musculoskeletal injuries often includes immobilization as part of the therapeutic regimen. This measure has been necessary to protect the injured tissue from disruptive forces during the early healing period. However, the deleterious effects of joint immobility on soft connective tissues are profound (12,18). The biomechanical properties of the ligaments and ligament insertion sites become significantly compromised following immobilization.

Increases in joint stiffness have been seen clinically following periods of joint immobilization, and the knee is no exception. This increase in stiffness is associated with proliferation of fibro-fatty connective tissue. In

S. L-Y. Woo, C. W. Wang, P. O. Newton, and R. M. Lyon: Orthopaedic Bioengineering Laboratory, Division of Orthopaedic Surgery, University of California, San Diego, School of Medicine, La Jolla, California 92093; and San Diego Veterans Administration Medical Center, La Jolla, California 92161.

337

cases of prolonged immobilization, this process can obliterate the joint space, as observed by Enneking (7), who studied human pathology specimens which were immobilized for many months. Resulting synovial adhesions may lead to tearing of the articular surface during forced manipulation. Evans (8) evaluated rat knee joints that had been immobilized for 15–90 days and observed, histologically, a proliferation of fatty connective tissue within the joint. Adhesions formed by this tissue were well established by 30 days and were felt to substantially contribute to the joint stiffness. Langenskiold (13) reported periarticular soft tissue thickening, which was evident after only 2 weeks of immobilization of rabbit knees in extension. They noted marked joint stiffness restricting knee motion to only 20–40° after 2–14 weeks of immobilization. However, it should be noted that most animal models evaluated up to 90 days have contracture which is not easily explained by gross adhesions and which is probably due to microfibrillar alterations at a microscopic level.

Clinically, joint stiffness is difficult to evaluate quantitatively; however, it has been accomplished experimentally in animals, using an instrument called the *arthrograph* (32). This device measures the amount of torque and energy required to cycle a rabbit knee joint through a range of motion. When the knee joint is cycled between 50° and 80° of flexion, a torque (T) versus angular rotation (θ) curve is generated. Energy is required to cycle the knee through this arc of motion and is represented by the area within the hysteresis loop (Fig. 17-1). The amount of torque required to extend the knee to a predetermined angle of flexion, such as 65° or 80°, represents joint stiffness. Our laboratory reported that after 9 weeks of immobilization, the rabbit knee joint required a manyfold increase in the amount of torque and energy necessary to extend the joint (Fig. 17-1). These increases in knee joint stiffness may be largely attributed to adhesions of the periarticular connective tissues (1,2). One possible hypothesis for the mechanism of contracture is that the new collagen fibrils, synthesized during the immobilization period, form interfibrillar contacts and restrict normal sliding of fibers in the extensible structures of the joint capsule. Normally, collagen fibers of the periarticular capsule are arranged in a cross-weave pattern; these fibers straighten and become parallel upon loading. This change in fiber alignment is dependent on fibers sliding independent of neighboring fibers and accounts for the initial high compliance normally seen in this tissue. Very little load is generated until the collagen fibers become parallel. Figure 17-2 illustrates this concept and demonstrates how interfibrillar crosslinking can cause joint contracture (1).

The structural properties of the femur–ligament–tibia complex of the knee also significantly change following immobilization. We have demonstrated drastic

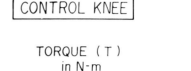
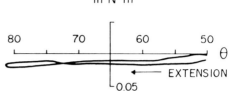
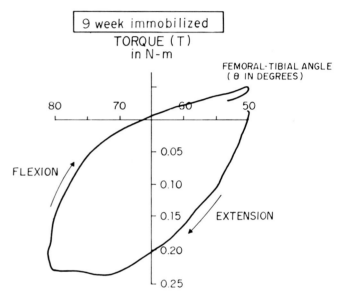

FIG. 17-1. Torque–angular-rotation curves of control and immobilized rabbit knees. (Modified from ref. 1.)

decreases in structural properties using a rabbit model after 9 weeks of knee joint immobilization (29). The femur–medial collateral ligament–tibia complex (FMTC) of the immobilized knee failed at a tensile load of only 29% of that of the contralateral nonimmobilized knee. Meanwhile, the energy absorbed at failure decreased to 16% of the contralateral controls (Fig. 17-3) (30). Other investigators have observed similar trends. Tipton (20) reported a 28% decrease in ultimate load of the rat bone–medial collateral ligament (MCL) complex after 6 weeks of plaster-cast immobilization. Studies of complexes involving the anterior cruciate ligament (ACL) show similar results. Larsen (15) found a 25% decrease in the ultimate load and linear stiffness of the femur–ACL–tibia complex (FATC) of rats after a period of 4 weeks of immobilization. Noyes (16) found similar decreases in the structural properties of the FATC of rhesus monkeys after 8 weeks of total body-cast immobilization.

The structural integrity of the bone–ligament–bone

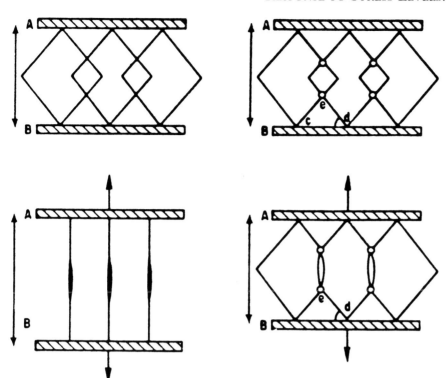

FIG. 17-2. Model demonstrating the loss of compliance when collagen fiber sliding in the connective tissue matrix (A,B) is prevented. **Left:** Normal fiber sliding. **Right:** Matrix-fiber attachments (c,d) and interfibrillar attachments (e) prevent sliding. (From ref. 32.)

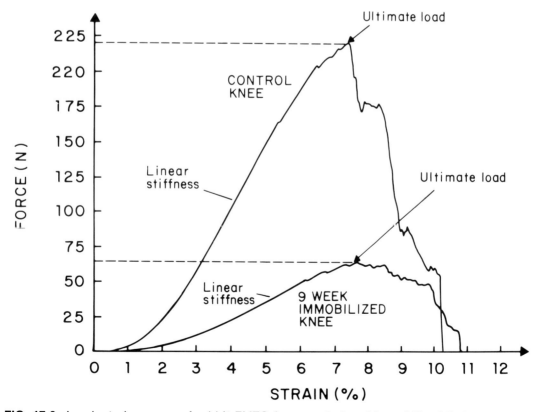

FIG. 17-3. Load–strain curves of rabbit FMTC from control and immobilized limbs. (Modified from ref. 30.)

complex has been found to be largely dependent on the quality of the attachment of the ligament to bone in a transition zone known as the *ligament insertion site*. The effects of joint immobility on the ligament insertion site are beginning to be better understood; they may be dependent on the specific site involved. For example, the tibial insertion of the MCL is much different from the femoral insertion (29). The subperiosteal (indirect) insertion into the tibia is made up of two layers: (i) a superficial layer in which fibers of the MCL join with the periosteum and (ii) a deep layer with fibers obliquely anchored into bone. In contrast, the ligament at the femoral insertion passes directly through zones of fibrocartilage, mineralized fibrocartilage, and bone. Our histological preparations demonstrated a clear disruption of the deep fibers inserting into bone at the tibial insertion of the MCL following immobilization. Osteoclasts were activated during immobilization, leading to resorption of subperiosteal bone and disruption of the attaching ligamentous collagen fibers. There were only minimal changes at the femoral (direct) insertion. As a result, the distal MCL was secured by its superficial periosteal attachment, and a large reduction in strength of the FMTC resulted after 9 weeks of immobilization (Fig. 17-3). Furthermore, the failure mode occurred exclusively by avulsion of the MCL at the tibial insertion (29). Similarly, Laros (14) reported that following knee joint immobilization, during tensile testing, the FMTC of dogs failed at the tibial attachment site. This occurrence was correlated with a histological demonstration of bone resorption at the tibial insertion site. Examining the ACL–bone complex, Noyes (16) found subperiosteal resorption in the tibia and femur of immobilized primates. The percentage of failures by ACL avulsion increased slightly with immobilization, and this investigator concluded that the loss of cortex immediately beneath the ligament insertion was responsible for reducing the strength of the ACL–bone junction. The nearly uniform failure of the FMTC by avulsion at the tibial insertion may be a reflection of the changes in the unique distal MCL attachment to the tibia following stress and motion deprivation. The less dramatic effects on the insertion sites of the ACL following immobilization may be due to the more stable nature of the direct type of insertion of the ACL into both the tibia and the femur.

Since changes in the structural properties of the bone–ligament–bone complex may be, in part, due to changes in the mechanical properties of either the bone, the ligament insertion sites, or the ligament substance, it is important to attempt to separate the effects of joint immobility on each of these components. Therefore, changes in the mechanical properties of the ligament substance are equally as important as the changes that have been demonstrated in the structural behavior of the bone–ligament–bone complex. Determination of the mechanical properties of a ligament requires generating a stress–strain relationship of its substance. Our laboratory has accomplished this and has measured ligament strain in a noncontact fashion using a video dimension analyzer (VDA) system (28). (Also see Chapter 7.) With this technique we found decreases in the tensile strength and tangent modulus (defined as the slope between 2% and 4% strain) for the rabbit MCL following 9 weeks of immobilization. Stress–strain curves demonstrating these changes are presented in Fig. 17-4 (29). Meanwhile, minimal histologic changes were noted in the middle of these ligaments. Normal parallel alignment of the collagen fibrils and periodic crimp pattern were maintained. Recent preliminary work in our laboratory suggests increased cellularity within portions of the immobilized MCL. Further investigation will be required to confirm these findings. Binkley (5) demonstrated similar changes in mechanical properties after immobilization in the rat MCL. He also observed a shift in the fibril cross-sectional area distribution, noting a significantly decreased proportion of small fibers, which he attributed to decreased synthesis and decreased degradation. From these observations he suggested that a relationship between ultrastructural properties and mechanical properties might exist. Gamble (10) demonstrated decreased cytoplasmic and mitochondrial enzymatic activity (of the MCL) after 4 weeks of immobilization. Increased lysosomal enzymatic activity, responsible for glycosaminoglycan (GAG) degradation, was also noted. In addition, this investigator reported histologic changes in the MCL after 8 weeks of immobilization which included loss of eosinophilic staining and widely spaced irregular collagen fascicles.

Amiel (3,4) demonstrated an increase in collagen turnover with immobility. The rate of degradation was matched by the rate of synthesis; therefore, after 9 weeks of immobilization, no significant changes in tissue mass were detected. With longer periods of immobilization (i.e., 12 weeks), degradation had outpaced synthesis, leading to ligament atrophy. The higher turnover of collagen may have a significant effect on the mechanical properties of MCL, since the new collagen synthesized during joint immobility would not be required to resist tensile loads or enhance joint motion. Also, the newly synthesized collagen fibers may be arranged haphazardly, and the crosslinking may be less efficient in resisting tensile force. Morphologic and chemical changes are discussed in more detail in Chapter 16. Decreases in GAG content could also significantly affect interfibrillar collagen interactions. However, many questions remain unanswered as to what cellular events are responsible for the decrease in the mechanical properties of immobilized ligaments. Further biochemical study of the collagen

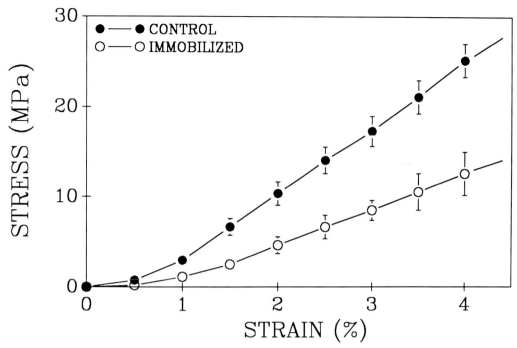

FIG. 17-4. Mechanical properties (represented by stress–strain curves) of normal and immobilized MCL from the rabbit knee. (Modified from ref. 29.)

structure of immobilized ligaments, as well as study of its ultrastructure using transmission electron microscopy, would help in the understanding of the changes seen in the mechanical properties of the ligament substance.

EFFECTS OF REMOBILIZATION

When a patient's knee is removed from a long leg cast (after a period of immobilization), what will be the future of these mechanically compromised ligaments and ligament insertion sites? This important question addresses the fact that immobilized joints are less able to resist applied loads and are therefore more susceptible to reinjury in the time after immobilization.

Several studies have been reported on the effects of reconditioning on ligament–bone complexes after immobilization and have found that increased activity, or remobilization, leads to a slow reversal of the immobilization effects on the structural properties of the bone–ligament complex. Noyes (16) subjected primates to 8 weeks of body-cast immobilization and demonstrated that a 12-month period of remobilization was required for the structural properties of the FATC to approach normal control values. Laros (14) studied remobilization effects in the canine MCL. After 6 weeks of immobilization of the lower extremity, 18 weeks of remobilization were required for the structural properties of the FMTC to return to normal. The

recovering ligament insertion sites demonstrated new bone formation, whereas prior to remobilization they had demonstrated bony resorption. In contrast, Larsen (15) examined rats that were retrained for 6 weeks with a swimming regimen, following a 4-week immobilization period. This short remobilization period was sufficient to return the stiffness and strength characteristics of the FATC to control levels. He also noted that avulsion failures at the insertion sites that prevailed in the immobilized group decreased in frequency after remobilization.

The above studies have presented only the structural properties of the bone–ligament–bone complexes and, as such, have not ascertained whether the prolonged recovery times apply to the insertion sites, the ligament substance, or both. Our laboratory has studied the MCL substance of rabbit knees remobilized for 9 weeks after 9 weeks of immobilization. The stress–strain relationship of the MCL substance in the remobilized limbs was similar to the controls after this period of increased motion (Fig. 17-5B). This observation demonstrates the relatively rapid return of the mechanical properties of the ligament substance to normal levels following remobilization (29). Structural properties of the FMTC, however, remained inferior (Fig. 17-5A). The ultimate load and energy absorbed at failure attained only 80% of the control values. Also, failures of the FMTC continued to occur at the ligament insertion sites. Histological examination of these insertion sites revealed incomplete reorganization

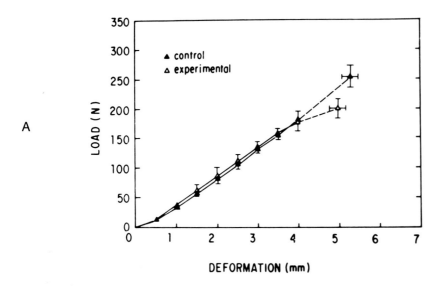

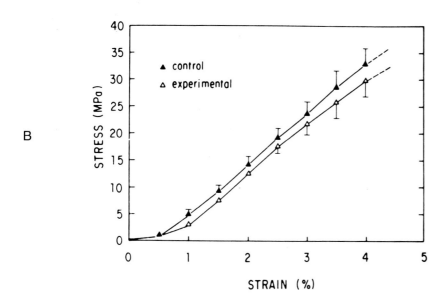

FIG. 17-5. Effects of 9 weeks of immobilization and 9 weeks of remobilization. **A:** Structural properties of the FMTC. **B:** Mechanical properties of the MCL substance. (Modified from ref. 29.)

after 9 weeks of cage activity. In comparison, a group of animals that had been allowed 52 weeks of cage activity after a period of 12 weeks of immobilization demonstrated complete reconstitution of the MCL insertion sites. Thus, the rapid decline in the structural properties of bone–ligament–bone complexes with immobilization are reversible with resumed motion. Unfortunately, the bone–ligament–bone structure remains weak for a significant period of time. A remobilization period of up to sixfold that of the time of immobilization may be required for recovery. These findings suggest that the patient treated with a long leg cast may have weakened ligament insertion sites for at least several months following an immobilization period as short as a few weeks. It appears that the

prolonged recovery time is due largely to the slow remodeling at the ligament insertion sites which occurs during joint remobilization. This slow process is asynchronous with respect to the more rapid recovery of the mechanical properties of the ligament substance.

EFFECTS OF INCREASED TENSION

While increased stress levels profoundly improve the biomechanical properties of previously immobilized ligaments, their effect on normal ligaments deserves equal attention. Numerous animal studies have suggested that elevated stress levels incurred by exercise improve normal ligament properties. We will discuss these changes later in the chapter. These results have important implications, especially when considering the frequency and circumstances of ligament injury. An increased tensile strength or stiffness, as a result of exercise training, will help to reduce the likelihood of ligamentous failure when subjected to strenuous physical activity. Routine exercise regimens might be prescribed, in turn, as a preventive measure for athletes or others participating in nonsedentary activities to reduce the chances of injury. Thus, an understanding of the effects of increased stress on ligaments is important.

In our laboratory, Gomez (11) studied the effect of increased tension on the rabbit MCL by inserting a stainless steel pin underneath the ligament. The pin was 9.5 mm in length and 1.6 mm in diameter and was placed perpendicular to the distal end of the ligament. The response to the added tension was evaluated at "zero time" in an *in vitro* model and at 6 and 12 weeks post-surgery in an *in vivo* model. In an earlier study (see Chapter 7), our laboratory had demonstrated that the strain, stress, and load in the rabbit MCL of an intact knee at 90° were 3.5%, 1 MPa, and 3.0 N, respectively (27). Regional changes in the stresses and strains across the width of the ligament were observed while extending the knee to 60° and flexing to 120°. For example, at 60° of flexion, the stresses ranged from 0.25 MPa in the anterior region to 4 MPa in the posterior region, while the strains varied from 2% (anterior region) to 5.4% (posterior region). In the *in vitro* model, insertion of the pin underneath the ligament increased the strain levels from 2.5% to 4% at 90° of flexion. At 60° and 120° of flexion, the strains in the

anterior and posterior regions were elevated by 1%. Meanwhile, the loads and stresses increased by 2- to 3.5-fold in each region of the MCL. At 90° of flexion, the load was elevated from 5.8 N to 18.0 N, while the stress in each region rose from 0.5 MPa to 1.6 MPa. The insertion of the pin was also responsible for significant increases in the loads at other angles of knee flexion. For 60° of flexion, the load increased from 10 N to over 20 N, whereas at 120°, it changed from 6 N to 15 N (Fig. 17-6).

Knowing the quantitative increases in stress and load levels in the MCL, the response of the ligament to the new level of stress was studied *in vivo* in a series of animals. Like the *in vitro* studies, a stainless steel pin was inserted surgically beneath the MCL of the left hind limb. The right hind limb was sham operated to serve as a control. The animals were sacrificed at 6 and 12 weeks post-surgery, during which time they were allowed free cage activity. At sacrifice, the strains in the MCL were measured in a manner similar to those in the *in vitro* samples, so that the load and stress in the MCL could be subsequently determined.

By 6 weeks post-surgery, load–deformation curves of the FMTC were similar up to 4 mm of deformation for normal ligaments with increased tension and without increased tension. Beyond this point the structural behavior of the two groups began to diverge. The FMTC with the increased tension failed at a 26% higher ultimate load than that of controls, whereas the ultimate deformation was 33% higher. However, by 12 weeks these differences diminished, and the load–deformation curves became similar for both groups (Table 17-1). Histologically, there was a reaction to

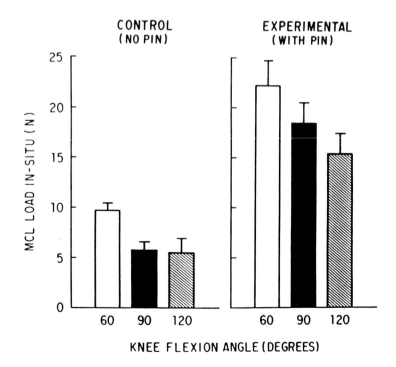

FIG. 17-6. *In situ* load in the rabbit MCL at different angles of flexion with and without increased tension. (From ref. 11.)

TABLE 17-1. *Structural properties of the rabbit FMTC in response to increased tension, 6 and 12 weeks post-surgery*

Property	6 weeks		12 weeks	
	Sham-op	Tension	Sham-op	Tension
MCL cross-sectional area (mm²)	4.0 ± 0.3	4.5 ± 0.4	4.5 ± 0.1	5.2 ± 0.9
Ultimate load (N)	140 ± 42	177 ± 40	248 ± 27	234 ± 67
Ultimate deformation (mm)	5.1 ± 0.4	6.8 ± 0.1[b]	6.8 ± 1.0	7.0 ± 0.8
Linear stiffness (N/mm) (3–4 mm deformation)	39 ± 9	29 ± 8	53 ± 10	48 ± 9

[a] From ref. 11.
[b] $p < 0.05$.

the pin, as noted by surrounding increased cellularity. Increasing the tension in the ligament induced remodeling of the collagen fibers. Regional changes in fiber alignment and a flattened crimp pattern were observed.

Comparison of the mechanical properties of the ligament substance at 6 weeks showed that for a given strain level, the stress was lower for the MCL under increased tension (i.e., a lower tangent modulus). However, by 12 weeks, this trend had reversed: The group with increased MCL tension exhibited higher stress values than the control group at a given strain level. A numerical analysis of the data was employed to compare the shapes of these curves. Constitutive equations characterizing the stress–strain relations were derived from a pseudo-strain energy density func-

tion formulated by Fung (9). Material constants in this equation were obtained by curve-fitting experimental data and subsequently were compared statistically to differentiate the stress–strain curves. The salient result of this study was that increased tension in the ligament led to improved biomechanical properties by 12 weeks post-surgery (Fig. 17-7). In view of these results, future studies should consider longer duration studies, comparable to studies of exercise training regimens, to be discussed next.

EFFECTS OF EXERCISE

Results of experimental animal studies suggest that exercise can indeed strengthen ligament structures. Bio-

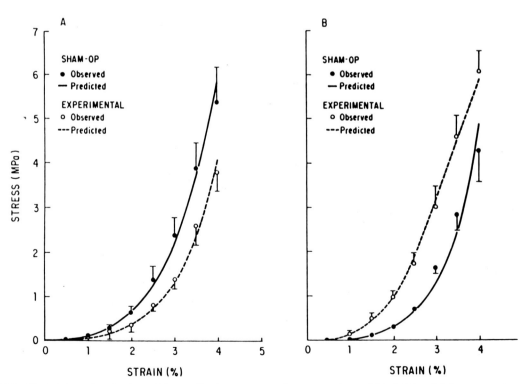

FIG. 17-7. Experimental and theoretical stress–strain curves for rabbit MCL with increased tension. **A:** Six weeks post-surgery. **B:** Twelve weeks post-surgery. (From ref. 11.)

mechanical properties of the ligament substance and the insertion sites are affected by exercise, and some histological changes have been documented as well. Laros (14) studied the effects of various activity levels on the strength of the canine MCL and on the morphological changes in the insertion sites. The ultimate load, normalized to body weight, correlated with the level of activity. The highest value occurred in the most active dogs (which were maintained in large pens), followed by caged dogs, then immobilized dogs. Histological examination of the insertion sites demonstrated resorption at some sites but not at others. Interestingly, this investigator noted that limited activity resulting from confinement in a cage for more than 6 weeks induced bone resorption at the MCL insertion into the proximal tibia. Tipton (22,24) also examined the effects of exercise on knee structures. Primates were trained on a treadmill for 20 weeks (22). The MCL weight/length ratio (an indirect method for determining cross-sectional area) increased significantly by 26%. Tensile strength measurements revealed an increase of over 30% in the patellar tendon but revealed no change in the MCL or in the lateral collateral ligament (LCL). The ultimate load of the FMTC *in situ* was not found to be affected by exercise.

Noyes (17), also using a primate model, analyzed the effects of various activity levels on the ACL. In one experimental group, the right lower limb was exercised daily, while the rest of the body was immobilized in a cast. The active exercise was found to be ineffective in preventing the detrimental effects of immobilization. Load–deformation curves of the exercised FATC were similar to those of the limbs immobilized by the casts. Bone resorption was evident at the insertion sites of both the exercised and the immobilized specimens. In contrast, Viidik (25) demonstrated positive effects of training on the structural properties of the rabbit ACL. The ultimate load, ultimate deformation, and energy absorbed at failure of the FATC were elevated significantly above control levels in response to 40 weeks of daily training. Thus, strengthening of the bone as a result of training was responsible for the observed structural changes. Viidik also found that the stress-relaxation behavior of the ligaments from the trained animals differed from that of the controls. The rate of relaxation was faster, and the amount of stress relaxation was higher (i.e., stress values were lowered). These findings indicate that the tensile properties of the ligament substance were altered as a result of the exercise training.

The differences in ligament responses to exercise might be attributed to the different animal species. However, it has been shown that other factors may influence the response of the ligament to increased stress levels. Zuckerman (33) subjected rats to 9 weeks of swimming or running (15 min/day, 5 days/week).

This forced physical activity accompanied by ad lib cage activity increased the ultimate load of the bone–ligament–bone complexes of the MCL and LCL by more than 35% over those of the untrained controls. Similarly, Tipton (20) demonstrated in the rat that 10 weeks of endurance training in treadmills significantly increased the ultimate load of the FMTC and the ultimate load/body weight ratio by 10%. The energy absorbed at failure of the trained animals was 20% higher than that of the untrained group. Other changes induced by the exercise included a 10% increase in ligament weight, indicating hypertrophy of the ligament. In contrast, sprint training had no effect on the strength of the FMTC but produced heavier ligaments. Also, the response to a single exercise bout was found to have no effect on any of the measured biomechanical characteristics of the MCL. The properties of the ligament were enhanced only when the animals were subjected to endurance exercise.

In another study, Tipton (21) compared two types of endurance exercise and found a 12% increase in the ultimate load of the FMTC as a result of running on a graded surface. Level running, however, did not affect the ultimate load of the FMTC. The authors attributed this observation to a lack of stimulation or stress imposed to knee structures while running on a flat surface. Frequency and duration of exercise may also play a role. Cabaud (6) examined the ACL of rats after 8 weeks of training on a treadmill. The animals were divided into exercise groups of varying duration (30 or 60 min/day) and frequency (3 or 6 days/week). Biomechanical properties assessed included linear stiffness, ultimate load, energy absorbed at failure, tangent modulus, tensile strength, and ultimate strain. Exercising 6 days/week proved to be more effective than 3 days/week at increasing each of these properties. Also, exercise periods of 30 min/day enhanced the linear stiffness, ultimate load, tangent modulus, and tensile strength more than 60 min/day. The higher frequency and shorter duration exercise regimen yielded the greatest changes in the ultimate load (17% increase), linear stiffness (7% increase), and energy absorbed at failure (31% increase). Tensile strength and ultimate strain of the ACL also were both elevated by approximately 20%.

Age and sex may also determine the response of ligaments to exercise. Tipton (23) showed that exercise significantly increased the tensile strength of the isolated LCL for 6- and 12-month-old rats but not for 18- and 24-month-old rats. In another study, Tipton (19) showed that male and female rats responded differently to 10–15 weeks of exercise. While males experienced a significant increase in ultimate load/body weight ratio of the FMTC, females showed no such increase. From these studies it is clear that multiple

TABLE 17-2. Structural properties of control and exercised swine FMTC[a]

Property	Control (n − 7)	Exercised (n − 10)
Ultimate load (N)	945.0 ± 74.0	1008.0 ± 83.0
Ultimate load/body weight (N/kg)	1.3 ± 0.1	1.8 ± 0.2[b]
Ultimate deformation (mm)	10.4 ± 0.3	10.0 ± 0.5
Linear stiffness (10^4 N/m)	10.8 ± 0.8	12.3 ± 0.6
Energy absorbed at failure (N-m)	4.3 ± 0.4	4.4 ± 0.6

[a] From ref. 31. Data are expressed as mean ± standard error.
[b] $p < 0.05$.

factors including age and sex must be controlled in exercise studies.

Changes induced by long-term exercise are equally important, but only limited data are available. Our laboratory studied the effects of prolonged exercise on the biomechanical properties of the FMTC (31). One-year-old swine were trained for 12 months on a schedule of 1 hr/day at 1.6 m/sec plus 0.5 hr every other day at 2.2 m/sec, based on a 5-day/week regimen. Age-matched control swine were allowed ad lib activity in 1.5- × 3-m cages during this time. At sacrifice the average body weights of the two groups were significantly different from each other; the exercised swine were 66 ± 6 kg, while the controls were 77 ± 16 kg. Tensile testing showed that this long-term exercise in-

duced some increases in the structural properties of the FMTC. As shown in Table 17-2, the ultimate load increased from 945 ± 74 N to 1008 ± 83 N. These values were not statistically different, but when normalized to body weight, a 38% increase was shown. There was also a 14% increase in the linear stiffness, while ultimate deformation remained unaffected. Figure 17-8 graphically displays the stress–strain characteristics of the MCL substance. It can be seen that the long-term exercise produced slight increases in tangent modulus (measured between 4% and 10% strain), a 20% increase in tensile strength, and a 10% increase in ultimate strain.

Also in our laboratory, the effects of a lifelong duration of exercise training on the biomechanical properties of the FMTC are being investigated. In a collaborative study with the University of Iowa (Dr. J. A. Albright, Dr. J. Buckwalter, and Dr. R. Martin), beagles were exercised on a treadmill for most of their life span (26). The training schedule involved running at a speed of 3 km/hr for 75 min/day, 5 days/week, for a total training period of 420–557 weeks. While exercising, the animals were also fitted with an 11-kg backpack. Age-matched control animals subjected to cage activity for the same duration were also studied. The FMTC of the control and trained animals were tested in tension using standard methodology previously described. Addressing the aging effects, the FMTC of young, skeletally mature beagles approximately 1 year of age also were tested.

Preliminary data suggest that the lifelong exercise training had little or no effect on the structural prop-

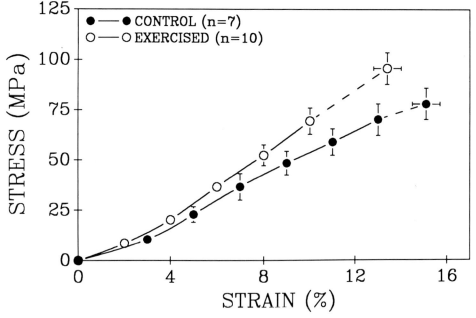

FIG. 17-8. Stress–strain curves of control and exercised swine MCL.

erties of the FMTC, as demonstrated by the similar load–deformation curves as well as specific structural parameters (Fig. 17-9A). The linear stiffness (taken between 2.5 and 5.0 mm deformation), ultimate load, ultimate deformation, and energy absorbed at failure were seemingly unaffected by the exercise (Table 17-3). Comparing these data to the biomechanical properties of the younger samples, values for linear stiffness, ultimate load, ultimate deformation, and energy absorbed at failure did not reflect significant differences. The mechanical properties of the MCL substance of the control and trained groups also were not shown to be statistically different from one another. Table 17-3 shows how the values for tangent modulus (measured between 4% and 8% strain), tensile strength, and ultimate strain were also similar for both groups. Figure 17-9B further demonstrates the similar stress–strain behaviors of both groups. The effect of age, however, had a pronounced effect on the mechanical properties. The younger samples failed at sig-

nificantly higher tensile strengths (40% higher) and ultimate strains (40% higher). The young samples were shown to have structural properties similar to those of their older counterparts. However, the mechanical properties of the MCL substance differed significantly from the aged animals, since the younger MCLs were much smaller and shorter. For the older animals, the lack of changes in the biomechanical properties after an intensive exercise regimen for their entire life span is indeed surprising. It was not possible to perform a time study in these animals, so interval effects are not known. Conceivably, processes of aging have taken effect and, as a result, have masked earlier positive effects of exercise. These findings suggest that a lifelong period of exercise training, in concert with the normal aging process, does not induce measurable changes in the biomechanical properties of the MCL. In order to determine the effects of each of these factors independently, future studies should be planned to include (a) shorter exercise periods (i.e., 2–3 years)

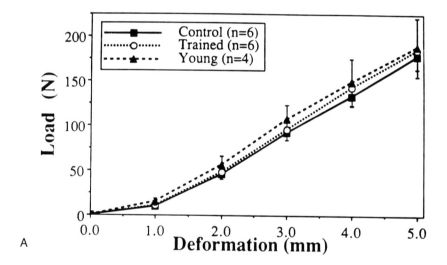

A

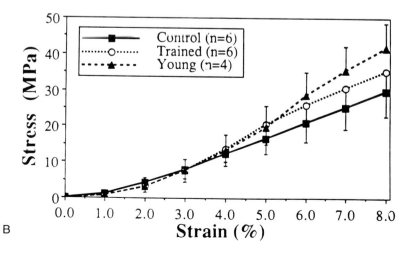

B

FIG. 17-9. Effects of long-term exercise on the canine MCL. A: Load–deformation curves depicting structural properties. B: Stress–strain curves illustrating mechanical properties. (From ref. 26.)

TABLE 17-3. *Structural and mechanical properties of control and exercised canine MCL[a]*

	Ultimate load (N)	Ultimate deformation (mm)	Stiffness (H/mm)	Energy absorbed (N-m)	Tangent modulus (MPa)	Tensile strength (MPa)	Ultimate strain (%)
Control (n = 6)	268.9 ± 29.2	8.0 ± 0.5	43.4 ± 3.6	1.10 ± 0.20	4.4 ± 0.9	57.4 ± 6.6[b]	12.4 ± 0.3[b]
Trained (n = 6)	295.1 ± 23.6	8.8 ± 0.9	45.2 ± 4.2	1.36 ± 0.29	6.0 ± 0.8	55.6 ± 5.2	12.0 ± 0.9
Young (n = 4)	290.6 ± 39.9	7.7 ± 0.4	41.9 ± 7.7	1.07 ± 0.19	7.1 ± 0.8	80.6 ± 5.0[c]	17.0 ± 1.1[d]

[a] From ref. 26.
[b] $n = 4$ due to two insertion-site failures.
[c] Different from control and trained groups at $p < 0.02$.
[d] Different from control and trained groups at $p < 0.01$.

and (b) the effects of aging through senescence, without exercise.

DISCUSSION

Clearly, different levels of stress, ranging from deprivation to enhancement, can produce a variety of effects on the biomechanical properties of knee ligaments and their insertion sites. These responses can be quantified by evaluation of changes in the structural properties of the bone–ligament–bone complex and in the mechanical properties of the ligament substance. Histological evaluation of these structures also reveals important corroborative information, since it suggests mechanisms by which the biomechanical changes are occurring. From the studies described in this chapter, a general trend of the responses of ligaments and their insertions to stress deprivation and enhancement emerges. This trend is depicted in Fig. 17-10, where the observations are schematically summarized (29). In general, immobilization quickly compromises the stiffness and strength of the bone–ligament–bone complex, and the weakening occurs most notably at the insertion sites. Ligaments, as well as their attachments to bone, become weaker, and failure under tensile loading occurs most frequently by ligament avulsion from bone. Histologic correlation with the biomechanical studies suggest that bony resorption by increased osteoclastic activity is the cause of insertion weakness following immobilization.

During remobilization, the biomechanical properties of the bone–ligament–bone complex may return to normal values, but only after a significant retraining period. However, one should note that the recovery rates of the components of the bone–ligament–bone complex are not the same (Fig. 17-10). The destruction of the insertion sites by immobilization is not readily overcome, since the repair processes of the insertion sites are slow. Such would not be the case for the ligament substance, since its recovery rate was found to mirror that during immobilization (Fig. 17-10). Thus, avulsion types of failure continue to occur. Nonethe-

less, this reversal of the immobilization effects is a remarkable phenomenon when considering the magnitude of the drop in the structural properties of the FMTC (50–70%) following immobilization.

The dramatic effect of remobilization, however, is very unlike the response of ligaments from animals which start from a normal, healthy baseline and are subjected to increased tension or exercise. Increasing the tension in the MCL by inserting a pin beneath it was effective in inducing increased stress levels in the ligament. While the biomechanical properties of the ligament were enhanced in response to this stress environment, the changes seen in load–deformation and stress–strain behavior were only mild improvements. Parameters such as ultimate load and deformation were significantly affected, but the magnitudes of these increases were noticeably smaller compared to immobilization changes. In the situation of exercise training, the effects on ligaments are less straightforward. Many factors are involved in determining the degree to which the tissue responds. These parameters include age, species, sex, exercise type, and exercise intensity. However, the cumulated data seem to indicate that increased stress levels enhance the structural and mechanical properties of ligaments. This effect is small, and a long duration of exercise is required (Fig. 17-10). To date, histological findings have been limited, and further studies along this avenue should be pursued. It is important, however, to consider the difficulties involved in these experiments. First, controlling the activity level in exercise studies is much more difficult than imposing no activity as in immobilization. Also, some exercise regimens may not involve enough motion or the appropriate movement patterns to extensively stress the knee structures. Hence, it is obvious that eliciting consistent responses would not be an easy task. Also, determination of normal homeostatic stress levels, necessary to maintain "normal qualities," are unknown and would be helpful for future exercise studies. Given the high incidence of knee injuries in conjunction with the high participation rate in athletic activities, the studies have major clinical relevance.

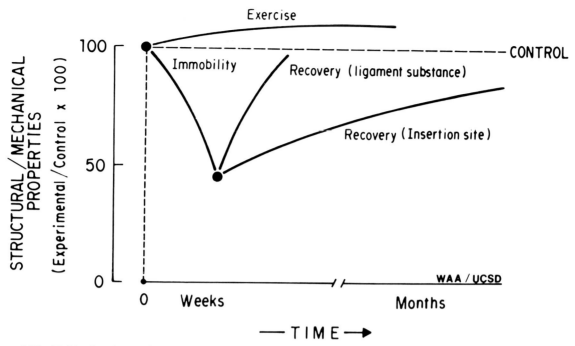

FIG. 17-10. A schematic representation of the time course and magnitude of effects of various stress levels on the structural and mechanical properties of ligaments. (From ref. 29.)

ACKNOWLEDGMENTS

We gratefully acknowledge the support of the following: Veterans Administration RR&D Grant A188-3RA; NIH Grants AR14918, AR33097, and AR34264; and the Malcolm and Dorothy Coutts Institute for Joint Reconstruction and Research.

REFERENCES

1. Akeson WH, Amiel D, Woo SL-Y. Immobility effects on synovial joints. The pathomechanics of joint contracture. *Biorheology* 1980;17:95–110.
2. Akeson WH, Woo SL-Y, Amiel D, Matthews JV. Biomechanical and biochemical changes in the periarticular connective tissue during contracture development in the immobilized rabbit knee. *Connect Tissue Res* 1974;2(4):315–323.
3. Amiel D, Akeson WH, Harwood FL, Frank CB. Stress deprivation effect on metabolic turnover of medial collateral ligament collagen. *Clin Orthop* 1983;172:265–270.
4. Amiel D, Woo SL-Y, Harwood FL, Akeson WH. The effect of immobilization on collagen turnover in connective tissue: a biochemical–biomechanical correlation. *Acta Orthop Scand* 1982; 53:325–332.
5. Binkley JM, Peat M. The effects of immobilization on the ultrastructure and mechanical properties of the medial collateral ligament of rats. *Clin Orthop* 1986;203:301–308.
6. Cabaud HE, Chatty A, Gildengorin V, Feltman RJ. Exercise effects on the strength of the rat anterior cruciate ligament. *Am J Sports Med* 1980;8(2):79–86.
7. Enneking WF, Horowitz M: The intra-articular effects of immobilization on the human knee. *J Bone Joint Surg [Am]* 1972;54A:973–985.
8. Evans EB, Eggers GWN, Butler JK, Blumel J. Experimental immobilization and remobilization of rat knee joints. *J Bone Joint Surg [Am]* 1960;42A(5):737–758.
9. Fung YC. Biorheology of soft tissues. *Biorheology* 1973;10:139–155.
10. Gamble JG, Edwards CC, Max SR. Enzymatic adaptation in ligaments during immobilization. *Am J Sports Med* 1984;12(3):221–228.
11. Gomez MA. The effect of tension on normal and healing medial collateral ligaments. Ph.D Thesis, University of California, San Diego, 1988.
12. Klein L, Player JS, Heiple KG, Bahniuk E, Goldberg VM. Isotopic evidence for resorption of soft tissues and bone in immobilized dogs. *J Bone Joint Surg [Am]* 1982;64A:225–230.
13. Langenskiold A, Michelsson JE, Videman T. Osteoarthritis of the knee in the rabbit produced by immobilization. *Acta Orthop Scand* 1979;50:1–14.
14. Laros GS, Tipton CM, Cooper RR. Influence of physical activity on ligament insertions in the knees of dogs. *J Bone Joint Surg [Am]* 1971;53A(2):275–286.
15. Larsen NP, Forwood MR, Parker AW. Immobilization and retraining of cruciate ligaments in the rat. *Acta Orthop Scand* 1987;58:260–264.
16. Noyes FR. Functional properties of knee ligaments and alterations induced by immobilization. A correlative biomechanical and histological study in primates. *Clin Orthop* 1977;123:210–242.
17. Noyes FR, Torvik PJ, Hyde WB, DeLucas JL. Biomechanics of ligament failure. *J Bone Joint Surg [Am]* 1974;56A(7):1406–1418.
18. Thaxter TH, Mann RA, Anderson CE. Degeneration of immobilized knee joints in rats. *J Bone Joint Surg [Am]* 1965;47A:567–585.
19. Tipton CM, Martin RK, Matthes RD, Carey RA. Hydroxyproline concentrations in ligaments from trained and nontrained rats. In: Howald H, Poortmans JR, eds. *Metabolic adaptation to prolonged physical exercise*. Basel: Birkhauser Verlag, 1975;262–267.
20. Tipton CM, Matthes RD, Maynard JA, Carey RA. The influence of physical activity on ligaments and tendons. *Med Sci Sports* 1975;7(3):165–175.
21. Tipton CM, Matthes RD, Vailas AC. Influences de l'exercise sur les structures ligamentaires. In: Lacour J, ed. *Facteurs lim-*

itant l'endurance humaine. Saint-Etienne Conference, 1977;103–114.

22. Tipton CM, Matthes RD, Vailas AC, Schnoebelen CL. The response of the Galago senegalensis to physical training. *Comp Biochem Physiol* 1979;63A:29–36.

23. Tipton CM, Vailas AC, Matthes RD. Experimental studies on the influences of physical activity on ligaments, tendons and joints: a brief review. *Acta Med Scand [Suppl]* 1986;711:157–168.

24. Vailas AC, Tipton CM, Matthes RD, Gart M. Physical activity and its influence on the repair process of medial collateral ligaments. *Connect Tissue Res* 1981;9:25–31.

25. Viidik A. Elasticity and tensile strength of the anterior cruciate ligament in rabbits as influenced by training. *Acta Physiol Scand* 1968;74:372–330.

26. Wang CW, Weiss JA, Albright JP, Buckwalter JA, Woo SL-Y. The effects of long term exercise on the structural and mechanical properties of the canine medial collateral ligament. *1989 ASME Biomech Symp AMD* 1989;98:69–72.

27. Weiss JA, Gomez MA, Hawkins DA, Woo SL-Y. The effect of epiphyseal closure on ligament *in situ* stresses and strains. In: *Proceedings of the 12th Annual Meeting of the ASB*. Urbana-Champaign, Illinois, 1988;106–107.

28. Woo SL-Y, Gomez MA, Seguchi Y, Endo CM, Akeson WH. Measurement of mechanical properties of ligament substance from a bone–ligament–bone preparation. *J Orthop Res* 1983;1:22–29.

29. Woo SL-Y, Gomez MA, Sites TJ, Newton PO, Orlando CA, Akeson WH. The biomechanical and morphological changes in the medial collateral ligament of the rabbit after immobilization and remobilization. *J Bone Joint Surg [Am]* 1987;69A(8):1200–1211.

30. Woo SL-Y, Gomez MA, Woo YK, Akeson WH. Mechanical properties of tendons and ligaments. II. The relationships of immobilization and exercise on tissue remodeling. *Biorheology* 1982;19:397–408.

31. Woo SL-Y, Kuei SC, Gomez MA, Winters JM, Amiel D, Akeson WH. The effect of immobilization and exercise on the strength characteristics of bone–medial collateral ligament–bone complex. *1979 ASME Biomech Symp AMD* 1979;32:67–70.

32. Woo SL-Y, Matthews JV, Akeson WH, Amiel D, Convery FR. Connective tissue response to immobility: correlative study of biomechanical measurements of normal and immobilized rabbit knees. *Arthritis Rheum* 1975;18:257–264.

33. Zuckerman J, Stull GA. Effects of exercise on knee ligament separation force in rats. *J Appl Physiol* 1969;26(6):716–719.

CHAPTER 18

The Response of Ligaments to Injury

Healing of the Collateral Ligaments

Savio L-Y. Woo, Shuji Horibe, Karen J. Ohland, and David Amiel

Torn collateral ligaments heal well, and clinical results following isolated collateral ligament injuries have generally been good (see Chapter 26). In order to improve healing and reduce recovery time, O'Donoghue (39) recommended surgical repair and subsequent immobilization. This concept of primary repair of torn collateral ligaments has been supported by several animal studies (8,40). Recently, however, Indelicato (22) and Hastings (21) reported good results following conservative treatment of patients with isolated collateral ligament tears. Experimental studies performed in our laboratory (15,62,66) have further demonstrated that conservative treatment of isolated medial collateral ligament (MCL) injury produced better results than surgical repair and immobilization.

EXPERIMENTAL TECHNIQUES FOR ASSESSMENT OF COLLATERAL LIGAMENT HEALING

In order to compare the relative success of different treatment regimens, it is essential that a multidisciplinary approach be used in evaluating the progress of healing, correlating histological, biochemical, and biomechanical results.

Histology

Hematoxylin and eosin (H&E) stain is used for routine histological evaluation of both cells (fibroblasts) and collagen fibers within the healing ligament. The degree of alignment of the collagen fibers and the "crimp" pattern reflect the stiffness and strength of the ligament and are, therefore, frequently examined. Polarized light microscopy is an effective way to visualize the "crimp" pattern and is helpful for evaluating the architecture of the injured ligament (56).

The characteristics of the cells in healing ligaments are also important to evaluate, since they indicate the

S. L-Y. Woo, S. Horibe, K. J. Ohland, and D. Amiel: Orthopaedic Bioengineering Laboratory, San Diego Veterans Administration Medical Center, San Diego, California, and University of California, San Diego, La Jolla, California 92093.

351

status of the various metabolic processes that are occurring within the ligament. One technique for examining cells involves immunological labeling such as the use of goat anti-rabbit fibronectin antibodies to label fibronectin containing cells within the ligament substance (31). In addition, electron microscopy permits more precise visualization of the structure of the fibroblast cells and collagen fibrils. Evaluation of the size of the collagen fibrils in the healing tissue may also be useful for assessing the maturation of the healing ligament (37).

Blood supply to the torn ligament is important in the early stages of healing, and revascularization is necessary during the remodeling phase. Microangiography permits (a) evaluation of the pattern of blood vessels at the repair site and (b) assessment of the extent of revascularization (5).

Biomechanics

Since the collateral ligaments are important supporting structures of the knee joint, assessment of the func-

tional status of the healing ligament should be part of the evaluative process. Therefore, a basic understanding of these biomechanical parameters (such as the structural properties of the bone–ligament–bone complex and the mechanical properties of the ligament substance), together with measurement of knee joint stability, is needed. We will discuss these biomechanical parameters below.

Measurement of Knee Joint Stability

Several methods have been developed to assess the role ligaments play in constraining joint motion. Some investigators have measured the force or moment produced by translation or rotation of a joint (18,46,49), whereas others have measured joint motion as a result of an externally applied load (23,35,36,62). However, the findings of these experimental studies have not been in agreement. The discrepancies may be due to the different species studied, the variety of testing protocols used, the constraints to knee motion inherent in the design of the experimental apparatus, or other un-

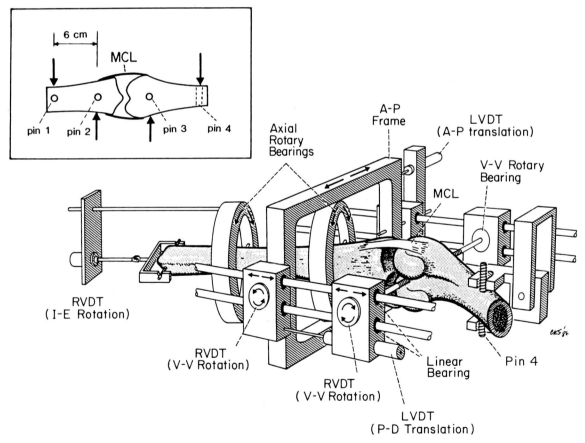

FIG. 18-1. The device used to measure the V–V rotation of the canine knee. The principle of four-point bending was used. This device allows the following: up to 5 DOF of knee motion during testing; three translations (anterior–posterior, proximal–distal, and medial–lateral); and two rotations (varus–valgus and internal–external). (From ref. 23.)

known factors. A normal knee has six degrees of free-dom (DOF) of motion: anterior–posterior, proximal–distal, and medial–lateral translations; and varus–val-gus, flexion–extension, and internal–external rota-tions. Therefore, measurement of knee stability with a device that does not permit normal knee motion may bias the experimental results. In our laboratory, we have investigated the influence of the number of DOF on varus–valgus (V V) knee rotation (23) using an ap-paratus designed to apply a V–V bending moment to canine knee joints fixed at a chosen angle of flexion (90°) (Fig. 18-1). The remaining 5 DOF, all three trans-lations and two rotations (V–V and internal–external), were permitted. In order to examine more constrained motion (e.g., 3 DOF), anterior–posterior translation and internal–external rotation were restricted. Valgus rotation was measured in both 3 and 5 DOF following transection of the MCL. We found that in the 3-DOF case after transection, the valgus rotation increased to 180% of that of the intact knee (23). When 5 DOF of motion was allowed, however, transection of the MCL had much less of an effect on the valgus rotation; that is, only a 21% increase over the intact knee was ob-served (Fig. 18-2). To assess the function of normal and/or healing MCL, therefore, measurement of valgus rotation by limiting the knee joint to 3 DOF is rec-ommended.

Tensile Testing

For evaluation of the biomechanical characteristics of the healing ligament, tensile testing of a bone–liga-ment–bone complex is usually performed. The exper-imental apparatus used is shown in Fig. 18-3. (For more details, see Chapter 7.) The results obtained from this testing procedure are the structural properties (i.e. the load–deformation curves), together with quanti-tative data on linear stiffness, ultimate load, ultimate deformation, and energy absorbed at failure (see Fig. 7-4A). Whereas structural properties reflect the bio-mechanical behavior of the ligament substance as well as that of the bone–ligament structure, the mechanical properties of the ligament reflect the biomechanical characteristics of the ligament substance alone. With the data on tensile load and the cross-sectional area of the ligament, the tensile stress within the ligament can be calculated. Also, the strain of the ligament is mea-sured using the video dimension analyzer (VDA) sys-tem. Therefore, the stress–strain curve, representing the mechanical properties of the ligament substance, can be plotted (61,63), and quantitative data on tangent modulus, tensile strength, and ultimate strain can be assessed (see Fig. 7-4B).

Although tensile testing is usually done *in vitro* (8,40,62), Tipton (52) developed a method for assessing

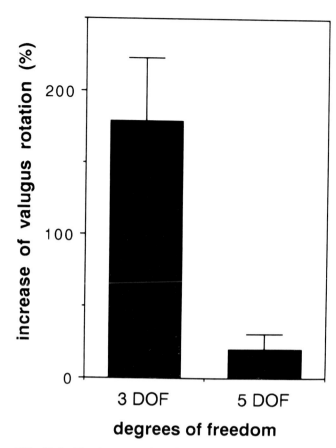

FIG. 18-2. The increase in valgus rotation after transec-tion of MCL. The data are plotted in terms of increased valgus rotation over that of the intact knee. When the knee was allowed 3 DOF, the valgus rotation increased significantly.

the structural properties of the femur–MCL–tibia complex (FMTC) of rats *in situ*. Anesthetized rats were placed on a loading platform and incisions made to expose the MCL with minimal disruption of the sur-rounding blood vessels. The popliteal artery was sev-ered just prior to testing and tensile load was applied along the axis of the MCL via fixation pins inserted transversely into the femur and tibia, until failure oc-curred. Although he reported small but significant dif-ferences in ultimate load and ultimate deformation be-tween isolated and *in situ* preparations, this author did not measure the stress and strain properties of the lig-ament substance.

Biochemistry

Biochemical analysis of the healing ligament, including measurements of water content, collagen content, col-lagen type and crosslinks, total glycosaminoglycans, and DNA concentration during the course of healing can further enhance our understanding of the ligament healing process. Total collagen is assessed by mea-

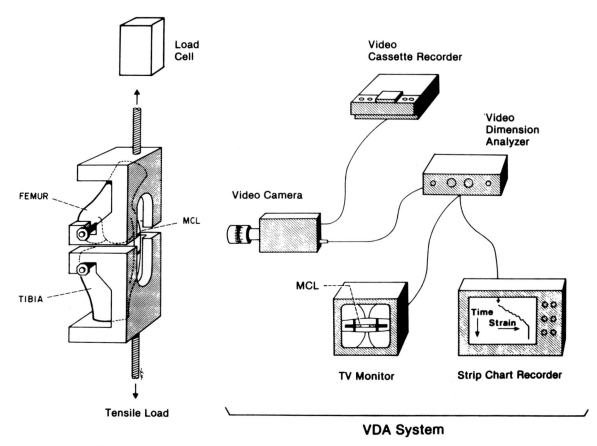

FIG. 18-3. The experimental apparatus used to measure the tensile characteristics of the FMTC with the video dimension analyzer (VDA) system; this setup can also be used to determine ligament strains. (From ref. 62.)

suring the hydroxyproline content (60). The relative amounts of Type I and Type III collagen are determined by separation of the peptides resulting from cyanogen bromide digestion of the tissue collagen (20, 33). A normal ligament has 90% Type I collagen with less than 10% Type III collagen. In the healing ligament, the percentage of Type III collagen is generally higher, reflecting increases in the amount of scar tissue. Increases or decreases in tissue cellularity are indicated by the concentration of DNA. Changes in the ratio of the intermolecular reducible Schiff-base crosslinks, as determined by cation-exchange liquid chromatography, are used to evaluate collagen maturation during repair (2,6). (For details, see Chapter 2.)

HEALING OF UNTREATED MEDIAL COLLATERAL LIGAMENTS

Although the ligament healing process is model-specific and is affected by various systemic (hormone levels, disease, nutrition, etc.) and local factors (severity of injuries, infection, circulation, etc.), it is important to understand the healing of collateral ligaments that have not received any treatment. In general, healing takes place in three overlapping phases: inflammation, repair, and remodeling (Fig. 18-4) (3).

Histology

Inflammatory Phase

Following complete midsubstance tear of a ligament, the ruptured gap fills with blood. The cellular and vascular reactions affect the whole ligament. Inflammatory cells proliferate from the surrounding tissue, convert the clot into granulation tissue, and begin forming new collagen fibrils. Cells and fibrils also migrate from the torn ends into the granulation tissue until the gap is bridged by new collagenous tissue (24). After 2 weeks, the granulation tissue is replaced by well-developed parallel collagen fibers of immature type, continuous with the original ligament fibers (24). By the end of this inflammatory phase, fibroblasts dominate the central scar region in a random and disorganized fashion and produce extracellular scar matrix (13).

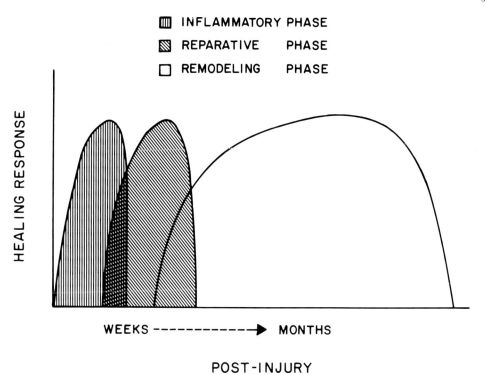

FIG. 18-4. Conceptual representation of the three phases of ligament healing. (From ref. 3.)

Reparative Phase

After the granulation tissue has been replaced by the parallel arrangement of immature collagen fibers, and the torn ends can no longer be distinguished, there is a decrease in the number of fibroblasts and inflammatory cells. The collagen fibers increase in size and strength and begin arranging into bundles.

Remodeling Phase

Over the course of several months, the collagen fibers begin to realign. The healed tissue gradually matures, becoming similar to normal tissue. Still, even after 1 year, the ligament does not mimic the typical uninjured ligament (13), and several years may be required for the ligament to return to its uninjured state. The duration of this phase is variable and is dependent on the method of treatment.

Biomechanics

Quantitative assessment of function of the healing ligament relative to normal ligaments, such as measurement of the biomechanical characteristics of the knee joint at different time periods, is important. In our laboratory (62,66), the healing of untreated MCL injuries was assessed in the canine by measuring knee joint stability, the structural properties of the FMTC, and

the mechanical properties of the MCL substance. Six weeks after the MCL was transected, the values for V–V rotation of the experimental knee were significantly higher than those of the contralateral sham-operated control knees. By 12 weeks postoperatively, the V–V rotation of the experimental knee had decreased to a level nearly the same as that of the control knee.

The load–deformation curves of the transected FMTC were below those for the controls at 6 weeks after surgery. By 12 weeks, the load–deformation curves and ultimate loads for the transected MCLs had become similar to those of the controls. This trend continued up to 48 weeks, where no significant differences between the structural properties of the transected and control FMTC were found.

At 6 weeks post-surgery, the stress–strain curves of the healing MCL substance were well below those of the controls. Despite significant increases in the tangent modulus and tensile strength of the healing MCLs at both 12 and 48 weeks postoperatively, the overall mechanical properties of the healing ligament remained inferior to those of the control group. These findings are similar to those of a previous study by our laboratory (15). In studies using the rabbit knee, the mechanical properties of transected MCL did not return to normal even 40 weeks after injury. Biomechanical study has shown, therefore, that although the knee with the healed MCL regains normal function in terms of its V–V rotation, the histological structure and mechanical properties of the healed MCL are not the same as those of normal ligament.

Biochemistry

During the inflammatory phase, increases in DNA content (reflecting the proliferation of cells) and in water content were observed (15). The values for Type III collagen and for reducible collagen crosslinks were also increased in the transected MCL (15,17). Collagen turnover studies demonstrated that active collagen synthesis and degradation occurred as a result of an increase in the synthesis of extracellular matrix (4).

Although the amount of Type III collagen, the number of reducible collagen crosslinks, and the rate of collagen turnover were still high during the reparative phase, collagen synthesis and cellularity were decreased. Water content, DNA content, and collagen concentration were also lowered during this phase (4,15,17). By 48 weeks, the amount of Type III collagen, the number of the reducible collagen crosslinks, and the rate of collagen turnover had returned to nearly normal values, indicating that remodeling of the ligament was progressing well.

REPAIR VERSUS NO REPAIR

Although investigators agree that the torn ACL does not heal without repair (32,41,57,58), controversy exists as to whether isolated tears of the collateral ligaments should be repaired. Several investigators have suggested that in the absence of surgical repair, the torn ends of the ligament may not remain in close apposition, creating a gap that is filled by scar tissue rather than by true ligament material (8,40). According to previous studies, sutured ligaments had a more normal histological appearance (cells and fibrils were more aligned) and failed at higher ultimate loads than did nonsutured ligaments (8,38,40). O'Donoghue (39) reported that surgical repair minimized the scar formation of the injured canine lateral collateral ligament (LCL). A biomechanical study by Clayton (8,9) demonstrated that sutured canine MCLs were stronger than unsutured controls at all postoperative time periods up to 9 weeks. Also, stress roentgenograms suggested that sutured ligaments resulted in less joint instability than did unsutured ligaments. Korkala (26) examined repaired and nonrepaired ligament injuries in rats at 4–5 weeks post-surgery. Using scanning electron microscopy, he found that the appearance of the nonrepaired ligament was less consistent, with extensive scarring visible in some cases. Although this investigator showed that suturing torn ligaments produced better histological results in the early stages, the

precise biomechanical properties and the long-term effects of suturing have not been examined.

Recently, we have performed a comparative study in which the healing of the transected MCL was examined histologically, biomechanically, and biochemically at 6, 12, and 48 weeks postoperatively in skeletally mature canines (66). Ligament injuries received either (a) conservative treatment with no repair or (b) surgical treatment with repair and 6 weeks of immobilization. At 6 weeks, histological sections of the healing site in both groups were similar in appearance. The tissue contained fibroblasts, some of which were aligned along the longitudinal axis of the ligament. At 12 weeks, the alignment of the fibroblasts in the longitudinal direction was more pronounced in the surgically repaired ligaments. This finding is similar to the results of previous studies (26,40). By 48 weeks, however, the healing tissues from both the repaired and nonrepaired groups had microscopic appearances similar to those of the normal MCL. Examination under polarized light microscopy, however, revealed that the orientation of the collagen fibers of MCL remained irregular.

The biomechanical properties of the nonrepaired ligaments exhibited the best results at all time periods. At 6 weeks, both groups showed higher V–V rotation than their controls, but there was no significant difference between the groups at this time. At 12 weeks, the V–V rotation values of the nonrepaired group knees had returned to normal, but the values of the repaired group knees had not returned to normal (Fig. 18-5). At 48 weeks, the V–V rotation for the nonrepaired group remained similar to normal, whereas that for the repaired group was still higher than that for the controls.

Load–deformation curves of the FMTC at 6 and 48 weeks are shown in Fig. 18-6. At 6 weeks, the curves for the nonrepaired and repaired FMTC were below the curve for the controls. At 48 weeks, curves for both groups were similar to the control curve; however, the structural properties of the nonrepaired group were nearer normal. Examination of the FMTC at 6 weeks revealed that for both groups the ultimate loads were lower than those of the controls. Although the average ultimate load for the nonrepaired FMTCs had returned to normal levels by 12 weeks, that for the repaired specimens had not. At 48 weeks, the ultimate load for the nonrepaired FMTCs remained at about the same level as that for the controls. In spite of a significant recovery from 12 weeks, the ultimate load for the repaired FMTCs was well below that for the controls.

For both groups, the stress–strain curves for the MCL substance demonstrated trends similar to those found for the load–deformation curves of the FMTC. However, the mechanical properties of the healing ligament did not improve as rapidly nor as completely.

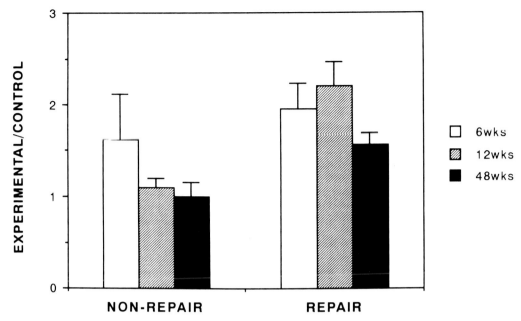

FIG. 18-5. The V–V rotation for nonrepaired and repaired canine MCL at 6, 12, and 48 weeks postoperatively. The data are normalized with respect to the contralateral control.

At 6 weeks, the stress–strain curves of both healing MCLs were similar, but stresses were well below those of the sham-operated controls for given strains. At 12 weeks, the average tangent modulus of the stress–strain curves of the healed MCLs increased, but no experimental group achieved properties similar to the sham-operated controls. The tensile strength of the nonrepaired MCL was only 63% of the control value at 48 weeks (Fig. 18-7). Biochemical analysis showed that there were no significant differences in collagen content, collagen types, or reducible crosslinks among the groups at any time period.

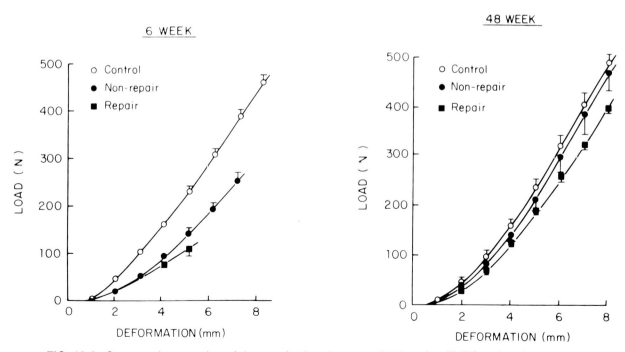

FIG. 18-6. Structural properties of the repaired and nonrepaired canine FMTC at 6 and 48 weeks postoperatively. The controls are shown for comparison.

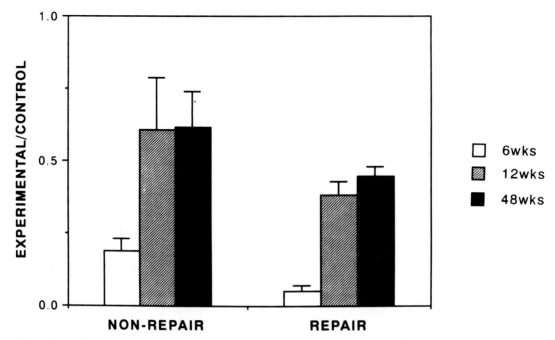

FIG. 18-7. The tensile strength for nonrepaired and repaired canine MCL at 6, 12, and 48 weeks postoperatively. The data are normalized with respect to the contralateral control.

OTHER FACTORS INFLUENCING LIGAMENT HEALING

Systemic and Local Factors

Systemic Conditions

Hormone levels have been demonstrated to play a role in ligament healing. In a study of the repair strength of the MCL from hypophysectomized rats, Tipton (51) reported that interstitial cell-stimulating hormone (ICSH) and testosterone replacement increased the ultimate load of the repaired ligament. However, adrenocorticotrophic hormone, somatotrophic hormone, thyroid-stimulating hormone, and thyroxine injections either diminished or had no effect on the ultimate loads. The author hypothesized that the increase in the strength of the repaired MCL following administration of ICSH and testosterone replacement may have been mediated by changes in collagen and glycosaminoglycan (GAG) synthesis or degradation rates. Diseases that alter endocrine and metabolic homeostasis such as diabetes mellitus, nutritional deficiency, and so on, may also affect ligament healing. Diabetes mellitus produces circulatory abnormalities that may impede ligament healing, and the absence of insulin has been demonstrated to alter collagen synthesis and cross-linking (54).

Local Conditions

During the inflammatory stage, inflammatory cells proliferate from the surrounding tissue and form new collagen fibrils. Local conditions, such as poor circulation and infection, may delay proliferation of the cells and thus prolong the inflammatory stage of ligament healing.

The severity of injury also affects ligament healing. Clinically, Grade I or II injuries heal very well. Recently, healing of Grade II MCL injury in sheep has been examined histologically and biomechanically (29). Compared to the studies described in the previous section which examined healing following Grade III injury of the MCL (8,40,66), the recovery of the Grade II MCL injury was more rapid. One week after injury, all of the "new" cells were fibroblasts; no inflammatory cells were observed. By 6 weeks, the fibroblasts were uniformly spindle-shaped and the collagen fibers were aligned along the longitudinal axis of the MCL. Valgus rotation values for the injured knee had decreased to normal by 6 weeks. Tensile testing of the bone–MCL–bone complex revealed that the ultimate load and stiffness of the injured ligament had also returned to normal by 6 weeks.

The healing of Grade III injuries is also influenced by local conditions. During Grade III injury the torn ends of the ligament become displaced, creating a gap. During the inflammatory phase this gap fills with blood, and later the hematoma is converted into granulation tissue. The size of the gap could also influence the time course of the healing. It is safe to assume that if the gap is wide, a large mass of granulation tissue is produced and more time may be required for healing and remodeling. However, no quantitative data are currently available.

Site of Injury

Ogata (43) has shown that ligament healing is ligament-specific. Unlike the MCL, the torn anterior cruciate ligament (ACL) and posterior cruciate ligament (PCL) do not heal well (10,42,45); this topic will be described in detail in Chapter 19. Variations in the healing ability of the different ligaments may be attributable to differences in blood supply and intra/extra-articular environment, as well as in structural and cellular characteristics (orientation of collagen fibers, fibroblast shape, etc.). Furthermore, differences in healing properties may be due, in part, to the differences between the cells of the ACL and MCL (31,34). Microscopic examination has demonstrated that these ligaments differ in their crimp pattern and cellular appearance. The MCL has a low-frequency crimp pattern and spindle-shaped fibroblasts. In contrast, the crimp pattern of the ACL is of higher frequency, and the fibroblasts are oval-shaped. Transmission electron microscopy has shown that the fibroblasts of the ACL have short cellular processes, whereas the fibroblasts of the MCL have long processes that are in close apposition with the collagen fibers (31). Biomechanically, the stress–strain relationships demonstrate that for a given strain, the ACL experiences less stress than the MCL (i.e., it has a lower tangent modulus). Furthermore, the variations in the healing response of the different ligaments may be due to other, as yet undescribed, anatomical and functional differences.

Complications of Associated Injuries

More than one ligament is frequently damaged when the knee is injured (Chapter 26). Unlike the favorable results that can be obtained following either operative or nonoperative treatment of isolated MCL injuries, the clinical outcome of combined ACL and MCL injuries is generally worse, regardless of the method of treatment selected (11).

The ability of the MCL to heal under conditions of associated ACL injury has been investigated in our laboratory. Our model examines the effect of partial and total transection of the ACL on the healing of a transected, unrepaired canine MCL (44). We have found that 6 weeks postoperatively, the V–V rotation of the experimental knees from both groups was significantly higher than that of their contralateral sham-operated controls. At 12 weeks, however, the V–V rotation for knees with partial transection of the ACL

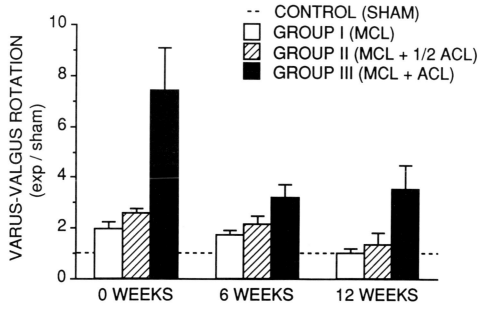

FIG. 18-8. The V–V rotation for three groups at 6 and 12 weeks postoperatively. The three groups are as follows: isolated MCL transection (intact ACL); MCL transection with section of the anteromedial portion of the ACL (partial ACL); and both ACL and MCL transection (total ACL). The data are normalized with respect to the contralateral control.

was similar to the control values (Fig. 18-8). In contrast, the normalized V–V rotation (defined as experimental/control) following total ACL transection was very high at both time periods. These results are in agreement with those obtained by Forbes (12). This investigator showed that rabbit knees with combined MCL and ACL injuries also demonstrated greater V–V rotation (medial joint opening with valgus stress) than the controls even after 14 weeks. Also, the structural properties for the canine FMTC from the experimental side for both groups became similar to the controls at 12 weeks (Fig. 18-9B). However, the mechanical properties of the healed MCL remained significantly different from those of the control ligament. The MCLs from the knees with a totally cut ACL showed the least recovery (Fig. 18-10B).

Immobilization Versus Mobilization

Torn ligaments have traditionally been immobilized to protect the healing tissue from motion and stress. In recent years, experimental studies have shown that immobilized ligaments exhibit a loss of collagen fiber orientation, a drastic change in the mechanical properties, and a decrease in the strength of the bone ligament complex as a result of bone resorption at the tibial insertion site (64,65). Histological examination of the FMTC from immobilized knees revealed (a) higher os-teoclastic activity and resorption of bone at the tibial insertion sites and (b) disruption of the normal attachment of the ligament to bone. As a result, following immobilization, the FMTC failed by tibial avulsion during tensile testing.

Tipton (50) reported that in canines whose legs had been immobilized for 6 weeks, the ultimate load of repaired MCLs was significantly lower than those of MCLs from nonimmobilized animals. Later, this author (51) further demonstrated that immobilization has a detrimental effect on the ultimate load of rat MCLs. He hypothesized that decreased blood flow was responsible for inhibition of repair during immobilization based on the finding of Rothman (48) that capillarization was diminished by immobilization. Vailas (55) found that 8 weeks of immobilization following transection and surgical repair of the rat MCL produced decreases in ligament weight and ultimate load as well as in the rate of new collagen synthesis. Measurement of DNA concentrations in the MCL indicated that long-term immobilization also hindered the restoration of cellularity levels to normal.

Two studies on the positive effects of passive motion on the healing MCL have been conducted. Fronek (16) examined the effect of passive motion on the healing of rabbit MCLs histologically and mechanically. Histological evaluation showed that 6 weeks of intermittent passive motion of the knee resulted in improved longitudinal alignment of the cells and collagen fibers

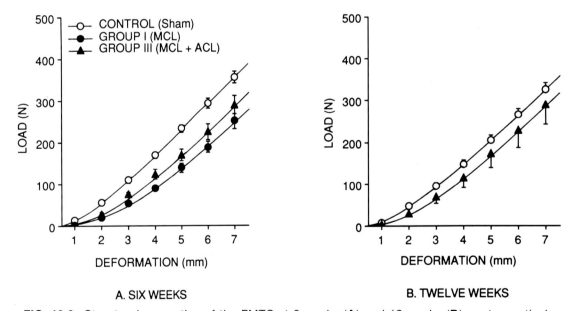

FIG. 18-9. Structural properties of the FMTC at 6 weeks (**A**) and 12 weeks (**B**) postoperatively. For the purpose of clarity, only the curves for Groups I and III are shown at 6 weeks. The curve for Group II was similar to that for Group III. At 12 weeks, the curves for the knees from all three experimental were similar, and only Group III is shown here with the controls. The three groups are as follows: I—isolated MCL transection (intact ACL); II—MCL transection with section of the anteromedial portion of the ACL (partial ACL); and III—both ACL and MCL transection (total ACL). The controls are shown for comparison.

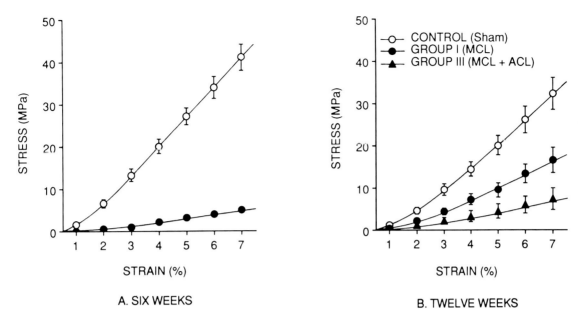

FIG. 18-10. Mechanical properties of the FMTC at 6 weeks (**A**) and 12 weeks (**B**) postoperatively. At 6 weeks the curves for the knees from all three experimental groups were similar; therefore, only the curve for Group I is shown here. The three groups are as follows: I—isolated MCL transection (intact ACL); II—MCL transection with section of the anteromedial portion of the ACL (partial ACL); and III—both ACL and MCL transection (total ACL). The controls are shown for comparison.

in the torn ligament. The ultimate load of the FMTC treated by intermittent passive motion was four times greater than that of immobilized ligaments. These results are in agreement with those obtained by Long (30). This study also demonstrated that matrix organization was improved and that the collagen concentration of healing ligaments was elevated. Histological and mechanical evaluation of healing rabbit MCLs revealed that passive motion produced structural properties of the FMTC superior to those subjected to immobilization during healing. In addition, their matrix organization was improved, and the collagen concentration of the healing ligaments was elevated.

The effect of immobilization in cases involving multiple ligament injuries has been studied by Piper (45). Anterior displacement and valgus rotation of the knee joint and ultimate load of the bone–MCL–bone complex were measured in canines 8 weeks after transection of both the MCL and the ACL. Two postoperative treatment regimens were used: (i) 6 weeks of immobilization followed by 2 weeks of remobilization and (ii) 8 weeks of unlimited motion. The knees that had undergone motion were found to be more stable than the immobilized knees. The bone–MCL–bone complexes of the mobilized knees failed at higher ultimate loads than did those of the immobilized knees. However, motion applied too early and excessively may elongate or even disrupt the newly formed tissue, leading to failure of the healed mass. Hart (19) examined

the level of motion with respect to the severity of the injury. With isolated MCL injury the ultimate loads of the bone–MCL–bone complexes from the mobilized knees were found to be higher than those from the immobilized knees. However, when the secondary restraints were also transected, the active motion had an adverse effect on the strength of the bone–MCL–bone complex.

Effects of Exercise

Tipton (50) examined the effect of exercise on the strength of repaired MCLs in canines and found increases in the ultimate loads. In a study involving both dogs and rats, the same author (51) found similar results at 12 weeks after surgery but stated that 15–18 weeks are needed before "normal" values are obtained. Vailas (55) examined rats in which the MCL had been transected, repaired, and immobilized for 2 weeks, followed by 6 weeks of either exercise or cage activity. He concluded that the healing process was enhanced by exercise as evidenced by the more rapid return of tissue DNA, collagen synthesis, and ultimate load to normal levels.

Timing of Repair

Many investigators have indicated that the timing of repair may have an effect on the healing response.

Warren (58) reported that when surgery was required following MCL injury, results were superior if the surgery was performed acutely. This is in agreement with O'Donoghue (39), who concluded that early surgical repair (within 2 weeks) is essential following complete rupture of any knee ligament. These conclusions are based on clinical experience, however, and no definitive experimental data are available. There remains a need to study the effects of delayed repair under more controlled conditions in a well-defined experimental model.

FUTURE STUDIES

Many questions regarding factors that may influence ligament healing still remain. These factors include the following: the effects of age, sex, and hormones; the choice of an experimental model of ligament injury; and the effectiveness of methods for accelerating the healing process. Although some of these questions have been addressed, the results obtained have not been definitive and much work remains to be done.

Studies have demonstrated that age and sex affect the biomechanical characteristics of normal ligaments (7,53,67) and, therefore, might influence ligament healing. In addition, the mode of injury has been shown to affect ligament healing. In most experimental studies conducted to date, the ligament was sharply transected. This model differs significantly from the ligament injuries observed clinically. Development of models that more closely approximate the "real life" situation is needed and would provide additional knowledge of ligament healing with greater clinical relevance. Recently, our laboratory has initiated a study to examine MCL healing in two different injury models. In one model, the MCL is cut in the shape of a "Z" to examine the ability of the MCL to heal in a shear plane as well as in a tensile plane. In the second model, the MCL is torn abruptly, producing shredding of the ligament substance at the site of the injury. This "mop-end tear" model was designed to mimic the more complex injury pattern seen clinically, and it involves damage to the insertion sites as well as to the ligament substance. A pilot study examining the gross appearances of ligaments at 3–4 weeks postoperatively revealed that scar formation was more pronounced following the "mop-end tear" procedure than after sharp transection.

In addition, certain treatments, including the use of electrical stimulation (25), hyaluronic acid (59), and systemic or local hormones (51), have been shown to improve the repair response of the ligament. Frank (14) examined the influence of electromagnetic stimulation on healing in rabbits MCL. Biomechanical testing revealed that the stiffness and strength of the stimulated

ligaments returned to control levels earlier than in the nonstimulated ligaments. Also, after 6 weeks, the collagen content of the stimulated ligaments was closer to control levels than that of the nonstimulated ligaments. Therefore, electrical stimulation was felt to influence the early stages of the healing process. Additional research is required in order to determine whether this early phenomenon persists.

Adams (1) examined surgically repaired rabbit MCLs after immobilization and invasive stimulation. At 35 days after repair, the ligaments that had been electrically stimulated failed at higher ultimate loads than ligaments that had not been stimulated. They also observed that electrical current produced a greater cellular reaction and a less random cellular organization in the early phases of healing. In light of this finding, further study of electrical current and ligament healing is suggested.

The effects of hormones on repair strength were discussed earlier, however, the number of hormones examined was limited and the mechanism of this interaction remains unknown. Additional research into the mechanism underlying this correlation, as well as the effects of other hormones is needed. Currently much attention has been focused on a class of peptides commonly called growth factors. Growth hormone and epidermal growth factor have been shown to accelerate healing of skin wounds (27,28,47). Based on this response, it has been suggested that these factors could play a similar role in ligament healing. Although there are numerous growth factors, including transforming growth factor-beta, epidermal growth factors, fibroblast growth factor, insulin-like growth factors, and platelet-derived growth factor, being investigated, their effects on accelerating ligament healing must be studied.

ACKNOWLEDGMENTS

The authors would like to acknowledge the financial support of the VA RR&D Grant A188-3RA, the NIH Grant AM14918, and the Malcolm and Dorothy Coutts Institute for Joint Reconstruction and Research.

REFERENCES

1. Adams EL, Bradford DS, Oegema TR. Early histological and biomechanical change in ligament healing under electrical stimulation. *Trans Orthop Res Soc* 1988;13:106.
2. Akeson WH, Amiel D, Mechanic GL, Woo SL-Y, Harwood FL, Hamer ML. Collagen cross-linking alterations in joint contractures: changes in the reducible cross-links in periarticular connective tissue collagen after nine weeks of immobilization. *Connect Tissue Res* 1977;5:15–19.
3. Akeson WH, Woo SL-Y, Amiel D, Frank C. The biology of ligaments. In: Hunter LY, Funk FJ, eds. *Rehabilitation of the injured knee*. St. Louis: CV Mosby, 1984;93–148.

4. Amiel DA, Frank CB, Harwood FL, Akeson WH, Kleiner JB. Collagen alteration in medial collateral ligament healing in a rabbit model. *Connect Tissue Res* 1987;16:357–366.
5. Arnoczky SP, Rubin RM, Marshall JL. Microvascularization of the cruciate ligaments and its response to injury: an experimental study in dogs. *J Bone Joint Surg* 1979;61A:1221–1229.
6. Bailey AJ, Bazin S, Delaunay A. Changes in the nature of collagen during development and resorption of granulation tissue. *Biochem Biophys Acta* 1973;328:383–390.
7. Booth FW, Tipton CM. Ligamentous strength measurements in pre-pubescent and pubescent rats. *Growth* 1970;34:177–185.
8. Clayton ML, Weir GJ. Experimental investigations of ligamentous healing. *Am J Surg* 1959;98:373–378.
9. Clayton ML, Miles JS, Abdulla M. Experimental investigations of ligamentous healing. *Clin Orthop* 1968;61:146–153.
10. Feagin JA, Curl WW. Isolated tear of the anterior cruciate ligament: five-year follow-up study. *Am J Sports Med* 1976;4:95–100.
11. Fetto JF, Marshall JL. Medial collateral ligament injuries of the knee: a rationale for treatment. *Clin Orthop* 1978;132:206–218.
12. Forbes I, Frank C, Lam T, Shrive N. The biomechanical effects of combined ligament injuries on the medial collateral ligament. *Trans Orthop Res Soc* 1988;13:196.
13. Frank C, Schachar N, Dittrich D. Natural history of healing in the repaired medial collateral ligament. *J Orthop Res* 1983;1:179–188.
14. Frank C, Schachar N, Dittrich D, Shrive N, deHaas W, Edwards G. Electromagnetic stimulation of ligament healing in rabbits. *Clin Orthop* 1983;175:263–272.
15. Frank C, Woo SL-Y, Amiel D, Harwood FL, Gomez M, Akeson WH. Medial collateral ligament healing—a multidisciplinary assessment in rabbits. *Am J Sports Med* 1983;11:379–389.
16. Fronek J, Frank C, Amiel D, Woo SL-Y, Coutts RD, Akeson WH. The effect of intermittent passive motion (IPM) in the healing of the medial collateral ligament. *Trans Orthop Res Soc* 1983;8:31.
17. Gomez MA, Woo SL-Y, Inoue M, Amiel D, Harwood F, Kitabayashi L. Medial collateral ligament healing subsequent to different treatment regimens. *J Appl Physiol* 1989;66:245–52.
18. Grood ES, Noyes FR, Butler DL, Suntay WJ. Ligamentous and capsular restraints preventing straight medial and lateral laxity in intact human cadaver knees. *J Bone Joint Surg* 1981;63A:1257–1269.
19. Hart DP, Dahners LE. Healing of the medial collateral ligament in rats. The effects of repair, motion and secondary stabilizing ligaments. *J Bone Joint Surg* 1987;69A:1194–1198.
20. Harwood FL, Amiel D. Semiquantitative HPLC analysis of types I and III collagen in soft tissues. *LC–GC Magazine of Chromatographic Science* 1986;4:122–126.
21. Hastings DE. The non-operative management of collateral ligament injuries of the knee joint. *Clin Orthop* 1980;147:22–28.
22. Indelicato PA. Non-operative treatment of complete tears of the medial collateral ligament of the knee. *J Bone Joint Surg* 1983;65A:323–329.
23. Inoue M, McGurk-Burleson E, Hollis JM. Treatment of the medial collateral ligament injury. 1. The importance of anterior cruciate ligament on the varus–valgus knee laxity. *Am J Sports Med* 1987;15:15–21.
24. Jack EA. Experimental rupture of the medial collateral ligament of the knee. *J Bone Joint Surg* 1950;32A:396–402.
25. Kenney TG, Dahners LE. The effect of electrical stimulation on ligament healing in a rat model. *Trans Orthop Res Soc* 1988;13:107.
26. Korkala O, Rusanen M, Groblad M. Healing of experimental ligament rupture: findings by scanning electron microscopy. *Arch Orthop Traumat Surg* 1984;102:179–182.
27. Kowalewski K, Young S. Effect of growth hormone and an anabolic steroid on hydroxyproline in healing dermal wounds in rats. *Acta Endocrinol* 1968;59:53–66.
28. Laato M, Ninikoski J, Gerdin B, Lebel L. Stimulation of wound healing by epidermal growth factor. *Ann Surg* 1986;203:379–381.
29. Laws G, Walton M. Fibroblastic healing of grade II ligament injuries: histological and mechanical studies in the sheep. *J Bone Joint Surg* 1988;70B:390–396.
30. Long ML, Frank C, Schachar NS, Dittrich D, Edwards GE. The effects of motion on normal and healing ligaments. *Trans Orthop Res Soc* 1982;7:43.
31. Lyon RM, Billings E Jr, Woo SL-Y, Ishizue KK, Kitabayashi L, Amiel D, Akeson WH. The ACL: a fibrocartilagenous structure. *Trans Orthop Res Soc* 1989;14:189.
32. McDaniel WJ Jr, Dameron TB Jr. Untreated anterior ruptures of the cruciate ligament: a follow-up study. *J Bone Joint Surg* 1980;62A:310–322.
33. Miller EJ, Rhodes RK, Furoto DK. Identification of collagen chains as a function of cyanogen bromide peptide patterns using gel permeation high performance liquid chromatography. *Coll Rel Res* 1983;3:79–87.
34. Newton PO, MacKenna DA, Lyon RM, Akeson WH, Woo SL-Y. Comparison of the mechanical properties of the medial collateral and anterior cruciate ligaments of the rabbit knee. Presented at the 3rd Joint ASCW/ASMW Mechanics Conference, San Diego, California, 1989.
35. Nielson S, Andersen CK, Rasmussen O, Andersen A. Instability of cadaver knees after transection of capsule and ligaments. *Acta Orthop Scand* 1984;55:30–34.
36. Nielson S, Rasmussen O, Ovesen J, Andersen K. Rotatory instability of cadaver knees after transection of collateral ligaments and capsule. *Arch Orthop Trauma Surg* 1984;103:165–169.
37. Oakes BW. Acute soft tissue injuries: Nature and management. *Aust Fam Physician* 1982;10(7 Suppl):3–16.
38. Odensten M, Hamberg P, Nordin M, Lysholm J, Gillquist J. Surgical or conservative treatment of the acutely torn anterior cruciate ligament: a randomized study with short-term follow-up observations. *Clin Orthop* 1985;198:87–93.
39. O'Donoghue DH. An analysis of end results of surgical treatment of major injuries to the ligaments of the knee. *J Bone Joint Surg* 1955;37A:1–12.
40. O'Donoghue DH, Rockwood CC Jr. Repair of knee ligaments in dogs. 1. The lateral collateral ligament. *J Bone Joint Surg* 1961;43A:1167–1178.
41. O'Donoghue DH, Rockwood CC Jr. Repair of the anterior cruciate ligament in dogs. *J Bone Joint Surg* 1966;48A:503–519.
42. O'Donoghue DH. Reconstruction for medial instability of the knee. Technique and results in sixty cases. *J Bone Joint Surg* 1973;55A:941–955.
43. Ogata K, Whiteside LA, Andersen DA. The intra-articular effect of various postoperative managements following knee ligament repair. An experimental study in dogs. *Clin Orthop* 1980;150:271–276.
44. Ohland KJ, Marcin JP, Young EP, Lin HC, Horibe S, Woo SL-Y. The effect of partial and total transection of the anterior cruciate ligament on medial collateral ligament healing in the canine knee. *Trans Orthop Res Soc* 1989;14:322.
45. Piper TL, Whiteside LA. Early mobilization after knee ligament repair in dogs. *Clin Orthop* 1980;150:277–282.
46. Piziali RL, Rastegar J, Nagel DA, Schurman DJ. The contribution of the cruciate ligaments to the load–displacement characteristics of the human knee joint *J Biomech Eng* 1980;102:277–283.
47. Prudden JF, Nishihara G, Ocampo L. Studies on growth hormone. III. The effect on wound tensile strength of marked postoperative anabolism induced with growth hormone. *Surg Gynecol Obstet* 1958;107:481–482.
48. Rothman RH, Slogoff S. The effect of immobilization on the vascular bed of tendon. *Surg Gynecol Obstet* 1967;124:1064–1066.
49. Seering WP, Piziali RL, Nagel DA, Schurman DJ. The function of the primary ligaments of the knee in varus–valgus and axial rotation. *J Biomech* 1980;13:785–794.
50. Tipton CM, James SL, Mergner, Tcheng T-K. Influence of exercise on strength of medial collateral ligaments of dogs. *Am J Physiol* 1970;218:894–902.
51. Tipton CM, Matthes RD, Maynard JA, Carey RA. The influence of physical activity on ligaments and tendons. *Med Sci Sports* 1975;7:165–175.
52. Tipton CM, Matthes RD, Sandage DS. *In situ* measurement of

junction strength and ligament elongation in rats. *J Appl Physiol* 1974;37:758–761.

53. Tipton CM, Schild RJ, Flatt AE. The measurement of ligamentous strength in rats. *J Bone Joint Surg* 1967;49A:63–72.

54. Tipton CM, Vailas AC, Matthes RD. Experimental studies on the influences of physical activity on ligaments, tendons and joints: a brief review. *Acta Med Scand [Suppl]* 1986;711:157–168.

55. Vailas AC, Tipton CM, Matthes RD, Gart M. Physical activity and its influence on the repair process of medial collateral ligaments. *Connect Tissue Res* 1981;9:25–31.

56. Viidik A. Simultaneous mechanical and light microscopic studies of collagen fibers. *Zeitschrift Für Anatomie und Entwicklungsgeschichte* 1972;136:204–212.

57. Warren RF, Marshall, JL. A retrospective analysis of clinical records—Part I. *Clin Orthop* 1978;136:191–197.

58. Warren RF, Marshall JL. Injuries of the anterior cruciate and medial collateral ligaments of the knee: a long term follow-up of 86 cases—Part II. *Clin Orthop* 1978;136:197–211.

59. Wiig ME, Amiel D, Harwood FL, Kitabayashi L, Woo SL-Y, Akeson WH. Anterior cruciate ligament healing: the effect of high molecular weight hyaluronan (hyaluronic acid). *Trans Orthop Res Soc* 1989;14:297.

60. Woessner JF. The determination of hydroxyproline in tissue and protein samples containing small proportions of this imino acid. *Arch Biochem Biophys* 1961;93:44–47.

61. Woo SL-Y, Akeson WH, Jemmott GF. Measurements of non-homogeneous, directional mechanical properties of articular cartilage in tension. *J Biomech* 1976;9:785–791.

62. Woo SL-Y, Gomez MA, Inoue M, Akeson WH. New experimental procedures to evaluate the biomechanical properties of healing canine medical collateral ligaments. *J Orthop Res* 1987;5:425–432.

63. Woo SL-Y, Gomez MA, Seguchi Y, Endo CM, Akeson WH. Measurement of mechanical properties of ligament substance from a bone–ligament–bone preparation. *J Orthop Res* 1983;1:22–29.

64. Woo SL-Y, Gomez MA, Sites TJ, Newton PO, Orlando CA, Akeson WH. The biomechanical and morphological changes in the medial collateral ligament of the rabbit after immobilization and remobilization. *J Bone Joint Surg* 1987;69A:1200–1211.

65. Woo SL-Y, Gomez MA, Woo Y-K, Akeson WH. Mechanical properties of tendons and ligaments. II. The relationships of immobilization and exercise on tissue remodeling. *Biorheology* 1982;19:397–408.

66. Woo SL-Y, Inoue M, McGurk-Burleson E. Treatment of the medial collateral ligament injury. 2. Structure and function of canine knees in response to differing treatment regimens. *Am J Sports Med* 1987;15:22–29.

67. Woo SL-Y, Orlando CA, Frank CB, Gomez MA, Akeson WH. Tensile properties of the medial collateral ligament as a function of age. *J Orthop Res* 1986;4:133–141.

Knee Ligaments: Structure, Function, Injury,
and Repair, edited by D. Daniel, et al.
© 1990 by Raven Press, Ltd. All rights reserved.

CHAPTER 19

Cruciate Ligaments

Response to Injury

David Amiel, Scott Kuiper, and Wayne H. Akeson

The poor healing potential of the anterior cruciate ligament (ACL) has been a recognized problem in orthopedics since the early 1900s. In 1938, Palmer (46) described the cruciate ligament healing problem, succinctly stating that "as a rule, total rupture of a cruciate band is probably incapable of healing spontaneously." He reported in a large series of patients that the transected ACL had absorbed following injury.

O'Donoghue (45) studied the reparative processes of the ACL using an ACL injury model that involved an ACL laceration at the tibial attachment site in dogs. The degree of healing was assessed after the ACL was (a) partially or completely transected with no repair, (b) transected completely with subsequent repair, or (c) excised and reconstructed with a portion of iliotibial band. An inflammatory reaction was noted in the partially transected ACLs and was characterized by an initial stage of necrosis followed by round-cell infiltration and early fibroblastic proliferation. There was little healing at the base of the incision at 10 weeks. The knees with fully transected ACLs had gross instability, and none of the ligament ends reunited. The cut ligament ends became rounded, and they either retracted or absorbed. By 2 weeks time, the amount of ligament

necrosis and absorption was such that any repair would have been impossible. In O'Donoghue's transection/repair group, poor healing was demonstrated in ligaments repaired with excessive tension. A variable but unpredictable percentage of ligaments would heal after accurate suturing of opposing ends with proper tension. Ligaments repaired under proper tension had defects filled with collagen but without excessive scar. Mechanical testing showed that the strength of the ligament never approached a normal level up to 1 year post-repair. This study was the first to critically study the healing process of the ACL and the factors that affect this process. It seems likely that in this model, transected at the attachment site, the healing response is mounted by cells from the adjacent bone.

A subsequent study was performed to examine what effects time, type of suture, and type of inflammatory reaction have on the ultimate tensile strength of an ACL repair (44). Repairs with wire increased in strength over a time period of 6 months to 4 years, whereas silk repairs did not. The progression of inflammatory reaction in wire-repaired ACLs correlated with the strength of the repairs as well. Again, resorption of repaired ligaments was not uncommon, since this occurred in 14 of 36 repairs.

Cabaud (12) confirmed O'Donoghue's results using dogs and Rhesus monkeys. Healing at both the tibial and femoral insertions was noted after primary repair,

D. Amiel, S. Kuiper, and W. H. Akeson: Department of Surgery, Division of Orthopedics and Rehabilitation, University of California, San Diego, School of Medicine, La Jolla, California 92093.

suggesting that improved results could be obtained if proper immobilization and meticulous surgical technique were carried out. Results from these studies were an impetus to continue performing primary repair of the ACL; however, controversy has continued to exist concerning the adequacy of results obtained from these procedures.

Skeptics of primary repair emphasize that studies by O'Donoghue and Cabaud utilize ACL laceration models that involve detachment of the ACL at either the tibial or femoral insertion sites. Healing in these models involves bony ingrowth and does not adequately represent healing of an interstitial tear of the ACL. Studies have shown that the majority of ACL tears (greater than 80%) are in the proximal 20% of the ligament, whereas 10% involve the midsubstance (mop-end tears); moreover, less than 5% are avulsion injuries, which these models most closely represent (61).

In 1972, Feagin (19) reported promising results of primary repair of "isolated" acutely torn ACLs in military cadets at early follow-up. After 2 years, 25 of 30 patients had good to excellent results. Long-term (5-year) follow-up of these patients, however, demonstrated progressive deterioration of the knee as evidenced by pain (71%), swelling (66%), stiffness (71%) and instability (94%) (20). A retrospective long-term follow-up by Balkfors (10) indicated that primary repair of the cruciate ligament was unrewarding. A large number of cases in these studies were treated as isolated tears, leaving open the possibility that "missed" associated injuries impaired results from these studies. In a separate study, however, Odensten (43) repaired all injured structures about the knee along with the ACL, and about half of these patients were unstable after 4 years.

Despite the controversy regarding clinical management of the patient with an acute ACL injury, most agree that the ACL has a poor capacity for healing. This healing deficiency has been the focus of numerous studies involving various ACL healing models (5,8,11,44,45). Numerous factors are present which may in some way detract from the ACL's ability to repair itself after the proper surgical intervention. In general, wound healing is affected by factors that are associated with the patient's condition, including age, activity level, nutrition, and associated disease states. Factors that solely affect the healing capacity of the cruciate ligaments include the complex anatomy of these structures (Chapter 4), biomechanical forces resulting from motion and muscle action (Chapters 10 and 11), the nutritional delivery system, the unique biological environment these ligaments reside in, and the intrinsic capacity of the cells to support the healing process.

ACL NUTRITION

The blood supply to various subsections of the cruciate ligament core is poor or limited (1,8). Alm (1) performed early vascularization studies on the anterior and posterior cruciate ligaments in dogs by means of microangiography and histology. A paraligamentous network of vessels was noted coursing through the synovial membrane. These vessels entered the ligaments transversely and anastomosed freely with endoligamentous vessels. The core of the midportion of the cruciate ligaments was less well vascularized than the proximal and distal cores. Arnoczky (8) reported similar findings for normal vascular anatomy of the cruciate ligaments, including less abundant vasculature in the central part of the midportion of both cruciate ligaments. The posterior cruciate ligament (PCL), however, was consistently surrounded by a greater density of vessels than the ACL.

A vascular response has been noted in the ACL after partial transection (8). Vascular proliferation occurred throughout the entire ligament in knees with intact synovial tissue and infrapatellar fat pad. The vascular response was especially pronounced at the lesion site. Histologic sections at 8 weeks revealed that the lesion was covered by synovial tissue, but the defect remained, indicating that the healing response was inadequate despite the vascular and fibroblastic response.

Synovial fluid, formed from an ultrafiltrate of blood (59), has been shown to be a physiologically important nutrient delivery pathway for the ACL (2) in addition to its blood supply. Studies of the nutrient pathway to flexor tendons suggest that diffusion is an important route of nutrient delivery to fibrous structures emersed in synovial fluid (36,49,50).

Recently our laboratory studied the role of synovial fluid in providing nutrition to rabbit knee ligaments and menisci by intraarticular injection of tritiated proline (a collagen precursor) (2). Measurement of the incorporated substrate, tritiated hydroxyproline ([^{3}H]hyp), was measured in the collateral ligaments, cruciate ligaments, and menisci. Autoradiography demonstrated concentration of the isotope ([^{3}H]proline) and its metabolite ([^{3}H]hyp) in and around fibroblasts of all these tissues. Measurements of [^{3}H]hyp incorporation showed that all knee structures tested utilized synovial-fluid-derived proline. The cruciate ligaments demonstrated the highest uptake of [^{3}H]hyp (Fig. 19-1). Control ligaments and menisci from the contralateral limb showed no detectable isotope. These findings indicate that these structures can derive nutrition from a synovial fluid source and that a major pathway of nutrient delivery is from synovial arterial capillaries to the synovial cavity, followed by trans-synovial bulk flow and diffusion to the knee ligaments and menisci.

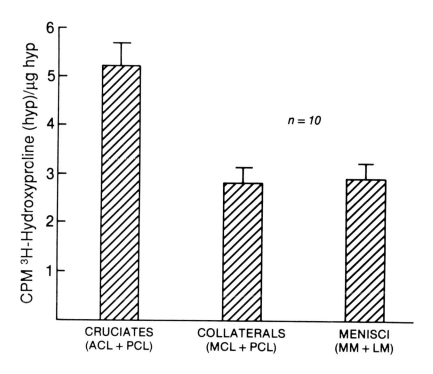

FIG. 19-1. Nutrient uptake of the various periarticular connective tissue structures. (From ref. 2.)

It is apparent, then, that the cruciate ligaments derive their nutrition from two sources: (i) its vascular supply, which courses from the middle geniculate artery and popliteal arteries to the synovial membrane and, finally, to the cruciate ligament structures and (ii) the synovial fluid, which continuously bathes the cruciates and allows for trans-synovial bulk flow and diffusion for nutrient delivery. Although a vascular response is noted after injury, the viability of these tissues post-injury and post-repair has been questioned. Ultimately the effectiveness of the synovial fluid delivery system depends on tissue metabolism, ligament thickness, permeability, and synovial nutrient concentration. Adequate nutrition is essential for any tissue to mount a healing response. Poor delivery of nutrients and metabolic substances could profoundly limit cruciate ligament healing capacity. The question remains whether the vascular response and synovial fluid diffusion are sufficient to support the injured ligament's healing response above its basic nutritional requirements.

BIOLOGICAL ENVIRONMENT

The cruciate ligaments reside in a unique environment. Both ligaments are intracapsular, and both are enveloped by a synovial membrane, effectively making them extrasynovial. The synovial membrane, which is only a few cells thick, separates the ACL and PCL from the synovial fluid that bathes the other intracapsular knee joint structures.

Of the many factors important in ligament healing such as mechanical forces, blood supply, and local environment, it is the local environment which has often been used as an explanation for the poor healing capacity of the cruciate ligaments (45). This local environment has been referred to as the "hostile" environment of the synovial joint space. During ACL injury the synovial membrane is usually torn, exposing the frayed ligament ends to a host of potentially destructive enzymes released by the breakdown of hemarthrosis fluid of the injured joint.

Synovial fluid has been shown to adversely affect ligament fibroblasts, which are crucial for ligament healing. Using tissue culture techniques, Andrish (7) demonstrated that ACL fibroblast proliferation was diminished when exposed to synovial fluid.

Rapid degeneration of the ACL occurs after acute rupture. This phenomenon was described clinically by Warren (66), who showed that ruptured ACL ligament substance can completely disappear 6 weeks after injury. Kohn (28) confirmed these results, noting either complete disappearance or only a remnant of the ACL in 32 patients arthroscoped 8 months to 20 years after injury. O'Donoghue (45), using a dog model of ACL injury, reported inflammatory changes in the unrepaired, released ligaments with significant shortening within 10 weeks of injury.

To test the hypothesis that ligament resorption following ACL injury represents a cellular response of intrinsic ligamentous cells to degrade their extracellular matrix, a rabbit model of ACL injury was created by our laboratory with the development of an *in vitro* assay for collagenase activity (5). A collagenase assay was utilized because collagen represents the major structural protein of the cruciate ligament. The left ACL was transected off its tibial insertion, while the right knee served as a sham-operated control. The ACL and menisci were harvested 10 days postoperatively, placed in tissue culture, and assayed for collagenase 3 days later. Results demonstrated a relatively large increase (82%) in injured ACL collagenase content as compared to control ACLs (Fig. 19-2). This was consistent with the average net loss of 34% in total collagen mass from the injured ACLs.

Collagenase release has been documented from other articular structures such as synovium (13,67) and articular cartilage (16,54). These structures synthesize and release a latent form of collagenase. The data from this experiment indicated that the ACL and menisci secrete only active enzymes which may be detrimental to the intraarticular structures (33).

In addition, the transected ACLs were swollen and retracted (Fig. 19-3). The free transected ligament ends displayed a relative hypocellularity and a loss of collagen matrix organization histologically confirming the observations of others (28,45,66) that, once ruptured, the free ends of the ACL undergo rapid degeneration (Fig. 19-4). The transected ACL tissue itself may be responsible for this degenerative process. Cells within the ACL may respond to injury by degrading their collagenous matrix.

Detractors from the "hostile environment" theory

emphasize that tendons are exposed to a fluid similar to synovial fluid in their sheath, and no evidence for poor tendon healing in these areas exists. Flexor tendon fibroblasts appear to utilize synovial fluid for nutrition. Tendon segments which were replaced within a synovial sheath chamber demonstrated histologically that peripheral fibroblasts survived and proliferated (17,34,38). While the cellular elements in tendon appear to show no adverse effects from synovial fluid, one must remember that we cannot validly compare tendons to ligaments in this manner. Tendons and ligaments have different histological and biochemical characteristics (4). They are strikingly similar but distinctly unique in composition. In addition, flexor tendon naturally exists within the synovial fluid-filled sheath, whereas the native environment of the cruciate ligaments is extrasynovial in location.

Following ACL injury, acute hemarthrosis fluid fills the joint space. Noyes (42) has shown that over 70% of patients presenting with acute hemarthrosis of the knee have an acute tear of the ACL. The sheath enveloping the ACL is generally torn, leaving the frayed ends of the ACL exposed to hemarthrosis fluid, which appears to have a deleterious affect on knee joint structures (23,55). In 1982, Fabry (18) proposed that degradative enzymes were responsible for the degenerative changes seen in hemophilic arthropathy. Pforringer (47) demonstrated a decrease in the mechanical properties of the femur–ACL–tibia complex, as well as histological changes in the ACL after acute

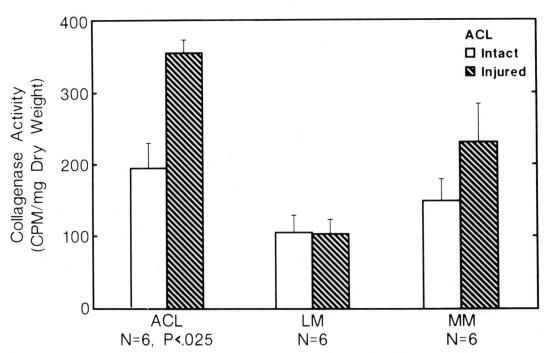

FIG. 19-2. Collagenase activity. Note significant increase in collagenase activity in injured ACLs. No differences were noted in menisci. (From ref. 5.)

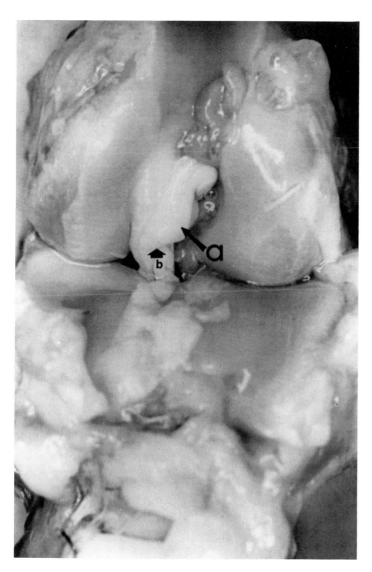

FIG. 19-3. Gross morphology showing transected ACL. Note swollen (a) and retracted (b) appearance. (From ref. 5.)

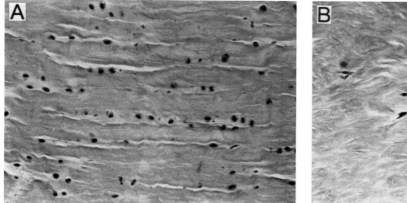

FIG. 19-4. Microscopic evaluation (final magnification: ×30). A: ACL in region of bony attachment (normal cellular organization). B: ACL near transected end of ligament. Note loss of cellularity and loss of organization. (From ref. 5.)

hemarthrosis (48). Further reduction in mechanical properties of the ACL after hemarthrosis were observed with injury to the synovial sheath.

Using a rabbit model of acute hemarthrosis, our own laboratory has shown that the menisci, which lack a synovial covering, demonstrated an increase in degradative activity assessed by levels of collagenase activity (26). Subsequent work found no significant effects of acute hemarthrosis on collagenase activity in the media from ACLs with intact synovium and controls (25). A proliferative synovitis was elicited and deposits of iron within synovial cells were noted; however, ACL with intact synovium showed no microscopic evidence of response to acute hemarthrosis.

Although inconclusive, the elevated levels of collagenase secreted by the menisci following acute hemarthrosis may reflect the reaction of meniscal tissue to an altered and potentially hostile environment. In contrast to the menisci, the ACL may be a privileged intraarticular structure, since it possesses a synovial covering that allows it to be protected from the intraarticular environment. With acute rupture of the ACL and resultant synovial injury, this protective barrier may be lost. Subsequent exposure of ligament substance to the intraarticular environment may produce changes in the ligament and may, in part, explain the poor results reported with attempts to primarily repair the ACL.

A STUDY OF THE INTRINSIC HEALING MECHANISM

Animal Model

To allow us to understand the ACL's intrinsic healing mechanism, a surgical model was developed after numerous surgical repair methods were studied (27).

Initial attempts to repair a complete laceration of the ACL were carried out on rabbits with complete midsubstance lacerations, using a technique described by Marshall (37). Six weeks postoperatively, none of the repaired ligaments showed evidence of healing; all ACLs were in the process of resorption, and a large gap spanned by suture was uniformly evident. A second group was operated on in a similar manner, except the sutures were placed prior to lacerating the ACL in an attempt to decrease the interstump gap. The same

COMPLETE LACERATION

A. Straight cut with Marshall type repair

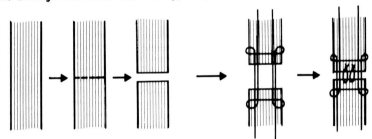

B. Z Step cut and repair

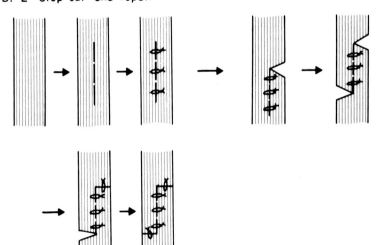

FIG. 19.5A & B.

resorptive process, as well as lack of healing response, was observed in all animals 6 weeks after surgery.

To limit stump retraction and ensure accurate approximation of the lacerated portions of the ACL, a Z-plasty repair was attempted. Six weeks later, no evidence of healing was observed. Failure of this technique was again related to the retraction of lacerated ACL stumps, followed by resorption of the exposed ligament ends.

Partial transection of the ACL has been attempted previously in animal models. O'Donoghue (45) described their poor results, and Arnoczsky (8) noted a vascular proliferation in the area of injury but detected no evidence of bridging of the gap. Arnoczsky concluded that the inability to heal may be related to the fact that he had lacerated the "anteromedial band" of the ACL, a portion of the ACL which is taut throughout the normal range of motion.

To obviate this problem, the posterolateral portion of the ACL was transected by our laboratory (Fig. 19-5C). An immediate retraction of the incised portion of the ligament was noted. In all animals, no evidence of gap reduction was shown. A modified Marshall procedure was then attempted to hold the edges of the partially transected ACL together (Fig. 19-5D). Six weeks after this operation, none of the animals revealed evidence of ACL wound healing. It became obvious that a stent of uncut tissue on one side of the laceration was insufficient to control retraction of the cut ends of the ligament. To circumvent this problem, a model was developed where only the midportion of the ligament was transected. This model minimally disturbs the biomechanical stability of the ligament by retaining lateral and medial ligament continuity. Thus, the lacerated ends stay in close proximity to each other during the postlaceration recovery period (Figs. 19-5E and 19-6).

The surface area of the ligament exposed to joint fluid is limited to the site of penetration into the ligament by a 2-mm-wide razor-thin square-edged Beaver blade. Access to the area of injury by enzymes contained in the synovial space is restricted. The model

PARTIAL LACERATION (Posterolateral band)

C. Simple side cut, and repair

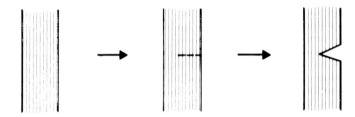

D. Side cut with Marshall type repair

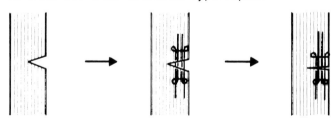

E. Straight cut center, 70%

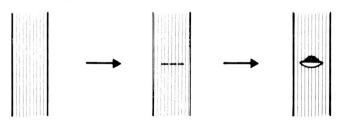

FIG. 19-5. Surgical models for the evaluation of ACL healing. **A** and **B**: Complete laceration models. (From ref. 6.) **C, D,** and **E**: Partial laceration models. (From ref. 6.)

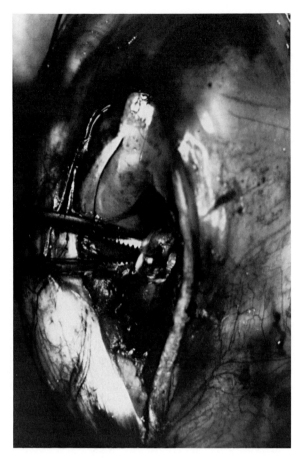

FIG. 19-6. Midsubstance partial laceration in rabbit ACL.

thereby largely, although not totally, eliminates two mechanisms proposed to be responsible for failure of ACL healing: (i) destabilizing biomechanical forces at the injury site and (ii) enzymatic degradation of ligament substance along with inhibition of fibroblast activity by synovial fluid. Using the surgical ACL laceration described herein, we have observed a partial healing response in a small percentage (5%) of ACLs tested in a reproducible fashion (Fig. 19-7).

Healing Response

While a few of the injured ligaments showed abortive attempts at healing, our laboratory failed to demonstrate improvement in ligament strength measured at 3-, 6- and 12-month intervals. The results of the healing response to this injury model strongly suggest that earlier explanations are insufficient in and of themselves to explain the limited healing response of the ACL.

The intrinsic healing capacity of the cruciates may be the limiting factor in their response to injury. Ultrastructural, histological, biochemical, and biomechanical differences have been described between the ACL and medial collateral ligament (MCL), tissues with strikingly different healing capacities (4,35). Light microscopy of the MCL reveals spindle-shaped cells aligned with the long axis of the ligament and interspersed throughout the collagen fiber bundles (4). The ACL cells are oval-shaped and aligned in columns between fiber bundles. Ultrastructurally, MCL collagen fibers are uniformly of large diameter (4,35). The fibroblasts have long cellular processes in close apposition to surrounding collagen fibrils. The ACL has a more heterogeneous population of fibril diameters. Oval-shaped cells are surrounded by an amorphous ground substance and have small microprocesses that are not in close apposition to collagen fibrils.

It appears that a spectrum of fibroblast phenotypes exists between (a) the spindle-shaped connective tissue fibroblast of dermis, tendon, and fascia and (b) the rounded, nested fibroblast of fibrocartilage. The ACL fibroblast seems to exist near the fibrocartilaginous end of the spectrum in terms of morphologic features. Quite possibly the morphological features of these fibroblasts are interrelated with cellular function and play a determinate role in their response to injury. The form/function suitable for survival in a synovial environment may not be sufficient for mounting and sustaining an effective healing response. The concept that the shape of a cell and its orientation with its environment are important factors in modulating its proliferative response to mitogens was mentioned by Wessels (68) in studies on skin. These observations were expanded by Gospodarowicz in a paper entitled "Cellular Shape Is Determined by the Extracellular Matrix and Is Responsible for the Control of Cellular Growth and Function" (21).

Fibronectin

Fibronectins are a class of high-molecular-weight glycoproteins proposed as a key element in the structural interrelationship of cells to matrix and to other cells (6,52,53). They are associated with an array of cellular functions, including cellular adhesion (both cell-to-cell and cell-to-substratum), intra- and extracellular matrix morphology, cell migration, and reticuloendothelial system function (i.e., phagocytosis and chemotaxis). By having adhesive domains specific to fibrin, actin, hyaluronic acid, collagen, heparin, and cell surface factors, they function to attract and couple key elements in normal, healing and growing organized tissue. In fact, fibronectin has been shown to facilitate wound healing (32,41) and to be required for normal collagen organization and deposition by fibroblasts *in vitro* (39).

The ACL, MCL, and meniscus have stained positive for fibronectin. Fibronectin is heavily concentrated in the amorphous ground substance surrounding ACL fibroblasts and meniscal cells, whereas in the MCL it is

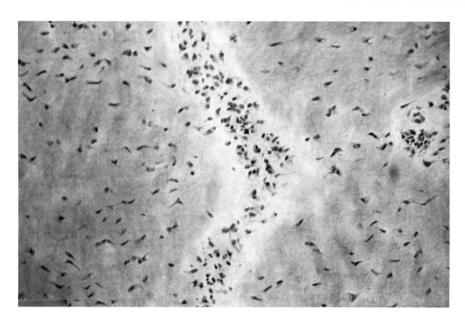

FIG. 19-7. Laceration site, 12 weeks post-operation (H&E, ×50). (From ref. 6.)

distributed evenly over the cellular membrane, even out along the long cellular processes (Fig. 19-8).

Fibronectin levels in rabbit periarticular soft tissues have also been quantitated (3). The amounts of total extractable fibronectin found to be present in ACL, PCL, MCL, and patellar tendon (PT), respectively, were 2.0, 1.9, 0.8, and 0.7 µg/mg of dry tissue. Whereas fibronectin quantities in ACL and PCL were found to be similar, they were over twice as high as the amounts found in either MCL or PT.

Although increased fibronectin levels have been observed in healing tissue (30,32,70), it is not known whether differences in the baseline levels of fibronectin affect the healing potential of a tissue such as cruciate ligament. Baseline levels of fibronectin in the cruciates are high compared to those in other periarticular tissues that have a better healing response. While the importance of fibronectin in various connective tissues is becoming more evident, much remains to be studied.

FUTURE DIRECTIONS

Hyaluronic Acid

Using the surgical model described above (i.e., midsubstance partial laceration), our laboratory has investigated the morphological and biochemical effects of hyaluronan, also known as hyaluronic acid (HA), on the early repair process of the ACL. HA is a linear polysaccharide that has been shown to affect cell proliferation and differentiation by influencing cell–cell and cell–matrix contacts (63–65,71,72). Following laceration of the ligament as described, and immediately after closure of the joint capsule, a single 0.4-ml vol-

ume of hyaluronan (molecular weight 3.6×10^6 daltons) was injected into one knee, with 0.4 ml of saline being injected into the contralateral knee. The repair sites were assessed 4 and 12 weeks post-surgery (69) (Fig. 19-9). Four weeks post-laceration, five of the HA-treated lacerations were completely covered, four were partially covered, and two were not covered. In the saline group, none of the lacerations were completely covered, only two were partially covered, and nine were not covered (Table 19-1). Paired evaluation of the lacerated ligaments showed that the HA-treated side received a healing grade higher than that of the saline side in eight of the 11 animals at 4 weeks post-laceration. At 12 weeks post-laceration the paired evaluation revealed that six of the 10 HA-treated ligaments received a healing grade higher than that of the saline side, and the remaining four of 10 ligaments had an equal healing grade. None of the saline-treated ligaments received a healing grade higher than an HA-treated ligament.

HA seems to have multifactorial effects on ACL healing. Its effect has been shown; however, its mechanism is unclear. We hypothesize that HA may stimulate fibroblasts and contribute to the structural scaffold necessary for repair.

Growth Factors

A vast and rapidly growing literature abounds on a class of peptides commonly called *growth factors*. Accelerated healing of skin wounds has been reported after local application of several growth factors (29,31,51).

After injury, the platelets travel to the wound site

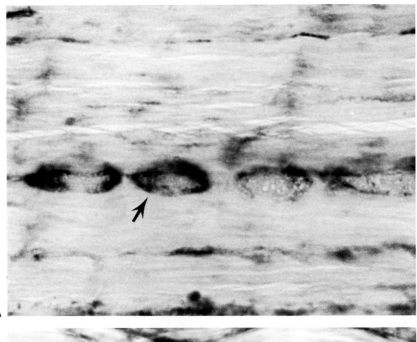

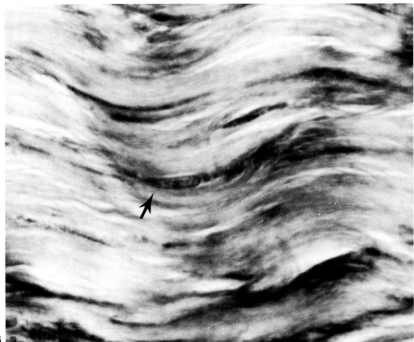

FIG. 19-8A & B.

and form a clot, and hemostasis is obtained. Platelets secrete peptides such as platelet-derived growth factor (PDGF) and transforming growth factor-beta (TGF$_\beta$). Both PDGF and TGF$_\beta$ play an important role in the initiation of repair processes after injury. These factors are chemotactic for inflammatory cells and appear to regulate proliferation and differentiation of fibroblasts (15,56,57,60,62). Inflammatory cells at the wound site then release other peptides such as basic fibroblast growth factor ($_b$FGF) and epidermal growth factor (EGF). $_b$FGF is multifunctional, since it can either stimulate proliferation and induce or delay differentia-

tion (22). Most importantly, $_b$FGF has demonstrated stimulatory effects on angiogenesis, urokinase-type plasminogen activator (implicated in the neovascular response), and wound healing (40).

Because the synovial fluid washes clot away from the ACL injury site, it is hypothesized that a deficiency of growth factor exists at the wound site. Without the necessary stimulus from growth factors and other clot-derived substances, the response to injury is poor.

Encouraging work in this area has been recently reported by Arnoczky (9), who was able to achieve meniscus healing in the central avascular zone by intro-

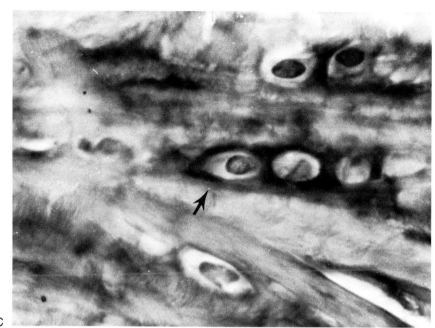

C

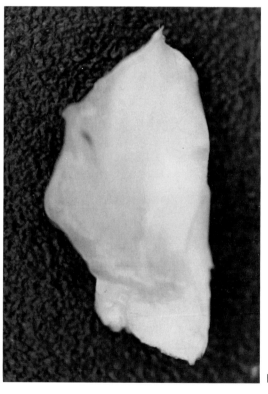

FIG. 19-8. A: ACL stained for fibronectin with goat antirabbit fibronectin antibody using substrate DAB-NiCl$_2$, counterstained with MGP ($\times$1250). Fibronectin is stained about the fibroblast cell membranes and the surrounding area of amorphous ground substance. B: MCL stained (same as above) ($\times$1250). Fibronectin is stained on fibroblast cell membrane on the cell body and along its long cellular processes. C: Medial meniscus stained (same as ACL) ($\times$1250). The staining for fibronectin is noted on cell membranes and about the lacunae in which they lie.

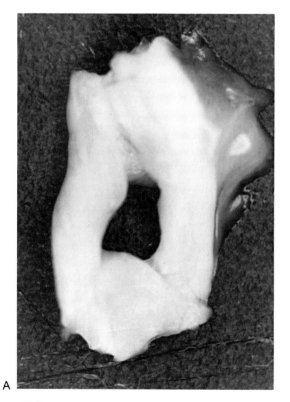

A

B

FIG. 19-9. A: Uncovered laceration (Grade 1), 12 weeks post-surgery (saline-treated). B: Completely covered laceration (Grade 3), 12 weeks post-surgery (hyaluronan-treated).

TABLE 19-1. *Gross observation of rabbit ACL laceration at 4 and 12 weeks post-surgery*

Weeks	Treatment	N	Grade 1 laceration (not covered)	Grade 2 laceration (partially covered)	Grade 3 laceration (completely covered)
4 weeks	Hyaluronan[a]	11	2	4	5
	Saline	11	9	2	0
12 weeks	Hyaluronan[a]	10	1	4	5
	Saline	10	7	2	1

[a] Hyaluronan (molecular weight: 3.6×10^6 daltons).

duction of a fibrin clot into a meniscus laceration. Growth factors in the clot were probably a contributing factor that helped this tissue, which normally has a poor healing capacity, to achieve a healing response. Addition of such a clot might similarly stimulate the healing response in the ACL by supplying growth factors locally as well as supplying a fibrinous scaffold on which healing can occur. Additional studies are required to explore this possibility.

ADHESIVE PROTEIN RECEPTORS

Recently, a superfamily of adhesion-mediating cell-surface glycoproteins (the integrins) has been identified and partially characterized (22). A major subfamily called the "very late antigens" (VLAs) appear to play a primary role in the adhesion of cells to components of the extracellular matrix, including fibronectin, collagen, and laminin.

The VLAs are transmembrane glycoproteins expressed on a wide variety of cells such as fibroblasts, epithelial cells, and various hematopoietic cells. A number of functional roles have been assigned to these adhesive protein receptors, including cell migration cell–matrix adhesions, wound contraction, and ligament "tensioning" (14).

The adhesive protein receptors of ligament tissue have received little attention to date. Generalizing from other fibroblast-containing structures, it is reasonable to expect that these receptors exist on cells of the cruciate ligaments and other periarticular tissues in a unique fashion. Recently, TGF_β has been found to (a) regulate the cell-surface display of VLAs on a variety of cell types and (b) modulate the interaction of cells with the extracellular matrix (24,58). These studies lead us to believe that cell-surface receptor distribution and expression may have profound effects on ligament healing capacity. Fundamental studies on these receptors are in progress in several laboratories.

REFERENCES

1. Alm A, Stromberg B. Vascular anatomy of the patellar and cruciate ligaments. A microangiographic and histologic investigation in the dog. *Acta Chir Scand [Suppl]* 1974;445:25–35.
2. Amiel D, Abel MF, Kleiner JB, Lieber RL, Akeson WH. Synovial fluid nutrient delivery in the diarthrial joint: an analysis of rabbit knee ligaments. *J Orthop Res* 1986;4:90–95.
3. Amiel D, Foulk RA, Harwood FL, Akeson WH. Quantitative assessment by competitive ELISA of fibronectin (fn) in tendons and ligaments. *Matrix* 1989;9(6), in press.
4. Amiel D, Frank C, Harwood FL, Fronek J, Akeson WH. Tendons and ligaments: a morphological and biochemical comparison. *J Orthop Res* 1984;1:257–265.
5. Amiel D, Ishizue KK, Harwood FL, Kitabayashi L, Akeson WH. Injury of the ACL: the role of collagenase in ligament degeneration. *J Orthop Res* 1989;7(4):486–493.
6. Amiel D, Kleiner JB. Biochemistry of tendon and ligament. In: Nimni M, Olsen B, eds. *Collagen, vol III: biotechnology*. Cleveland: CRC Press, 1988;223–251.
7. Andrish J, Holmes R. Effects of synovial fluid on fibroblasts in tissue culture. *Clin Orthop* 1979;138:279–283.
8. Arnoczky SP, Rubin RM, Marshall JL. Microvasculature of the cruciate ligaments and its response to injury. *J Bone Joint Surg* 1979;61A:1221–1229.
9. Arnoczky SP, McDevitt CA, Warren RF, Spivak J, Allen A. Meniscal repair using an exogenous fibrin clot. *Trans Orthop Res Soc* 1986;11:452.
10. Balkfors B. The course of knee ligament injuries. *Acta Orthop Scand [Suppl]* 1982;198(53):1–99.
11. Butler DL, Noyes FR, Grood ES, Olmstead ML, Hohn RB. The effects of vascularity on the mechanical properties of primate anterior cruciate ligament replacements. *Trans Orthop Res Soc* 1983;8:93.
12. Cabaud HE, Rodkey WG, Feagin JA. Experimental studies of acute anterior cruciate ligament injury and repair. *Am J Sports Med* 1979;7:18–22.
13. Cheung HS, Halverson PB, McCarty DJ. Release of collagenase, neutral protease, and prostaglandins from cultured mammalian synovial cells by hydroxyapatite and calcium pyrophosphate dihydrate crystals. *Arthritis Rheum* 1981;24:1338–1344.
14. Dahners LE. Ligament contraction-a correlation with cellularity and actin staining. *Trans Orthop Res Soc* 1986;11:56.
15. Deuel TF, Senior M, Huang JS, Griffin GL. Chemotaxis of monocytes and neutrophils to platelet-derived growth factor. *J Clin Invest* 1982;69:1046–1049.
16. Ehrlich MG, Mankin HJ, Jones H, Wright R, Crispen C, Vigliani G. Collagenase and collagenase inhibitors in osteoarthritic and normal cartilage. *J Clin Invest* 1977;59(2):226–233.
17. Eiken O, Lundborg G, Rank F. The role of the digital synovial sheath in tendon grafting. *Scand J Plast Reconstr Surg* 1975;9:182–189.
18. Fabry G. Early biochemical and histological findings in experimental haemarthrosis in dogs. *Arch Orthop Trauma Surg* 1982;100:167–173.
19. Feagin JA, Abbott HG, Rokous JA. The isolated tear of the ACL [Abstract]. *J Bone Joint Surg* 1972;54A:1340.
20. Feagin JA Jr, Curl WW. Isolated tear of the ACL: 5-year followup study. *Am J Sports Med* 1976;4:95–100.
21. Gospodarowicz D, Neufeld G, Schweigerer L. Cellular shape is determined by the extracellular matrix and is responsible for the control of cellular growth and function. *Mol Cell Endocrinol* 1986;46(3):187–204.
22. Hemler ME, Huang C, Schwartz L. The VLA protein family. *J Biol Chem* 1987;262:3300–3309.
23. Hough AJ, Barfield WO, Sokoloff L. Cartilage in hemophilic

arthropathy; ultrastructural and microanalytical studies. *Arch Pathol Lab Med* 1976;100:91–96.

24. Ignotz RA, Massague J. Cell adhesion protein receptors as targets for transforming growth factor-β action. *Cell* 1987;51:189–197.

25. Ishizue KK, Amiel D, Lyon R, Woo SL-Y. Acute hemarthrosis; a histological, biochemical and biomechanical correlation of effects on the ACL in a rabbit model. *J Orthop Res* 1990; in press.

26. Ishizue KK, Lyon R, Amiel D, Woo SL-Y, et al. Hemarthrosis: a biochemical and mechanical evaluation of effects on the ACL and menisci. *Trans Orthop Res Soc* 1988;13:55.

27. Kleiner JB, Roux RD, Amiel D, Woo SL-Y, Akeson WH. Primary healing of the ACL. *Trans Orthop Res Soc* 1986;11:131.

28. Kohn D. Arthroscopy in acute injuries of anterior cruciate-deficient knees: fresh and old intraarticular lesions. *Arthroscopy* 1986;2:98–102.

29. Kowalewski K, Yong S. Effect of growth hormone and an anabolic steroid on hydroxyproline in healing dermal wounds in rats. *Acta Endocrinol* 1968;59:53–66.

30. Kurkinen M, Vaheri AV, Roberts PJ, Stenman S. Sequential appearance of fibronectin and collagen in experimental granulation tissue. *Lab Invest* 1980;43(1):47–51.

31. Laato M, Niinikoski J, Lebel L, Gerdin B. Stimulation of wound healing by epidermal growth factor. *Ann Surg* 1986;203:379–381.

32. Lehto M, Duance VC, Restall D. Collagen and fibronectin in a healing skeletal muscle injury. *J Bone Joint Surg* 1985;67B:820–828.

33. Lindy S, Turto H, Sorsa T, Halme J, Lauhio A, Suomalainen K, Utto VJ, Wegelius O. Increased collagenase activity in human rheumatoid meniscus. *Scand J Rheumatol* 1986;15:237–242.

34. Lundborg G, Myrhage R, Rydevik B. Original communication: the vascularization of human flexor tendons within the digital synovial sheath region, structural and functional aspects. *J Hand Surg* 1977;2:417–427.

35. Lyon RM, Billings E Jr, Woo SL-Y, Ishizue KK, Kitabayashi L, Amiel D, Akeson WH. The ACL: a fibrocartilaginous structure. *Trans Orthop Res Soc* 1989;14:189.

36. Manske PR, Whiteside LA, Lesker PA. Nutrient pathways to flexor tendons using hydrogen washout technique. *J Hand Surg* 1978;3:32–36.

37. Marshall JL, Rubin RM, Wang JB, et al. The anterior cruciate ligament. The diagnosis and treatment of its injuries and their serious prognostic implication. *Orthop Rev* 1978;7:35–46.

38. Matthews P. The fate of isolated segments of flexor tendons within the digital sheath—a study in synovial nutrition. *Br J Plast Surg* 1978;29:216–224.

39. McDonald JA, Kelley DG, Broekelmann TJ. Role of fibronectin in collagen deposition: Fab' to the gelatin-binding domain of fibronectin inhibits both fibronectin and collagen organization in fibroblast extracellular matrix. *J Cell Biol* 1982;92(2):485–492.

40. Montesano R, Vassalli JD, Baird A, Guillemin R, Orci L. Basic fibroblast growth factor induces angiogenesis *in vitro*. *Proc Natl Acad Sci* 1986;83:7297–7301.

41. Nagelschmidt M, Becker D, Bonninghoff N, Engelhardt GH. Effect of fibronectin therapy and fibronectin deficiency on wound healing: a study in rats. *J Trauma* 1987;27(11):1267–1271.

42. Noyes FR, Bassett RW, Grood ES, Butler DL. Arthroscopy in acute traumatic hemarthrosis of the knee. *J Bone Joint Surg* 1980;62A:687–695.

43. Odensten M, Lysholm J, Gillquist J. Suture of fresh ruptures of the ACL. *Acta Orthop Scand* 1984;55:272–280.

44. O'Donoghue DH, Frank GR, Jeter GL, Johnson W, Zeiders JW, Kenyon R. Repair and reconstruction of the anterior cruciate ligament in dogs. *J Bone Joint Surg* 1971;53A(4):710–718.

45. O'Donoghue DH, Rockwood CA Jr, Frank GR, Jack SC, Kenyon R. Repair of the ACL in dogs. *J Bone Joint Surg* 1966;48A:503–519.

46. Palmer I. On the injuries of the ligament of the knee joint: a clinical study. *Acta Chir Scand [Suppl]* 1938;53:1–282.

47. Pforringer W. Hamarthros and kreuzbander—biomechanische untersuchangen teil 1. *Unfallchirugie* 1982;8:353–367.

48. Pforringer W. Hamarthros and kreuzbander—morphologische untersuchangen teil 2. *Unfallchirugie* 1982;8:368–378.

49. Potenza AD. Critical evaluation of flexor tendon healing and adhesion formation with artificial digital sheaths: an experimental study. *J Bone Joint Surg* 1963;45A:1217–1233.

50. Potenza AD. The healing of autogenous tendon grafts within the flexor digital sheaths in dogs. *J Bone Joint Surg* 1964;46A:1462–1484.

51. Prudden JF, Nishihara G, O'Campo L. Studies on growth hormone. III. The effect on wound tensile strength of marked postoperative anabolism induced with growth hormone. *Surg Gynecol Obstet* 1958;107:481–482.

52. Ruoslahti E, Pierschbacher, MD. Arg-Gly-Asp: a versatile cell recognition site. *Cell* 1986;44:517–518.

53. Ruoslahti E, Pierschbacher, MD. New perspectives in cell adhesion: RGD and integrins. *Science* 1987;238:491–497.

54. Ridge SC, Oransky AL, Kerwar SS. Induction of the synthesis of latent collagenase and latent neutral protease in chondrocytes by a factor synthesized by activated macrophages. *Arthritis Rheum* 1980;23:448–454.

55. Rippey JJ, Hill RR, Lurie A, Sweet M, Thonar E, Handelsman JE. Articular cartilage degradation and the pathology of haemophilic arthropathy. *S Afr Med J* 1978;54:345–351.

56. Roberts AB, Anzano MA, Lamb LC, Smith JM, Sporn MB. New class of transforming growth factors potentiated by epidermal growth factor: isolation from non-neoplastic tissues. *Proc Natl Acad Sci USA* 1981;78:5339–5343.

57. Roberts AB, Sporn MB, Assoian RK, Smith JM, Roche NS, Wakefield LM, Heine UI, Liotta LA, Falanga V, Kehrl JH, Fauci AS. Transforming growth factor type β: rapid induction of fibrosis and angiogenesis *in vivo* and stimulation of collagen formation *in vitro*. *Proc Natl Acad Sci USA* 1986;83:4167–4171.

58. Roberts CJ, Birkenmeier TM, McQuillan JJ, Akiyama SK, Yamada SS, Chen W-T, Yamuda KM, McDonald JA. Transforming growth factor β stimulates the expression of fibronectin and of both subunits of the human fibronectin receptor by cultured human lung fibroblasts. *J Biol Chem* 1988;263(10):4586–4592.

59. Ropes MW, Bennett GA, Bauer W. The origin and nature of normal synovial fluid. *J Clin Invest* 1939;18:351–372.

60. Seppa H, Grotendorst G, Seppa S, Schiffmann E, Martin GR. Platelet-derived growth factor is chemotactic for fibroblasts. *J Cell Biol* 1982;92:584–588.

61. Sherman MF, Bonamo JR. Primary repair of the anterior cruciate ligament. *Clin Sports Med* 1988;7(4):739–750.

62. Sporn MB, Roberts AB, Wakefield LM, Assoian RK. Transforming growth factor β: biological function and chemical structure. *Science* 1986;233:532–534.

63. Toole BP. Hyaluronate and hyaluronidase in morphogenesis and differentiation. *Am Zool* 1973;13:1061–1065.

64. Toole BP. Glycosaminoglycans in morphogenesis. In: Hay E, ed. *Cell biology of extracellular matrix*. New York: Raven Press, 1981;259–294.

65. Turley EA, Bowman P, Kytryk MA. Effects of hyaluronate and hyaluronate-binding proteins on cell motile and contact behaviour. *J Cell Sci* 1985;78:133–145.

66. Warren RF. Primary repair of the anterior cruciate ligament. *Clin Orthop* 1983;172:65–70.

67. Werb Z, Reynolds JJ. Stimulation by endocytosis of the secretion of collagenase and neutral proteinase from rabbit synovial fibroblasts. *J Exp Med* 1974;140:1482–1497.

68. Wessels NK. *Tissue interactions and development*. Menlo Park, CA: Benjamin-Cummings, 1977;213–229.

69. Wiig ME, Amiel D, VandeBerg J, Kitabayahsi L, Harwood FL, Arfors KE. The early effect of high molecular weight hyaluronan (hyaluronic acid) on ACL healing. *J Orthop Res* 1990;8.

70. Williams IF, McCullagh KG, Silver IA. The distribution of types I and III collagen and fibronectin in the healing equine tendon. *Connect Tissue Res* 1984;12:211–227.

71. Yoneda M, Yamagata M, Suzuki S, Kimata K. Hyaluronic acid modulates proliferation of mouse dermal fibroblasts in culture. *J Cell Sci* 1988;90:265–273.

72. Yoneda M, Shimuzu S, Nishi Y, Yamagata M, Suzuki S, Kimata, K. Hyaluronic acid-dependent change in the extracellular matrix of mouse dermal fibroblasts that is conductive to cell proliferation. *J Cell Sci* 1988;90:275–286.

Knee Ligaments: Structure, Function, Injury, and Repair, edited by D. Daniel, et al.

CHAPTER 20

Experimental Studies on Anterior Cruciate Ligament Grafts

Histology and Biochemistry

David Amiel and Scott Kuiper

The biochemical, histological, and vascular changes that take place in an anterior cruciate ligament (ACL) graft ultimately determine the graft's viability, as well as its ability to act as a functional replacement for the ACL. This review of grafts utilized in ACL reconstruction will concentrate primarily on patellar tendon (PT) tissue (autografts and allografts) because this graft tissue has been characterized very thoroughly.

The natural history of the ACL autograft of PT origin has been documented using histological, biochemical, and microvascular techniques. Studies have shown that the PT graft undergoes dramatic changes in its structure, effectively transforming itself into a ligamentous tissue. These changes can be divided into four stages: (i) avascular necrosis, (ii) revascularization, (iii) cellular proliferation, and (iv) remodeling (4,20). Several investigations of PT substitution for the ACL in both human and animal models demonstrate long-term graft viability and suggest that successfully grafted tissue has the same histological appearance as ''normal ligament'' (7,9,17,24).

Investigators first noted morphological changes in PT autografts when they correlated clinical and morphological findings at various intervals after reconstruction of the ACL with a PT autograft in canine and human subjects (1). Biopsy specimens of transplants ranging from 3 months to $5\frac{1}{2}$ years post-surgery were obtained from 16 patients. The biopsy specimens, which were taut *in situ*, were all histologically organized, and some resembled normal ligamentous tissue at the light-microscopic level. The arrangement of collagen fibers, fibrocytes, and vascular elements in autografts from canine specimens (16–20 weeks postoperatively) resembled the structure of a normal ligament. Other investigators similarly observed that ACL autografts of PT origin appeared histologically like a normal ligament with dense, longitudinally oriented collagen bundles (4).

The interpretation of these histological studies was based solely on subjective impressions. No definition for normal tendon or ligament existed at that time. Recently, however, it has been concluded that, despite their gross similarities, tendons and ligaments have unique histological and biochemical characteristics (Chapter 5) (2).

The natural history of the ACL autograft after ACL

D. Amiel and S. Kuiper: Department of Surgery, Division of Orthopedics and Rehabilitation, University of California, San Diego, School of Medicine, La Jolla, California 92093.

reconstruction using the medial one-third of the quadriceps/patellar tendon in rabbits has been described (3). ACL autografts, native ACL, and control PT were evaluated histologically as well as biochemically with respect to time to determine the graft's response to its new intrasynovial milieu and new physical forces.

MORPHOLOGY

Gross Morphology

Native PT and ACL were similar at gross inspection: Both structures were white, glistening, and firm to palpation. Autografts were evaluated 2, 3, 4, 6, and 30 weeks postoperatively. Two weeks postoperatively the autografts were noted to be a dull white color, frayed, and necrotic-appearing, without adherent synovium. At 4 weeks postoperatively, the autografts were swollen two to three times their original size, glistening, and still without evidence of a synovial sheath. At 6 weeks post-surgery, the autografts showed diminished swelling and a thin synovial envelope. The autografts at 30 weeks were similar to those at 6 weeks. None of the autografts had grossly visible blood vessels. Similar gross morphological results have been reported by others (10) after experimental replacement of the ACL. Hypertrophy of the intraarticular segment of the PT autograft was noted and this continued for up to a year post surgery. Additionally, development of a covering of synovial membrane of this newly created ligament had occurred by 8 weeks postoperatively.

Histology

The four stages of autograft transformation (avascular necrosis, revascularization, cellular proliferation, and remodeling) are quite evident in histologic studies. PT autografts examined as early as 2 days postoperatively revealed a relative decrease in tissue cellularity as compared to the tissue of origin (18). The autograft fibroblasts had become noticeably round when compared to the spindle-shaped cells of the PT. Seven days postoperatively the cellular population diminished even further, to the point that fibroblasts were only observed sporadically in the tissue midsubstance and periphery. The autograft was notable for its midsubstance acellularity at 14 days post surgery. A peripheral rim of fibroblasts constituted the entire cellular population.

Two weeks postoperatively the autografts showed the normal PT crimp, but no fibroblasts were seen centrally (Fig. 20-1C) (3). However, round to ovoid cells were visible on the peripheral margin of the grafts (Fig. 20-1D). Three weeks postoperatively the tissue's crimp pattern remained similar to that of PT. However, the peritendineum areas showed a marked cellular proliferation, with cells spilling out into the collagenous matrix. The tissue was hypocellular relative to normal PT, but a mixture of cells, some rod-like, others ovoid, were present and orientated longitudinally (Fig. 20-1E). Autografts obtained at the 4-week period maintained a longitudinal axis, but crimping was much less distinct (Fig. 20-1F). The number of cells had increased dramatically, approximating the relative cellularity of the normal ACL. Cells were no longer focally concentrated and had spread homogeneously throughout the matrix of the graft. Nuclei present in the 4-week autografts were very similar to those of the ACL (Fig. 20-1F). The cells were, for the most part, ovoid, plump, and occasionally rod-like, resembling cells in the ACL. Few spindle-shaped nuclei were seen. At 6 weeks postsurgery the autografts maintained a longitudinal axis, although the crimping pattern was present only in some sections (Fig. 20-1G). Cellularity was greater than either ACL or PT, and ovoid cells very similar to native ACL predominated. At the 30-week postoperative time period (Fig. 20-1H), cellular size and shape were similar to those seen at the 6-week time point. The longitudinal orientation of the cells was predominant, and the relative cell number had decreased to that of the native ACL.

An earlier study by Clancy (11) demonstrated that 8-week autografts have a small area of central acellularity. Leading cells in the zones of cellular invasion appeared to have plump, ovoid nuclei that would correspond to cells similar to those in the ACL described previously (2). At 9 and 12 months, however, it was reported that the individual fibroblasts resumed their narrowed spindle shape. Despite this cellular change, the birefringent pattern remained typical of mature ACL collagen bundles.

In a similar investigation by Arnoczky (4), PT autografts used to replace ACLs in dogs were studied, using both histology and tissue clearing techniques. The PT graft had a normal appearance at 2 weeks post-surgery. At 4 weeks post-surgery, evidence of avascular necrosis was noted with cell death, hypocellularity, and collagen fragmentation, particularly in the central core, with a surrounding zone of cells undergoing fibrocartilaginous metaplasia. A proliferation of mesenchymal cells was noted at 6 weeks post-surgery. At 16 weeks a marked proliferation of cells was seen, whereas at 26 weeks the graft appeared less proliferative. At 52 weeks the autograft was histologically like a ''normal-appearing ligament with dense, longitudinally orientated collagen bundles.''

Thus, it is apparent that the autograft initially undergoes necrosis (although the time sequence varied slightly between studies), revascularization (which will be discussed further in the section entitled ''Vascular

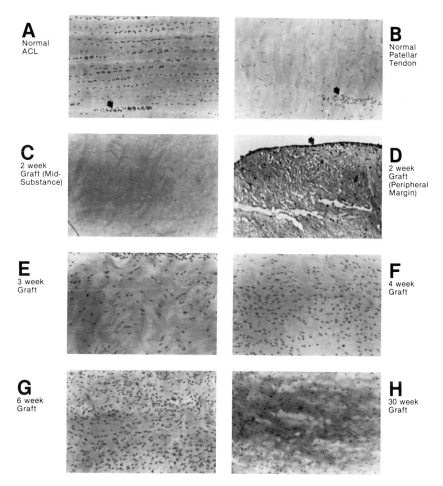

FIG. 20-1. Histology of normal ACL, PT and PT autografts (H&E, ×50). **A:** Note rounded fibroblasts, fine fibrillar crimp, and cluster of potential reserve cells (*arrow*). **B:** Note spindle-shaped fibroblasts, coarse fibrillar crimp, and peritendineum (*arrow*). **C:** Acellular central portion of 2-week autograft. **D:** Rounded fibroblasts inhabit peripheral portions of 2-week autograft (*arrow*). **E:** Focal areas of proliferation are evident in the 3-week autograft with cells spilling into unoccupied matrix. **F:** Homogeneous distribution of fibroblasts in the 4-week graft. **G:** Relative hypercellularity and rare crimping pattern in 6-week autograft. **H:** Cellular appearance and number in the 30-week autograft is similar to those in the normal ACl. (From ref. 3.)

Studies''), cellular repopulation, and, finally, tissue remodeling into a structure similar to the ACL histologically.

Replacement Cell Origin

Histological observations of PT autografts used in ACL reconstruction showed (a) central acellularity with a peripheral rim of cells at 2 weeks postoperatively and (b) a cellular invasion culminating with cellular homogeneity at 4 weeks postoperatively (3). Because graft necrosis precedes cellular proliferation, the early events of graft incorporation were studied to determine the origin of the cellular replacement population (19). Selective destruction of native PT cells with liquid N_2 immersion prior to ACL reconstruction was performed to study the extrinsic contribution of cells. The intrinsic contribution of cells was evaluated by sequestration of the PT autograft in a semipermeable membrane before it was used to reconstruct the ACL. Histological analysis of liquid N_2-treated PT tissue, used as an autograft and then harvested 3 weeks postsurgery, revealed fibroblastic incorporation of the graft. In contrast, no cells were observed in autografts sequestered in a semipermeable membrane. These findings suggest that autogenous ACL autografts of PT origin are repopulated by cells from an extrinsic origin, and not by cells from an intrinsic source (such as the autograft itself).

The most likely source for these cells is the synovial membrane, which has a combination of macrophage-like cells (Type A cells), fibroblast-like cells (Type B cells), and undifferentiated cells (Type C cells) (12).

These cells are adapted for survival in synovial fluid and are present in the joint fluid throughout the postoperative period.

The source of replacement cells has obvious and important implications. If cells that inhabit the autograft are of PT origin, a strong case would be made for procedures that maintain a blood supply to the graft in an attempt to maintain viability of native PT fibroblasts (4,21). However, because this study demonstrates that the cells which repopulate the autograft are from a source other than the autograft (extrinsic), then the necessity of maintaining a blood supply to the graft tissue at the time of surgery is questionable.

Early Metabolic Assessment

During the first 3 postoperative weeks, the PT fibroblasts die and are replaced by cells from an extrinsic source. To evaluate the metabolic activity of replacement cells following native cell drop-out, a study of the *in vivo* cellular biochemistry of the autograft was undertaken (18). Results from this study revealed that the native autograft cell population rapidly necroses, as evidenced by (a) the loss of its ability to synthesize collagen, (b) its low metabolic activity, and (c) cell drop-out as early as day 2. Explanations put forth for

this include (a) a lack of sufficient nutrition from the synovial fluid or (b) a possible toxic effect of synovial fluid on these cells. Interestingly, the 7-day autografts revealed increased metabolic activity with a further decrease in the cell population (Fig. 20-2). This can be interpreted as an expression of the ingrowth of a metabolically active replacement population. This trend continued through the 14th day postoperatively. At 3 weeks post-surgery a proliferative histological pattern correlated well with the high specific activity of the tissue at that time point. It is of special interest that the cell proliferation and heightened metabolism are not limited by the lack of autograft vascularity, which was evident with vascular injection studies 3 weeks after surgery. The fibroblasts that repopulate the graft are adapted for survival in synovial fluid and have a high synthetic capacity.

BIOCHEMISTRY

Biochemical Transformations

To confirm whether PT autografts biochemically transform into a ligament-like substance, PT autografts were analyzed using three parameters with respect to time, namely, collagen crosslinking, collagen typing,

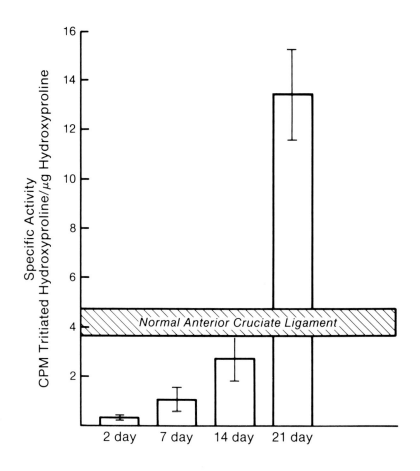

FIG. 20-2. Specific activity of autografts of PT origin and of the normal ACL. (From ref. 18.)

and total glycosaminoglycan (GAG) (3). Earlier studies demonstrated measurable differences between tendon and ligament when these tissues were characterized biochemically using these parameters (2). If the autograft actually transforms from a tendinous material to a ligamentous material, one would expect these biochemical parameters in the autograft to change as well.

Collagen crosslinking characteristics of the ACL autografts changed dramatically as a function of time during the postsurgical period of recovery. As reported previously, normal PT and ACL have very distinct reducible crosslink patterns (2). Most notably, the ACL contains a high concentration of dihydroxylysinonorleucine (DHLNL) and relatively little histidinohydroxymerodesmosine (HHMD) and hydroxylysinonorleucine (HLNL). The PT exhibits just the opposite pattern (i.e., much HHMD and HLNL, with little DHLNL). Because of these differences, collagen crosslinking changes provide an important index of tissue transformation.

Such a transformation had already begun to appear by 2 weeks post-surgery, since the amount of DHLNL was seen to have increased relative to HHMD (Fig. 20-3). One can see that by 4 weeks, DHLNL had increased dramatically, although HHMD was still quite high. As the time period increased to 30 weeks, the relative amounts of DHLNL and HHMD appeared to be very similar to those observed for normal ACL. Perhaps most significant was the observation that by 30 weeks the concentration of HHMD (very high in normal PT) had dropped to levels normally found in ACL. Table 20-1 summarizes the relative amounts of the reducible crosslinks found in ACL, PT, and PT autograft at different postsurgical time intervals.

In addition to the reducible collagen crosslinks, a stable nonreducible crosslink, 3-hydroxypyridinium, was present in those tissues. The concentration of 3-hydroxypyridinium has been found to be four to five times higher in ACL than in PT (2). Autografts at 30 weeks post-surgery demonstrated 3-hydroxypyridi-

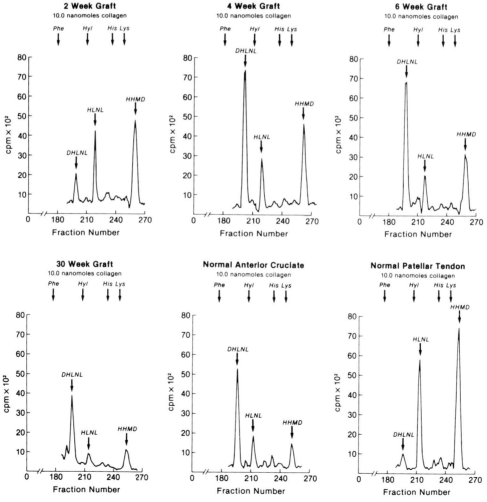

FIG. 20-3. Radioactive elution profile of reducible collagen crosslinks from PT, ACL, and PT autografts. (From ref. 3.)

TABLE 20-1. *Relative amounts of collagen crosslinks in patellar tendon (PT), anterior cruciate ligament (ACL), and PT autografts[a]*

Tissue	DHLNL/HLNL[b]	DHLNL/HHMD[b]
Normal PT	0.23 ± 0.05	0.15 ± 0.03
2-week graft	0.53 ± 0.07	0.25 ± 0.05
4-week graft	2.95 ± 0.15	1.60 ± 0.20
6-week graft	5.23 ± 0.92	2.56 ± 0.87
30-week graft	4.40 ± 0.80	3.50 ± 0.62
Normal ACL	3.28 ± 0.35	3.65 ± 0.47

[a] From ref. 3.

[b] DHLNL, dihydroxylysinonorleucine; HLNL, hydroxylysinonorleucine; HHMD, histidinohydroxymerodesmosine.

nium at a concentration that averaged a little more than half that found in normal ACL (Fig. 20-4).

Collagen typing of the tissues provided another valuable parameter for characterizing time-dependent changes in the autograft. PT and ACL have been found to exhibit different collagen-type characteristics (2). Whereas PT had no detectable Type III collagen, ACL contained about 10% Type III. The predominant type of collagen in both tissues was Type I. High-pressure liquid chromatography (HPLC) separation of the CNBr peptides from PT, ACL, and PT autografts at various stages of recovery following surgery is illustrated in Fig. 20-5. Marker peptides representative of Type I collagen are designated under Peak A, and the

Type III marker peptides are designated under Peak B. These chromatograms show that Type III collagen was detected in the PT autografts as early as 2 weeks post-surgery. The amount of Type III collagen reached a maximum at 6 weeks, and it decreased only slightly by 30 weeks after operation. The estimated amount in the PT autograft at 30 weeks was comparable to that found in normal ACL. Table 20-2 summarizes the approximate proportions of Type I and Type III collagen found in the different tissues.

The normal GAG content of ACL and PT are statistically different. The ACL contains more than twice the amount of GAG as that contained in PT (2). As early as 2 weeks post-surgery the PT autografts had an increase in the amount of GAG when compared to native PT (Table 20-3). Concentrations of GAG were increased significantly ($p < 0.05$) when comparing autografts obtained at 4-, 6-, and 30-week periods to their original structure (PT). After 4 weeks post-surgery the amount of GAG remained constant, and no statistical significance was found when the autografts at 4, 6, and 30 weeks were compared to the GAG concentration of the ACL.

Biochemical/Histological Assessment Summary

The histological and biochemical data demonstrate a remarkable metamorphosis: Tissue that was originally

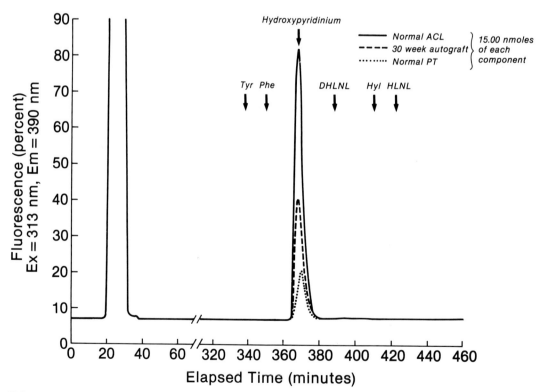

FIG. 20-4. Isolation of the hydroxypyridinium crosslink by cation-exchange liquid chromatography of the tissue hydrolysates. (From ref. 3.)

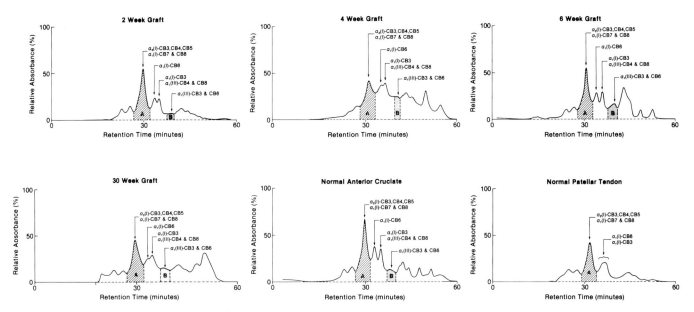

FIG. 20-5. HPLC of the CNBr peptides from PT, ACL, and PT autografts. **Top row:** Type I marker peptides. **Bottom row:** Type III marker peptides. (From ref. 3.)

PT transformed to a substance very similar to normal ACL. The general process of tissue transformation was recognized by Wilhelm Roux in 1905 (26). Roux's "law of functional adaption," which states that "an organ will adapt itself structurally to an alteration, quantitative or qualitative in function" seems to hold true for PT autografts. However, as was described in detail in Chapter 18, most of the animal studies on ACL reconstruction with autografts from various sources show stiffness and ultimate load values of only 30–40% of controls 8–24 months after transplantation. The discrepancy between this rather disappointing outcome compared to the good to excellent functional results following autografting for reconstruction of human knees has not been explained.

TABLE 20-2. *Proportions of Type I and Type III collagen in patellar tendon (PT), anterior cruciate ligament (ACL) and PT autografts*[a]

Tissue	Percent Type I	Percent Type III
PT	>95	—
2-week graft	92–95	5–8
4-week graft	87–90	10–13
6-week graft	82–85	15–18
30-week graft	84–88	12–16
ACL	86–89	11–14

[a] From ref. 3.

TABLE 20-3. *Total glycosaminoglycan (GAG) content (mg of hexosamine/g dry tissue) in patellar tendon (PT), anterior cruciate ligament (ACL) and PT autografts*[a]

Tissue	GAG
Patellar tendon (PT)	3.92 ± 0.16
Anterior cruciate ligament (ACL)	9.89 ± 0.56
ACL reconstruction	
2-week graft	5.62 ± 0.82
4-week graft	10.72 ± 1.12
6-week graft	11.71 ± 1.24
30-week graft	11.42 ± 0.93

[a] From refs. 2 and 3. Note: All results are mean values ± SE.

VASCULAR STUDIES

Long-term viability of transplanted autologous PT is necessary if the graft is to behave as a functional replacement for the ACL. Revascularization of the graft is required if the graft is to remain a viable substitute for the ACL. The primary contributors to the revascularization process appear to be the soft tissues of the infrapatellar fat pad, the proximal remnant of the excised ligament, and the endosteal vasculature of the femoral attachment (1). Additionally, the importance of the posterior synovial fold for revascularization of PT autografts used to reconstruct ACLs has been emphasized (11).

The viability of the transplanted autogenous PT was first studied by Alm (1), who performed ACL reconstructions in dogs. He evaluated PT autografts using segmental microangiography from 1 to 20 weeks postsurgery. Revascularization of the paraligamentous and endoligamentous blood supply to the graft was by contributions from (a) the infrapatellar fat pad (which was sutured around the graft), (b) the proximal remnant of the excised ACL, and (c) the endosteal vessels at the femoral attachment site. From 2 to 6 weeks the avascular proximal end of the graft was invaded by the endoligamentous vessels from the middle portion of the graft. By the 8th week the grafts were completely revascularized. From that point, up to the 20th week, the tissue remodeled to the extent that the collagen bundle arrangement and vascularity resembled the pattern in a normal ligament.

Clancy (11) performed ACL reconstructions with autogenous PT in monkeys and noted revascularization of grafts at 8 weeks also, even though the fat pad was not sutured around the graft. His study emphasized the importance of the vascular contribution from the posterior synovial fold. He described abundant vascularity at 8 weeks, made up of paraligamentous and endoligamentous vessels originating mainly from the posterior synovial fold, with additional contributions from the femoral endosteal vessels proximally and the tibial endosteal vessels distally.

Other investigators (4) evaluating PT autografts have noted that the transplanted graft is surrounded by a vascular synovial sheath as early as 6 weeks postoperatively and has evidence of intrinsic vessels at 8–10 weeks after transfer. Revascularization was not complete, however, until 20 weeks postoperatively. These results demonstrate that the time course of graft revascularization is variable. The effect this avascular period has on the graft is not completely known. Prior to completion of the revascularization process the graft is an avascular scaffold on which cells can proliferate and form a new collagenous matrix. Although the early replacement cells are not dependent on the vascular supply for their nutrition, the graft tissue may be vulnerable to stretch, rupture, or alteration in its material properties during this avascular period (18).

ALLOGRAFT STUDIES

PT autografts are avascular at the time of transfer and are therefore free grafts (4,11). For this reason, PT and ACL allografts have been evaluated by several investigators as possible graft alternatives (5,15,23,27,28). The use of allograft material for reconstruction is advantageous because it eliminates the need to disrupt periarticular supporting structures of the knee, thereby reducing postoperative functional disability (29). Allografts are, in addition, readily available and can be stored indefinitely by deep-freezing. Biologically, the PT allograft would seem capable of providing the same biological "scaffold" as a PT autograft has been shown to provide. Whichever type of graft is used must become vascularized and maintain or develop an orientated pattern of collagen fibers.

Several issues must be addressed for successful allotransplantation. These include biocompatibility of the graft, preservation of the tissue prior to transplantation, and finally, sterilization of the allograft before transplantation.

Freeze-drying and deep-freezing techniques have been shown to be effective methods for rendering connective tissue allografts less antigenic, probably by killing cells and denaturing the histocompatibility antigens on their surface (8,13,14,22). However, antidonor antibodies have been detected in the synovial fluid of dogs receiving frozen bone–ligament–bone ACL allografts indicating immunogenicity of the allograft even though systemic antibodies were not detected (28). Whether this is clinically significant has not been thoroughly studied. Changes in the material properties of deep-frozen ligaments are not statistically different from those of fresh controls (6). Sterilization procedures must be tested more thoroughly for allografts. Proteins degenerate on heating, and neither irradiation nor gas sterilization by ethylene oxide provide certain sterility. Ethylene oxide sterilization of allografts resulted in an inflammatory response in the human knee sufficient to require that this procedure be discontinued (16,25).

Shino (27) evaluated the revascularization and remodeling of PT allografts used to replace the ACL in the canine knee. Central portions of PTs were harvested aseptically from donor dogs and preserved at −20°C for at least 2 weeks. These were subsequently thawed in saline and used to reconstruct the ACL in 26 dogs. Six reconstructions were performed using PT autograft for comparison. After the 15th postoperative week, all the knees showed some degree of anterior laxity. However, no significant degenerative disease or meniscal tears were seen. Macroscopically, all reconstructed ligaments appeared viable and were adherent to the infrapatellar fat pad. Microangiographic studies revealed that after 3 weeks, half the graft was already revascularized. The anterodistal portion of the graft was hypervascular, whereas the posterior half of the distal third remained essentially avascular. At 6 weeks, abundant vascularity in and about the graft was noted, with major contributions from the infrapatellar fat pad and the proximal synovial folds. The central portion of the allograft remained relatively less vascular. At 15 weeks the graft was less vascular than at 6 weeks; by 30 weeks the vascular response had subsided, leaving the graft adequately vascularized. Fifty-two weeks postoperatively the vascular pattern of the PT allografts was similar to that of the normal ACL, suggesting that the allograft had matured as a functional ligament.

Histological studies revealed that spindle-shaped mesenchymal cells invaded the allograft as early as 3 weeks postoperatively. By 15 weeks, most of the PT allograft was invaded by proliferating cells. However, small areas remained which appeared relatively acellular and nonviable. These areas disappeared by 30 weeks post-surgery: The graft showed peripheral hypercellularity and central normal cellularity with spindle-shaped nuclei and longitudinally arranged collagen bundles. By 52 weeks the allograft appeared histologically similar to a mature ligament.

Arnoczky (5) replaced the ACL in 25 dogs with fresh and frozen medial-third PT allografts and evaluated these grafts using routine histological and vascular injection techniques from 2 weeks to 1 year postoperatively. A marked inflammatory reaction was noted in fresh PT allografts, characterized by perivascular cuffing and lymphocyte invasion as early as 2 weeks postoperatively. Frozen grafts had no such reaction. Four weeks postoperatively the histological evaluation revealed an avascular tissue surrounded by a vascular synovial membrane. The periphery of the graft was only beginning to be populated with cells. At 8 weeks the graft had not changed significantly, except that the synovial tissue was extremely vascular and thickened. By 12 weeks, intrinsic revascularization was accompanied by cellular proliferation. These changes progressed such that at 6 months the PT allograft resembled a normal ligament, with dense, longitudinally oriented collagen bundles and a normal cell population.

Deep-frozen PT allografts and fresh PT autografts appear to undergo a similar transformation into a ligamentous tissue. Some investigators have found the revascularization process in allografts to be complete by the 6th postoperative week (earlier than that of the autografts) (27). Others have noted the revascularization time to be similar to that of the PT autografts (5). There remains, however, a long period between transplantation and revascularization during which the graft may sustain stretch, rupture, or alteration of its material properties. Indeed, two studies have demonstrated increased laxity of the joint over time (5,27). Neither demonstrated degenerative changes within the joint over the first postoperative year.

Similar allotransplantation studies have been undertaken using ACL allografts to replace the ACL (5,23,28). One such study (23) found that ACL allografts appear to be partially revascularized by 8 weeks, with (a) vascularity at the femoral and tibial attachments and (b) hypovascularity in the mid-zone. By 24 and 36 weeks postoperatively, the endoligamentous and periligamentous patterns were more organized. No differences were noted between the vascular patterns of the normal and transplanted ligaments at 18 months. Fibroblastic proliferation in the periligamentous portion of the graft was noted at 8 weeks, whereas the central area had diminished cellularity. By 16 weeks the central area had become rich with cells as well. By 18 months the specimens had a normal collagen bundle orientation and a vascular and cellular appearance.

Biochemical, histological, and vascular studies indicate that autografts and allografts used for ACL reconstruction transform themselves into a tissue similar to the ACL. The body uses the tendinous collagen framework to regenerate a functional ligament replacement. The tissue appears viable with complete revascularization. There is a lag period, however, before revascularization is complete. During this time, the graft is an avascular collagenous scaffold that must be protected to allow this process to occur.

ACKNOWLEDGMENTS

Support from NIH Grants AR34264 and the Malcolm and Dorothy Coutts Institute for Joint Reconstruction and Research is acknowledged.

REFERENCES

1. Alm A, Stromberg B. Vascular anatomy of the patellar and cruciate ligaments: a microangiographic and histologic investigation in the dog. *Acta Chir Scand [Suppl]* 1974;445:25–35.
2. Amiel D, Frank C, Harwood F, Fronek J, Akeson WH. Tendons and ligaments: a morphological and biochemical comparison. *J Orthop Res* 1984;1:257–265.
3. Amiel D, Kleiner JB, Roux RD, Harwood FL, Akeson WH. The phenomenon of "ligamentization": anterior cruciate ligament reconstruction with autogenous patellar tendon. *J Orthop Res* 1986;4:162–172.
4. Arnoczky SP, Tarvin GB, Marshall JL. ACL replacement using patellar tendons. *J Bone Joint Surg* 1982;64A:217–224.
5. Arnoczky SP, Warren RF, Ashock MA. Replacement of the anterior cruciate ligament using a patellar tendon allograft. *J Bone Joint Surg* 1986;68A(3):376–385.
6. Barad S, Cabaud HE, Rodrigo JJ. The effect of storage at −80°C as compared to 4°C on the strength of rhesus monkey anterior cruciate ligament. *Trans Orthop Res Soc* 1982;7:378.
7. Cabaud HD, Feagin JA, Rodkey WG. Anterior cruciate ligament injury and augmented repair. *Am J Sports Med* 1980;8:395–401.
8. Cameron RR, Conrad RH, Sell KW, Latham WD. Freeze-dried composite tendon allografts: an experimental study. *Plast Reconstr Surg* 1971;47:39–46.
9. Campbell WC. Reconstruction of the ligament of the knee. *Am J Surg* 1939;43:473–480.
10. Chiroff RT. Experimental replacement of the anterior cruciate ligament. *J Bone Joint Surg* 1974;57A(8):1124–1127.
11. Clancy WC, Narenchania RG, Rosenberg TD, Gmeiner JG, Wisnefski DD, Lange TA. Anterior and posterior cruciate ligament reconstruction in rhesus monkeys. *J Bone Joint Surg* 1981; 63A:1270–1284.
12. Dunphy JE. *Wound healing*, New York: Medcom Press, 1974.
13. Friedlaender GE, Strong DM, Sell KW. Studies on the antigenicity of bone. I. Freeze-dried and deep-frozen bone allografts in rabbits. *J Bone Joint Surg* 1976;58A:854–858.
14. Graham WC, Smith DA, McGuire MP. The use of frozen stored tendons for grafting. An experimental study. *J Bone Joint Surg* 1955;37A:624.
15. Jackson DW, Grood ES, Arnoczky SP, Butler DL, Simon TM. Freeze dried anterior cruciate ligament allografts. *Am J Sports Med* 1987;15(4):295–303.
16. Jackson DW, Simon TM, Windler G. Intraarticular reaction following reconstruction of the anterior cruciate ligament with ethylene oxide sterilized bone–patella-bone allograft. Presented at the AOSSM Meeting, Las Vegas, 1989.
17. Jones KG. Reconstruction of the anterior cruciate ligament: A technique using the central one-third of the patellar ligament. *J Bone Joint Surg [Am]* 1963;45:925–932.
18. Kleiner JB, Amiel D, Harwood FL, Akeson WH. Early histo-

logic, metabolic and vascular assessment of anterior cruciate ligament autografts. *J Orthop Res* 1989;7:235–242.

19. Kleiner JB, Amiel D, Roux RD, Akeson WH. Origin of replacement cells for the anterior cruciate ligament autograft. *J Orthop Res* 1986;4:466–474.

20. Kondo M. An experimental study on reconstructive surgery of the anterior cruciate ligament. *J Jpn Orthop Assoc* 1979;53:521–533.

21. Leeson TS, Leeson CR. *A brief atlas of histology*. Philadelphia: WB Saunders, 1979.

22. Minami A, Ishii S, Ogino T, Oikawa T, Kobayashi H. Effect of the immunological antigenicity of the allogenic tendons on tendon grafting. *Hand* 1982;14:111–119.

23. Nikolaou PK, Seaber AV, Glisson RR, Ribbeck BM, Bassett FH. Anterior cruciate ligament allograft transplantation. *Am J Sports Med* 1986;14(5):348–360.

24. Nimni ME. Collagen: structure, function and metabolism in normal and fibrotic tissues. *Semin Arthritis Rheum* 1983;13:1–85.

25. Roberts TS, Drez DJ, McCarthy W, Pain R. ACL reconstruction using freeze-dried ethylene oxide sterilized bone–patella-bone allograft. Presented at the AAOS 56th Meeting, Las Vegas, 1989.

26. Roux W. *Die Entwicklungsmechanic*. Leipzig, 1905.

27. Shino K, Kawasaki T, Hirose H, Gotoh 1, Inoue M, Ono K. Replacement of the anterior cruciate ligament by an allogeneic tendon graft. *J Bone Joint Surg* 1984;66B(5):672–681.

28. Vasseur PB, Rodrigo JJ, Stevenson S, Clark G, Sharkey N. Replacement of the anterior cruciate ligament with a bone–ligament–bone anterior cruciate ligament allograft in dogs. *Clin Orthop* 1987;219:268–277.

29. Webster DA, Werner FW. Freeze-dried flexor tendons in anterior cruciate ligament reconstruction. *Clin Orthop* 1983;181:238–243.

Knee Ligaments: Structure, Function, Injury,
and Repair, edited by D. Daniel, et al.
© 1990 by Raven Press, Ltd. All rights reserved.

CHAPTER 21

Experimental Studies on Anterior Cruciate Ligament Autografts and Allografts

Mechanical Studies

Peter O. Newton, Shuji Horibe, and Savio L-Y. Woo

Several autogenous and allogeneic tissues have been used in anterior cruciate ligament (ACL) reconstruction (11,12,19,26,33,38,49,65). These tissue grafts undergo a change in their biomechanical properties when placed into the intraarticular environment of the knee, and precise knowledge of the remodeling process is necessary. The graft remodeling process, as described in Chapter 20, consists of ischemic necrosis followed by progressive graft revascularization and cellular repopulation. Collagen fiber alignment and crimp pattern of the graft become disorganized initially, but with time, progressive realignment occurs. Histologic characteristics begin to resemble those of the normal ligament after roughly 1 year of remodeling. Experimental studies investigating the structural properties of the femur–graft–tibia complex have found that the linear stiffness (henceforth called *stiffness*) and strength (or ultimate load) of the graft is initially very low (4,7,13,15,27,32,35,36,40,48,50,52,58,64,66–68,70,74,75). Exposure of the graft material to exces-

sive tension while it is weak, early in the remodeling process, may result in disruption of the graft. Therefore, it is important to know the changes in the biomechanical characteristics of the graft throughout the remodeling period. In this chapter we will discuss several factors that have an influence on this process. These include the method of graft placement and fixation, initial graft tension, and postsurgical rehabilitation. We will review the experimental animal studies on autograft and allograft ligament reconstruction and will discuss the biomechanical aspects of graft remodeling as a function of time postoperatively.

AUTOGRAFT RECONSTRUCTIONS

Autograft reconstructions in experimental animals have been performed in order to quantify changes in the biomechanical properties of the graft tissues with respect to time. Until recently, most studies have placed emphasis on the ultimate load of the femur–ACL–tibia complex (FATC), while other important structural parameters such as stiffness of the FATC and measures of joint kinematics have largely been ignored.

P. O. Newton, S. Horibe, and S. L-Y. Woo: Orthopaedic Bioengineering Laboratory, University of California, San Diego, La Jolla, California 92093, and Malcolm and Dorothy Coutts Institute for Joint Reconstruction and Research, San Diego, California.

Types of Autografts

Fascia Lata/Iliotibial Tract

The fascia lata, or fascia of the proximal lateral thigh, forms a condensed fibrous band distally which inserts into the lateral aspect of the proximal tibia. The distal thickened portion is called the *iliotibial tract* (ITT) (39). Hey Groves (25,26) used a free graft of proximal fascia lata to perform the first ACL autograft reconstruction. The strength (ultimate load) of this tissue has been demonstrated to be comparable to the ITT (628 N and 769 N, respectively) (55). However, the proximal fascia lata has subsequently received little attention because of the large surgical exposure required to harvest this tissue.

The distal ITT is a structure that has also been used in several ways subsequent to Hey Groves' method. O'Donoghue (58) used the ITT as a free graft in a canine model. The ultimate load of the femur–graft–tibia complex was 157 N (23% of the control FATC value) after 4 years of implantation. In these knees, joint instability and arthritic changes were noted. More recently, the use of ITT for reconstructing the ACL has been studied by Holden (27) in a goat model. This author fashioned a free graft from the distal 13 cm of the fascia lata/ITT. The graft was placed through a tibial tunnel and was then placed over the top of the lateral femoral condyle. Structural properties of the donor ITT as determined by tensile testing found the stiffness to be 179 N/mm (22% of the control FATC) and found the ultimate load to be 1128 N (41% of the control FATC). These values for the ITT graft decreased after implantation. The ultimate load of the experimental femur–graft–tibia complex dropped to less than 10% of the control FATC value at the time of reconstruction, with failure occurring at the graft fixation site in 11 of 12 specimens. The ultimate load rose to only 15% of the control FATC after 8 weeks, with all failures now occurring within the graft substance. Anterior-posterior (A–P) joint translation of the grafted knee was five times greater than the control knee throughout the 8-week follow-up period (27).

Thorson (66) evaluated a distal ITT reconstruction of ACL-deficient canine knees 4 months after implantation. The average stiffness and ultimate load of the femur–graft–tibia complex was found to be 10% and 40% of the control FATC, respectively. In 1986, van Rens (67) reported a 1-year follow-up in a canine model in which a pedicled ITT graft was placed through tibial and femoral bone tunnels. The stiffness and ultimate load values of the graft–bone complex were, respectively, 45% and 40% of the control FATC. Butler (7) and Hulse (31) evaluated a combined reconstruction in the dog using both fascia lata and patellar tendon. A–P joint translation of the experimental knee was 154% of the control leg immediately after reconstruction, increasing to 306% after 4 weeks. At 26 weeks the A–P translation was 153% of the control value (31). Stiffness of the femur–graft–tibia complex increased from 9%, at the time of reconstruction, to 31% after 26 weeks relative to the control. Ultimate load values increased similarly from 14% to 28% (7).

Patellar Tendon

The patellar tendon (PT) has been one of the most widely used autograft tissues in ACL reconstruction since Jones (38) originally described its use in 1963. This is also the autograft that has been the most extensively studied in experimental models. The PT is a thick fibrous structure on the anterior aspect of the knee joint. Both the central and medial thirds of this structure are commonly used in ACL reconstruction. Widely varying biomechanical properties of PT autografts have been reported (Tables 21-1 and 21-2). The general trend, however, is for PT graft remodeling such that stiffness and ultimate load values reach approximately one-third of the control ACL value after as long as 24 months. Furthermore, most reconstructed joints demonstrated some degree of increased A–P joint translation and articular degeneration.

Early work by Ryan (62) examined the method of ACL reconstruction described by Jones 3 years earlier. In the 1966 study, the central third of the PT was passed along a groove made in the tibia and through a tunnel in the lateral femoral condyle in a canine model. Biomechanical testing of the graft after 2–22 weeks of implantation revealed graft strength to be less than 15% of the normal ACL, although no statistical correlation between the ultimate load and postoperative time could be made. Shino (64) used a free central PT autograft in a canine model. They noted the ultimate load and energy absorbed to failure of the PT graft–bone complex to be approximately 30% of the control FATC after 30 weeks. Also, "some degree of anterior laxity" was appreciated; however, "no significant degenerative disease" was found. McPherson (50) demonstrated patellofemoral degenerative changes in all goat ACL-deficient knees reconstructed using a central-third PT autograft after 3–24 months. Increased A–P joint translation, assessed subjectively, was found in all experimental knees. Biomechanical evaluation showed that the stiffness of the femur–graft–tibia complex was only 7.1 N/mm at the time of surgery, increasing to a maximum of 97 N/mm at 12 months, as compared to 275 N/mm for the controls. After 24 months, however, the value had reduced slightly to 83 N/mm. Ultimate load values followed similar trends. The maximum stiffness and ultimate load values of the autografts, which occurred at 12

TABLE 21-1. *Autograft stiffness, experimental/control (%)*

Investigator	Tissue[a]	Experimental animal	Weeks post-op				
			0	6–8	12–16	26–30	52–104
Holden	ITT	Goat	2	9	—	—	—
Thorson	ITT	Canine	—	—	10	—	—
van Rens	ITT	Canine	—	—	—	—	45
Butler	ITT/PT	Canine	9	—	23	31	—
Clancy	PT	Primate	—	—	39	—	47
McPherson	PT	Goat	3	—	15	33	35
Yoshiya	PT	Canine	11	—	22	—	—
McFarland	PT	Canine	—	—	15	—	—
Ballock	PT	Rabbit	15	11	—	24	13

[a] ITT, iliotibial tract; PT, patellar tendon.

months, were 35% and 45% of the control FATC, respectively (Fig. 21-1A and B) (50).

Clancy (13) used the medial third of the PT for ACL reconstruction. He passed a free PT autograft through tibial and femoral tunnels in reconstructing ACL-deficient knees of the Rhesus monkey. Evaluation 3–12 months after surgery demonstrated less than 1 mm increase in anterior tibial translation, with no degenerative joint changes. Stiffness values of the PT graft–bone complex increased from 39% of the control value at 3 months to 47% at 12 months. Ultimate load similarly increased from 26% at 3 months to 52% at 12 months. Clancy noted that in this model the PT graft was initially weaker than the control ACL. This is not the case in humans (55). However, at 12 months the graft had 82% of its original strength (13).

Yoshiya (74,75), in a canine model, demonstrated PT graft strength (tested as a tibia–patellar tendon–patella complex) to have ultimate load values of 937 N (72% of the control FATC). However, when the femur–PT graft–tibia complex was tested immediately

after reconstruction, the complex failed at a load that was only 10% that of the control PT. This was due to weakness at the fixation sites. After 3 months, this value increased to 20% of the control FATC, and specimens failed in the graft substance. Although the stiffness of the PT graft and control ACL were similar *in vitro*, the graft stiffness decreased to 11% of the control value after reconstruction (Fig. 21-2). After 3 months of implantation, the stiffness increased to 22%. A–P knee translation was nearly three times that of control knees 3 months after surgery (2.6 ± 0.3 mm and 7.4 ± 1.1 mm, respectively) (74,75). In contrast, longer-term results from this investigator showed that after 20 months the A–P translation was reduced to only 1.1 mm greater than that of controls. However, the ultimate load remained less than 32% of that of the controls. Also, moderate to severe degeneration of articular cartilage was present in the patellofemoral compartments, with minimal changes in the medial and lateral compartments (32). McFarland (48) also demonstrated inferior structural properties of medial-

TABLE 21-2. *Autograft ultimate load, experimental/control (%)*

Investigator	Tissue[a]	Experimental animal	Weeks post-op				
			0	6–8	12–16	26–30	52–104
Holden	ITT	Goat	6	15	—	—	—
O'Donoghue	ITT	Canine	—	—	—	—	23
Thorson	ITT	Canine	—	—	40	—	—
van Rens	ITT	Canine	—	—	—	—	40
Butler	ITT/PT	Canine	14	—	23	28	—
Clancy	PT	Primate	—	—	26	—	52
McPherson	PT	Goat	1	—	15	38	45
Shino	PT	Canine	—	—	—	30	—
Yoshiya	PT	Canine	7	—	20	—	—
Hurley	PT	Canine	—	—	—	—	<32
McFarland	PT	Canine	—	—	23	—	—
Ballock	PT	Rabbit	7	7	—	15	11
Kennedy	ST	Rabbit	—	—	—	13	—
Collins	M	Canine	—	~5	~35	~35	—
Mitsou	M	Rabbit	—	8	—	—	23

[a] ITT, iliotibial tract; PT, patellar tendon; ST, semitendinosus tendon; M, meniscus.

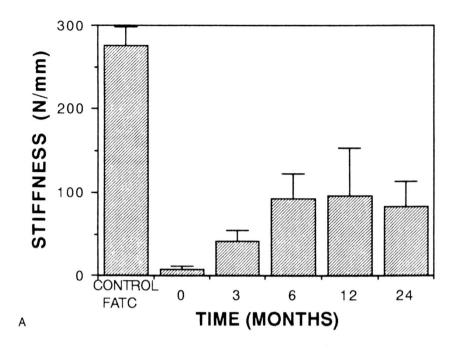

A

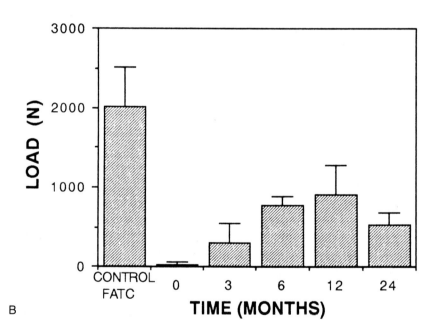

B

FIG. 21-1. **A:** Linear stiffness of control FATC and PT-reconstructed femur–graft–tibia complex after 0–24 months of implantation in a goat model. Linear stiffness of the reconstructed graft–bone complex reach approximately one-third of the control FATC value (From ref. 50.) **B:** Ultimate load of control FATC and PT graft–bone complex. Graft strength improved during the first year of implantation.

third PT grafts in dogs after reconstruction. At 4 months, the stiffness was 15% of the control value, whereas the ultimate load was 23% of the control FATC (48).

PT autograft reconstruction of the ACL has also been studied in rabbit models. Kondo (41) found steady improvement in free PT autografts between 1 and 8 months. At 8 months, stiffness values reached 83% of the control FATC, whereas ultimate load and energy absorbed at failure reached 74% and 73%, respectively. In contrast, our laboratory found lower stiffness and ultimate load values after a similar PT autograft

reconstruction in rabbits. After 52 weeks, these values were only 13% and 11% of the control FATC, respectively (4). It is important to point out that the data for the control FATC reported by our laboratory were more than double those reported by Kondo. We have demonstrated the importance of the axis of tensile loading on the structural properties of the FATC (Chapter 13). The stiffness and ultimate loads, when the FATC was tested along the ACL axis, were up to 170% and 270% higher than those tested along the tibial axis, respectively (Fig. 21-3) (72). Figgie (20) also demonstrated a 60–70% reduction in the ultimate load of

A

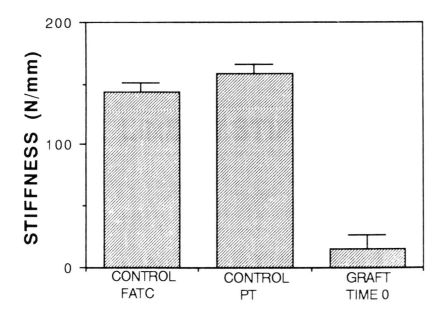

B

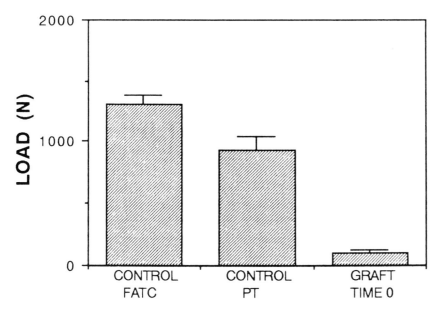

FIG. 21-2. A: Linear stiffness of canine control FATC and control femur–PT–patella complex, compared to that of the reconstructed femur–PT graft–tibia complex. Immediately after the reconstruction, there is a marked reduction in stiffness (From ref. 75.). **B:** Ultimate load values of control ACL–bone and PT–bone complex are similar and much greater than the initial femur–PT graft–tibia complex value.

the canine FATC if the knee was flexed between 45° and 90°, compared to 0°, when tension was applied along the longitudinal axis of the tibia (20). Thus, the difference in the results of these two studies may be due to variations in testing methods.

Other Autogenous Tissue Grafts

Other structures used for ACL reconstruction include the semitendinosus tendon (12,45,53,76) and medial meniscus (19,34,69). The semitendinosus tendon has been advocated for use in reconstruction of the ACL

by Cho (12) and later by Mott (53). Experimental animal studies evaluating this reconstruction are limited. In a rabbit model, the ultimate load of the semitendinosus graft was found to be less than 30% of the ACL. After 26 weeks of implantation, this autograft reconstruction was found to fail at loads less than 15% of the control FATC. Additionally, degenerative arthritic changes were apparent in all knees (40). Collins (15) used the medial meniscus for ACL reconstruction in a dog model. Six months postoperatively, the graft failed at an ultimate load of approximately 30% of the control (15). Mitsou (52) found similar results in a rabbit model. This procedure has received little attention,

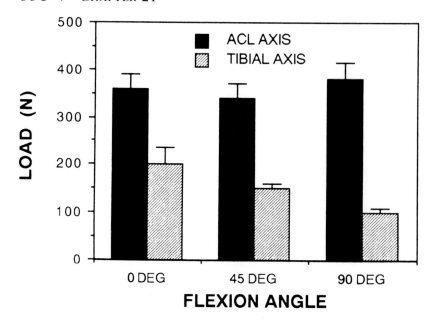

FIG. 21-3. Ultimate load of rabbit FATC. The importance of the axis of ACL loading is demonstrated. If the load is applied along the axis of the ACL, then the ultimate load is independent of knee flexion angle. However, if the axis of loading is along the tibia, then ultimate load is dependent on knee flexion angle and is a smaller value. (From ref. 72.)

since the detrimental effects of meniscectomy are significant.

Summary

In experimental studies, the ITT, PT, semitendinosus tendon, and meniscus autografts have all demonstrated similar behavior when placed intraarticularly in the knee as an ACL replacement. In most cases, the stiffness and ultimate load of the femur–graft–tibia complex were roughly 30–40% of the control FATC after 8–24 months of implantation (Tables 21-1 and 21-2). Differences in methods of testing may change the stiffness and strength of the control FATC and, therefore, may significantly alter the results when expressed in terms of a percentage (i.e., experimental versus control). However, these discrepancies notwithstanding, the outcome of autogenous tissues used for ACL reconstruction in animal models has generally been poor, with biomechanical properties of the grafts being far below normal. Normal knee kinematics have not been restored, and, in many cases, articular cartilage degeneration progressed despite the reconstruction.

ALLOGRAFT RECONSTRUCTIONS

Graft processing has been accomplished by deep-freezing and freeze-drying (35,36,54,64,70), and the biomechanical properties of these tissues are nearly retained (16,21,71,73). Additional processing is necessary for tissue sterilization. Ethylene oxide and gamma irradiation are possible methods for sterilizing allograft tissue. Although preliminary studies evaluating these techniques are not in complete agreement,

it appears that the biomechanical properties of the allografts are affected by these sterilizing processes (10,21,22,24,37,56).

Sources of allogeneic graft material for use as an ACL substitute can be grouped into two categories. The first group includes those in which bony insertion sites are maintained and a bone–graft–bone complex is transplanted. The second group includes those made up of only soft tissue. The advantages of transplanting a graft with bone plugs are similar to those of autogenous graft use. Better graft fixation can be achieved at the time of surgery, and the complex nature of the ligament–bone transition zone is preserved. However, because of the increased number of cellular components, transfer of bone may increase problems related to immunological graft rejection (30). Experimental studies evaluating the biomechanical aspects of ACL reconstruction using fresh-frozen bone–ACL–bone allografts in reconstructing dog knees have been performed by Vasseur (68) and Nikolaou (54). The ultimate load values of the femur–ACL allograft–tibia complex at 9 months were similar (163 N and 94 N respectively). However, the values for the control FATC were markedly different. The control ultimate load values reported by Vasseur (1202 N) were more than 10 times greater than those reported by Nikolaou (104 N). Control canine FATC ultimate load values reported in the literature are generally greater than 1000 N (7,20,48,75). The differences in control FATC values obtained by Vasseur and Nikolaou led to vastly different conclusions about the success of allograft reconstructions. Vasseur reported allograft complex ultimate loads of 14% of control, whereas Nikolaou reported values that were 89% of control. Difficulties with the control specimens of Nikolaou's study were

TABLE 21-3. *Allograft stiffness, experimental/control (%)*

Investigator	Tissue	Experimental animal	Weeks post-op				
			0	6–8	12–16	24–40	52
Jackson	ACL[a]	Canine	—	—	—	—	35
Vasseur	ACL	Canine	—	—	—	30	—

[a] ACL, anterior cruciate ligament.

related to premature failure of the tibial insertion site of the ACL. Avulsion failure at low loads may have been caused by stress deprivation due to decreased activity (Chapter 17) or by application of the tensile load during testing off the longitudinal axis of the ligament (20,72). Jackson (35,36) studied an allogeneic ACL bone complex treated using the freeze-drying method in mature goats. One year after implantation, the A–P knee translation was significantly greater in the reconstructed knees (3.8 ± 0.6 mm) than in the control knees (1.0 ± 0.1 mm). The stiffness and ultimate load values of the femur–allograft–tibia complex were only 35% and 25% of control values, respectively (35,36).

Several additional studies have been performed using allogeneic fibrous tissues without bony insertions. At 1 year, Shino (64) demonstrated fresh-frozen PT allografts with ultimate load values of 35% of the control FATC. Webster (70) evaluated freeze-dried flexor tendons in canine ACL reconstructions and found ultimate loads that were 29% of the control FATC 9 months postoperatively. Curtis (16) used freeze-dried fascia lata in a similar model and obtained somewhat better results. The ultimate load of the allograft–bone complex was less than 20% of the control at 6 weeks but increased to 67% after 24 weeks.

The experimental studies evaluating allograft reconstruction of the ACL yield results similar to those obtained with autogenous grafts. It appears that allografts undergo a remodeling process similar to autografts with progressive revascularization, cellular repopulation, and eventual collagen fiber reorganization (2,16,54,63,64,71). However, the stiffness and ultimate load of the allograft–bone complex during tensile test-

ing continue to be much lower than those for the normal FATC (Tables 21-3 and 21-4).

FACTORS INFLUENCING GRAFT REMODELING

Attempts have been made to isolate determinants that affect long-term results of autograft and allograft reconstructions. The effects of graft placement and fixation, graft tension, augmentation, maintenance of a vascular pedicle, and postoperative rehabilitation are being studied.

Graft Placement

The complex geometry and anatomy of the ACL are not reproduced by placing an autograft into the knee even if the graft insertion sites are located anatomically. However, near-ideal graft placement is important if some semblance of normal knee kinematics is to be achieved. Various methods of graft placement have been evaluated in order to maintain graft isometry (i.e., "constant" graft length and tension when the knee is moved through a range of motion). A method of graft placement known as "over the top" refers to attaching the graft to the femur after routing the graft through the intercondylar notch and over the posterior surface of the lateral femoral condyle (46). After this procedure, increases in graft length with knee extension of up to 10 mm have been reported in human cadaveric specimens (29,57,60). However, if a trough is made in the posterior intracondylar region of the lateral femoral condyle, isometry of the graft can be approximated (51,60). Alternatively, the graft may be placed through osseous tunnels created in both the tibia and

TABLE 21-4. *Allograft ultimate load, experimental/control (%)*

Investigator	Tissue[a]	Experimental animal	Weeks post-op				
			0	6–8	12–16	24–40	52
Curtis	FL	Canine	—	15	17	63	—
Jackson	ACL	Canine	—	—	—	—	25
Shino	PT	Canine	—	—	—	35	35
Vasseur	ACL	Canine	—	—	—	14	—
Webster	DFT	Canine	—	—	—	29	—

[a] ACL, anterior cruciate ligament; FL, fascia lata; PT, patellar tendon; DFT, digital flexor tendon.

femur, and this is called the "anatomic reconstruction." In this case, isometric graft placement is possible (23,29,44,51,57,60).

The concept of isometry is obviously an oversimplification, since the ACL is not isometric. In fact, the bundles of the ACL change in length with normal knee motion (8,28). This length change is also associated with a change in tension. The necessity of reproducing anatomic conditions in graft reconstruction is clear; however, at this point it seems reasonable to accept the concept of isometric placement in order to achieve consistent graft placement (Chapter 2).

Graft Fixation

Graft fixation to bone has been performed using sutures, staples, and screws with spiked washers or plates (Chapter 2). Robertson (61) evaluated these methods and demonstrated higher initial fixation strength with the screw and spiked plate combination. Holden (27) compared two methods of graft fixation to bone with respect to postoperative time. In the first case, the graft was stapled twice. In the second case, polypropylene braided reinforcement was sewn into the graft before it was fixed to the bone with a cancellous screw. The reinforced grafts secured with a screw were stronger during the initial 2 weeks postoperatively. After that time the graft substance became weaker than the fixation sites regardless of the fixation method, and thus the strength of fixation could not be evaluated.

Graft fixation, in the case of the anatomic reconstruction, has been accomplished in several ways. If the graft is left attached to a bone plug, this plug may be rigidly fixed to the femur or tibia using a cancellous interference screw (43). In a human cadaver study, Kurosaka (42) demonstrated that Lambert's technique of interference screw fixation (43) was stronger than stapling or suturing the graft over buttons. Additionally, a large 9.0-mm-diameter screw performed better than a standard 6.5-mm AO screw (42).

Graft Tension

Immediately after ACL reconstruction, anterior tibial translation is dependent on the initial graft tension (5,23,74). However, Yoshiya (74,75) found no difference in A–P joint translation 3 months postoperatively in dogs undergoing PT autograft reconstruction, with initial graft tension of either 1 N or 39 N. In both cases, the A–P translation was significantly increased. Structural properties of the femur–graft–tibia complex at 3 months were also similar. Stiffness values for grafts tensioned to 1 N and 39 N were 47 N/mm and 42 N/mm ($p > 0.05$), while ultimate load values were 277 N

and 315 N ($p > 0.05$), respectively. Grafts initially fixed at a tension of 39 N, however, had poor vascularity and greater collagen fiber disorganization as compared to those at 1 N.

As the knee is flexed and extended after reconstruction (and initial graft tensioning), the graft "settles," leading to a marked decrease in tension. The fact that grafts are viscoelastic material may also result in a loss of graft tension as the material undergoes stress relaxation (56). With graft remodeling, it is also likely that effects of initial graft tension may become diminished. Therefore, the most appropriate initial graft tension remains unclear.

Graft Augmentation

Initial graft weakness has led to concern that the graft may fail early in the postoperative period, even if subjected to minimal loading. This concern has prompted the use of ligament augmentation devices as an internal "splint" for the tissue grafts. Recent *in vitro* studies have demonstrated improved initial anterior joint stability when an augmentation device is added to the reconstruction. In addition, loads in the graft are reduced compared to those in the nonaugmented case (18,47). McPherson (50) reported on the use of the 3M ligament augmentation device (LAD) made of polypropylene (a synthetic material) together with a PT autograft for ACL reconstruction in a goat model. In the postoperative period, the femur–graft/LAD–tibia complex had a greater initial ultimate load value (364 N) than the complex without a LAD (26 N). However, 3 months after reconstruction, no significant difference in the ultimate load was demonstrated (50). Yoshiya (74) found similar results for canine PT autograft reconstructions with and without a dacron augmentation device. Immediately after the reconstruction, those knees with a dacron device had significantly greater ultimate load values. However, at 3 months, these differences were no longer significant. Stiffness values demonstrated similar trends, and graft vascularity was found to be decreased when a dacron device was present (74). Andrish (1) actually found a detrimental effect of the presence of the augmentation device. Ultimate load values of PT reconstructions with and without augmentation were 149 N and 210 N, respectively, after 6 months of implantation (1). In a goat model, however, Jackson (35,36) demonstrated the LAD to be beneficial in an ACL allograft reconstruction after 1 year of follow-up. The stiffness of the augmented allograft–bone complex was 364 N/mm as compared to 238 N/mm for the nonaugmented complex. Ultimate load and energy absorbed at failure were similarly increased when a LAD was utilized. However, the stiffness, ultimate load, and energy absorbed at failure re-

TABLE 21-5. *Ultimate load of augmented Graft–bone complex*

Investigator	Experimental animal	Load (N)				Months
		Initial (time 0)[a]		After implantation[a]		
		+ LAD	− LAD	+ LAD	− LAD	
McPherson	Canine	364	26	841	528	24
Yoshiya	Canine	370	100	245	250	3
Andrish	Canine	—	—	149	210	6
Jackson	Goat	—	—	1052	571	12

[a] + LAD, with ligament augmentation device; − LAD, without ligament augmentation device.

mained substantially lower than those of the controls (53%, 43%, and 39% of the controls, respectively). At 1 year, the LAD had a minimal effect on the A–P joint translation (3.1 mm with LAD versus 3.8 mm without LAD versus 1.0 mm intact ACL) (35,36). A summary of these data is presented in Table 21-5, and it appears that many questions remain with regard to the long-term efficacy of graft augmentation.

Other Parameters

Since graft remodeling is a relatively slow process, maintaining graft vascularity has been explored. This has been done in the hope of obviating the need for complete graft remodeling and, therefore, of achieving improved structural properties of the graft. Paulos (59) documented a technique for maintaining the vascularity of a medial PT graft and commented on the demanding nature of the procedure. Several experimental studies attempting to validate this extra effort have been made (9,14,17). Both vascularized and nonvascularized grafts demonstrate complete vascularization after 8–12 weeks. After 26–52 weeks, no differences in the structural properties of the femur–graft–tibia complex have been demonstrated. Although the data are preliminary, it appears that the beneficial effect of maintaining a vascular pedicle, if any, is minimal.

Rehabilitation after ACL reconstruction is likely to be very important in determining the outcome of the procedure. Unfortunately, rehabilitation is a parameter that is difficult to control in most experimental animal studies. The postoperative care used in the various studies discussed in this chapter have varied from several weeks of immobilization to immediate unrestricted activity. Experimental animal studies comparing various rehabilitation methods with regard to the biomechanical outcome of the graft are limited. Bair (3) demonstrated no difference in the biomechanical properties of grafts from knees that were casted for 6 weeks or that were allowed immediate free motion. The detrimental effects of joint immobility on normal ligaments have been discussed in Chapter 17; however, these effects on a hypovascular remodeling graft

are not clear. Concern that the graft will stretch or fail at the fixation sites in the early postoperative period if subjected to stresses associated with early joint motion has been raised (6). Currently, the timing and intensity of imposed graft stress have little or no scientific basis.

SUMMARY

Experimental animal studies in which autograft or allograft ACL reconstruction have been performed yielded structural properties of the graft–bone complex far different from those of the normal femur–ACL–tibia complex. At periods of up to 1 year after reconstruction, the stiffness and ultimate load of the graft–bone complexes reached approximately 30–40% of the control values (Tables 21-1 through 21-4). The experimental studies cited in this chapter are all limited with respect to the number of animals and ability to control postoperative rehabilitation. For these reasons, it is not possible to make direct conclusions relating to clinical practice. These studies do, however, provide insight into the mechanisms of autograft and allograft remodeling.

REFERENCES

1. Andrish JT, Woods LD. Dacron augmentation in anterior cruciate ligament reconstruction in dogs. *Clin Orthop* 1984;183:298–302.
2. Arnoczky SP, Warren RF, Ashlock MA. Replacement of the anterior cruciate ligament using a patellar tendon allograft. *J Bone Joint Surg* 1986;68A:376–385.
3. Bair GR. The effect of early mobilization versus casting on anterior cruciate ligament reconstruction. *Trans Orthop Res Soc* 1980;5:108.
4. Ballock RT, Woo SL-Y, Lyon RM, Hollis JM, Akeson WH. Use of patellar tendon autograft for anterior cruciate ligament reconstruction in the rabbit: a long term histological and biomechanical study. *J Orthop Res* 1989;in press.
5. Burks RT, Daniel DM. Anterior cruciate graft preload and knee stability. *Orthop Trans* 1984;8:52.
6. Burks RT, Daniel DM, Losse G. The effect of continuous passive motion on anterior cruciate ligament reconstruction stability. *Am J Sports Med* 1984;12:323–327.
7. Butler DL, Hulse DA, Kay MD, Grood ES, Shires PK, D'Ambrosia R, Shoji H. Biomechanics of cranial cruciate ligament

reconstruction in the dog. II. Mechanical properties. *Vet Surg* 1983;12:113–118.

8. Butler DL, Martin ET, Kaiser AD, Grood ES, Chun KJ, Sodd AN. The effects of flexion and tibial rotation on 3-D orientations and length of human anterior cruciate ligament bundles. *Trans Orthop Res Soc* 1988;13:59.

9. Butler DL, Noyes FR, Grood ES, Olmstead ML, Hohn RB. The effects of vascularity on the mechanical properties of primate anterior cruciate ligament replacements. *Trans Orthop Res Soc* 1983;8:93.

10. Butler DL, Noyes FR, Walz KA, Gibbons MJ. Biomechanics of human knee ligament allograft treatment. *Trans Orthop Res Soc* 1987;12:128.

11. Campbell W. Reconstruction of the ligaments of the knee. *Am J Surg* 1939;43:473–480.

12. Cho KO. Reconstruction of the anterior cruciate ligament by semitendinosus tenodesis. *J Bone Joint Surg* 1975;57A:608–612.

13. Clancy WG, Narechania RG, Rosenberg TD, Gmeiner JG, Wisnefske D, Lange TA. Anterior and posterior cruciate ligament reconstruction in Rhesus monkeys. *J Bone Joint Surg* 1981;63A:1270–1284.

14. Clancy WG, Thomsen E, Dueland RT, Wilson JM, Vanderby R, Graft BK. Anterior cruciate and posterior cruciate ligament reconstruction with patellar tendon using a medial vascularized graft, lateral vascularized graft and free patellar tendon graft. *Am J Sports Med* 1987;15(4):399–400.

15. Collins HR, Hughston JC, Dehaven KE, Bergfeld JA, Evarts CM. The meniscus as a cruciate ligament substitute. *Am J Sports Med* 1974;2(1):11–21.

16. Curtis RJ, Delee JC, Drez DJ. Reconstruction of the anterior cruciate ligament with freeze dried fascia lata allografts in dogs. A preliminary report. *Am J Sports Med* 1985;13:408–414.

17. deKorompay VL, Dessouki E. Vascularized versus nonvascularized patellar tendon for intraarticular cruciate reconstruction. Histological and biomechanical analysis in dogs. *Am J Sports Med* 1987;15(4):399.

18. Engebretsen L, Lew WD, Lewis JL, Hunter RE. Knee joint motion and ligament force in non-augmented and augmented primary repairs of ACL ruptures. *Trans Orthop Res Soc* 1989;14:512.

19. Ferkel RD, Fox JM, DelPizzo W, Friedman MJ, Synder SJ, Dorey F, Kasimian D. Reconstruction of the anterior cruciate ligament using a torn meniscus. *J Bone Joint Surg* 1988;70A(5):715–723.

20. Figgie HE, Bahniuk EH, Heiple KG, Davy DT. The effects of tibial–femoral angle on the failure mechanics of the canine anterior cruciate ligament. *J Biomech* 1986;19(2):89–91.

21. France PE, Paulos LE, Rosenberg TD, Harner CD. The biomechanics of anterior cruciate allografts. In: Friedmand MJ, Ferkel RD, eds. *Prosthetic ligament reconstruction of the knee*. Philadelphia: WB Saunders, 1988;180–185.

22. Gibbons MJ, Butler DL, Grood ES, Chun KJ, Noyes FR, Bukovec DB. Dose-dependent effects of gamma irradiation on the material properties of frozen bone–patellar tendon–bone allografts. *Trans Orthop Res Soc* 1989;14:513.

23. Grood ES, Hefzy MS, Butler DL, Noyes FR. Intra-articular vs. over the top placement of anterior cruciate ligament substitute. *Trans Orthop Res Soc* 1986;11:79.

24. Haut RC, Powlison AC. Order of irradiation and lyophilization on the strength of patellar tendon allografts. *Trans Orthop Res Soc* 1989;14:514.

25. Hey Groves EW. Operation for the repair of the crucial ligaments. *Lancet* 1917;2:674–675.

26. Hey Groves EW. The crucial ligaments of the knee-joint: their function, rupture and the operative treatment of the same. *Br J Surg* 1920;7:505–515.

27. Holden JP, Grood ES, Butler DL, Noyes FR, Mendenhall HV, VanKampen CL, Neidich RL. Biomechanics of fascia lata ligament replacements: early postoperative changes in the goat. *J Orthop Res* 1988;6:639–647.

28. Hollis JM, Marcin JP, Horibe S, Woo SL-Y. Load determination in ACL fiber bundles under knee loading. *Trans Orthop Res Soc* 1988;13:58.

29. Hoogland T, Hillen B. Intraarticular reconstruction of the anterior cruciate ligament. *Clin Orthop* 1984;185:197–202.

30. Horowitz MC, Friedlander GE. Analysis of the immune response to bone allografts. *Trans Orthop Res Soc* 1989;14:267.

31. Hulse DA, Butler DL, Kay MD, Noyes FR, Shires PK, D'Ambroisia R, Shoji H. Biomechanics of cranial cruciate ligament reconstruction in the dog. I. *In vivo* laxity testing. *Vet Surg* 1983;12:109–112.

32. Hurley PB, Andish JT, Yoshiya S, Manley M, Kurosaka M. Tensile strength of the reconstructed canine anterior cruciate ligament: a long term evaluation of the modified Jones technique. *Am J Sports Med* 1987;14(4):393.

33. Insall J, Joseph DM, Aglietti P, Campbell RD. Bone-block iliotibial-band transfer for anterior cruciate insufficiency. *J Bone Joint Surg* 1981;63A(4):560–569.

34. Ivey FM, Blazina ME, Fox JM, del Pizzo W. Intraarticular substitution for anterior cruciate insufficiency. *Am J Sports Med* 1980;8:405–410.

35. Jackson DW, Grood ES, Arnoczky SP, Butler DL, Simon TM. Freeze dried anterior cruciate ligament allografts. Preliminary studies in a goat model. *Am J Sports Med* 1987;15:295–303.

36. Jackson DW, Grood ES, Arnoczky SP, Butler DL, Simon TM. Cruciate reconstruction using freeze dried anterior cruciate ligament allograft and a ligament augmentation device (LAD). *Am J Sports Med* 1987;15:528–538.

37. Jackson DW, Grood ES, Wilcox P, Butler DL, Simon TM, Holden JP. The effects of processing techniques on the mechanical properties of bone–anterior cruciate ligament–bone allografts. *Am J Sports Med* 1988;16:101–105.

38. Jones KG. Reconstruction of the anterior cruciate ligament. *J Bone Joint Surg* 1963;45A(5):925–932.

39. Kaplan EB. The iliotibial tract. *J Bone Joint Surg* 1958;40A(4):817–832.

40. Kennedy JC, Roth JH, Mendenhall HV. Presidential Address: Intraarticular replacement in the anterior cruciate ligament-deficient knee. *Am J Sports Med* 1980;8(1):1–8.

41. Kondo M. An experimental study on reconstructive surgery of the anterior cruciate ligament. *J Jpn Orthop Assoc* 1979;53:521–533.

42. Kurosaka M, Yoshiya S, Andrish JT. A biomechanical comparison of different surgical techniques of graft fixation in anterior cruciate ligament reconstruction. *Am J Sports Med* 1987;15:225–229.

43. Lambert KL. Vascularized patellar tendon graft with rigid internal fixation for anterior cruciate ligament insufficiency. *Clin Orthop* 1983;172:85–89.

44. Larson RV, Sidles JA, Matsen FA, Garbini L. Isometric ligament insertions in the knee. *Am J Sports Med* 1987;15:394.

45. Lipscomb AB, Johnston RK, Synder RB, Brothers JC. Secondary reconstruction of anterior cruciate ligament in athletes by using the semitendinosus tendon. *Am J Sports Med* 1979;7(2):81–84.

46. MacIntosh DL. The anterior cruciate ligament: "over the top" repair. *J Bone Joint Surg* 1974;56B(3):591.

47. McCarthy JA, Van Kampen CL, Walt MJ, Moore RD, Steadman JR. Changes in knee kinematics and graft strain with LAD augmentation. *Trans Orthop Res Soc* 1989;14:27.

48. McFarland EG, Morrey BF, An KN, Wood MB. The relationship of vascularity and water content to tensile strength in a patellar tendon replacement of the anterior cruciate in dogs. *Am J Sports Med* 1986;14:436–448.

49. McMaster JH, Weinert CR, Scranton P. Diagnosis and management of isolated anterior cruciate ligament tears: a preliminary report on reconstruction with gracilis tendon. *J Trauma* 1974;14:230–235.

50. McPherson GK, Mendenhall HV, Gibbons DF, et al. Experimental, mechanical and histologic evaluation of the Kennedy ligament augmentation device. *Clin Orthop* 1985;196:186–195.

51. Melhorn JM, Henning LE. The relationship of the femoral attachment site to the isometric tracking of the anterior cruciate ligament graft. *Am J Sports Med* 1987;15(6):539–542.

52. Mitsou A, Villianatos P, Piskopakis N, Nikolaou P. Cruciate ligament replacement using a meniscus. *J Bone Joint Surg* 1988;70B:784–786.

53. Mott HW. Semitendinosus anatomic reconstruction for cruciate ligament insufficiency. *Clin Orthop* 1983;172:90–92.

54. Nikolaou PK, Seaber AV, Glisson RR, Ribbeck BM, Bassett FH. Anterior cruciate ligament allograft transplantation. *Am J Sports Med* 1986;14(5):348–360.

55. Noyes FR, Butler DL, Paulos LE, Grood ES. Intra-articular cruciate reconstruction, I: perspectives on graft strength, vascularization and immediate motion after replacement. *Clin Orthop* 1983;172:71–77.

56. O'Brien WR, Friederich NF, Muller W, Henning CE. The effects of stress relaxation on initial graft loads during anterior cruciate ligament reconstruction. *Trans Orthop Res Soc* 1989;14:213.

57. Odensten M, Gillquist J. Functional anatomy of the anterior cruciate ligament and rationale for reconstruction. *J Bone Joint Surg* 1985;67A(2):257–262.

58. O'Donoghue DH, Frank GR, Jeter GL, Johnson W, Zeiders JW, Kenyon R. Repair and reconstruction of the anterior cruciate ligament in dogs: factors influencing long term results. *J Bone Joint Surg* 1971;53A:710–718.

59. Paulos LE, Butler DL, Noyes FR, Grood ES. Intra-articular cruciate reconstruction. *Clin Orthop* 1983;172:78–84.

60. Penner DA, Daniel DM, Wood P, Mishra D. An *in-vitro* study of anterior cruciate ligament graft placement and isometry. *Am J Sports Med* 1988;16(3):238–243.

61. Robertson DB, Daniel DM, Biden E. Soft tissue fixation to bone. *Am J Sports Med* 1986;14(5):398–403.

62. Ryan JR, Droupp BW. Evaluation of tensile strength of reconstructions of the anterior cruciate ligament using the patellar tendon in dogs. *South Med J* 1966;59:129–134.

63. Shino K, Inoue M, Horibe S, Nagano J, Ono K. Maturation of allograft tendons transplanted into the knee. An arthroscopic and histological study. *J Bone Joint Surg* 1988;70B:556–560.

64. Shino K, Kawasaki T, Hirose H, Gotoh I, Inoue M, Ono R. Reconstruction of the anterior cruciate ligament by allogenic tendon graft: an experimental study in the dog. *J Bone Joint Surg* 1984;66B:672–681.

65. Shino K, Kimura T, Hirose H, Inoue M, Ono K. Reconstruction of the anterior cruciate ligament by allogenic tendon graft. *J Bone Joint Surg* 1986;68B:739–746.

66. Thorson EP, Rodrigo JJ, Vasseur PB, Sharkey NA, Heitter DO. Comparison of frozen allograft versus fresh autogenous anterior cruciate ligament replacement in the dog. *Trans Orthop Res Soc* 1987;12:65.

67. van Rens TJG, van den Berg AF, Huiskes R, Kuypers W. Substitution of the anterior cruciate ligament: a long-term histologic and biomechanical study with autogenous pedicled grafts of the iliotibial band in dogs. *Arthroscopy* 1986;2(3):139–154.

68. Vasseur PB, Rodrigo JJ, Stevenson S, Clark G, Sharkey N. Replacement of the anterior cruciate ligament with a bone–ligament–bone anterior cruciate ligament allograft in dogs. *Clin Orthop* 1987;219:268–277.

69. Walsh JJ. Meniscal reconstruction of the anterior cruciate ligament. *Clin Orthop* 1972;89:171–177.

70. Webster DA, Werner FW. Freeze-dried flexor tendons in anterior cruciate ligament reconstruction. *Clin Orthop* 1983;181:238–243.

71. Webster DA, Werner FW. Mechanical and functional properties of implanted freeze-dried flexor tendons. *Clin Orthop* 1983;180:301–309.

72. Woo SL-Y, Hollis JM, Roux RD, et al. Effects of knee flexion on the structural properties of the rabbit femur–anterior cruciate ligament–tibia complex (FATC). *J Biomech* 1987;20:557–564.

73. Woo SL-Y, Orlando CA, Camp JF, Akeson WH. Effects of postmortem storage by freezing on ligament tensile behavior. *J Biomech* 1986;19:399–404.

74. Yoshiya S, Andrish JT, Manley MT, Bauer TW. Graft tension in anterior cruciate ligament reconstruction. An *in vivo* study in dogs. *Am J Sports Med* 1987;15(5):464–470.

75. Yoshiya S, Andrish JT, Manley MT, Kurosaka M. Augmentation of anterior cruciate ligament reconstruction in dogs with prostheses of different stiffness. *J Orthop Res* 1986;4(4):475–485.

76. Zaricznyj B. Reconstruction of the anterior cruciate ligament using free tendon graft. *Am J Sports Med* 1983;11(3):164–176.

Knee Ligaments: Structure, Function, Injury, and Repair, edited by D. Daniel, et al.
© 1990 by Raven Press, Ltd. All rights reserved.

CHAPTER 22

Animal Models for Knee Ligament Research

Steven Paul Arnoczky

The last decade has seen an increased interest in the basic science investigation of ligaments, especially those in and around the knee. Although anatomical and biomaterial characterizations of human knee ligaments have been carried out in cadaveric specimens, the biological evaluation of these tissues necessitates the use of some *in vivo* system in which to examine and study the physiology of ligaments and their response to various stimuli. To this end, research scientists have utilized animal models to investigate ligament biology *in vivo*.

The first recorded use of animals in biomedical research dates back to the fourth century B.C. when Aristotle studied anatomical differences among various animal species by dissecting them (40). Since that time, research in animals has resulted in significant advances in all areas of medicine (15,16,35,36,40).

Central to the acceptance of animals as models of human physiology and pathology is the belief that all animals are so closely linked by the bonds of kinship that information gained from one is applicable to others (51). However, when one examines the vast heterogeneity that exists in the animal kingdom, such a generalization seems implausible. A more tempered concept was forwarded in 1929 by the distinguished Danish physiologist August Krogh (32), who wrote, "For a large number of problems there will be some animal of choice, or a few such animals, in which it can be most conveniently studied." This has become known as the "August Krogh Principle" and has served as a rationale for the use of animal models in biomedical research. Although the development and recognition of accepted animal models for the study of specific biologic phenomena have given support to the Krogh Principle, it also has been noted that the uncritical application of this principle may lead to fallacious generalizations, because extrapolating findings from one species to another is not invariably valid (30,31). Thus, the researcher is left with the dilemma of which animal model(s) most accurately represent(s) the human condition being investigated and to what extent can the results obtained from these models be extrapolated to humans.

In ligament research a variety of species have been used to investigate various aspects of anatomy, function, injury, and repair; these include the rat, rabbit, dog, cat, goat, sheep, and monkey. While these studies have contributed greatly to our understanding of ligament biology and function, no unanimity of opinion exists as to what animal species, if any, provides the most valid system in which to investigate ligament biology or to evaluate ligament prostheses.

This chapter will examine some of the considera-

S. P. Arnoczky: Laboratory of Comparative Orthopaedic Research, The Hospital for Special Surgery, New York, New York 10021.

tions involved in choosing animal models for knee ligament research and will discuss the scientific and ethical obligations of investigators using these models.

SELECTING AN ANIMAL MODEL

General Considerations

The selection of an animal model for biomedical research is based on many criteria that encompass a wide variety of factors. Some of these considerations include the appropriateness (analogy) of the model to the human condition, the background data available on the model, the "generalizability" of the data obtained from the model, the ease of experimental manipulation, the cost and availability of the specific animal, and the ethical implications of using animals in biomedical research (35).

In selecting an animal model the investigator must evaluate the overall fidelity and distinctiveness of the model to the human condition, since even the most carefully designed experiment can be vitiated by an animal model lacking in integrity (15). *Fidelity* refers to the overall faithfulness of the animal model to the human condition, and *distinctiveness* means that the animal model possesses a distinguishing characteristic(s) that mimics a particular property in the human condition. In knee ligament research there does not appear to be any one animal model that duplicates the exact anatomy and biomechanics of the human knee. However, in very general terms, the femoral–tibia joint of the more commonly used animal models (dog, rabbit, goat, sheep, and primate) is anatomically and physiologically analogous (see section entitled "Specific Considerations") to its human counterpart and appears to be an acceptable system in which to compare certain biological aspects of ligaments (24,49).

The degree to which the ligaments of the femoral–tibial joint of an animal are analogous to that of humans depends on what "level" we wish to compare them. As noted previously, the acceptance of animal models in biomedical research must be predicated on the fundamental belief that, at some level, the information gained from one species is applicable to others. This belief stems from the concept that since life is evolutionary, all animals share certain common features; the more basic the feature or function, the more common (and similar) its occurrence among species. (For example, the blood clotting mechanism is essentially the same in all warm-blooded animals.) Thus, when comparing various levels of biological phenomena among species, it is often concluded that the more basic the feature, function, or response being studied, the more valid the comparison. Conversely, the more the function or response is directly affected by species-dependent variables, the less the results can be (or should be) extrapolated. For example, on a molecular level the synthesis of Type I collagen by a fibroblast in a rat anterior cruciate ligament (ACL) should be comparable to a similar process in the human ACL. However, on a clinical level the ability of a prosthetic ACL to provide functional joint stability and prevent degenerative changes in a goat does not necessarily imply similar results in humans. It is important to recognize that in the latter example the results are influenced not only by the anatomical and functional (kinematic) differences between the species but also by the experimental variable of surgical technique. Therefore, when evaluating the validity of a particular animal model, the investigator must determine not only the level of comparison the specific aims of the study wish to achieve but also to what degree the results will be directly affected by species-dependent variables.

As noted previously, the following rule is generally accepted among the more commonly used animal models in ligament research: The more basic the level of comparison, the more valid the comparison of the results to the human condition being studied. Although, in theory, this may be true, the ultimate validation of any animal model is the confirmation that the results obtained in a model (or the processes observed in that model) are exactly the same as those seen in the human. In addition, the level(s) (molecular, physiologic, functional, etc.) at which these results are comparable must also be determined. Although such precise validation is not always possible in the human, enhanced clinical follow-up in the form of "second-look" arthroscopies and postoperative biopsies has provided increasing evidence that certain biological phenomena observed in animal models directly parallel those seen in the human. In the area of knee ligament research, these findings include the biological remodeling of autografts (1,4,11,20,21) and allografts (12,43,44), as well as the biological response to synthetic replacements (13,46), for the ACL.

In the absence of any direct human data, an alternative method of validating the "generalizability" of results obtained from an animal model is the comparison of the results to those obtained from other animal models. Similar results obtained in several animal models would suggest a common physiologic or pathologic pathway among species. Such a finding would provide strong support for the cautious extrapolation of the results to the human species. An example of this would be the similar remodeling process of patellar tendon (PT) grafts used to reconstruct the ACL observed in dogs (1,11,12,20,44), rabbits (4), and monkeys (21). Based on these findings, a similar remodeling process was postulated in the human. This process was later validated in the human through postoperative biopsies (43).

Thus the validation of a specific animal model can be done directly through comparison to available human data or indirectly through the demonstration of a common biological process among several species. In addition, it must be remembered that an animal model may only be valid at a specific level of comparison. The investigator must carefully identify this (these) level(s) and make comparisons and/or extrapolations within the limits of the model.

The selection of specific animal models for ligament research (or, for that matter, any biomedical research) is not always based on compelling scientific grounds. Oftentimes other factors such as cost, availability of animals and animal housing, ease of handling, or the size of the animal are the determining factors in why one species is chosen over another. For example, rats and rabbits are less expensive to purchase and house than dogs. On the other hand, larger animals such as goats and sheep provide the size necessary to implant ligament prostheses and augmentations that are designed (and sized) for the human knee. Another important consideration in the selection of an animal model is the animal welfare movement, which has strongly discouraged the use of certain animals (dogs, cats, primates) in medical research. Although these considerations do not justify the selection of an inappropriate animal model for a specific investigation, they are valid issues and therefore play an important role in the selection criteria.

Specific Considerations

In knee ligament research it is doubtful that any single animal species can precisely duplicate all the anatomical, physiological, and biomechanical aspects of the human knee. In addition, it appears that the general physiological responses (i.e., injury, healing, and remodeling) of ligaments among various species is comparable (1,2,4,10–12,19–22,26–29,44). Because of this fact there is no compelling scientific support for choosing one species over another for the study of ligament biology. The investigator must therefore base his or her decision on the aforementioned general considerations and a fundamental knowledge of the anatomy, function, and physiology of the animal species.

Anatomical Considerations

"Dogs don't have knees!"
Snoopy[1]

The femoral–tibial joint, while known as the *knee joint* in humans, is termed the *stifle* in animals. Al-

though many animals have four "legs," only the rear, or hind, limbs are homologous to the pelvic limbs of humans; thus the concept of tetrapedal animals having four "knees" is fallacious.

The stifle joint of animals is analogous to the knee joint of humans, in that their overall design is quite similar (24,49). However, although the stifle has many of the structural components of its human counterpart (cruciate ligaments, collateral ligaments, menisci), subtle differences do exist between species. The most striking difference (other than mere size) is the variance in the bony geometry of the stifle (Fig. 22-1). This variation in geometry is most likely related to the conformation, posture, and gait pattern of the individual species.

The general ligamentous anatomy of the stifle joint is similar to that observed in the human knee and varies only slightly among species (49). As an example, the ligamentous anatomy of the dog will be described. Anatomical descriptions for specific species are available in various veterinary and laboratory animal texts (6,34,45,49).

Cruciate Ligaments

The ACL of the dog attaches to a fossa on the posterior aspect of the medial side of the lateral femoral condyle (Fig. 22-2). The ACL courses anteriorly, medially, and distally across the intercondylar fossa and attaches to the anterior intercondyloid area of the tibia. The tibial attachment of the ACL is comma-shaped and has a general anteroposterior orientation (Fig. 22-3). The ACL passes beneath the intermeniscal ligament and has no attachment to either meniscus. Because of the orientation of the fibers on its femoral and tibial attachment, the ACL had a proximal-to-distal outward spiral of about 90°. As the stifle is flexed, the ACL becomes wound and twisted on itself (Fig. 22-4) (9). Because the stifle of the dog (and most other tetrapods) is flexed 30–50° during normal stance, the ACL makes a very acute angle with the tibial plateau (Fig. 22-5). This is a very important anatomical consideration when reconstructing/replacing the ACL in these animals. The tendency is to drill the tibial tunnel too vertically (too perpendicular to the plane of the tibial plateau). When this is done, the graft will exit the tibial tunnel too vertically and the normal weight-bearing orientation of the stifle will place stress on the posterior aspect of the reconstruction as it exits the tibial drill hole (Fig. 22-6). This may result in fraying and failure at that point. Thus, when replacing the ACL in animals, care should be taken to orient the tibial drill hole with the normal stifle angulation of the specific species taken into consideration.

The posterior cruciate ligament (PCL) is attached to

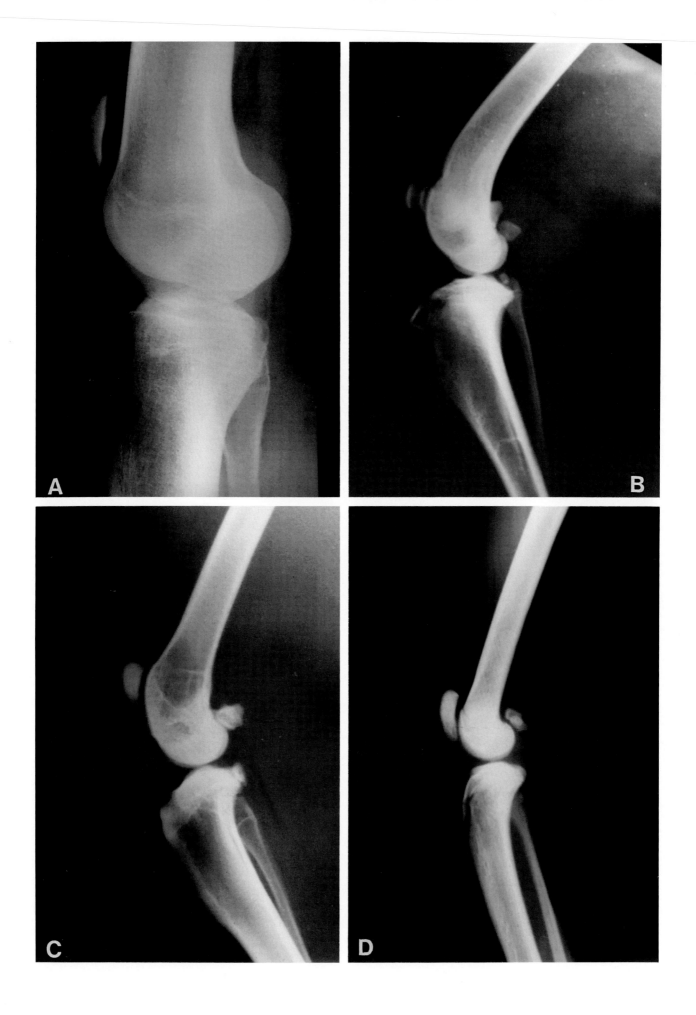

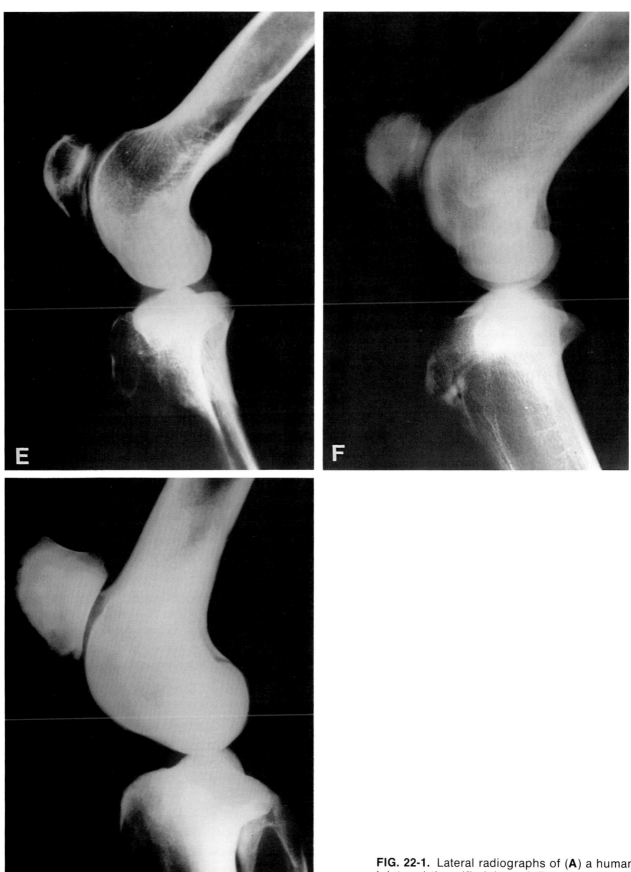

FIG. 22-1. Lateral radiographs of (**A**) a human knee joint and the stifle joints of (**B**) a dog, (**C**) a rabbit, (**D**) a cynomolgus monkey, (**E**) a goat, (**F**) a sheep, and (**G**) a pig. (Note: The size of the joints is not to scale, and the position of the joint does not necessarily reflect its normal functional angle.)

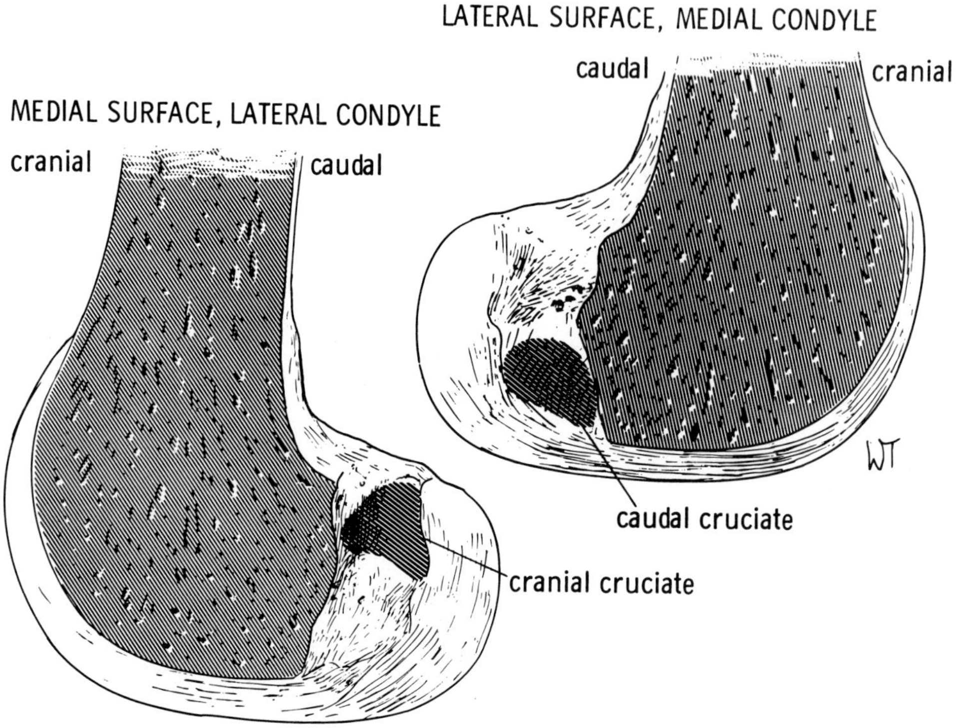

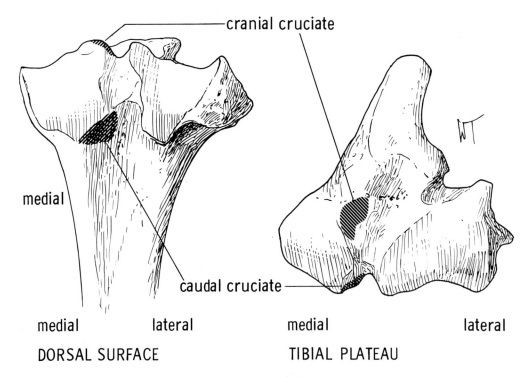

LATERAL SURFACE, MEDIAL CONDYLE

caudal · cranial

MEDIAL SURFACE, LATERAL CONDYLE

cranial | caudal

caudal cruciate

cranial cruciate

FIG. 22-2. Left: Drawing of the medial aspect of the lateral femoral condyle of a dog, showing the area of attachment of the anterior (cranial) cruciate ligament. **Right:** Drawing of the lateral aspect of the medial femoral condyle, showing the area of attachment of the posterior (caudal) cruciate ligament. (From ref. 8.)

cranial cruciate

medial

caudal cruciate

medial   lateral   medial   lateral

DORSAL SURFACE   TIBIAL PLATEAU

FIG. 22-3. Drawing of the tibial plateau of a dog, showing the area of attachment of the anterior (cranial) and posterior (caudal) cruciate ligament. (From ref. 8.)

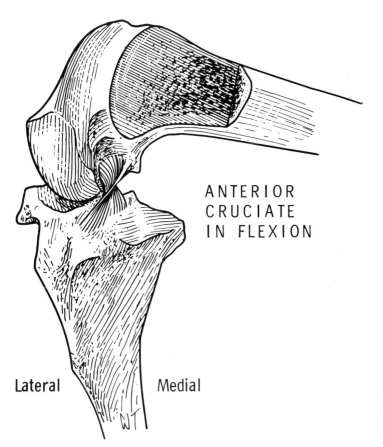

ANTERIOR
CRUCIATE
IN FLEXION

Lateral   Medial

FIG. 22-4. Drawing showing the ACL of a dog with the stifle in flexion. Note that the anterior fibers remain tense, whereas the posterior bulk of the ligament loosens. (From ref. 9.)

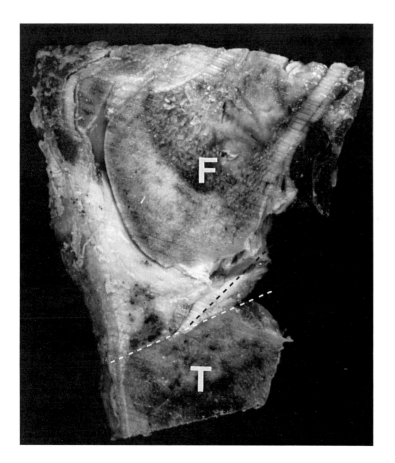

FIG. 22-5. Sagittal section of a sheep stifle, showing the orientation of the ACL with the limb in a functional position. Note how the ACL makes an acute angle with the tibial plateau when the limb is in a functional position. F, femur; T, tibia.

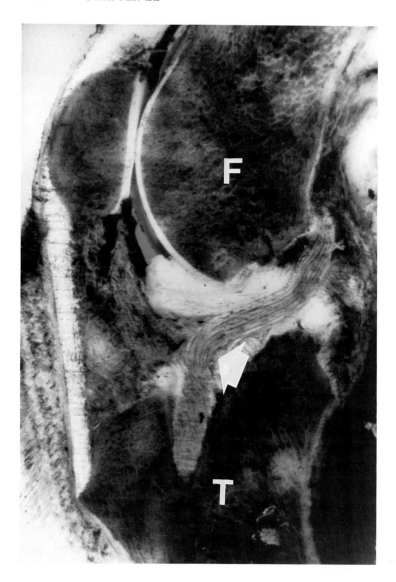

FIG. 22-6. Sagittal section of a dog's stifle, showing improper placement of a graft to replace the ACL. The vertical orientation of the tibial drill hole may cause the posterior aspect of the graft to fray as it exits the tibial tunnel (*arrow*). F, femur; T, tibia.

a fossa in the inferior aspect of the lateral side of the medial femoral condyle (Fig. 22-2). The femoral attachment of the PCL is somewhat elliptic, with its long axis oriented in a horizontal plane and the inferior convexity parallel to the lower articular margin of the medial femoral condyle. In a high percentage of dogs the femoral attachment of the PCL will also contain fibers from the meniscal femoral ligament of the lateral meniscus. The PCL passes from its femoral attachment in a posterior, inferior direction to the medial aspect of the popliteal notch (Fig. 22-3). No attachment of the PCL to the menisci has been reported. The orientation of the femoral and tibial attachment of the PCL causes it to spiral slightly (Fig. 22-7) (9).

In general, the PCL is slightly longer and broader than the ACL. The PCL lies medial and crosses posterior to the ACL. In flexion, both ligaments twist on themselves and on each other. The ACL and PCL are covered with synovium; thus while they are intraarticular, they are also extrasynovial (9).

The cruciate ligaments of the dog function in a manner similar to that of their human counterpart. Because of their anatomical relationship, the cruciate ligaments twist on each other as the stifle is flexed, and the tibia internally rotates on the femur (Fig. 22-8A and B). This twisting action limits the amount of normal internal rotation of the tibia. Thus both ligaments work together to limit internal rotation of the tibia in flexion. The cruciate ligaments are also responsible for the anteroposterior stability of the stifle. The ACL prevents anterior displacement of the tibia on the femur (anterior drawer motion), whereas the PCL prevents posterior displacement of the tibia on the femur (posterior drawer motion). Finally, the ACL also serves as the primary check against hyperextension of the stifle joint (9).

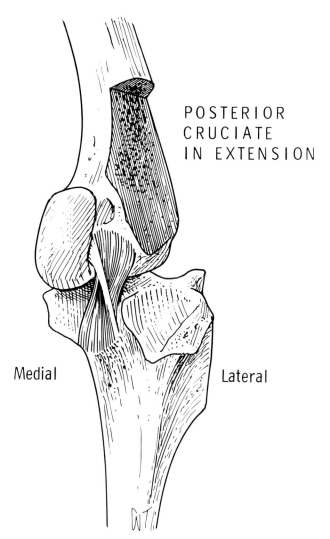

POSTERIOR
CRUCIATE
IN EXTENSION

Medial

Lateral

FIG. 22-7. Drawing of the PCL of a dog with the stifle in extension. Note how the ligament spirals slightly as it courses from the femur to the tibia. (From ref. 9.)

Collateral Ligaments

The origin of the lateral collateral ligament (LCL) is an oval roughened area, just proximal to the tendon of origin of the popliteal muscle on the lateral femoral epicondyle (Fig. 22-9). From this discrete origin, the ligament passes superficial to the popliteal tendon and extends posteriorly and distally as a strong fibrous band to insert on the fibular head. The fibers of the ligament are oriented longitudinally and maintain a fairly constant width. Loose connective tissue joins the ligament to the joint capsule. There are no reported attachments between the LCL and the lateral meniscus. The LCL has a superficial component that arises from the area of the lateral femorofabellar ligament and contributes to the prominent caudal border of the ligament. This superficial band merges with the major

component of the ligament as it crosses the joint surface, and then it separates to insert diffusely over the fascia of the fibularis longus muscle. The LCL is taut in extension but relaxes in flexion to allow internal rotation of the tibia on the femur (Fig. 22-10). As in the human, the LCL of the dog is important for the stability of the lateral aspect of the joint. This structure, along with the lateral joint capsule, popliteal tendon, and cruciate ligaments, acts to check varus stress in various degrees of flexion (50).

The medial collateral ligament (MCL) arises from an oval area of the medial femoral epicondyle (Fig. 22-9). The ligament extends distally and blends with the joint capsule, forming a strong attachment to the capsule and the medial meniscus. The fibers of the ligament are longitudinally oriented and maintain a uniform width. As the ligament extends distally across the medial tibial condyle, it passes superficial to the tibial insertion of the semimembranosus muscle and inserts over a large rectangular area of the proximal medial tibia. A bursa is located between the ligament and the tibia (50).

The MCL remains taut throughout the range of motion but appears to be most taut in extension (Fig. 22-11). The MCL is the prime stabilizer of the medial side of the stifle and acts as a check against valgus stress (50).

Functional Considerations

The ligaments of the stifle joint of animals function to stabilize the joint in much the same way as do the knee ligaments in humans. However, the stifle joint of most tetrapedal animals is said to be ACL-dependent. This is inferred from the angulation of the femur and tibia during normal stance. For example, in the normal standing position of the dog the articulating surface of the tibial plateau is sloped posteriorly (Fig. 22-12). Thus a weight-bearing force across the joint has the natural tendency to cause a posterior translation of the femur on the tibia (this can also be viewed as an anterior translation of the tibia on the femur). This tendency is, of course, countered by the stabilizing effect of an intact ACL (41). The ACL dependency of the stifle has also been inferred from studies that consistently demonstrate a progression of degenerative joint disease following ACL transection in the dog (33). In contrast, however, isolated transection of the PCL does not result in such marked degenerative changes (39).

Obviously, the extent to which the stifle of a specific animal is ACL-dependent is directly related to the anatomical orientation of the joint, the kinematics of the joint, and the gait pattern of the individual animal. Al-

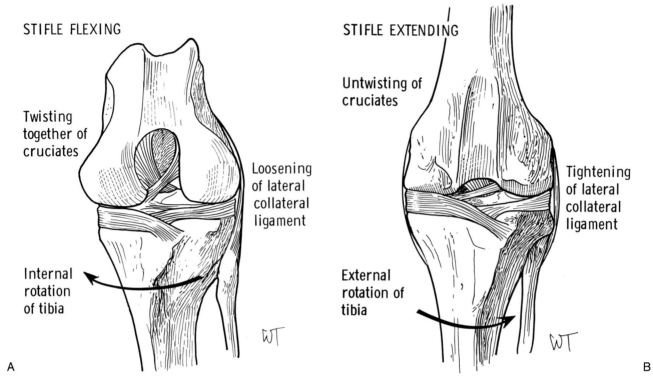

STIFLE FLEXING

Twisting together of cruciates

Loosening of lateral collateral ligament

Internal rotation of tibia

A

STIFLE EXTENDING

Untwisting of cruciates

Tightening of lateral collateral ligament

External rotation of tibia

B

FIG. 22-8. A: Drawing of the stifle of a dog in flexion. In this position the lateral collateral ligament (LCL) loosens, thereby allowing internal rotation of the tibia on the femur. The cruciate ligaments twist on each other to limit this internal rotation. **B:** Drawing of the stifle of a dog in extension. As the stifle extends, the LCL tightens and the tibia rotates externally, thereby untwisting the cruciate ligaments.

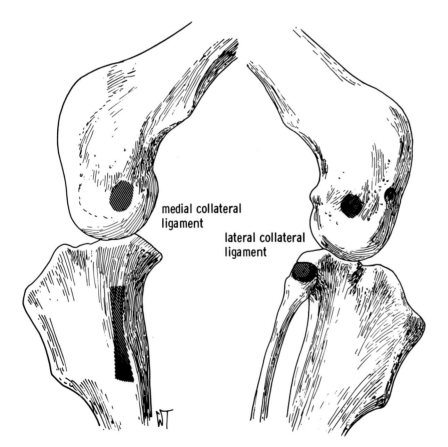

medial collateral ligament

lateral collateral ligament

FIG. 22-9. Drawing of the stifle of a dog, showing the areas of attachment for the medial and lateral collateral ligaments. (From ref. 50.)

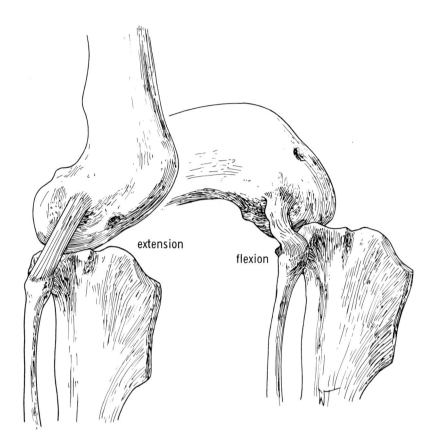

extension

flexion

FIG. 22-10. Drawing of the lateral aspect of the stifle joint of a dog, showing the LCL in flexion and extension. (From ref. 50.)

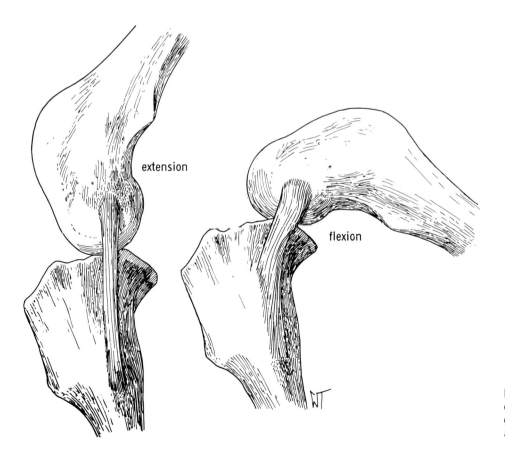

extension

flexion

FIG. 22-11. Drawing of the medial aspect of the stifle joint of a dog, showing the MCL in flexion and extension. (From ref. 50.)

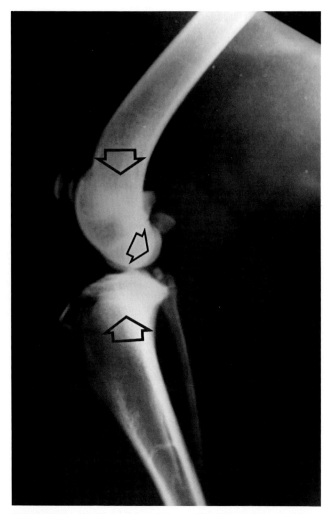

FIG. 22-12. Radiograph of the stifle joint of a dog in a functional position. The force of weight-bearing in this position will compress the stifle joint and cause the femur to want to slide posteriorly (or the tibia to displace anteriorly) on the sloping articular surface of the tibia. The presence of the ACL prevents this from happening.

though some information is available on the normal gait (i.e., force-plate analysis) of some breeds of dog (17,18), variations in size and gait within this species make generalizations difficult. The same holds true for other species where even the normal angulation of the stifle joint may vary several degrees, depending on the size and breed of the animal.

There does not appear to be an animal model that precisely duplicates the forces and kinematics of the human knee. Because of this, investigations that test the efficacy of a particular technique or prosthesis in stabilizing the stifle will not accurately reflect the conditions encountered in the human. For example, the success of a given ligament prosthesis in stabilizing the stifle of a sheep does not necessarily imply similar results in a human. Therefore, interpretations of these studies should be done with caution and should per-

haps be limited to more appropriate comparisons such as the physiologic reaction of the joint to a synthetic prosthesis or the remodeling response of a biologic graft.

Physiologic Considerations

In general terms, the morphology, physiology, and biochemistry of ligaments appear to be comparable across species lines. The generic description of dense regularly oriented connective tissue made up of fibroblasts in an extracellular matrix of collagen, proteoglycan, and water holds true for the ligaments of humans and animals (3,9,23,24). Although some biochemical data are available on specific animal ligaments (3), further studies are required to determine valid levels of comparison for these parameters.

Data from a variety of animal models suggest a common physiologic response in the healing of ligaments and the remodeling of ligament autografts and allografts (1,2,4,10–12,19–22,26–29,38,44). As noted previously, the existence of such common physiologic pathways among animals makes a strong case for the careful extrapolation of these pathways to humans. However, continued investigation on all levels is necessary to totally validate these comparisons.

SPECIFIC ANIMAL MODELS

In selecting an animal model, many investigators are quite naturally biased toward the animal(s) with which they worked during their early training in the field. Although this is an understandable prejudice, it should not prevent the consideration of other species in their research. The prudent scientist should evaluate each animal model on its strengths and weaknesses and utilize the model(s) that are the most valid for a specific area of study.

Dogs

The dog has been one of the more popular animal models for ligament research (14). This popularity is based on several factors, including ease of handling in a laboratory setting, a variety of available sizes, and the large information base available from the veterinary literature (6,7,9,34,37). Because cruciate ligament rupture is a common clinical problem in the dog, the veterinary literature abounds with the results of various surgical techniques, prosthetic implants, and postoperative management regimes designed to treat this problem (6,7,37). Therefore, investigators utilizing the dog as an experimental model already have a great deal of data available with which to compare and contrast their results. Although the dog is an excellent model for ligament research, increasing pressure from animal welfare groups has begun to limit its use in certain areas.

Rabbits

The rabbit is becoming a very popular model in knee ligament research. Because of their size and the relatively small expense (as compared to other species) of purchasing and housing these animals, the rabbit can be easily (and economically) maintained in large numbers. Although small in size, the rabbit has an adequate amount of ligamentous tissue available for manipulation and evaluation. This is especially true of the MCL. Whereas the position and kinematics of the rabbit stifle are markedly different from those of the human knee, the physiologic environment of the ligaments is the same as for other species. Extensive biochemical and biomechanical characterization of the ligaments of the rabbit stifle have provided a large data base for these species, and they should continue to be an excellent model to study the physiologic response of ligaments to various stimuli.

Goats and Sheep

The use of goats and sheep in ligament research has increased over the last 5 years. This is partially due to the pressures of local animal welfare groups that have vigorously objected to the use of dogs in biomedical research. Additionally, the larger size of these animals allows for the implantation of prosthetic ligaments designed (and sized) for use in the human knee. (It should be noted that even in these animals the size of the stifle joint is still much smaller than that of an average human.) Although the stifle joint of the goat and sheep is held in less flexion than that of the rabbit and some breeds of dog, it is still ACL-dependent. There is no scientific information available which would suggest that stifle function in these species is more comparable to the human knee than to the stifle of the dog.

One disadvantage of these species is that they are often less compliant than dogs and generally do not tolerate postoperative immobilization as well. In addition, housing these animals in an institutional setting requires specially designed facilities and is often expensive. Because of this, these animals are often shipped to farms where they are kept in group pens and/or open pastures. Although this is usually a less expensive housing arrangement, daily monitoring of animals and their limb function is not always possible. These limitations notwithstanding, the goat and sheep are excellent models for studying various aspects of knee ligament; furthermore, as the data base for these

animals increases, so will their use in biomedical research.

Primates

There is a natural anthropomorphic attraction to the subhuman primate species in medical research. This is especially true in musculoskeletal research, where anatomical similarities between humans and monkeys provide convenient comparison. However, close scrutiny of the movements of most laboratory primates reveals that their knees are habitually held in varying degrees of flexion, and although their ambulation is in the semierect position, it is, for the most part, tetrapedal. The close relationship between humans and monkeys on the evolutionary scale notwithstanding, there is nothing in the scientific literature to suggest that nonhuman primates are any more valid a model for ligament biology or function than some of the four-legged animals. In addition, the exorbitant cost of purchasing and maintaining these animals, along with the fact that some primates are on the endangered species list, makes their future availability for biomedical research questionable.

ETHICAL CONSIDERATIONS IN THE USE OF ANIMAL MODELS FOR BIOMEDICAL RESEARCH

Government Policy

The use of animals in biomedical research is a topic of passionate debate in today's society. Although each investigator must justify the use of animals in his or her own mind, there are certain ethical considerations that must be taken into account whenever animals are utilized in biomedical research. These considerations have been set forth in the forth of federal regulations and standards for the care and use of laboratory animals.

The Animal Welfare Act (originally passed in 1966 and subsequently amended in 1970, 1976, and 1985) is the federal statutory authority for inspection of research facilities and has set specific standards for the care and use of animals in biomedical research (5). These standards have been incorporated into the Public Health Service (PHS) Policy on the Humane Care and Use of Laboratory Animals (47). Although this policy is intended to govern institutions conducting U.S. PHS-supported research, it provides an excellent guideline for all facilities conducting research involving animals. The National Institutes of Health (NIH) has published a comprehensive guide that outlines these requirements (NIH Guide for the Care and Use of Laboratory Animals) (48). This text not only details the requirements for the housing and care of laboratory animals but also covers the requirements of analgesia, anesthesia, surgery, and postoperative care. All investigators utilizing animals in their research should be thoroughly familiar with its contents. In addition, the investigator should be familiar with specific state and local regulations governing the use of animals in biomedical research (25).

Conservation of Laboratory Animals

Although investigators have the ethical obligation to adhere to the regulations and standards set forth for the care and use of animals, they should also have a moral obligation to seek ways of limiting the number of animals used in their scientific studies. This idea of conserving the numbers of animals required in experimental studies was set forth by Russell and Burch in their book entitled *The Principles of Humane Experimental Technique* (42). To encourage the conservation of laboratory animals, they put forth the concepts of the three R's: replacement, reduction, and refinement.

Replacement refers to the obligation of the investigator to seek alternatives to the use of animals. This would include the use of computer modeling or tissue/organ culture techniques to achieve the information being sought.

If the use of an animal model is the only means of obtaining the desired information, then the reduction in the number of animals used is another very important concept that should be practiced by the scientist. This involves (a) the use of statistics (i.e., power study) to determine the minimum number of animals necessary to produce significant results and/or (b) small "pilot studies" to evaluate the appropriateness of a given hypothesis or technique. The use of the "team approach" in which many disciplines (pathology, biochemistry, biomechanics) collaborate to optimize the value of the results obtained is another way to reduce duplication and thus minimize the number of animals used.

Finally, the concept of refinement refers to development of new equipment and techniques to improve the procedures in which animals are used. Through these advances, the quantity and quality of data obtained from animals may also be improved. Hopefully, this would ultimately lead to a decrease in the number of animals needed for a specific study.

Although the debate over the use of laboratory animals in biomedical research is certain to continue, one fact is axiomatic: Investigators utilizing animals in their research are bound by ethical standards and moral obligations to conduct those studies in the most humane and scientifically rigorous methods possible.

SUMMARY

It was not the purpose of this discussion to attack or defend the use of specific animal models in ligament research but rather to provide investigators with an overview of the general considerations involved with the selection and use of animals in ligament research. In terms of microstructure, physiology, and material properties, there is no evidence to suggest that one animal model is the best for the study of ligament biology. No matter what animal model is used, it is the responsibility of the investigator to carefully define the valid levels of comparison for each model and to interpret the results within these established confines. As the data base for each animal model increases and as more information becomes available from the evaluation of human material, the validity of the animal model in knee ligament research will be more clearly defined.

REFERENCES

1. Alm A, Stromberg B. Transposed medial third of patellar ligament in reconstruction of the anterior cruciate ligament: a surgical and morphologic study in dogs. *Acta Chir Scand [Suppl]* 1974;445:37–49.
2. Amiel D, Abel MF, Kleiner JB, et al. Synovial fluid nutrient delivery in the diarthrodial joint: an analysis of rabbit knee ligaments. *J Orthop Res* 1986;4:90–95.
3. Amiel D, Frank C, Harwood FJ, Akeson WH. Tendons and ligaments: a morphological and biochemical comparison. *J Orthop Res* 1984;1:257–265.
4. Amiel D, Kleiner JB, Akeson WH. The natural history of the anterior cruciate ligament autograft of patellar tendon origin. *Am J Sports Med* 1986;14:449–462.
5. Animal Welfare Act (Title 7 U.S.C. 2131–2156), as amended by P.L. 99-198, December 23, 1986.
6. Archibald J, Catcott EJ. *Canine surgery,* 1st edition. Santa Barbara, CA: American Veterinary Publications, 1984.
7. Arnoczky SP. Cranial cruciate ligament repair, In: Bojrab MJ, Crane SW, Arnoczky SP, eds. *Current techniques in small animal surgery.* Philadelphia: Lea & Febiger, 1983.
8. Arnoczky SP. Cruciate ligament rupture and associated injuries. In: Newton CD, Nunamaker DM, eds. *Textbook of small animal orthopaedics.* Philadelphia: JB Lippincott, 1985;925–935.
9. Arnoczky SP, Marshall JL. The cruciate ligaments of the canine stifle: an anatomical and functional evaluation. *Am J Vet Res* 1977;38:1807–1814.
10. Arnoczky SP, Rubin RM, Marshall JL. Microvasculature of the cruciate ligaments and its response to injury. *J Bone Joint Surg* 1979;61A:1221–1229.
11. Arnoczky SP, Tarvin GB, Marshall JL. Anterior cruciate ligament replacement using patellar tendon: an evaluation of graft revascularization in the dog. *J Bone Joint Surg* 1982;64A:271–224.
12. Arnoczky SP, Warren RF, Ashlock MA. Anterior cruciate ligament replacement using a patellar tendon allograft: an experimental study in the dog. *J Bone Joint Surg* 1986;68A:376–385.
13. Arnoczky SP, Warren RF, Minei JP. Replacement of the anterior cruciate ligament using a synthetic prosthesis: an evaluation of graft biology in the dog. *Am J Sports Med* 1986;14:1–6.
14. Arnoczky SP, Wilson JW. Experimental surgery of the skeletal system. In: Gay WI, Heavner JE, eds. *Methods of animal experimentation, vol VII: research surgery and care of the research animal.* New York: Academic Press, 1986;67–108.

15. Balls M, Riddell RJ, Worden AN. *Animals and alternatives in toxicology testing*. New York: Academic Press, 1983.
16. Bernard C. *An introduction to the study of experimental medicine* (English translation). New York: Dover Publications, 1957.
17. Budsberg SC, Verstraete MC, Soutas-Little RW, et al. Force plate analysis of the walking gait in healthy dogs. *Am J Vet Res* 1987;48:915–918.
18. Budsberg SC, Verstraete MC, Soutas-Little RW, Flo GL, Probst CW. Force plate analysis before and after stabilization of canine stifles for cruciate injury. *Am J Vet Surg* 1988;49:1523–1524.
19. Cabaud HE, Rodkey WG, Feagin JA. Experimental studies of acute anterior cruciate ligament injury and repair. *Am J Sports Med* 1979;7:18–22.
20. Chiroff RT. Experimental replacement of the anterior cruciate ligament: a histological and microangiographic study. *J Bone Joint Surg* 1975;57A:1124–1127.
21. Clancy WG Jr, Narechania RG, Rosenberg TD, Gmeiner JG, Wisnefske DD, Lange TA. Anterior and posterior cruciate ligament reconstruction in rhesus monkeys. *J Bone Joint Surg* 1981;63A:1270–1284.
22. Clayton ML, Weir GJ. Experimental investigations of ligamentous healing. *Am J Surg* 1959;98:373–378.
23. Danylchuk KD, Findlay JB, Krcek JP. Microstructure organization of human and bovine cruciate ligaments. *Clin Orthop* 1978;131:294–298.
24. DePalma AF. *Diseases of the knee*. Philadelphia: JB Lippincott, 1954.
25. Foundation for Biomedical Research. *The biomedical investigator's handbook: for researchers using animal models*. Washington, DC, 1987.
26. Frank C, Schachar N, Dittrich D. The natural history of healing in the repaired medial collateral ligament. A morphologic accessment in rabbits. *J Orthop Res* 1983;1:179–188.
27. Frank C, Woo SL-Y, Amiel D, Gomez MA, Harwood FL, Akeson WH. Medial collateral ligament healing. A multidisciplinary assessment in rabbits. *Am J Sports Med* 1983;11:379–389.
28. Ginsberg JH, Whiteside LA, Piper TL. Nutrient pathways in transferred patellar tendon used for ACL reconstruction. *Am J Sports Med* 1980;8:15–18.
29. Jack EA. Experimental rupture of the medial collateral ligament of the knee. *J Bone Joint Surg* 1950;32B:396–402.
30. Krebs HA. The August Krogh Principle: "For many problems there is an animal on which it can be most conveniently studied." *J Exp Zool* 1975;194:221–226.
31. Krebs HA, Krebs JR. The "August Krogh Principle." *Comp Biochem Physiol* 1980;67B:379–380.
32. Krogh A. Progress of physiology. *Am J Physiol* 1929;90:243–251.
33. Marshall JL. Periarticular osteophytes–initiation and formation in the knee of the dog. *Clin Orthop* 1969;62:37–47.
34. Miller ME. *Miller's anatomy of the dog*, 2nd ed. Philadelphia: WB Saunders, 1979.
35. National Research Council. *Models for biomedical research—a new perspective*. Washington, DC: National Academy Press, 1985.
36. National Research Council. *Use of laboratory animals in biomedical and behavioral research*. Washington, DC: National Academy Press, 1988.
37. Newton CD, Nunamaker DM. *Textbook of small animal orthopaedics*, 1st ed. Philadelphia: JB Lippincott, 1985.
38. O'Donoghue DH, Rockwood CA Jr, Zaricznyj B, Kenyon R. Repair of knee ligaments in dogs. I. The lateral collateral ligament. *J Bone Joint Surg* 1961;43A:1167–1178.
39. Pournaras J, Symeonides PP, Karkavelas G. The significance of the posterior cruciate ligament in the stability of the knee: an experimental study in dogs. *J Bone Joint Surg* 1983;65B:204–209.
40. Prichard RW. Animal models in human medicine. In: *Animal models of thrombosis and hemorrhagic diseases*. Washington, DC: US Department of Health, Education, and Welfare (No. 76-982), 1976;169–172.
41. Rubin RM, Marshall JL, Wang J. Prevention of knee instability. Experimental model for prosthetic anterior cruciate ligament. *Clin Orthop* 1975;113:212–236.
42. Russell WMS, Burch RL. *The principles of humane experimental technique*. Springfield, IL: Charles C Thomas, 1959.
43. Shino K, Kimura T, Hirose H, Inoue M, Ono K. Reconstruction of the anterior cruciate ligament by allogenic tendon graft. *J Bone Joint Surg* 1986;68B:739–746.
44. Shino K, Kawaski T, Hirose H, et al. Replacement of the anterior cruciate ligament by an allogenic tendon graft: an experimental study in the dog. *J Bone Joint Surg* 1984;66B:672–681.
45. Sisson S, Grossman JD. *The anatomy of the domestic animals*. Philadelphia: WB Saunders, 1968.
46. Thomas NP, Turner IG, Jones CB. Prosthetic anterior cruciate ligaments in the rabbit. *J Bone Joint Surg* 1987;69B:312–316.
47. U.S. Department of Health and Human Services, National Institutes of Health, Office for the Protection from Research Risks. Public Health Service Policy on Humane Care and Use of Laboratory Animals, revised September 1986, pursuant to Health Research Extensions Act of 1985 (P.L. 99-158, No. 495, November 20, 1985).
48. U.S. Department of Health and Human Services, Public Health Service, National Institutes of Health. *Guide for the care and use of laboratory animals*, NIH No. 85-23, 1985.
49. Van Sickle DC, Kincaid SA. Comparative arthrology. In: Sokoloff L, ed. *The joints and synovial fluid*, vol I. New York: Academic Press, 1978;1–47.
50. Vasseur PB, Arnoczky SP. Collateral ligaments of the canine stifle: anatomic and functional analysis. *Am J Vet Res* 1981;42:1133–1137.
51. Warbasse JP. *The conquest of disease through animal experimentation*. New York: D Appleton, 1910.

SELECTED REFERENCES

Cattle

Danylchuk KD, Finlay JB, Krcek JP. Microstructural organization of human and bovine cruciate ligaments. *Clin Orthop* 1978;131:294–298.

Dog

Alm A, Stromberg B. Transposed medial third of patellar ligament in reconstruction of the anterior cruciate ligament: a surgical and morphologic study in dogs. *Acta Chir Scand [Suppl]* 1974;445:37–49.

Amstutz HC, Caulson WR, David E. Reconstruction of the canine achilles and patella tendons using dacron mesh silicone prosthesis. *J Biomed Mater Res* 1976;10:47–59.

Andrish JT, Woods LD. Dacron augmentation in anterior cruciate ligament reconstruction in dogs. *Clin Orthop* 1984;183:298–302.

Aragona J, Parsons JR, Alexander H, Weiss AB. Medial collateral ligament replacement with a partially absorbable tissue scaffold. *Am J Sports Med* 1983;11:228–233.

Arnoczky SP, Marshall JL. The cruciate ligaments of the canine stifle: an anatomical and functional evaluation. *Am J Vet Res* 1977;38:1807–1814.

Arnoczky SP, Rubin RM, Marshall JL. Microvasculature of the cruciate ligaments and its response to injury. *J Bone Joint Surg* 1979;61A:1221–1229.

Arnoczky SP, Tarvin GB, Marshall JL. Anterior cruciate ligament replacement using patellar tendon: an evaluation of graft revascularization in the dog. *J Bone Joint Surg* 1982;64A:217–224.

Arnoczky SP, Torzilli PA, Warren RF, Allen AA. Biologic fixation of ligament prostheses and augmentations. An evaluation of bone ingrowth in the dog. *Am J Sports Med* 1988;16:106–112.

Arnoczky SP, Warren RF, Ashlock MA. Anterior cruciate ligament replacement using a patellar tendon allograft: an experimental study in the dog. *J Bone Joint Surg* 1986;68A:376–385.

Arnoczky SP, Warren RF, Minei JP. Replacement of the anterior cruciate ligament using a synthetic prosthesis: an evaluation of graft biology in the dog. *Am J Sports Med* 1986;14:1–6.

Brody GA, Eisinger M, Arnoczky SP, Warren RF. *In vitro* fibroblast seeding of prosthetic anterior cruciate ligaments: a preliminary study. *Am J Sports Med* 1988;16:203–208.

Butler DL, Hulse DA, Kay MD, Grood ES, Shires PK, D'Ambrosia R, Shoji H. Biomechanics of cranial cruciate reconstruction in the dog. II. Mechanical properties. *Vet Surg* 1983;12:113–188.

Cabaud HE, Feagin JA, Rodkey WG. Acute anterior cruciate ligament injury and augmented repair. *Am J Sports Med* 1980;8:395–401.

Cabaud HE, Feagin JA, Rodkey WG. Acute anterior cruciate ligament injury and repair reinforced with a biodegradable intraarticular ligament. *Am J Sports Med* 1982;10:259–265.

Cabaud HE, Rodkey WG, Feagin JA. Experimental studies of acute anterior cruciate ligament injury and repair. *Am J Sports Med* 1979;7:18–22.

Chiroff RT. Experimental replacement of the anterior cruciate ligament: a histological and microangiographic study. *J Bone Joint Surg* 1975;57A:1124–1127.

Clayton ML, Weir GJ Jr. Experimental investigations of ligamentous healing. *Am J Surg* 1959;98:373–378.

Cooper RR, Misol S. Tendon and ligament insertion—a light and electron microscopic study. *J Bone Joint Surg* 1970;52A:1–20.

Curtis RJ, Delee JC, Drez DJ Jr. Reconstruction of the anterior cruciate ligament with freeze-dried fascia lata allografts in dogs: a preliminary report. *Am J Sports Med* 1985;13:408–414.

Emery MA, Rostrup O. Repair of the anterior cruciate ligament with 8mm tube teflon in dogs. *Can J Surg* 1960;4:111–115.

Ginsberg JH, Whiteside LA, Piper TL. Nutrient pathways in transferred patellar tendon used for ACL reconstruction. *Am J Sports Med* 1980;8:15–18.

Gupta BN, Brinker WO. Anterior cruciate ligament prosthesis in the dog. *J Am Vet Med Assoc* 1969;154:1586–1588.

Hulse DA, Butler DL, Kay MD. Biomechanics of cranial cruciate ligament reconstruction in the dog. I. *In vitro* laxity testing. *Vet Surg* 1983;12:109–112.

Laros GS, Tipton CM, Cooper RR. Influence of physical activity on ligament insertions in the knees of dogs. *J Bone Joint Surg* 1971;53A:275–286.

Marshall JL, Olsson SE. Instability of the knee: a long-term experimental study in dogs. *J Bone Joint Surg* 1971;53A:1561–1570.

McFarland EG, Morrey BF, Wood MB. The relationship of vascularity and water content to tensile strength in a patellar tendon replacement of the anterior cruciate in dogs. *Am J Sports Med* 1986;14:436–448.

McMaster WC. A histologic assessment of canine anterior cruciate substitution with bovine xenograft. *Clin Orthop* 1985;196:196–201.

McMaster WC. Bovine xenograft collateral ligament replacement in the dog. *J Orthop Res* 1985;3:492–498.

Mendenhall HV, Roth JH, Kennedy JC, Winter GD, Lumb WV. Evaluation of the polypropylene braid as a prosthetic anterior cruciate ligament replacement in the dog. *Am J Sports Med* 1987;15:543–546.

Mendes DG, Iusim M, Angel D, Rotem A, Roffman M, Grishkan A, Mordohohvich, Boss J. Histologic pattern of biomechanic properties of the carbon fiber-augmented ligament tenon. *Clin Orthop* 1985;196:51–60.

Meyers JF, Grana WA, Lesker PA. Reconstruction of the anterior cruciate ligament in the dog. *Am J Sports Med* 1979;7:85–90.

Nikolaou PK, Seaber AV, Glisson RR, Ribbeck BM, Bassett FH. Anterior cruciate ligament allograft transplantation: long-term function, histology, revascularization, and operative technique. *Am J Sports Med* 1986;14:348–360.

O'Donoghue DH, Frank CG, Jeter GL, Johnson W, Zeiders JW, Kenyon R. Repair and reconstruction of the anterior cruciate ligament in dogs: factors influencing long term results. *J Bone Joint Surg* 1971;53A:710–718.

O'Donoghue DH, Rockwood CA Jr, Frank GR, Jack SC, Kenyon R. Repair of the anterior cruciate ligament in dogs. *J Bone Joint Surg* 1966;48A:503–519.

O'Donoghue DH, Rockwood CA Jr, Zaricznyj B, Kenyon R. Repair of knee ligaments in dogs. I. The lateral collateral ligament. *J Bone Joint Surg* 1961;43A:1167–1178.

Ogata K, Whiteside LA, Andersson DA. The intra-articular effect of various postoperative managements following knee ligament repair. An experimental study in dogs. *Clin Orthop* 1980;150:271–276.

Oretorp N, Alm A, Ekstrom H, Gillquist J. Immediate effects of meniscectomy of the knee joint: the effects of tensile load on knee joint ligaments in dogs. *Acta Orthop Scand* 1978;49:407–415.

Park JP, Grana WA, Chitwood JS. A high-strength dacron augmentation for cruciate ligament reconstruction. *Clin Orthop* 1985;196:175–185.

Pournaras J, Symeonides PP, Karkavelas G. The significance of the posterior cruciate ligament in the stability of the knee. An experimental study in dogs. *J Bone Joint Surg* 1983;65B:204–209.

Rubin RM, Marshall JL, Wang J. Prevention of knee instability-experimental model for prosthetic anterior cruciate ligament. *Clin Orthop* 1975;113:212–236.

Ryan JR, Drompp BW. Evaluation of tensile strength of reconstructions of the anterior cruciate ligament using the patellar tendon in dogs. *South Med J* 1966;59:129–131.

Shino K, Kawaski T, Hirose H. Replacement of the anterior cruciate ligament by an allogenic tendon graft: an experimental study in the dog. *J Bone Joint Surg* 1984;66B:672–681.

Tipton CM, James SL, Mergner W, Tcheng T-K. Influence of exercise on strength of medial collateral knee ligaments of dogs. *Am J Physiol* 1970;218:894–902.

van Rens TJG, van den Berg AF, Huiskes R. Substitution of the anterior cruciate ligament: a long-term histologic and biomechanical study with autogenous pedicled grafts of the iliotibial band in dogs. *Arthroscopy* 1986;2:139–154.

Vasseur PB, Arnoczky SP. Collateral ligaments of the canine stifle joint: anatomic and functional analysis. *Am J Vet Res* 1981;42:1133–1137.

Woo SL-Y, Gomez MA, Akeson WH. The time- and history-dependent viscoelastic properties of the canine medial collateral ligament. *J Biomech Eng* 1981;103:293–295.

Woo SL-Y, Gomez MA, Inoue M, Akeson WH. New experimental procedures to evaluate the biomechanical properties of healing canine medial collateral ligaments. *J Orthop Res* 1987;5:425–432.

Woo SL-Y, Gomez MA, Seguchi Y, Endo CM, Akeson WH. Measurement of mechanical properties of ligament substance from a bone–ligament–bone preparation. *J Orthop Res* 1983;1:22–29.

Yoshiya S, Andrish JT, Manley MT, Bauer TW. Graft tension in anterior cruciate ligament reconstruction: an *in vivo* study in dogs. *Am J Sports Med* 1987;15:464–470.

Yoshiya S, Andrish JT, Manley MT, Kuroska M. Augmentation of anterior cruciate ligament reconstruction in dogs with prostheses of different stiffnesses. *J Orthop Res* 1986;4:475–485.

Goat

Holden JP, Grood ES, Butler DL, Noyes FR, Mendenhall HV, Van Kampen CL, Neidich RL. Biomechanics of fascia lata ligament replacements: early postoperative changes in the goat. *J Orthop Res* 1988;6:639–647.

Jackson DW, Grood ES, Arnoczky SP, Butler DL, Simon TM. Freeze-dried anterior cruciate ligament allografts: preliminary studies in a goat model. *Am J Sports Med* 1987;15:295–303.

Jackson DW, Grood ES, Arnoczky SP, Butler DL, Simon TM. Cruciate reconstruction using freeze-dried anterior cruciate ligament allograft and a ligament augmentation device (LAD). An experimental study in a goat model. *Am J Sports Med* 1987;15:528–538.

Jackson DW, Grood ES, Wilcox P, Butler DL, Simon TM, Holden JP. The effect of processing techniques on the mechanical properties of bone–anterior cruciate ligament–bone allografts. An experimental study in goats. *Am J Sports Med* 1988;16:101–105.

McPherson GK, Mendenhall HV, Gibbons DF, et al. Experimental mechanical and histologic evaluation of the Kennedy ligament augmentation device. *Clin Orthop* 1985;196:186–195.

Cat

Jack EA. Experimental rupture of the medial collateral ligament of the knee. *J Bone Joint Surg* 1950;32B:396–402.

Rabbit

Amiel D, Abel MFR, Kleiner JB. Synovial fluid nutrient delivery in the diarthrodial joint: an analysis of rabbit knee ligaments. *J Orthop Res* 1985;4:90–95.

Amiel D, Akeson WH, Harwood FL, Frank CB. Stress deprivation effect on metabolic turnover of the medial collateral ligament collagen. *Clin Orthop* 1983;172:265–270.

Amiel D, Frank C, Harwood F, Fronek J, Akeson W. Tendons and ligaments: a morphological and biochemical comparison. *J Orthop Res* 1984;1:257–265.

Amiel D, Kleiner JB, Akeson WH. The natural history of the anterior cruciate ligament autograft of patellar tendon origin. *Am J Sports Med* 1986;14:449–462.

Amiel D, Kleiner JB, Roux RD, Harwood FL, Akeson WH. The phenomenon of "ligamentization": anterior cruciate ligament reconstruction with autogenous patellar tendon. *J Orthop Res* 1986;4:162–172.

Amis AA, Kempson SA, Campbell JR, Miller JH. Anterior cruciate ligament replacement-biocompatibility and biomechanics of polyester and carbon fiber in rabbits. *J Bone Joint Surg* 1988;70B:628–634.

Frank C, Edwards P, McDonald D, Bodie D, Sabiston P. Viability of ligaments after freezing: an experimental study in a rabbit model. *J Ortho Res* 1988;6:95–102.

Frank C, Schachar N, Dittrich D, Shrive N, deHaas W, Edwards G. Electromagnetic stimulation of ligament healing in rabbits. *Clin Orthop* 1983;175:263–272.

Frank C, Schachar N, Dittrich D. The natural history of healing in the repaired medial collateral ligament. A morphological assessment in rabbits. *J Orthop Res* 1983;1:179–188.

Frank C, Woo SL-Y, Amiel D, Gomez MA, Harwood FL, Akeson W. Medial collateral ligament healing. A multidisciplinary assessment in rabbits. *Am J Sports Med* 1983;11:379–389.

Goodship AE, Wilcock SA, Shah JS. The development of tissue around various prosthetic implants used as replacements for ligament and tendons. *Clin Orthop* 1985;196:61–68.

Horwitz MT. Injuries of the ligaments of the knee joint. An experimental study. *Arch Surg* 1989;38:946–954.

Kappakas GS, Brown TD, Goodman MA, Kikuike A, McMaster JH. Delayed surgical repair of ruptured ligaments. A comparative biomechanical and histologic study. *Clin Orthop* 1978;135:281–286.

Kleiner JB, Amiel D, Roux RD, Akeson WH. Origin of replacement cells for the anterior cruciate ligament autograft. *J Orthop Res* 1986;4:466–474.

McMaster WC, Liddle S, Anzel SH, Waugh TR. Medial collateral ligament replacement in the rabbit. A preliminary report. *Am J Sports Med* 1975;3:271–276.

Miltner LJ, Hu CH, Fang HC. Experimental joint sprain. *Arch Surg* 1937;35:234–240.

Mitsou A, Vallianatos P, Piskopakis N, Nicolaou P. Cruciate ligament replacement using a meniscus: an experimental study. *J Bone Joint Surg* 1988;70B:784–786.

Parsons JR, Bhayani S, Alexander H, Weiss AB. Carbon fiber debris within the synovial joint. *Clin Orthop* 1985;196:69–76.

Thomas NP, Turner IG, Jones CB. Prosthetic anterior cruciate ligaments in the rabbit. A comparison of four types of replacement. *J Bone Joint Surg* 1987;69B:312–316.

Torzilli PA, Arnoczky SP. Mechanical properties of the lateral collateral ligament: effect of cruciate instability in the rabbit. *J Biomech Eng* 1988;110:208–212.

Woo SL-Y, Gomez MA, Seguchi Y, Endo CM, Akeson WH. Measurement of mechanical properties of ligament substance from a bone–ligament–bone preparation. *J Orthop Res* 1983;1:22–29.

Woo SL-Y, Orlando CA, Gomez MA, Frank CB, Akeson WH. Tensile properties of the medial collateral ligament as a function of age. *J Orthop Res* 1986;4:133–141.

Sheep

Bercovy M, Goutallier D, Voisin MC, Geiger D, Blanquaert D, Gaudichet A, Patte D. Carbon-PGLA prostheses for ligament reconstruction. *Clin Orthop* 1985;196:159–168.

Bolton CW, Bruchman WC. The GORE-TEX expanded polytetrafluoroethylene prosthetic ligament. *Clin Orthop* 1985;196:202–213.

Claes L, Neugebauer R. *In vivo* and *in vitro* investigation of the long-term behavior and fatigue strength of carbon fiber ligament replacement. *Clin Orthop* 1985;196:99–111.

Porcine (Pig)

Woo SL-Y, Gomez MA, Seguchi Y, Endo CM, Akeson WH. Measurement of mechanical properties of ligament substance from a bone–ligament–bone preparation. *J Orthop Res* 1983;1:22–29.

Primate

Butler DL, Grood ES, Noyes FR, et al. Mechanical properties of primate vascularized vs. nonvascularized patellar tendon grafts; changes over time. *J Orthop Res* 1989;7:68–79.

Clancy WG Jr, Narechania RG, Rosenberg TD, Gmeiner JG, Wisnefske DD, Lange TA. Anterior and posterior cruciate ligament reconstruction in rhesus monkeys: a histologic, microangiographic, and biomechanical analysis. *J Bone Joint Surg* 1981;63A:1270–1284.

Noyes FR. Functional properties of knee ligaments and alterations induced by immobilization: a correlative biomechanical and histological study in primates. *Clin Orthop* 1977;123:210–242.

Noyes FR, DeLucas JL, Torvik PJ. Biomechanics of anterior cruciate ligament failure: an analysis of strain-rate sensitivity and mechanisms of failure in primates. *J Bone Joint Surg* 1974;54A:236–253.

Noyes FR, Grood ES. The strength of the anterior cruciate ligament in humans and rhesus monkeys. Age and species-related changes. *J Bone Joint Surg* 1976;58A:1074–1082.

Noyes FR, Grood ES, Nussbaum NS, Cooper SM. Effect of intraarticular corticosteroids on ligament properties. A biomechanical and histological study in rhesus knees. *Clin Orthop* 1977;123:197–209.

Noyes FR, Nussbaum N, Torvik PJ, Cooper SM. Biomechanical and ultrastructural changes in ligaments and tendons after local corticosteroid injections. *J Bone Joint Surg* 1975;57A:876.

Noyes FR, Torvik PJ, Hyde WB, DeLucas JL. Biomechanics of ligament failure. II. An analysis of immobilization, exercise, and reconditioning effects in primates. *J Bone Joint Surg* 1974;56A:1406–1418.

Rat

Adams A. Effect of exercise upon ligament strength. *Res Q* 1966;37:163–167.

Booth FW, Tipton CM. Ligamentous strength measurements in prepubescent and pubescent rats. *Growth* 1970;34:177–185.

Cabaud HE, Chatty A, Gildengorin V, Feltman RJ. Exercise effects on the strength of the rat anterior cruciate ligament. *Am J Sports Med* 1980;8:79–86.

Tipton CM, Matthes RD, Martin RK. Influence of age and sex on the strength of bone–ligament junctions in knee joints of rats. *J Bone Joint Surg* 1978;60A:230–234.

Tipton CM, Schild RJ, Flatt AE. Measurement of ligamentous strength in rat knees. *J Bone Joint Surg* 1967;49A:63–72.

PART V

Clinical Studies

Knee Ligaments: Structure, Function, Injury, and Repair, edited by D. Daniel, et al.
© 1990 by Raven Press, Ltd. All rights reserved.

CHAPTER 23

Instrumented Measurement of Knee Motion

Dale M. Daniel and Mary Lou Stone

Ligaments limit joint motion. *In vitro* ligament sectioning studies have documented that disruption of a specific ligament results in a characteristic change in motion (Chapter 9). One indicator of a successful ligament repair or reconstruction is the reestablishment of the normal motion limits. Instrumented measurement of joint motion (a) assists the clinician in diagnosing ligament disruptions by detecting pathologic motion, (b) documents the amount of pathologic motion, and (c) measures the success of ligament surgery to reestablish the normal motion limits. This chapter will discuss the principles of instrumented measurement of knee motion. Chapter 24 presents the technique of measuring anterior–posterior displacement with the KT-1000 arthrometer and discusses our experience with that instrument.

Motion measurements consist of:

1. positioning the limb in a specified manner;
2. applying a displacing force; and
3. measuring the resultant joint motion.

The testing devices may perform one, two, or all of the above tasks. The early reports of instrumented testing consisted of positioning the limb, applying a standard displacement force, and documenting change in joint position by comparing photographs (20) or radiographs (10,11,22,23) taken of the unstressed and stressed knee. Though stress radiography techniques are widely known to the clinician, they have not been widely used. This may be due to (a) a concern about the resultant radiation exposure, (b) the expense of multiple roentgenograms, and (c) the attention to detail needed when positioning the patient and when measuring the films. Stress radiography is discussed in Chapter 25.

Instrumented measurement systems that document anterior–posterior (A–P) tibial displacement by tracking the tibial tubercle in relation to the patella have become popular in the orthopedic community relatively recently. Markolf (USA) (14), Shino (Japan) (19), and Edixhoven (Netherlands) (8) developed stationary testing systems. Portable testing systems commercially available were developed by Cannon and Lamoreux (Knee Laxity Tester, Stryker Ligament Tester) and by Malcom and Daniel (KT-1000, MEDmetric, San Diego, California) (7,12). More recently, commercial devices have been introduced which simultaneously measure motion in several directions (Genucom, Faro Medical Technologies, Champlain, New York and KSS, Acufex, Norwood, Massachusetts).

TESTING VARIABLES

Motion measurements depend on:

1. joint position at the initiation of the test;

D. M. Daniel: Department of Orthopedic Surgery, University of California, San Diego, School of Medicine, La Jolla, California 92037; and Kaiser Permanente Medical Center, San Diego, California 92120.
 M. L. Stone: Department of Orthopedics, Kaiser Hospital of San Diego, San Diego, California 92120.

422 / CHAPTER 23

2. motion constraints imposed by the testing system;
3. displacing force;
4. measurement system;
5. muscle activity; and
6. the passive motion constraints.

The role of the testing device is to minimize the variability between factors 1 through 5 so that the difference in measurements between two knees or one knee tested at time intervals indicates a true change in the passive motion constraints. Examples of how variables 1 through 5 may affect the displacement measurements are presented below.

Joint Starting Position

Flexion

The joint flexion angle will affect the orientation of the ligament with respect to the applied force and may affect the distance between the ligaments' attachment sites. The changing orientation of the cruciate ligaments with joint flexion is illustrated in Fig. 10-6. From a review of these figures it may be noted that the anterior cruciate ligament (ACL) is better oriented to resist an anterior displacement force when the knee is flexed to 90° than when the knee is extended. The posterior cruciate ligament (PCL) is better oriented to resist a posterior displacement force with the knee in full extension than it is in 90° of flexion.

This observation correlates with the clinical experience that anterior tibial displacement is less at 90° of flexion than at 30° (14,16,21). However, when the ACL is disrupted, there is a greater increase in anterior displacement with the knee in 30° of flexion than in 90° of flexion (15,16,21). When the PCL is disrupted, there is a greater increase in displacement at 90° of flexion than at 30° of flexion (6). With the cruciates sectioned, other structures become the primary A–P displacement constraints. The effects of joint position on these structures vary. For example, the anterior fibers of the medial collateral ligament (MCL) tighten with knee flexion (Fig. 10-30). If the menisci are intact and the tibia is displaced anteriorly, the femoral condyles ride up on the wedge-shaped meniscus and tension the capsule and collateral ligaments (15), thereby constraining anterior tibial displacement.

As illustrated in Fig. 11-5, the anterior displacement force is resisted by tensile forces in the ligaments and by joint surface compression forces. This may be compared to the supportive forces on a tent, with (a) compression through the central pole and (b) tension in the guy ropes. Lengthening the guy ropes or shortening the central pole both render the guy ropes lax and result in greater tent motion when the wind blows.

Likewise, disruption of the ligaments or destruction of the joint surface will alter the joint motion limits.

Rotation

Rotation of the tibia affects (a) the distance between the ligaments' attachment sites and (b) anterior displacement measurements (1,15,17). Markolf (14,15) reported that 15° of external rotation results in the greatest anterior knee laxity *in vivo*.

Sagittal Plane Translation

Flexion of the knee relaxes the posterior capsule. In a supine patient the PCL then supports the weight of the leg. If the PCL is disrupted, the tibia will sag posteriorly (Fig. 1-2). When the patient is prone, the tibia translates anteriorly and the ACL supports the leg. The joint resting position depends on patient position and intact structures.

Markolf (14,15) reported sagittal plane translation as total A–P translation. Others have divided the motion into anterior and posterior excursions. Shino (19) reported anterior translation as anterior motion from the knee resting position. Daniel (5) and Edixhoven (8) have referenced measurements to the position of the limb after a posterior displacing force is applied and then released. Before assuming that the joint resting position in a supine patient is a physiologic position, the *quadriceps active test* may be used (Chapter 24) to confirm that the PCL is intact.

MOTION CONSTRAINTS IMPOSED BY THE TESTER OR THE TESTING SYSTEM

An unconstrained testing system allows 6 degrees of freedom (DOF), that is, rotation around and translation along each of the three axes (Fig. 8-2). Many motions are linked or coupled to one another. For example, anterior translation and internal rotation are normally paired, as are posterior translation and external rotation (Fig. 23-1). When motions are coupled, constraint of one of the motions will limit the other. This concept is illustrated in Fig. 23-2.

The comparison of two *in vitro* ACL sectioning studies demonstrates the effect of the testing apparatus on anterior displacement measurements. In a 1-DOF system the anterior displacement after sectioning the ligament was 5 mm (3), whereas in a 5-DOF system the tibial displacement was 15 mm (21).

In vivo, a 1-DOF measurement system is probably neither desirable nor attainable. In the modestly constrained A–P testing system reported by Edixhoven (8), pulling the tibia anteriorly resulted in 6–11° of knee

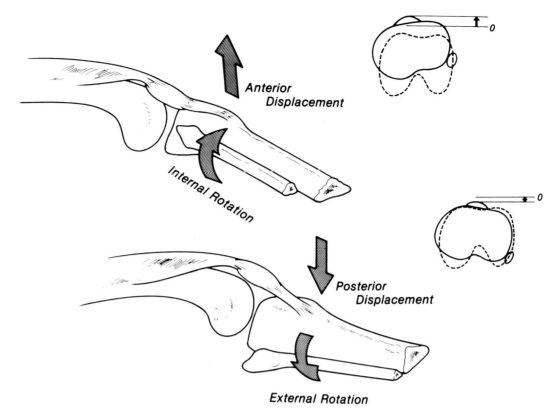

FIG. 23-1. Coupled motion. Anterior drawer testing shows combined anterior translation and internal rotation. Posterior drawer shows combined posterior translation and external rotation.

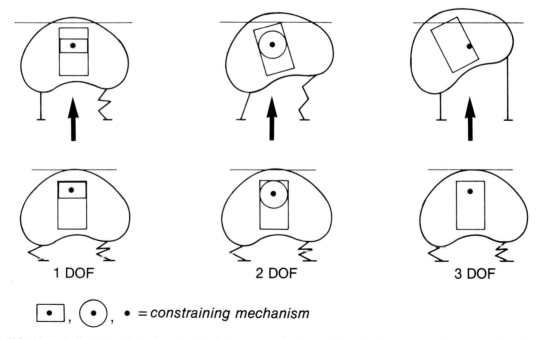

1 DOF   2 DOF   3 DOF

▢•, ⊙, • = constraining mechanism

FIG. 23-2. Influence of motion constrains on anterior translation in structures with two restraining tethers of different lengths. A structure shaped like the surface of the tibia is drawn with a central rectangular window. When the structure is placed over a rectangular peg the same width of the window, the structure can only translate anteriorly and posteriorly, and there is 1 DOF. When the structure is placed over a large circular peg, it has 2 DOF, A–P translation, and rotation about the peg. When the structure is placed over a small peg, there is A–P translation, medial–lateral translation, and rotation around the peg (3 DOF). The anterior translation of the structure is restrained by two tethers of different lengths. When there is only 1 DOF the structure can move only as far as the shorter tether will allow. When the structure has 2 DOF, the anterior translation increases; when there is 3 DOF, the structure can move forward until the two tethers are taut.

flexion and 11–13° of internal tibia rotation. The KT-1000 testing system was designed to minimally constrain knee motion while measuring A–P translation. Perhaps one of the reasons that Sherman (18) measured greater displacements with the KT-1000 than with the UCLA testing device is because the UCLA device provides greater limb constraint.

DISPLACEMENT FORCE

Magnitude

The soft tissue constraints of the knee lengthen when loaded. The greater the displacement force, the greater the displacement. Figure 23-3 illustrates factors to consider when calculating the displacing force. The ligaments are viscoelastic tissues; therefore the rate of load application will affect joint displacement. However, Markolf (14) and Edixhoven (8) have reported that the rate of load application in clinical testing did not affect the force–displacement curve. Edixhoven recommends that one testing cycle be performed to condition the joint prior to measuring displacement.

Direction

If the displacement load is directed so that in addition to imparting an anterior force, a joint distraction or compression force or a rotational movement is applied, the resulting anterior displacement will be affected. An internal rotation moment on the tibia will increase anterior joint displacement, whereas an external rotational moment will increase posterior joint displacement. A joint compression force will increase joint stiffness (9,13,18).

Point of Application

The anterior force applied to a proximal point on the leg results in a moment that rotates the leg about the foot and ankle. The rotational moment is dependent on the distance of the point of force application from the ankle. In Fig. 23-3 the rotational moment about the ankle is applied through a 31-cm moment arm. The closer the applied load is to the knee joint, the greater the moment and therefore the greater the anterior displacement.

MEASUREMENT SYSTEM

Measurement Location

A–P knee displacement has been evaluated by stabilizing the femur and measuring A–P displacement of the tibial tubercle (14,18) or by measuring the differential displacement between the patella and the tibial

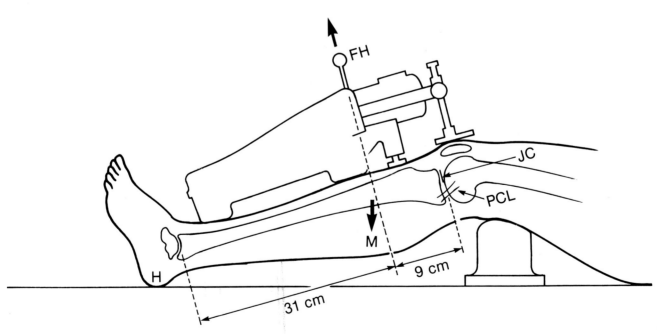

FIG. 23-3. The patient is supine. The testing instrument is mounted on the front of the leg. The mass of the leg and testing device (M) is supported by tension in the soft tissues, represented by the posterior cruciate ligament (PCL), compression force at the joint surface (JC), and compression at the heel (H). When an anterior force is applied through the force handle (FH), the weight of the leg and testing device is first lifted to unload the joint structures and then as further force is applied the anterior constraining soft tissues are placed under tension.

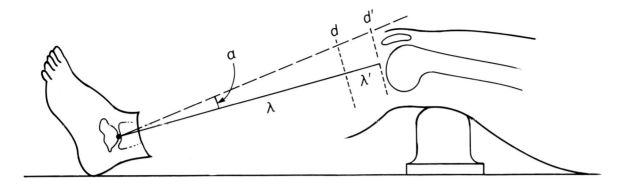

$$tangent\ a \cdot \lambda = d$$
$$tangent\ a\ (\lambda + \lambda') = d'$$

FIG. 23-4. An anterior force applied to the proximal tibia rotates the tibia about the ankle. The anterior tibial displacement is dependent on the change in flexion angle and on the distance from the ankle that the displacement is measured. The greater the distance, the greater the measured displacement.

tubercle (5,8,12,19). During a standard A–P displacement test, the patella and femur are maintained in a constant position and the foot rests on the examining table. When a displacement force is applied to the proximal segment of the leg, the leg rotates about the foot and ankle. The displacement measurement is dependent upon the distance at which the measurement is taken with respect to the ankle (Fig. 23-4). Most devices display the displacement at the tibial tubercle (4,8,14,18,19). The KT-1000 displays the displacement

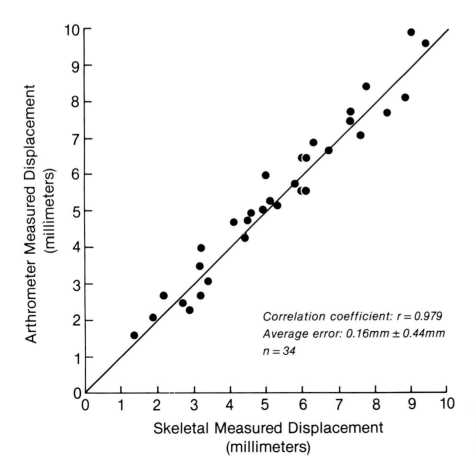

Correlation coefficient: $r = 0.979$
Average error: $0.16mm \pm 0.44mm$
$n = 34$

FIG. 23-5. Arthrometer measurement (KT-2000) versus skeletally mounted measurement system in two cadaver specimens.

occurring at the site of the arrow on the device that should be placed on the joint line. In a subject with a tibia 40 cm in length, the A–P displacement measured at the tibial tubercle (4,8,18,19) 5 cm distal to the joint line will be 15% less than the displacement measured at the joint line (KT-1000).

The precision of A–P displacement measurements are dependent on a standardized method of placing the measuring device on the leg and securely stabilizing the patella in the femoral trochlea as described in Chapter 24 (Fig. 24-2).

Soft Tissue Motion

A–P displacement measurement is performed by tracking the tibial tubercle motion in relation to the patella. There is a relatively thin layer of soft tissue between these structures and the skin. *In vitro* studies by Daniel (Fig. 23-5) (5) and Edixhoven (8) documented little discrepancy between displacements measured by skeletal pin motion (5) or radiographic techniques (8). In contrast, Shino (19) reported relatively large measurement errors secondary to soft tissue deformation. The measurement of varus–valgus and internal–external rotations with surface-placed testing devices pose a significantly greater potential error from soft tissue motion. The technique for dealing with the soft tissue deformation utilized by the Genucom system (2) is to measure the stiffness of the soft tissue sleeve of the thigh and then, with computer assistance, subtract the predicted soft tissue motion from the measured motion.

MUSCLE ACTIVITY

Muscle activity is probably the most significant variable in the measurement of motion limits (6,8,14,19). Activities in muscles crossing the joints not only increase the joint stiffness but also affect the joint resting position (6,8). Testing should be comfortable and conducive to muscle relaxation. The tester should continually monitor muscle tone and encourage patient relaxation.

ACKNOWLEDGMENTS

Support from the following sources is gratefully acknowledged: MEDmetric Corporation, San Diego, California 92121.

REFERENCES

1. Bargar WL, Moreland JR, Markolf KL, Shoemaker SC. The effect of tibia–foot rotatory position on the anterior drawer test. *Clin Orthop* 1983;173:200–203.
2. Baxter MP. Assessment of normal pediatric knee ligament laxity using the Genucom. *J Pediatr Orthop* 1988;8:546–550.
3. Butler DL, Noyes FR, Grood ES. Ligamentous restraints to anterior–posterior drawer in the human knee. A biomechanical study. *J Bone Joint Surg* 1980;62A:259–270.
4. Cannon D. Personal communication.
5. Daniel DM, Malcom LL, Losse G, Stone ML, Sachs R, Burks R. Instrumented measurement of anterior laxity of the knee. *J Bone Joint Surg* 1985;67A:720–726.
6. Daniel DM, Stone ML, Barnett P, Sachs R. Use of the quadriceps active test to diagnose posterior cruciate ligament disruption and measure posterior laxity of the knee. *J Bone Joint Surg* 1988;70A:386–391.
7. Daniel DM, Stone ML, Sachs R, Malcom L. Instrumented measurement of anterior knee laxity in patients with acute anterior cruciate ligament disruption. *Am J Sports Med* 1985;13:401–407.
8. Edixhoven P, Huiskes R, de Graaf R, van Rens TJ, Slooff TJ. Accuracy and reproducibility of instrumented knee-drawer tests. *J Orthop Res* 1987;5:378–387.
9. Hsieh HH, Walker PS. Stabilizing mechanisms of the loaded and unloaded knee joint. *J Bone Joint Surg* 1976;58A:87–93.
10. Jacobsen K. Stress radiographical measurement of the anteroposterior, medial and lateral stability of the knee joint. *Acta Orthop Scand* 1976;47:335–344.
11. Kennedy JC, Fowler PJ. Medial and anterior instability of the knee. An anatomical and clinical study using stress machines. *J Bone Joint Surg* 1971;53A:1257–1270.
12. Malcom LL, Daniel DM, Stone ML, Sachs R. The measurement of anterior knee laxity after ACL reconstructive surgery. *Clin Orthop* 1985;196:35–41.
13. Markolf KL, Bargar WL, Shoemaker SC, Amstutz HC. The role of joint load in knee stability. *J Bone Joint Surg* 1981;63A:570–585.
14. Markolf KL, Graff-Radford A, Amstutz HC. *In vivo* knee stability. A quantitative assessment using an instrumented clinical testing apparatus. *J Bone Joint Surg* 1978;60A:664–674.
15. Markolf KL, Kochan A, Amstutz HC. Measurement of knee stiffness and laxity in patients with documented absence of the anterior cruciate ligament. *J Bone Joint Surg* 1984;66A:242–252.
16. Nielsen S, Kromann-Andersen C, Rasmussen O, Andersen K. Instability of cadaver knees after transection of capsule and ligaments. *Acta Orthop Scand* 1984;55:30–34.
17. Noyes FR, Keller CS, Grood ES, Butler DL. Advances in the understanding of knee ligament injury, repair, and rehabilitation. *Med Sci Sports Exerc* 1984;16:427–443.
18. Sherman OH, Markolf KL, Ferkel RD. Measurements of anterior laxity in normal and anterior cruciate absent knees with two instrumented test devices. *Clin Orthop* 1987;215:156–161.
19. Shino K, Inoue M, Horibe S, Nakamura H, Ono K. Measurement of anterior instability of the knee. *J Bone Joint Surg* 1987;69B:608–613.
20. Sprague RB, Asprey GM. Photographic method for measuring knee stability: a preliminary report. *Phys Ther* 1965;45:1055–1058.
21. Sullivan D, Levy IM, Sheskier S, Torzilli PA, Warren RF. Medial restraints to anterior–posterior motion of the knee. *J Bone Joint Surg* 1984;66A:930–936.
22. Torzilli PA, Greenberg RL, Hood RW, Pavlov H, Insall JN. Measurement of anterior–posterior motion of the knee in injured patients using a biomechanical stress technique. *J Bone Joint Surg* 1984;66A:1438–1442.
23. Torzilli PA, Greenberg RL, Insall JN. An *in vivo* biomechanical evaluation of anterior–posterior motion of the knee. Roentgenographic measurement technique, stress machine and stable population. *J Bone Joint Surg* 1981;63A:960–968.

Knee Ligaments: Structure, Function, Injury, and Repair, edited by D. Daniel, et al.

CHAPTER 24

KT-1000 Anterior–Posterior Displacement Measurements

Dale M. Daniel and Mary Lou Stone

We have used the KT-1000 arthrometer in our clinic to measure anterior–posterior (A–P) displacement since 1982. Measurements are routinely performed on patients with acute injuries and chronic instabilities. Patients who have knee ligament surgery are measured (a) in the clinic at the time of their preoperative examination, (b) under anesthesia prior to surgery, and (c) under anesthesia after wound closure. Postoperative displacement measurements are performed at 6 weeks, 3 months, 6 months, and 1 and 2 years. We have used instrumented measurements to diagnose a cruciate ligament disruption, to document the amount of pathologic laxity, and to evaluate the success of cruciate ligament reconstruction surgery. Testing technique and testing results will be presented in this chapter.

TESTING TECHNIQUE

The arthrometer is placed on the anterior aspect of the leg and held with two circumferential Velcro straps (Fig. 24-1). There are two sensor pads: One is in contact with the patella, and the other is in contact with the tibial tubercle. These move freely in the A–P plane in relation to the arthrometer case. The instrument de-

tects the relative motion (in millimeters) between the two sensor pads; therefore, motion of the arthrometer case (as the calf compresses under the Velcro straps) does not affect the instrument output. Displacement loads are applied through a force-sensing handle that is located 10 cm distal to the joint line.

The precision of A–P displacement measurements are dependent on a standardized method of placing the measuring device on the leg and securely stabilizing the patella in the femoral trochlea. With adequate patellar stabilization, tibial tubercle motion relative to the patella accurately reflects the motion of the tibia relative to the femur. It is necessary to flex the knee 20–30° in order to engage the patella in the femoral trochlea. In patients with patella alta or lateral tracking patella, the knee may need to be flexed to 40°. The patella is stabilized in the femoral trochlea by direct pressure that should be oriented to seat the patella (Fig. 24-2). The patellar stabilization pressure must remain constant. Altering the patellar pressure may result in motion of the patellar sensor, especially in subjects with a joint effusion or patellar chondromalacia. The hand stabilizing the patella in the femoral trochlea should rest on the thigh and prevent the instrument from rotating during the test. To facilitate patellar stabilization, the femur should be positioned so the patella is facing up or in slight external rotation. If there is excessive rotation, the thigh should be supported with a thigh strap (Fig. 24-3). The foot support should be used not to internally rotate the leg but, simply, to support the feet.

  D. M. Daniel: Department of Orthopedic Surgery, University of California, San Diego, School of Medicine, La Jolla, California 92037; and Kaiser Permanente Medical Center, San Diego, California 92120.

  M. L. Stone: Department of Orthopedics, Kaiser Hospital of San Diego, San Diego, California 92120.

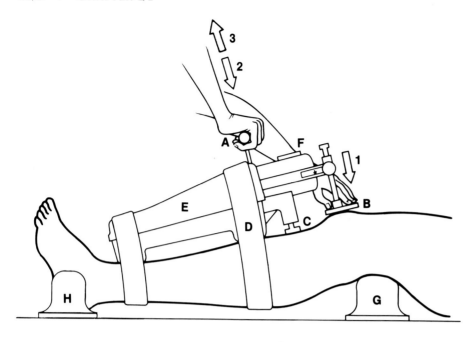

FIG. 24-1. KT-1000 arthrometer. (A) Force handle (posterior force [2] or anterior force [3] is applied). (B) Patellar sensor pad (a constant force [1] is applied to stabilize the patellar sensor pad). (C) Tibial sensor pad. (D) Velcro straps. (E) Arthrometer body. (F) Displacement dial. (G) Thigh support. (H) Foot support.

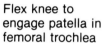

Flex knee to engage patella in femoral trochlea

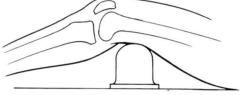

Support thigh to place patella facing up

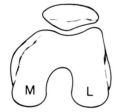

Apply pressure to stabilize patella

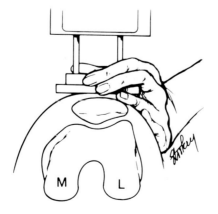

FIG. 24-2. The knee is supported in a flexed position to engage the patella in the femoral trochlea. In some patients the thigh support must be raised an additional 3–6 cm to provide sufficient knee flexion to engage the patella in the femoral trochlea. This may be done by placing a board under the thigh support. The thigh should be supported so that the patella is facing up. Occasionally a thigh strap is used to accomplish this task (Fig. 24-3). The examiner stabilizes the patellar sensor with manual pressure. The stabilizing hand should rest against the lateral thigh and should apply 2–5 lb of pressure on the patellar sensor pad. The hand position, patellar sensor position, and patellar sensor pressure must remain constant throughout the test. Varying the pressure on the patellar sensor pad and rotating the pad is a common cause of measurement error.

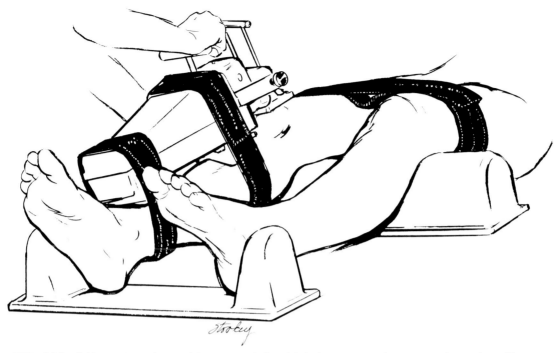

FIG. 24-3. A 7-cm strap is used to support the thigh from excessive external rotation. The optimum limb position places the patella facing upward or in slight external rotation as shown in this figure. The foot support should not be used to internally rotate the limb; it is simply to support the feet.

Posterior Cruciate Screen

Prior to performing 30° displacement measurements, the 90° active quadriceps test is performed to determine if there is posterior tibial subluxation. The examination is performed with the patient supine. The examiner sits lightly on the patient's foot to stabilize the limb, with the knee flexed 90° as when performing a 90° drawer test. The arthrometer is placed on the leg. With the hand stabilizing the arthrometer patellar sensor pad, the examiner also supports the patient's knee so that the patient may completely relax the leg musculature (Fig. 24-4A). When examining larger patients, we frequently have an assistant sit by the side of the table and support the limb (Fig. 24-4B). It is critical that the muscles crossing the knee are completely relaxed. The testing reference position is established: In this case, it is the resting position after a 20-lb posterior force is applied and then released. The patient then performs an isolated quadriceps contraction. We have found that the most helpful command to tell the patient is, "Gently try to slide your foot down the examining table." The examiner palpates the hamstring tendons to confirm that there is no hamstring contraction. The test is repeated until the patient performs an isolated quadriceps contraction without concomitant knee extension. The arthrometer documents the anterior or posterior tibial displacement. Anterior tibial motion

greater than 1 mm is abnormal and probably indicates a posterior cruciate ligament (PCL) injury. If the anterior tibial motion is greater than 1 mm, then the quadriceps neutral angle test should be performed. This is described later in this chapter. If there is no anterior tibial motion, the tibial position is normal and the examination should proceed to the 30° tests.

Passive 30° Tests

An anterior cruciate ligament (ACL) disruption is best revealed by testing the patient with the knee in slight flexion (16,19,24). To minimize measurement errors secondary to patellar motion, it is necessary to engage the patella in the femoral trochlea. This requires 20–40° of knee flexion (Fig. 24-2).

An 11-cm thigh support and a footrest are used to position both limbs in an equal position of flexion (30 ± 5°) and limb rotation (10–30° of external rotation). If insufficient flexion is obtained by the thigh support to stabilize the patella in the femoral trochlea, further knee flexion is obtained by placing a board under the thigh support. The lateral aspect of the foot rests against the foot support. If the limb lies in an externally rotated position with the patella facing laterally, the thigh should be internally rotated and supported with a restraining strap, to face the patella anteriorly (Fig.

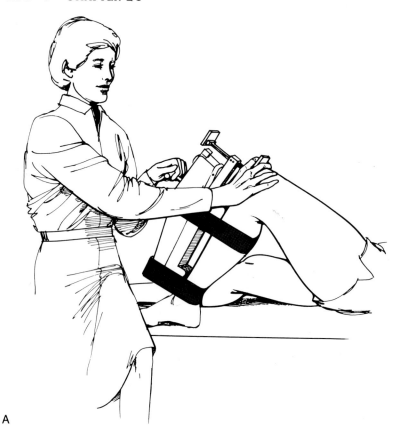

A

FIG. 24-4. Measurement of anterior and posterior displacement using a knee-ligament arthrometer and an 89-N displacing force. **A:** The examiner supports the subject's limb by sitting lightly on the foot and stabilizing the knee laterally.

24-3). Positioning the limb to place the patella anteriorly while the patella is engaged in the femoral trochlea optimizes stabilization of the patella in the femoral trochlea. The limb must not be held in an internally rotated position by the foot support because this places an internal rotation moment on the knee.

The patient should be comfortable and relaxed. Gentle manual A–P oscillation may assist in obtaining muscle relaxation (Fig. 24-5). The arthrometer is applied to the leg and oriented in a position so that pressure on the patellar sensor pad will stabilize the patella within the femoral trochlea (Fig. 24-2). This usually places the force handle parallel to the foot axis. Constant firm pressure is then applied to the patellar sensor pad and is maintained throughout the test. The patellar pad pressure must remain constant during the test because variation in the patellar pad pressure will alter the position of the patellar sensor pad secondary to soft tissue and cartilage compression and will result in spurious displacement measurements. A 20-lb A–P cycle is performed to condition the joint. The measurement reference position is then obtained by repeatedly applying and releasing a 20-lb posterior load until a reproducible unloaded knee position is obtained. The instrument dial is then set at 0. A 30-lb anterior force, followed by a 20-lb posterior force, is applied; then the displacements are read directly off the dial.

After each anterior load cycle is performed and a 20-lb posterior force is applied and released, the dial should return to 0 ± 0.5 mm to confirm that the instrument orientation on the leg has not been altered and that the quadriceps is relaxed. Confirmation of a stable reference position should be performed after the manual maximum test, the quadriceps active test, and those tests where the anterior load is applied through the force handle. The mean of three tests rounded to 0.5 mm is recorded as the measurement.

Five passive displacement measurements are recorded for each limb at 30°:

1. **20-lb (89-N) posterior displacement.** The posterior excursion from the measurement reference position with a 20-lb push.
2. **15-lb (67-N) anterior displacement.** The anterior excursion from the measurement reference position with a 15-lb pull.
3. **20-lb (89-N) anterior displacement.** The anterior excursion from the measurement reference position with a 20-lb pull.
4. **30-lb (134-N) anterior displacement.** The anterior excursion from the measurement reference position with a 30-lb pull.
5. **The manual maximum anterior displacement.** The anterior displacement with a high anterior force applied directly to the proximal calf just distal to

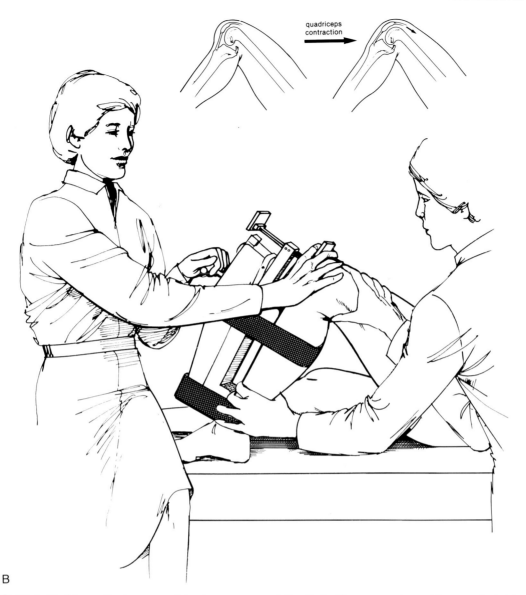

FIG. 24-4. B: Alternatively, an assistant may support the limb. The support must be comfortable to ensure complete relaxation. The quadriceps neutral angle in the normal knee is located and measured. Anterior and posterior displacement are measured at this angle using the displacing force. The injured knee is then supported at the angle that has been identified as the quadriceps neutral angle in the normal knee. A posterior displacing force is applied and released to establish a reproducible reference position. Anterior and posterior displacement from the reproducible reference position are measured using the displacement force. The quadriceps active test is used to measure posterior subluxation of the tibia at the reproducible reference position.

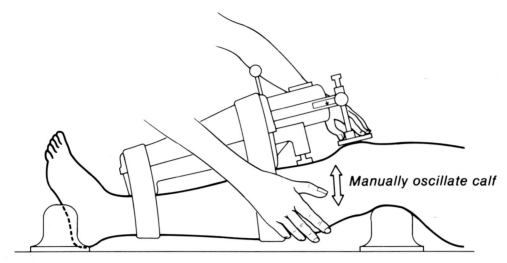

FIG. 24-5. Gentle manual oscillation of the leg may assist in obtaining muscle relaxation.

the knee joint line (Fig. 24-6). The manual maximum test produces greater displacement because of a higher applied load and a more proximally applied load (see section entitled "Displacement Force" in Chapter 23). In our clinic, manual loads applied are estimated to be 30–40 lb.

Anterior joint compliance may be measured by calculating the anterior displacement between any two load levels recorded in the same cycle (e.g., the displacement difference between the 15- and 20-lb anterior load as illustrated in Fig. 24-7).

When testing the anesthetized patient, additional care must be taken to adequately stabilize the patella in the femoral trochlea. The lower limbs usually lie in an externally rotated position in the anesthetized patient. A thigh strap is required to internally rotate the limbs and position the patella anteriorly (Fig. 24-3). In many patients the knee must be flexed 35–40° to stabilize the patella (17).

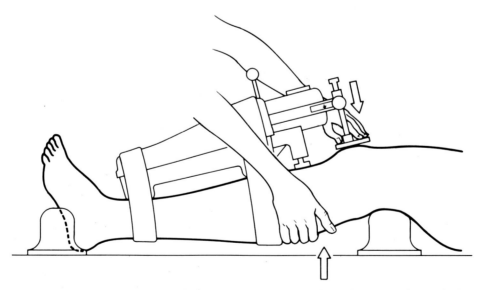

FIG. 24-6. The limbs are positioned with the support system, the arthrometer is applied, and the testing reference position is obtained in the standard way. While the patellar sensor pad is stabilized with one hand, the other hand applies a strong anterior displacement force directly to the proximal calf to produce the maximum anterior displacement. Care is taken that the knee is not extended. The tibial displacement is read off the dial.

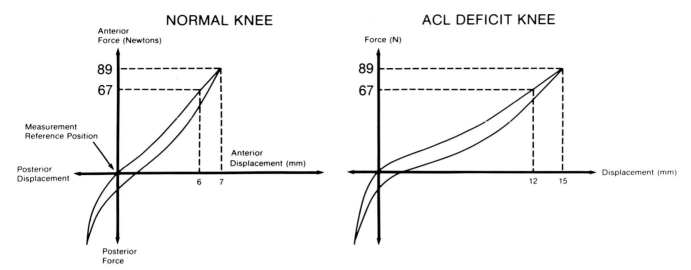

FIG. 24-7. Force–displacement curves for normal knees (**left**) and for ACL-deficit knees (**right**). The compliance index is obtained by measuring the displacement between the 67- and 89-N anterior-force levels. On this curve, the compliance index for the normal knee is 1 mm; for the knee with an ACL deficit, it is 3 mm.

Displacement measurements in normal subjects are presented in Fig. 24-8. There is a small side-to-side difference between a subject's two normal knees. Therefore, an evaluation should always include testing of both limbs so that side-to-side differences may be calculated. The figure also presents measurements on a group of patients with a chronic unilateral ACL disruption. The usual relationship between the various measurements is noted in Fig. 24-9.

It is important to establish the precision of a testing system prior to utilizing it in decision-making. The manufacturer recommends monthly monitoring of the KT-1000 instrument to confirm accuracy of the load-sensing handle and the displacement sensors. The important indicator of pathology is side-to-side difference. The same machine must be used on both sides to minimize the significance of small calibration errors in the machine itself. The crucial element in the testing process is to duplicate on the second knee the testing technique that was used on the first knee. Important points are:

1. muscle relaxation;
2. similar limb orientation;
3. similar arthrometer placement on the leg with respect to the instrument marker at the joint line, as well as similar instrument rotation with respect to the patella;
4. consistent patellar pad pressure technique and establishing the testing reference position;
5. establishing the testing reference position; and
6. similar speed of force application.

The two greatest sources of measurement error with the arthrometer are (i) lack of muscle relaxation and (ii) inability to stabilize the patellar sensor pad.

Anterior Testing Results

Normal Subjects

In the published report of A–P displacement testing with the KT-2000 (5), L. L. Malcolm measured (a) 338 normal subjects (150 females and 188 males) between the ages of 15 and 45 and (b) 87 patients with a unilateral ACL-disrupted knee. In the normal population there was no significant difference between age and sex groups as illustrated in Fig. 24-10. Testing results of normal subjects with the KT-1000 have been reported by Sherman (22), Daniel (7), and Bach (2). For all tests reported by these investigators, greater than 95% of normal subjects had a right–left difference of less than 3 mm. Six different examiners each examined 20 normal subjects between the ages of 15 and 45 (10 males and 10 females) to produce the values for 120 normal subjects tested with the KT-1000 reported by Daniel (Table 24-1, Fig. 24-11A and B) (7). One hundred sixteen of the 120 patients (97%) had a right–left (R–L) difference of less than 3 mm on all anterior displacement tests (20-lb, manual maximum, and quadriceps active).

To document the test/retest variation by a single skilled examiner, author MLS examined 10 normal subjects on five different days without reference to her

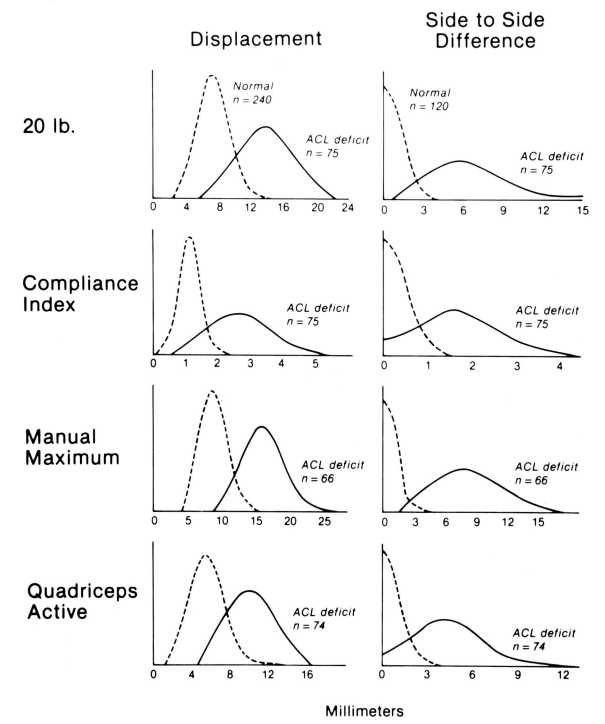

Displacement

Side to Side Difference

20 lb.

Normal
n = 240

ACL deficit
n = 75

0 4 8 12 16 20 24

Normal
n = 120

ACL deficit
n = 75

0 3 6 9 12 15

Compliance Index

ACL deficit
n = 75

0 1 2 3 4 5

ACL deficit
n = 75

0 1 2 3 4

Manual Maximum

ACL deficit
n = 66

0 5 10 15 20 25

ACL deficit
n = 66

0 3 6 9 12 15

Quadriceps Active

ACL deficit
n = 74

0 4 8 12 16

ACL deficit
n = 74

0 3 6 9 12

Millimeters

FIG. 24-8. Anterior displacement measurements for 120 normal subjects (240 knees) and for a group of patients with a chronic ACL disruption. Frequency distribution; 30° of knee flexion.

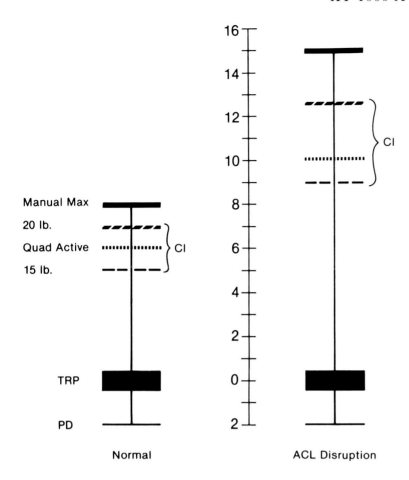

FIG. 24-9. The relationship between displacement measurements in a typical patient with a unilateral ACL disruption. CI, compliance index; 30° A–P displacement.

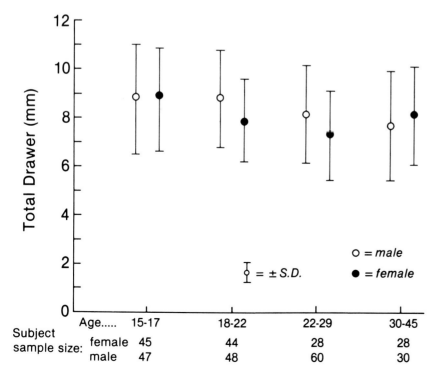

FIG. 24-10. Total A–P displacement with an 89-N (20-lb) displacement force, in the normal population. Measurements were obtained with the KT-2000. The device is similar to the KT-1000. The displacement is printed on an X–Y plotter as a load–displacement curve.

TABLE 24-1. *Normal A–P displacement measurements*

| Test | Range | | Mean | S.D.[a] | 95% Cutoff |
	Low	High			
Displacement (*n* = 240)					
20-lb posterior	1	6	2.8	0.9	4.5
20-lb anterior	3	14	7.2	2.0	10
20-lb A–P	5	18	10.0	2.4	12
Manual maximum anterior	4.5	15	8.6	2.1	12
Quadriceps active displacement	2	12.5	5.7	1.8	9
Right minus left (*n* = 120)					
20-lb posterior	0	2	0	0.7	1.0[b]
20-lb anterior	−0.2	−3.5	2	1.0	2.0[b]
20-lb A–P	−4	4	0.2	0.9	2.5[b]
Manual maximum anterior	−4	3	−0.3	1.1	2.0[b]
Quadriceps active displacement	−3	2	−0.4	1.0	2.0[b]

[a] S.D., standard deviation.
[b] Right–left difference.

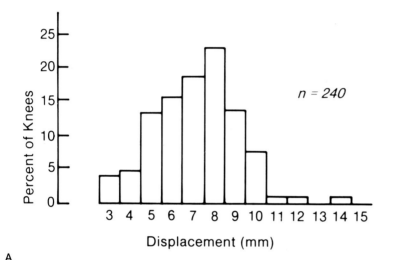

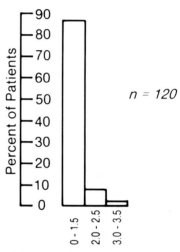

A

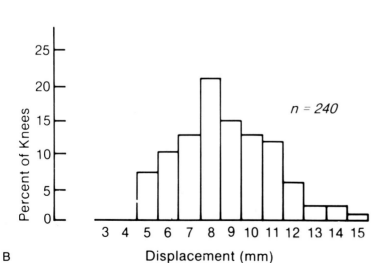

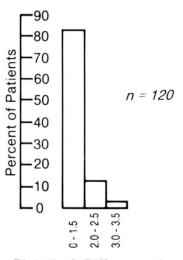

B

FIG. 24-11. Displacement measurements in normal subjects. Six examiners each examined different patients: 10 normal males and 10 normal females between the ages of 15 and 45. There were a total of 120 normal subjects. **A:** 30°/20-lb anterior displacement. **B:** 30°/manual maximum test.

previous examinations. The test/retest variations were seldom greater than 1 mm (Fig. 24-12A and B). MLS has tested patients with a unilateral ACL disruption at 6- to 12-month intervals for a period of 3 years. The first examination was performed within 2 weeks of injury. Table 24-2 presents the test/retest variation of the displacement in the normal knee between the patients first examination and last examination. The test/retest variation is less than 2.5 mm in 87% of patients with the 20-lb test and in 83% of subjects with the manual maximum test.

Authors DMD and MLS each independently examined a 34-player high-school football team (Table 24-3). MLS consistently recorded higher displacements than did DMD. All three examinations (20-lb anterior displacement, manual maximum anterior dis-

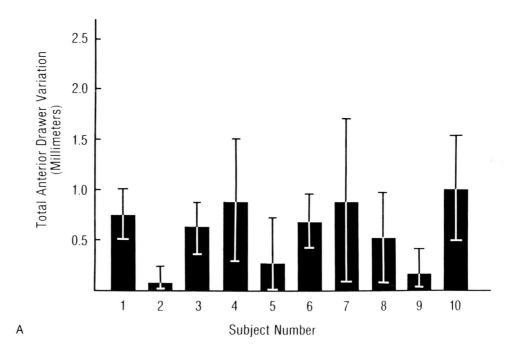

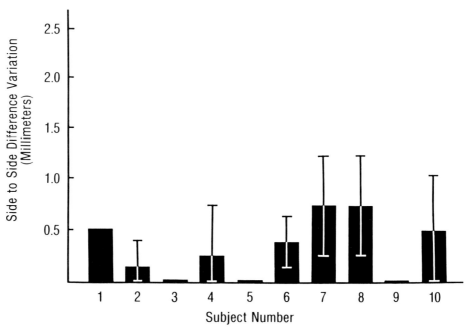

FIG. 24-12. A single examiner (MLS) tested 10 normal subjects once a day on five different days. **A:** The 30°/20-lb anterior displacement test/retest variation for each subject. **B:** The 30°/20-lb anterior displacement R–L difference test/retest variation for each subject.

TABLE 24-2. *Test/retest variation of the displacement in the normal knee in ACL-injured patients[a]*

Millimeters of difference	Percent of patients	
	20-lb test	Manual maximum test
≤1.0	60	59
≤2.0	87	83
≤3.0	97	94
≤4.0	100	100

[a] The test interval was 6–36 months; n = 134.

placement, quadriceps active test) were performed by both examiners on all patients. No subject had an R–L difference of greater than 2.5 mm in more than one examination by either examiner. MLS did record an R–L difference of greater than 2.5 mm

TABLE 24-3. *Evaluation of 34 high-school football players: Comparison of two examiners' displacement measurements[a]*

Test	Millimeters of displacement (mean ±S.D.)	
	Examiner MLS	Examiner DMD
Right 20-lb posterior	3.5 ± 1.0	3.6 ± 0.8
Right 20-lb anterior	8.1 ± 1.2	5.7 ± 1.4
Right manual maximum anterior	8.8 ± 1.4	6.9 ± 1.7
Right quadriceps active	6.1 ± 1.6	5.2 ± 1.4
Mean right minus left difference		
20-lb posterior	−0.4 ± 1.2	0.2 ± 0.7
20-lb anterior	−1.1 ± 1.6	−0.7 ± 0.7
Manual maximum anterior	−1.0 ± 1.2	−0.5 ± 1.0
Quadriceps active	−1.0 ± 1.2	−1.4 ± 1.0
Number of subjects with R–L difference >2.5 mm (no subject had R–L difference >3.5 mm)		
20-lb anterior	3	0
Manual maximum anterior	2	1
Quadriceps active	1	2
Right minus left difference between examiners		
20-lb anterior		0.9 ± 0.8
Manual maximum anterior		1.1 + 0.9
Quadriceps active		1.0 ± 0.6

[a] Measurements were obtained with the KT-1000. The knee flexion angle was 20–35°.

on six examinations, and DMD did so on three examinations.

Unilateral Chronic ACL Disruption

A number of authors have reported the results of instrumented testing of ACL-injured patients with commercially available devices. Some of the reports are presented in Table 24-4. Table 24-5 presents the results of two examiners (authors DMD and MLS) who independently tested patients with a unilateral ACL dis-

TABLE 24-4. *Unilateral chronic ACL disruption: injured minus normal (I − N) displacement difference[a]*

Clinic examination and author	n	Mean	Percent ≥3.0
20-lb test			
Anderson[b]	35	4.3	—
Bach	153	—	79
KSD[d]	177	5.2	85
Drez[e]	19	6.3	—
3M LAD[f]	297	6.1	89
Sherman (19)	19	5.1	95
Manual maximum test			
Bach	153	—	72
KSD	177	8.5	99
Drez	19	7.6	—
3M LAD	297	7.8	96
Quadriceps active test			
KSD	177	4.3	70
3M LAD	258	4.4	76
Examination under anesthesia prior to reconstruction			
20-lb Test			
KSD	223	5.6	87
3M LAD	297	6.9	96
Manual maximum test			
KSD	223	8.9	97
3M LAD	297	8.9	99
Examination under anesthesia after reconstruction			
20-lb (I − N) test			
KSD	223	−1.4	5

[a] The knee flexion angle was 20–35°.
[b] A. Anderson, *personal communication.*
[c] B. Bach, *personal communication.*
[d] KSD, Kaiser San Diego. Preoperative measurements of patients with a unilateral chronic ACL disruption.
[e] D. J. Drez, *personal communication.*
[f] Preoperative measurements of patients with a unilateral chronic ACL disruption scheduled for surgery in the multicenter 3M LAD study. Data were pooled from 10 centers and were provided by the 3M Company, St. Paul, Minnesota.

TABLE 24-5. Evaluation of 29 patients with a unilateral ACL injury: Comparison of two examiners' displacement measurements[a]

Test	Millimeters of anterior displacement (mean ± S.D.)	
	Examiner MLS	Examiner DMD
Normal 20-lb	6.9 ± 2.5	6.6 ± 2.1
Injured minus normal		
20-lb	4.2 ± 2.2	4.4 ± 2.5
Manual maximum	6.8 ± 3.5	6.7 ± 3.3
Quadriceps active	3.7 ± 2.2	3.9 ± 2.7
Subjects with R–L difference >2.5 mm		
20-lb	25 (86%)	22 (76%)
Manual maximum	29 (100%)	29 (100%)
Quadriceps active	21 (72%)	21 (72%)
Injured minus normal difference between examiners		
20-lb	1.2 ± 0.9	
Manual maximum	1.5 ± 1.7	
Quadriceps active	1.1 ± 1.1	

[a] The knee flexion angle was 20–35°.

ruption. Both examiners recorded an R–L difference of >2.5 mm on all patients by at least one examination. The recorded mean R–L displacement differences were similar. The same two examiners also examined independently 23 patients with a unilateral ACL disruption that had been reconstructed (Table 24-6). The mean R–L differences and number of patients with a R–L difference of greater than 2.5 mm for the two examiners were similar. We have routinely tested patients having ACL surgery in the clinic at the time of their preoperative evaluation (Fig. 24-14) and again under anesthesia prior to surgery. Data from our clinic, along with data from 10 centers participating in the ligament augmentation device (LAD) ACL reconstruction study, are presented in Table 24-4. At the con-

clusion of the surgical procedure, after wound closure, we repeated the displacement measurements (Table 24-4).

Unilateral Acute ACL Disruption

We routinely perform KT-1000 measurements in the clinic on patients with suspected ACL disruptions. To allow better stabilization of the patella, we aspirate the knee prior to testing if we estimate that the patient has an effusion of greater than 50 cc. Frequently, the examiner must spend a little time coaching the patient to relax and demonstrating that the examination is not going to be painful. Patients who have received an injury to the patella may not tolerate the pressure needed to stabilize the patellar sensor. The normal knee is tested prior to testing the injured knee. Data on 125 confirmed acute ACL disruptions are presented in Fig. 24-13A and B. In a report from The Hospital for Special Surgery, Bach (2) reported that the clinic measurements of 107 acute ACL disruptions revealed a side-to-side difference of 3 mm or greater in 69% of patients on the 20-lb test and in 87% of subjects on the manual maximum test. We recently added a 30-lb displacement test to our testing routine. This test reveals greater displacement than the 20-lb test but shows less displacement than the manual maximum test (Table 24-7). If the injured minus normal knee displacement difference on any of the four tests routinely performed (20-lb, 30-lb, manual maximum, and quadriceps active test) is 3 mm or greater, the likelihood of a cruciate ligament disruption is greater than 95%. Both an ACL-injured knee and a PCL-injured knee may result in an

TABLE 24-6. Evaluation of 23 ACL-reconstructed patients: Comparison of two examiners' displacement measurements[a]

Test	Millimeters of anterior displacement (mean ± S.D.)	
	Examiner MLS	Examiner DMD
20-lb		
Reconstructed knee	11.0 ± 2.5	8.7 ± 2.7
Contralateral knee	8.3 ± 1.9	6.3 ± 2.5
R–L difference	2.7 ± 1.8	2.4 ± 2.7
Number >2.5 mm	13 (56%)	10 (43%)
Manual maximum		
R–L difference	3.7 ± 2.1	3.2 ± 2.3
Number > 2.5 mm	15 (65%)	16 (70%)

[a] Measurements were obtained with the KT-1000. The knee flexion angle was 20–35°.

TABLE 24-7. Patients with an acute unilateral ACL disruption measured without anesthesia within 14 days of injury (n = 37)

	Mean	Cutoff	n	Percent
Normal				
20-lb	5.6	<11	37	100
30-lb	6.8	<12	37	100
Manual maximum	7.4	<13	36	100
Injured				
20-lb	7.9	<11	35	95
30-lb	10.9	<12	22	59
Manual maximum	13.6	<13	15	42
Injured minus normal				
20-lb	2.2	<3	19	51
30-lb	4.0	<3	7	19
Manual maximum	5.6	<3	1	3
Compliance index				
Injured minus normal				
15- to 20-lb	0.9	<1.5	19	51
15- to 30-lb	2.6	<1.5	8	22
20- to 30-lb	1.5	<1.5	15	37

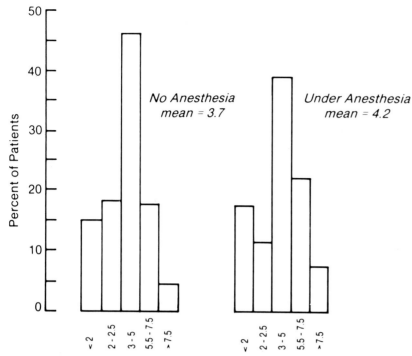

A   Right/Left Difference (mm)

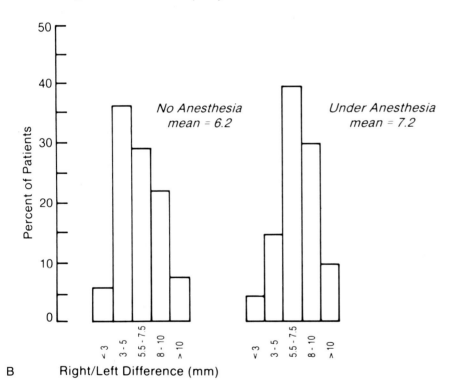

B   Right/Left Difference (mm)

FIG. 24-13. Examination of 125 patients with a unilateral acute ACL disruption confirmed at arthroscopy. **A:** 30°/20-lb displacement force. **B:** 30°/manual maximum displacement force.

Acute R-L difference (mm)
mean = 2.7mm

Follow up R-L difference (mm) mean = 3.4mm	< 2	2.0-2.5	3-5	5.5-7.5	> 7.5
< 2	26	5	2		
2.0-2.5	10	4	9		
3-5	6	10	33	9	
5.5-7.5	3	3	11	8	
> 7.5				2	2

Acute R-L difference (mm)
mean = 4.9mm

Follow up R-L difference (mm) mean = 5.0mm	< 3	3-5	5.5-7.5	8-10	> 10
< 3	29	5			
3-5	3	17	13	6	2
5.5-7.5	1	12	17	6	3
8-10	1	5	4	7	2
10	1	2	3	3	1

FIG. 24-14. One hundred forty-three patients with a unilateral acute knee injury. Measurements were made in the clinic within 14 days of injury. Follow-up measurements were made 6–60 months after injury (mean = 19 months). The R–L difference measured acutely is compared to the R–L difference measured at follow-up. **Top:** 20-lb test. **Bottom:** Manual maximum test.

increased anterior displacement measured from the supine 30° resting position (6). An ACL-injured knee will have an increased anterior compliance, and a PCL-injured knee will have an increased posterior compliance. The most diagnostic sign of a PCL disruption is demonstration of posterior sag in 90° of flexion and demonstration of an increased posterior displacement from the anatomic position at or near the quadriceps neutral angle. Figure 24-14 presents follow-up examinations on 143 patients with acute traumatic hemarthrosis. Not all of the patients had an ACL tear, and none have been reconstructed. Note that 85% (65/76) with an acute 20-lb R–L difference of 3 mm or greater acutely had a R–L difference of 3 mm or greater at follow-up. Ninety-five percent (103/108) on a manual maximum R–L difference of 3 mm or greater acutely had a follow-up R–L difference of 3 mm or greater. Foreman (9) reviewed 30 patients with arthroscopically confirmed partial ACL tears from our clinic. On acute examination, 14 patients had normal displacement measurements (the R–L difference on the 20-lb, manual maximum, and quadriceps active tests was less than 3 mm on all tests), and 16 had pathologic displacement measurements (on at least one test, the R–L difference was 3 mm or greater). Follow-up measurements 1 year after injury revealed that 13 of 14 patients with normal acute displacement measurements had normal measurements at follow-up, and all patients with pathologic measurements acutely had pathologic measurements at follow-up. The function in the patients with normal measurements was better than those with pathologic measurements (Chapter 27). In Fig. 24-15A and B, the displacement measurements in patients who are "coping" with an ACL disruption are compared to the displacement measurements in those who are not "coping." The 20-lb (89-N) load was selected as a standard test by Malcom and Daniel in 1980 (5) because it was a low load which, in cadaveric studies, consistently revealed an increase in anterior tibial displacement after the ACL was disrupted (Fig. 9-1). A low load was selected to make the examination easy to perform and to ensure comfort for the patient, as well as to minimize the risk of injury to repaired or reconstructed structures. However, a greater displacement force will reveal a greater level of pathology. Especially in the acutely injured patient with a large limb, greater than a 20-lb anterior displacement force is often needed to reveal pathology. At follow-up after knee ligament surgery, a low displacement force of 20 lb will not reveal the extent of pathologic motion that will be revealed by larger loads (Table 24-8).

Further testing has revealed to us that a 178-N (40-lb) anterior displacement force applied through the KT-1000 handle frequently lifts the foot off of the table, producing measurement error. A 134-N (30-lb) load, we have found, improves anterior displacement diagnostic accuracy and is well-tolerated by the testing system, tester, and patient. We continue to use the manual maximum test. Manual application of force to the proximal calf is more proximal than the force applied by pulling through the arthrometer handle. A more prox-

TABLE 24-8. *Patient with unilateral ACL reconstruction (n = 132)*[a]

	Mean	Percent less than
Displacement, reconstructed knee		
20-lb	9.0	<11 = 78%
30-lb	10.4	<12 = 66%
Manual maximum	12.2	<13 = 62%
Quadriceps active	8.4	<10 = 67%
Displacement, injured minus normal		<3 <5.5
20-lb	2.3	60% 92%
30-lb	2.6	52% 89%
Manual maximum	3.5	37% 80%
Quadriceps active	2.3	56% 87%

[a] Time since surgery = 1–3 years (mean 1.7 years).

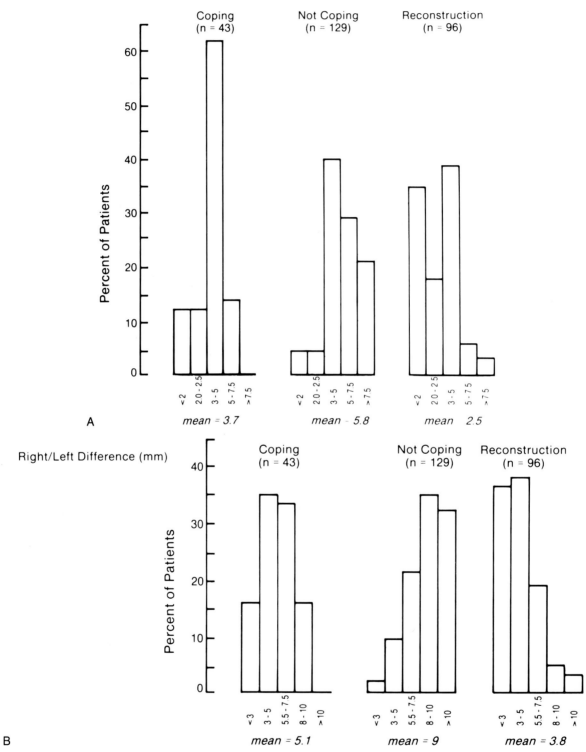

FIG. 24-15. Measurements in three populations with a chronic ACL disruption. **A:** 20-lb test. **B:** Manual maximum test. The "coping" patients are patients with a unilateral chronic ACL disruption who are participating in a running sport, having no or infrequent giving way episodes, and are not asking for an ACL reconstruction. The "not coping" patients have a chronic unilateral ACL disruption and are asking for a reconstruction. The "reconstruction" patients are 2 years post-ACL reconstruction. Note that most coping patients have a 20-lb R–L difference of 0–5 mm and a manual maximum R–L difference of 0–7.5 mm. In contrast, half of the "not coping" patients have a 20-lb R–L difference of greater than 5 mm, and the majority have a manual maximum R–L difference of greater than 7.5 mm. (Presented at the annual meeting of the AOSSM, Palm Desert, California, 1988 and at the AOA annual meeting, Hot Springs, Virginia, 1988.)

imally applied load provides a greater rotation moment and therefore a greater anterior displacement. The examiner applies the force until either the displacement stops, the knee begins to extend, or the patient begins to tighten the limb musculature. Performed by an experienced clinical examiner, the test produces the greatest anterior displacement of the standard arthrometer tests. However, the precise test load is not known, and there is greater risk of inadvertently applying axial rotation moments to the limb than when loads are applied through the force handle.

Quadriceps Active Tests

Orthopedic surgeons have routinely evaluated the integrity of knee ligaments by estimating or measuring the amount and direction of motion between the tibia and femur resulting from manually applied external forces such as drawer tests, varus and valgus stress tests, and pivot shift tests (12). These are *passive* tests, since the displacing force is applied by the examiner. Another method of assessing ligamentous and capsular integrity is to measure the change in joint position which results from active contraction of the patient's muscles. These are *active* tests, since the patient's muscle contraction provides the joint displacement force.

At full extension, as the patellar tendon (PT) runs from the tibial tubercle to the patella, it lies anterior to a reference line drawn perpendicular to the surface of the tibial plateau and passing through the tibial tubercle (4,11,12,15,18,20,23). As the knee flexes, the femur rolls posteriorly on the tibia, guided by the cruciate ligaments (10). The orientation of the PT changes continuously from anterior to posterior with respect to the reference line (Fig. 24-16) (14,20,21,23). Thus, the

resultant shear force produced by the pull of the PT on the tibial tubercle also changes from anterior to posterior with increasing flexion angle. The crossover from anterior to posterior shear occurs between 60° and 90° in the normal knee (3,4,20,21,23). The angle of flexion at which the crossover occurs in the normal knee is termed the "quadriceps neutral angle" and is defined as the angle of flexion at which the tibia does not shift anteriorly or posteriorly when the quadriceps is contracted in the normal knee. At this angle, the force in the PT is parallel to the reference line; therefore, no net shear occurs at the tibiofemoral interface.

At angles less than the quadriceps neutral angle, quadriceps contraction produces anterior movement of the tibia as a result of an anteriorly angled PT that may be constrained by the ACL. Similarly, at angles greater than the quadriceps neutral angle, quadriceps contraction produces backward motion of the tibia as a result of a posteriorly angled PT that may be constrained by the PCL (Fig. 24-17).

Anterior subluxation of the tibia with contraction of the quadriceps in the ACL-deficient knee can be documented with the 30° quadriceps active test. The limbs are supported with the thigh support and footrest as performed for the 30° passive tests. The testing reference position is established, and the instrument dial is set at 0. The patient is then asked to gently lift his or her heel off of the table. The anterior displacement as the heel leaves the table is recorded (Fig. 24-18). Thirty-degree quadriceps active data are presented in Fig. 24-8 and in Tables 24-1, 24-3, 24-4, 24-5, and 24-7.

A PCL rupture is diagnosed by using the quadriceps active test to demonstrate the posterior tibial subluxation. At 90° of flexion, the PT in the normal knee is oriented slightly posterior to the reference line, and

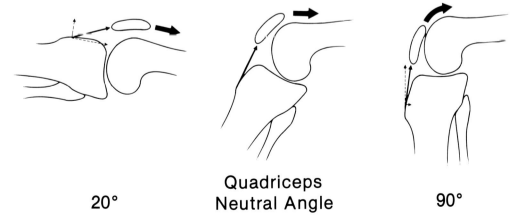

Quadriceps
20°　　　　**Neutral Angle**　　　　90°

FIG. 24-16. The PT force can be resolved into two components: (i) a normal component that is perpendicular to the tibial plateau and (ii) a shear component that is parallel to the tibial plateau. When the PT is anterior, the shear component tends to slide the tibia forward on the femur; when directed posteriorly, it tends to slide the tibia backwards on the femur.

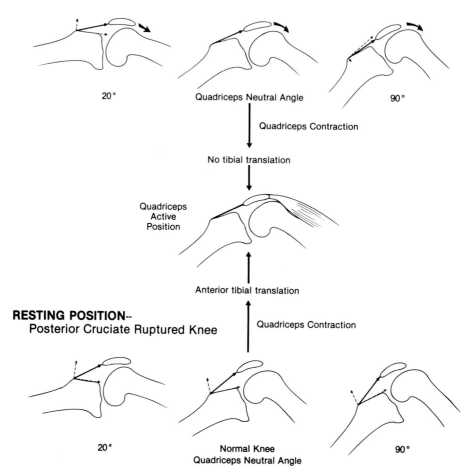

FIG. 24-17. At the quadriceps neutral angle, the quadriceps active position (tibial femoral position when the quadriceps is contracted) is independent of the cruciate ligaments.

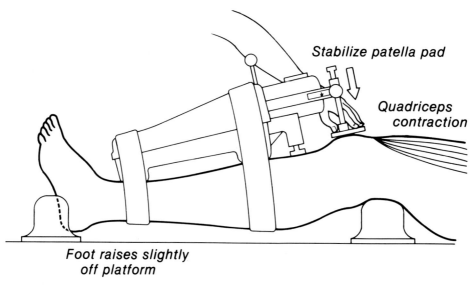

FIG. 24-18. The thigh is supported in about 30° of flexion. The patellar sensor pad is stabilized, and the testing reference position is established by pushing with a 20-lb load posteriorly and then releasing the force. The patient is then asked to "gently lift his or her heel off the table." The anterior displacement as the heel lifts off the table is recorded.

INJURED KNEE

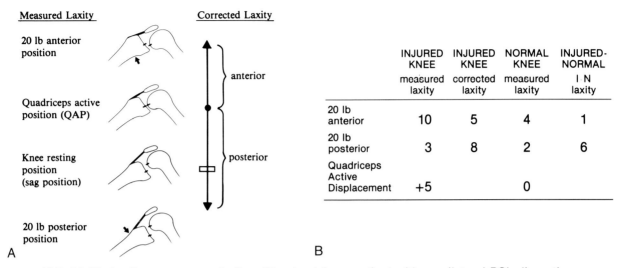

Measured Laxity

20 lb anterior position

Quadriceps active position (QAP)

Knee resting position (sag position)

20 lb posterior position

Corrected Laxity

anterior

posterior

A

B

	INJURED KNEE measured laxity	INJURED KNEE corrected laxity	NORMAL KNEE measured laxity	INJURED-NORMAL I N laxity
20 lb anterior	10	5	4	1
20 lb posterior	3	8	2	6
Quadriceps Active Displacement	+5		0	

FIG. 24-19. Laxity measurements (in millimeters) for a patient with a unilateral PCL disruption, measured at the quadriceps neutral angle. **A:** In the injured knee, the measured anterior tibial displacement is the distance from the resting position (*rectangle*) to the superior arrowhead (10 mm). The measured posterior displacement is from the resting position to the inferior arrowhead (3 mm). With contraction of the quadriceps, the tibia moves forward from the resting position to the quadriceps active position (*dark circle*). **B:** Determinations of the laxity are calculated from the quadriceps active position (corrected laxity).

	Passive Posterior Displacement	Testing Reference Position	Quadriceps Active Position	Passive Anterior Displacement
Normal				
Anterior Cruciate Disruption				
Posterior Cruciate Disruption				

FIG. 24-20. Measurements at the quadriceps neutral angle ($x = 70°$). Note that the quadriceps active test position (at the quadriceps neutral angle) is the only condition in which the joint is in the same position for all three states: the normal knee, the ACL-injured knee, and the PCL-injured knee.

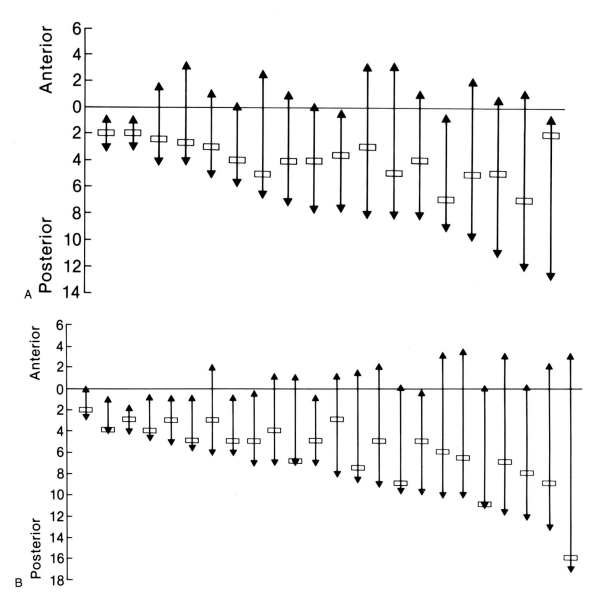

FIG. 24-21. R–L displacement difference for patients with a PCL disruption. **A:** Unilateral acute PCLs (*n* = 18). **B:** Unilateral chronic PCLs (*n* = 24). Each vertical line represents one patient. The zero mark is the knee neutral position (quadriceps active test position at the quadriceps neutral angle). The rectangle indicates the injured limb resting position, or posterior sag position. Note that in many of the patients there was only a small posterior displacement from the resting position.

contraction of the quadriceps results in no movement or a slight posterior shift. If the PCL is ruptured, the tibia "sags" into posterior subluxation and the PT is then directed anteriorly (Fig. 24-17). Contraction of the quadriceps in the PCL-deficient knee results in an average anterior shift of the tibia of 6 mm in the chronic PCL-injured knee and of 4.2 mm in the acute PCL-injured knee (6). The test is qualitative. No shift or a slight posterior shift of the tibia on contraction of the quadriceps indicates an intact PCL, whereas an anterior shift of the tibia from its "sagging"

position of posterior subluxation indicates a ruptured PCL.

The quadriceps active test is used to establish the quadriceps neutral position of the knee (the anatomic position) from which anterior and posterior tibial displacement can be observed or measured. This is determined by first locating and measuring the quadriceps neutral angle in the *normal* knee. To determine the quadriceps neutral angle, the patient is placed on the examining table in the supine position with the uninjured knee flexed to about 70°. To facilitate maximum patient muscle relaxation, the examiner supports the limb as shown in Fig. 24-4B. The quadriceps is actively contracted, and the tibial motion is observed. The angle of knee flexion is adjusted until there is no observable tibial shift. This is "the quadriceps neutral angle." The quadriceps neutral angle ranges from 60° to 90°, with a mean of 71° (6). Having determined the quadriceps neutral angle in the normal knee, the injured knee is then positioned at that angle.

Anterior and posterior passive tibial displacement are measured in the normal knee and contralateral injured knee at the normal knee quadriceps neutral angle. The quadriceps is contracted, and the amount of forward displacement of the tibia is determined. This distance is added to the measured posterior tibial displacement in the injured knee and subtracted from the measured anterior tibial displacement in the injured knee to reference the measurements to the quadriceps active position (Fig. 24-19). Figure 24-20 presents a normal, ACL-disrupted knee and a PCL-disrupted knee tested at the quadriceps neutral angle. The quadriceps active position is common in all three conditions.

The R–L displacement difference for patients with a PCL disruption is presented in Fig. 24-21A and B.

SUMMARY

KT-1000 measurements may be used to document the A–P knee motion and to diagnose cruciate ligament disruptions. The test begins with the assessment of posterior tibial sag at 90° of flexion, which indicates a PCL disruption. If the PCL is disrupted, measurements are then performed at the quadriceps neutral angle. If the PCL is intact, measurements are performed at 30° of flexion to evaluate the ACL. Measurements at 30° of flexion are performed under five loading conditions: 15 lb, 20 lb, 30 lb, manual maximum, and quadriceps contraction to lift the weight of the leg and testing device. In a unilaterally injured patient, a R–L difference of less than 3 mm is classified as *normal motion,* and a R–L difference on any test of 3 mm or greater is classified as *pathologic.* To obtain the greatest diagnostic accuracy as well as the greatest testing reproducibility, the patient must be relaxed, the instrument must be properly positioned, the patellar sensor must be stabilized against the patella, and the patella must be in the femoral trochlea. After each test, a posterior load is applied and then released, after which the knee should return to the zero resting position. It is recommended that physicians, nurses, therapists, and technicians who plan to do KT-1000 testing receive formal instruction in KT-1000 testing, and it is also suggested that they document their own test/retest reproducibility by testing a number of patients on different days.

ACKNOWLEDGMENTS

Support from the following sources is gratefully acknowledged: MEDmetric Corporation, San Diego, California 92121.

REFERENCES

1. Anderson A, personal communication.
2. Bach Bernard, personal communication.
3. Barnett P, Daniel D, Biden E, Stone ML, Lafferty C. Posterior cruciate ligament/quadriceps interaction. *Orthop Trans* 1984; 8:258.
4. Daniel DM, Lawler J, Malcom LL, Biden E, O'Connor JJ, Goodfellow JW. The quadriceps anterior cruciate interaction. *Orthop Trans* 1982;6:199–200.
5. Daniel DM, Malcom LL, Losse G, Stone ML, Sachs R, Burks R. Instrumented measurement of anterior laxity of the knee. *J Bone Joint Surg* 1985;67A:720–726.
6. Daniel DM, Stone ML, Barnett P, Sachs R. Use of the quadriceps active test to diagnose posterior cruciate ligament disruption and measure posterior laxity of the knee. *J Bone Joint Surg* 1988;70A:386–391.
7. Daniel DM, Stone ML, Sachs R, Malcom LL. Instrumented measurement of anterior knee laxity in patients with acute anterior cruciate ligament disruption. *Am J Sports Med* 1985; 13:401–407.
8. Drez DJ, personal communication.
9. Foreman K, Daniel DM, Stone ML. Determining the prognosis of partial tears of the ACL by anterior displacement measurements. Presented at the annual meeting of the AOSSM, Palm Desert, California, June 1988.
10. Goodfellow J, O'Connor J. The mechanics of the knee and prosthesis design. *J Bone Joint Surg* 1978;60B:358–369.
11. Grood ES, Suntay WJ, Noyes FR, Butler DL. Biomechanics of the knee-extension exercise. Effects of cutting the anterior cruciate ligament. *J Bone Joint Surg* 1984;66A:725–734.
12. Hennings CE, Lynch MA, Glick KR Jr. An *in vivo* strain gage study of elongation of the anterior cruciate ligament. *Am J Sports Med* 1985;13:22–26.
13. Hughston JC, Andrews JR, Cross MJ, Moschi A. Classification of knee ligament instabilities, Part I. The medial compartment and cruciate ligaments. *J Bone Joint Surg* 1976;58A:159–172.
14. Kapandji IA. *The Physiology of the joints: annotated diagrams of the mechanics of the human joints,* 2nd ed. (Honore LH, translator). London: E & S Livingstone, 1970–1974.
15. Lindahl O, Movin A. The mechanics of extension of the knee joint. *Acta Orthop Scand* 1967;38:226–234.
16. Markolf KL, Graff-Radford A, Amstutz HC. *In vivo* knee stability. A quantitative assessment using an instrumented clinical testing apparatus. *J Bone Joint Surg* 1978;60A:664–674.
17. Moore HA, Larson RL. Posterior cruciate ligament injuries. Results of early surgical repair. *Am J Sports Med* 1980;8:68–78.
18. Morrison JB. Bioengineering analysis of force actions transmitted by the knee joint. *Biomed Eng* 1968;3:164–170.
19. Nielsen S, Kromann-Andersen C, Rasmussen O, Andersen K. Instability of cadaver knees after transection of capsule and ligaments. *Acta Orthop Scand* 1984;55:30–34.
20. Nisell R. Mechanics of the knee. A study of joint and muscle load with clinical applications. *Acta Orthop Scand* [*Suppl*] 1985;216:1–42.
21. O'Connor JJ, Goodfellow JW, Young SK, Biden E, Daniel DM. Mechanical interactions between the muscles and the cruciate ligaments in the knee. *Trans Orthop Res Soc* 1985;9:271.
22. Sherman OH, Markolf KL, Ferkel RD. Measurements of anterior laxity in normal and anterior cruciate absent knees with two instrumented test devices. *Clin Orthop* 1987;215:156–161.
23. Smidt GL. Biomechanical analysis of knee flexion and extension. *J Biomech* 1973;6:79–92.
24. Sullivan D, Levy IM, Sheskier S, Torzilli PA, Warren RF. Medical restrains to anterior–posterior motion of the knee. *J Bone Joint Surg* 1984;66A:930–936.

CHAPTER 25

Stressradiography

Measurements of Knee Motion Limits

Hans-Ulrich Stäubli

The limits of knee motion *in vivo* have been evaluated by (a) the physical examination, (b) clinical knee testing devices using external transducers (2,4) (Chapters 23 and 24), (c) stressradiography with bony landmarks and reference lines, and (d) multiplanar roentgenstereophotogrammetry with tantalum markers, bony landmarks, and reference lines (3,5,8,13,20,21). In Europe, stressradiography has been used widely to document knee instability in the sagittal and frontal planes (1,6,7,10–12,16,17). Parallel to the development of stressradiography, Selvik (13) developed a method to study the kinematics of the skeletal system.

Lateral stressradiography with the knee tested at 90 degrees of flexion was reported by Kennedy and Fowler (9), Jacobsen (7), and Torzilli et al (18) to evaluate anterior-posterior (A-P) motion of the knee. Stäubli and colleagues (15,16) reported stressradiography with the knee in extension to measure the A-P motion limits. Varus and valgus stressradiographs to document collateral ligament injuries, as well as joint space narrowing, have been advocated by Kennedy and Fowler (9), Jacobsen (6,7), and Tria et al (19).

This chapter will describe the stressradiographic techniques for measuring valgus and varus and A-P motion near extension. One of the values of stressradiography is that it provides a method to document medial and lateral compartment displacements. The results of stressradiography studies will be presented and the clinical applications will be discussed.

STRESSRADIOGRAPHIC TECHNIQUE

Varus and valgus stress tests with the knee in extension may be performed manually or with a Telos unit (Fa. Telos, Medizinisch-Technische Geräte GmbH, D-6103 Griesheim, Federal Republic of Germany) as shown in Fig. 25-1. Another type of stress device is shown in Fig. 3-5. Coupled motions occur during varus and valgus stress testing. A valgus moment results in lateral compression, medial distraction, lateral translation, and axial rotation (Fig. 25-2A). A varus stress test results in medial compression, lateral distraction, medial translation, and axial rotation (Fig. 25–2B). Although there may be some errors in measurement accuracy as a result of these induced coupled motions, stressradiography in the frontal plane can document varus and valgus joint space openings at the tension site and compartmental cartilage width at the compression site of the knee joint. Acute and chronic knee joint changes after ligamentous, meniscal, and cartilaginous injuries may be documented (Fig. 25-3).

Posterior and anterior stressradiographic techniques with the knee near extension are shown in Figs. 25-4 and 25-5, and the measurement technique is described in Figs. 25-6 and 25-7.

H-U Stäubli: Chefarzt Orthopädie und Traumatologie, Tiefenau-spital der Stadt und der Region Bern; CH-3004 Bern, Switzerland.

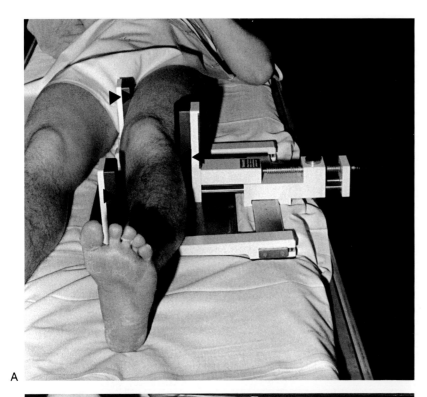

FIG. 25-1. A: Valgus stress test applied with Telos unit. An 89-N force is applied just above the joint line on the lateral femoral condyle.

A

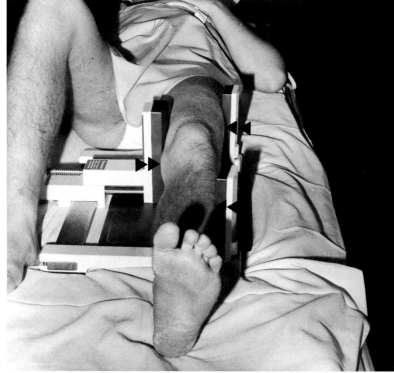

B

FIG. 25-1. B: Varus stress test with force applied just above the joint on the medial femoral condyle.

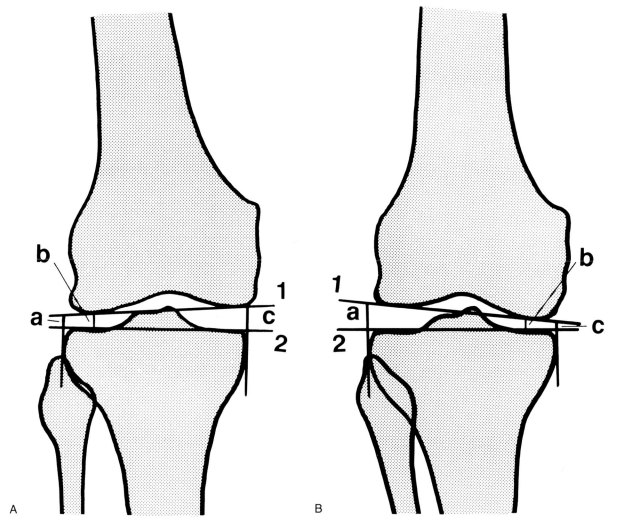

FIG. 25-2. Diagram of right knee, frontal plane. One line is drawn tangent to the femoral condyles, and a second line is drawn tangent to the tibial condyles. Two perpendicular lines are drawn tangent to the lateral and medial aspects of the tibial plateau. **A:** The medial joint space opening on the valgus stress test is defined as "c" minus "a". Line "b" indicates joint space width of the lateral compartment under compression. **B:** The lateral joint space opening on the varus stress test is defined as "a" minus "c". Line "b" indicates joint width of the medial compartment under compression.

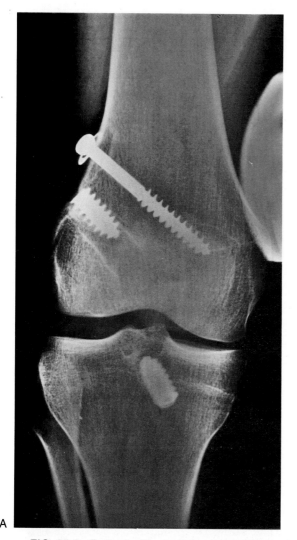
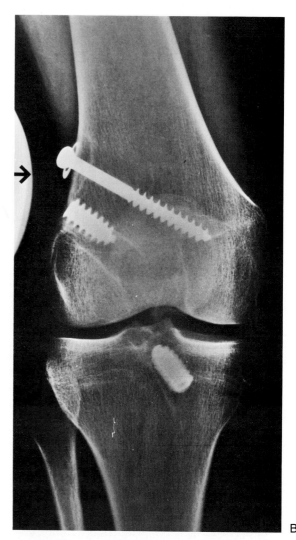

A   B

FIG. 25-3. Patient with medial compartment pain 1 year after patellar tendon ACL reconstruction. Varus **(A)** and valgus **(B)** stressradiographs with Telos unit, knee in 0 degrees flexion. Note pressure pad position (arrows). A 178-N *posterior* force is applied anteriorly to the distal thigh. The varus stressradiography reveals narrowing of the medial compartmental joint space **(A)**.

FIG. 25-5. Anterior stressradiograph. A support measuring 7.5 cm in diameter is positioned under the mid-tibia. A roentgen cassette is placed vertically adjacent to the medial side of the knee at a film focus distance of 120 cm. The foot is stabilized against the test platform. A 178-N force is applied *posteriorly* to the distal thigh. After the limb is loaded for 5 seconds, the lateral stressradiogram is obtained.

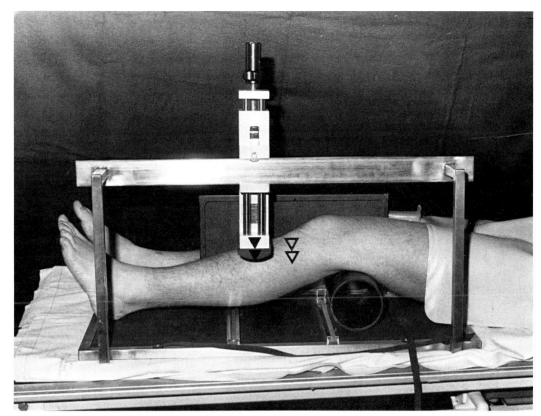

FIG. 25-4. Posterior stressradiograph. A thigh support measuring 11.5 cm in diameter is placed under the posterior aspect of the distal femur 10 cm proximal to the joint line. This places the knee near extension. The roentgen cassette (20 × 40 cm) is placed vertically adjacent to the medial side of the knee at a film focus distance of 120 cm. The joint is loaded with the Telos unit with a 178-N posteriorly directed force. After 5 seconds of posterior loading, the lateral radiograph is obtained with the stressradiographic tube oriented 6–8 degrees craniolaterally to caudomedially. The central ray is directed over the superimposed posterior contours of the femoral condyles. While learning the technique, fluoroscopy can be used to orient the condyles in respect to the central ray.

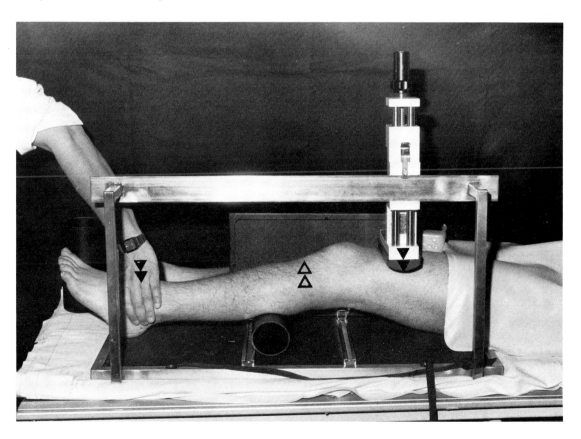

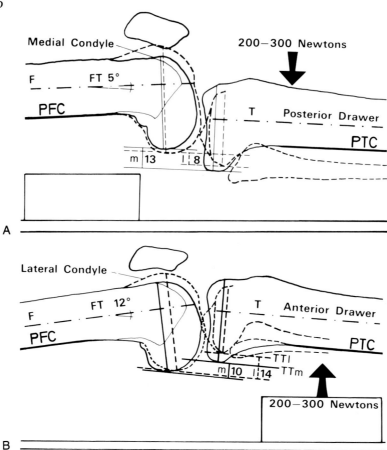

FIG. 25-6. Measurement technique to determine anterior-posterior compartmental displacements on posterior **(A)** and anterior **(B)** diagrams of stressradiographs. The posterior cortex of the midshaft of the tibia (PTC) is the reference line. Parallel to this reference line, tangent lines are constructed to the most posterior aspect of the medial and lateral femoral condyles and to the most posterior aspect of the medial and lateral tibial plateaus. When the tangent lines of both the medial and lateral compartments coincide, the knee joint is in neutral anatomical compartmental alignment as far as translation and rotation are concerned. F, femur; T, tibia; FT, femorotibial flexion angle; FTl, posterior tangent to lateral femoral condyle; FTm, posterior tangent to medial femoral condyle; TTl, tibial tangent to lateral plateau; TTm, tibial tangent to medial plateau; m, medial compartmental displacement (in millimeters); l, lateral compartmental displacement (in millimeters); PTC, posterior tibial cortex (i.e. reference measurement line); PFC, posterior femoral cortex. **A:** Diagram of posterior stressradiograph. Posterior displacement (PD) of medial compartment is +13 mm; PD of lateral compartment is +8 mm; central tibial displacement is 10.5 mm (medial plus lateral, divided by two). **B:** Diagram of anterior stressradiograph. Anterior displacement (AD) of medial compartment is +10 mm; AD of lateral compartment is +14 mm; central tibial displacement is 12 mm (medial plus lateral, divided by two).

CLINICAL APPLICATION OF STRESSRADIOGRAPHY

Diagnosis of a Collateral Ligament Injury

Varus and valgus stressradiography may be used to demonstrate a collateral ligament disruption. The primary restraints to medial and lateral joint line opening are the medial collateral ligament (MCL) and lateral collateral ligament (LCL), respectively (Chapter 9). Secondary restraints are the cruciate ligaments. Tria

et al (19) performed stressradiography on 32 patients with a Grade III MCL disruption and on 38 patients with a combined MCL-ACL disruption. They reported that the medial joint space opening on valgus stress testing was greater in patients with a combined MCL and anterior cruciate ligament (ACL) disruption than in those with only an MCL disruption. Stressradiography discriminates between (a) angular deformity resulting from joint space narrowing and (b) angular deformity resulting from ligament elongation (Fig. 25-3). This information is useful in planning limb alignment and ligament reconstructive procedures.

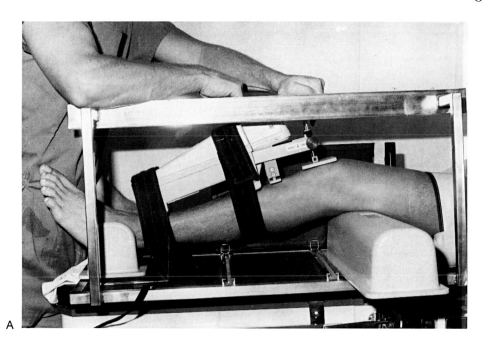

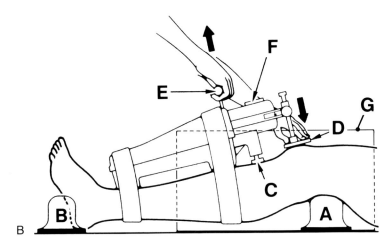

FIG. 25-7. Lateral stressradiograms were obtained with the knee in the resting position and while applying a 20-lb (89-N) anterior displacement force with the handle of the KT-1000. **A:** The patellar pad was stabilized with the examiner's hand on the top of the patellar sensor mechanism to minimize radiation exposure. **B:** Diagram of the KT-1000. Instructions for use of the KT-1000 recommend that the examiner place his hand on the patellar sensor pad for optimum stabilization. A = thigh support; B = foot support; C = tibial tuberosity sensor; D = patellar sensor; E = KT-1000 Arthrometer handle; F = dial.

Evaluation of the ACL-Injured Knee

Anterior displacement of the tibia in relation to the femur is evaluated by the clinician to diagnose an ACL disruption. The clinician may use instrumented testing during the evaluation process such as the KT-1000 that measures displacement of a patellar sensor relative to the displacement of a tibial tubercle sensor. The patellar sensor is stabilized against the femoral trochlea. The relative motion between the two sensors is a measure of patellotibial A-P displacement. By stressradiography, the displacement of the tibia relative to the femur under load is measured.

Using the two techniques, Staübli and Jakob (14) evaluated the results in a test series. They measured anterior knee displacement during manually applied stress with the KT-1000 and simultaneously documented the displacement of the tibia in relation to the femur (unstressed and stressed) with lateral stressra-diographs. The study group consisted of 16 patients each with a documented unilateral chronic ACL-injured knee. There were nine women and seven men, with an age range of 16–53 years (mean 28.4 ± 10 years). Patients were measured under peridural anesthesia. The testing technique is illustrated in Fig. 25-7. Measurements were obtained on both knees, flexed to 20 degrees, with an applied anterior force of 89 N. The lateral stressradiographs allowed measurement of compartmental displacements. The sum of the compartmental displacements is divided by two to obtain the anterior tibial displacement (Fig. 25-8).

Mean KT-1000 displacement measurements and stressradiographic measurements are presented graphically in Fig. 25-9 for 16 ACL-deficient knees and 16 ACL-intact knees. The difference between the KT-1000 measurements and the KT-1000/stressradiographic measurements is presented in Fig. 25-10. Both methods revealed a significant increase (p < 0.01)

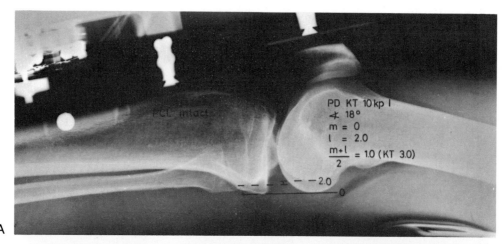

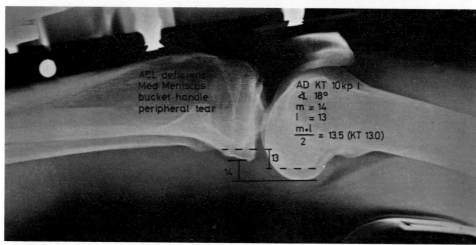

FIG. 25-8. Lateral stressradiographs. **A:** Stressradiographic view obtained during posterior drawer (89-N force) measurements. **B:** Stressradiographic view of anterior displacement of tibia in relation to femur when an 89-N anterior displacement force was applied through the KT-1000 force handle. Technique for measuring the anterior-posterior compartmental displacement is described in the legend of Fig. 25-6.

in anterior displacement in the ACL-deficient knee. The scattergrams representing paired values of simultaneous KT-1000 measurements and stressradiographic displacements showed slight correlation in ACL-deficient knees (Fig. 25-11A) but no correlation in ACL-intact knees (Fig. 25-11B).

Evaluation of the PCL-Injured Knee

Posterior tibial subluxation tests and posterior tibial position on stressradiography help to differentiate posterior cruciate ligament (PCL) injuries from ACL injuries. To determine the diagnostic value of clinical tests designed to measure posterior tibial subluxation in patients with acute PCL injuries, we studied 20 patients with PCL disruption (15). All patients had intact ACLs. After evaluating the uninvolved knee, the gravity test near extension and active reduction of posterior

tibial subluxation were performed without anesthesia. Under peridural anesthesia the following tests were performed: posterior tibial subluxation, reduction of posterior tibial subluxation, external rotational recurvatum, and reverse pivot shift. All 20 knees revealed a positive gravity sign, 18 had positive active reduction, and all patients had posterior subluxation under anesthesia. Posterior stressradiographs showed mean central posterior tibial displacement of 10.4 mm in the PCL-deficient group compared to 3.7 mm in the PCL-intact group.

Compartmental Displacement Measurements

Motion of the femur in the soft tissue sleeve of the thigh musculature makes it difficult to measure compartmental motion manually or with noninvasive instruments. Stressradiography provides an opportunity

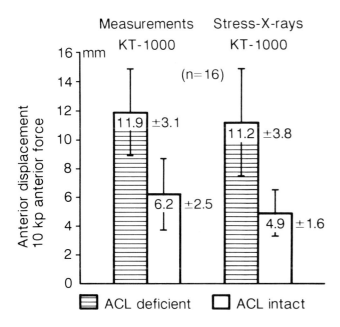

FIG. 25-9. Simultaneous KT-1000 and stressradiographic measurements of 16 ACL-deficient knees. Graph shows displacement measurements (mean +/− standard deviation) of the patients' ACL-intact and displacement of the ACL-deficient (involved) knees (14). Reproduced by permission, American Journal of Sports Medicine.

to measure compartmental motion limits. The displacement in both compartments, the medial tibial plateau relative to the medial femoral condyle and the lateral tibial plateau relative to the lateral femoral condyle, can be measured from the stressradiograph (Fig. 25-8).

A coupled anterior translation and internal rotation is recorded if the anterior displacement of the lateral tibial plateau is greater than the anterior displacement of the medial tibial plateau (Fig. 25-6B). A coupled anterior translation/external rotation is recorded if the anterior displacement of the medial tibial plateau is greater than the anterior displacement of the lateral tibial plateau (Fig. 25-8B). A coupled posterior translation/external rotation is recorded if the posterior displacement of the lateral tibial plateau is greater than the posterior displacement of the medial tibial plateau. A coupled posterior translation/internal rotation is recorded if the posterior displacement of the medial tibial plateau is greater than the posterior displacement of the lateral tibial plateau (Fig. 25-6A). Stressradiographic measurements of 85 ACL-incompetent knees and 53 ACL-competent knees are presented in Fig. 25-12.

Stressradiographic measurements of compartmental displacement in 24 PCL-disrupted knees revealed a medial compartment posterior displacement of 10.7 ± 2.4 mm and a lateral compartment posterior displacement of 10.0 ± 3.9 mm. In 114 PCL-intact knees the mean medial tibial plateau posterior displacement was

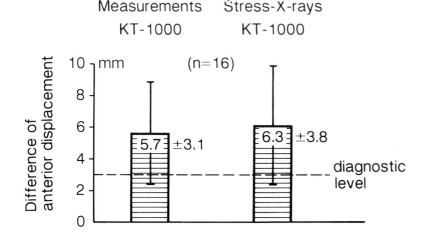

FIG. 25-10. The differences in the measurements of simultaneous KT-1000 and stressradiographic procedures are presented graphically (14). Reproduced by permission, American Journal of Sports Medicine.

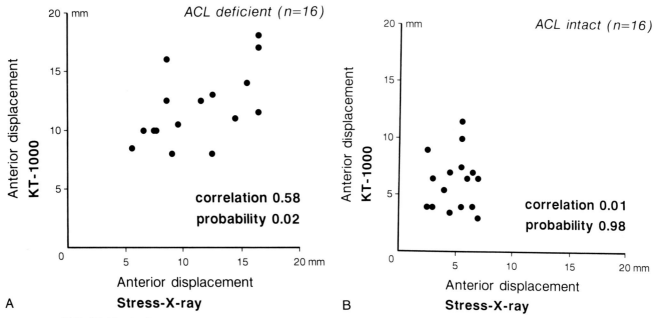

FIG. 25-11. A: Scattergram of results from simultaneous measurements (stressradiographic and KT-1000) of 16 unilateral ACL-disrupted knees (14). **B:** Scattergram of results from simultaneous measurements (stressradiographic and KT-1000) of 16 uninjured knees (14). Reproduced by permission, American Journal of Sports Medicine.

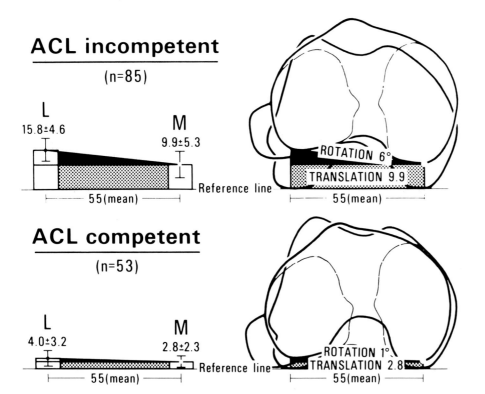

FIG. 25-12. Graphic representation of the mean compartmental displacement on anterior stress-radiograph of 85 ACL-incompetent knees and 53 ligament-intact (competent) knees. Measurements (in millimeters) of the coupled anterior translation/rotation are shown.

4.0 ± 3.0 mm and the lateral tibial plateau posterior displacement was 3.3 ± 2.6 mm (15).

SUMMARY

Stressradiography is an adjunct to the clinical examination and instrumented evaluation of knee motion. On stressradiographs the examiner can (a) Measure the A-P displacement limits and the medial and lateral joint space openings, including the relative position between the two compartments, (b) Define the anterior and posterior motion segments in relation to the neutral anatomical alignment in the sagittal plane, (c) Diagnose knee ligament injuries, and (d) Document knee subluxations in acute and chronic cruciate ligament-deficient knees.

ACKNOWLEDGMENT

Chr. Langenegger (AUM) of the University of Bern prepared the graphic illustrations.

REFERENCES

1. Böhler J. Röntgenologische Darstellung von Kreuzbandverletzungen. *Chirurg* 1944;16:136–138.
2. Daniel DM, Stone ML, Sachs R, Malcom LL. Instrumented measurement of anterior knee laxity in patients with acute anterior cruciate ligament disruption. *Am J Sports Med* 1985; 13:401–407.
3. Edixhoven Ph, Huiskes R, de Graaf R, van Rens ThJG, Slooff TJ. Accuracy and reproducibility of instrumented knee-drawer tests. *J Orthop Res* 1987;5:378–387.
4. Forster IW, Warren-Smith CD, Tew M. Is the KT1000 knee ligament arthrometer reliable? *J Bone Joint Surg [Br]* 1989; 71B:843–847.
5. Huiskes R, van Dijk R, de Lange A, Woltring HJ, van Rens ThJG. Kinematics of the human knee joint. In: Berne N, Engin AE, Correla da Silva KM, eds. *Biomechanics of normal and pathological human articulating joints.* NATO ASI Series, Series E: 93. Dordrecht: Martinus Nijhoff, 1985:165–187.
6. Jacobsen K. Stress radiographical measurement of anteroposterior, medial and lateral stability of the knee joint. *Acta Orthop Scand* 1976;47:335–344.
7. Jacobsen K. Gonylaxometry. Stress radiographic measurement of passive stability in the knee joints of normal subjects and patients with ligament injuries. Accuracy and range of application. *Acta Orthop Scand* 1981;52(Suppl 194):1–263.
8. Kärrholm JK, Selvik G, Elmqvist L-G, Hansson LI, Jonsson H. Three-dimensional instability of the anterior cruciate deficient knee. *J Bone Joint Surg [Br]* 1988; 70B:777–783.
9. Kennedy JC, Fowler PJ. Medial and anterior instability of the knee. An anatomical and clinical study using stress machines. *J Bone Joint Surg* 1971;53A:1257–1260.
10. Lenggenhager K. Über Genese, Symptomatolgie und Therapie des Schubladensymptoms des Kniegelenkes. *Zentbl Chir* 1940;67:1810–1825.
11. Levén H. Determination of sagittal instability of the knee joint. *Acta Radiolog [Diagn]* 1977;18:689–697.
12. Nyga W. Röntgenologische Darstellung von Kreuzbandverletzungen des Kniegelenkes. *Z Orthop* 1970;107:340–344.
13. Selvik GA. Roentgenstereophotogrammetric method for the study of the kinematics of the skeletal system. Dissertation, University of Lund, 1974.
14. Stäubli HU, Jakob RP. Anterior knee motion in chronic anterior cruciate ligament deficient knees. Arthrometry and stressradiography. A prospective comparison. *Am J Sports Med* 1990 in press.
15. Stäubli HU, Jakob RP. Posterior instability of the knee near extension. A clinical and stressradiographic analysis of acute injuries of the posterior cruciate ligament. *J Bone Joint Surg [Br]* 1990;72B:225–230.
16. Stäubli HU, Noesberger B, Jakob RP. The drawer sign of the knee in extension. A prospective study. Transactions of the 29th Annual Meeting of the International Society of the Knee. Orthopaedic Transactions. *J Bone Joint Surg [Am]* 1983:585.
17. Stedtfeld H-W, Strobel M. Ein Neues Haltegerät für die Anfertigung gehaltener Röntgenaufnahmen des Kniegelenkes. [A new device for stress-X-rays of the knee joint.] *Unfallheilkunde [Traumatology]* 1983;86:230–235.
18. Torzilli PA, Greenberg RL, Insall JN. An in vivo biomechanical evaluation of anterior-posterior motion of the knee. Roentgenographic measurement technique, stress machine, and stable population. *J Bone Joint Surg* 1981;63A:960–968.
19. Tria AJ, McBride M, Zawaksky JP. Medial injuries. A new roentgenographic index. Scientific Exhibit, AAOS Annual Meeting, 1985.
20. van Dijk R. The Behaviour of the Cruciate Ligaments of the Human Knee. A roentgen stereophotogrammetric study of the length patterns of the cruciate ligaments and of the three dimensional kinematic behaviour of the knee during flexion-extension and endo-exorotation. (Translated by: Th. van Winsen). Amsterdam: Rodopi, 1983.
21. van Dijk R, Huiskes R, Selvik G. Roentgen stereophotogrammetric method for evaluation of the three dimensional kinematic behaviour and cruciate ligament length patterns of the human knee. Technical Note. *J Biomechanics* 1979;12:727–731.

Knee Ligaments: Structure, Function, Injury, and Repair, edited by D. Daniel, et al.
© 1990 by Raven Press, Ltd. All rights reserved.

CHAPTER 26

Diagnostic Imaging of Ligamentous Injuries of the Knee

Jean P. Schils, Donald Resnick, and David J. Sartoris

Acute or chronic ligamentous injuries of the knee remain a difficult diagnostic imaging challenge. Conventional radiography is the most important method for initial evaluation. During the last 25 years, however, arthrography has become a popular and accurate diagnostic imaging technique for the characterization of meniscal lesions. Its value in defining abnormalities of the collateral and cruciate ligaments is more limited. Computed tomography (CT) has also become a reliable diagnostic tool for a broad spectrum of disorders affecting the musculoskeletal system. This technique, when combined with arthrography, has been used to evaluate the menisci and cruciate ligaments, although its precise value in this regard is not widely accepted. Ultrasound is noninvasive, requires no ionizing radiation, and is relatively inexpensive when compared to CT. It is a useful technique for the detection and characterization of abnormalities of the popliteal fossa as well as those of the quadriceps and patellar tendons, and it has been applied with some success to the evaluation of ligaments, menisci, and hyaline cartilage in the knee. Magnetic resonance (MR) imaging has recently shown great promise for the diagnostic assessment of the musculoskeletal system, particularly the bone marrow, supporting soft tissue, and articular structures. With recent advancement in this technology, ultrasonography and CT have assumed less importance in the assessment of the injured knee.

This chapter is divided into two parts: The first part will review the application of conventional radiography and arthrography as well as CT to the evaluation of acute or chronic ligamentous injuries of the knee; the second part will address the promising role of MR in assessing such injuries.

CONVENTIONAL RADIOGRAPHY

Acute Ligamentous Injuries

The radiologic examination of the knee consists of multiple projections (4). In evaluating acute knee injuries, the anteroposterior and lateral views are routinely obtained. Complete assessment may require supplementary projection, including tunnel, Merchant, oblique, and cross-table lateral views. In some injuries, such as fractures of the tibial plateau, conventional (or computed) tomography also may be required for accurate diagnosis.

Routine radiographs, by themselves, do not usually allow direct visualization of injured ligaments or tendons, unless they are surrounded by fat. It is the as-

J. P. Schils, D. Resnick, and D. J. Sartoris: Department of Radiology, University of California, San Diego, School of Medicine, La Jolla, California 92093; and Department of Radiology, San Diego Veterans Administration Medical Center, La Jolla, California 92037.

sociated alterations in the bone or soft tissue (or both) that more commonly provide important clues in allowing accurate diagnosis of ligamentous injuries. Stress views for acute ligamentous injuries of the knee frequently are cited as being important, but they are difficult to obtain following acute trauma (49). In this situation, the orthopedic surgeon generally prefers to assess the stability of the knee under general anesthesia.

Soft tissue abnormalities that may accompany tendinous or ligamentous injury of the knee include swelling, effusion, and change in contour or configuration of the tendon or ligament itself. Any soft tissue swelling must be noted, especially in the vicinity of the patellar or quadriceps tendon on the lateral radiographic projection. Soft tissue swelling in the medial part of the knee is often the only radiological finding in cases of injuries of the medial collateral ligament (MCL). A bloody effusion, often associated with intraarticular ligament damage, is detected as a soft tissue density in the suprapatellar pouch on the lateral projection. The presence of fat in the effusion, a *lipohemarthrosis*, suggests an osseous injury and is identified as a fat–fluid level on a cross-table lateral projection. Although fat globules are occasionally seen in many other types of effusion, the accumulation of fat is much greater in cases of trauma (41).

Extensive fractures about the knee are readily demonstrated by standard radiography, but careful analysis may be required to detect avulsion injuries at the attachment sites of any ligament or tendon. This is particularly true among children, in whom cruciate injuries are commonly of the avulsion type. An avulsion of the insertion of the anterior cruciate ligament (ACL) is diagnosed on the lateral view by identification of the displaced fragment superior and anterior to the tibial spines (Fig. 26-1); the fragment also can be observed on the tunnel view (33). In cases of a posterior cruciate ligament (PCL) injury, a radiograph may demonstrate avulsion of its tibial attachment in the posterior intercondylar area (Fig. 26-2). The fragment may consist of a thin flake or a large piece of bone. Conventional tomography is useful for better delineation of the avulsed fragment.

The radiographic findings of lateral ligamentous damage are represented by an avulsed fragment of the fibular head at the site of the biceps femoris or fibular collateral ligament (Fig. 26-3), or by a Segond fracture located posterior to Gerdy's tubercle (Fig. 26-4) (9,44,50). The latter fracture, located far superior and anterior to the fibular head, is vertically oriented. Although variable in size, it is usually several millimeters in diameter. It results from excessive tension on the lateral capsular ligament of the knee. The fragment is

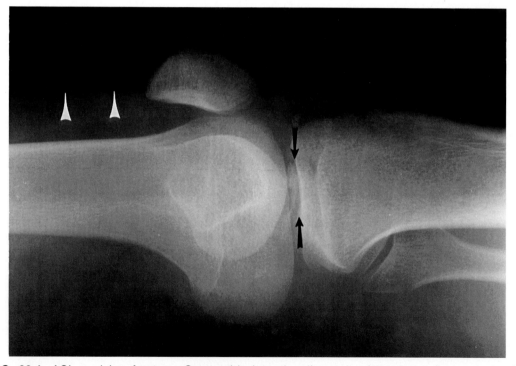

FIG. 26-1. ACL avulsion fracture. Cross-table lateral radiograph of the knee demonstrates lipohemarthrosis in the suprapatellar pouch (*white arrowheads*). An osseous density is identified in the femorotibial joint space (*black arrows*). At surgery, a large osseous fragment at the tibial insertion of the ACL was identified with an intact ligament.

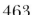

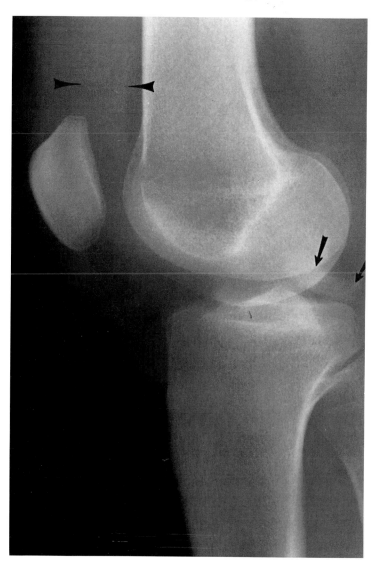

FIG. 26-2. PCL avulsion fracture. A lateral view of the knee demonstrates an osseous fragment at the tibial insertion of the PCL (*arrows*), associated with an effusion in the suprapatellar pouch (*arrowheads*).

identified lateral to the tibial condyle on the anterior–posterior (A–P) radiograph. The Segond fracture, or the lateral capsular sign, is invariably associated with an ACL injury, and an avulsed fracture fragment at the site of tibial attachment of the ACL may be apparent. Infrequently, an avulsed fragment of the femoral attachment of the MCL or LCL is identified on the frontal projection (Fig. 26-5).

Chronic Ligamentous Injuries

A careful history and physical examination are the most crucial elements in the diagnosis of chronic instability of the knee. The purpose of radiography in this clinical situation is to allow identification of the sequelae of an unstable knee and to assist the surgeon in determining the most appropriate treatment.

Most authors agree that if untreated, the unstable knee secondary to a ligamentous injury will develop

osteoarthritic change. No prospective study of the evolution of the traumatized knee has firmly established this relationship, however (11,20,25,43,45). According to McDaniel (25), there appears to be a definite relationship between varus deformity, medial meniscectomy, and the development of medial joint narrowing and osteoarthritis on radiographs in cases of untreated ACL rupture. In an extensive clinical and radiographic study of 127 ACL injuries of the knee, the effect of meniscal injury, meniscectomy, or both, in the presence of ligamentous insufficiency, was correlated with radiographic signs. It has been shown that the degree of degeneration appears to be influenced by the absence of the meniscus and associated collateral ligament damage and that progressive functional deterioration correlates with radiographic evidence of degenerative change (45). In another study related to the natural evolution of ACL-deficient knees, osteoarthritis involved the medial femorotibial compartment with genu varum and, in advanced cases, lateral sub-

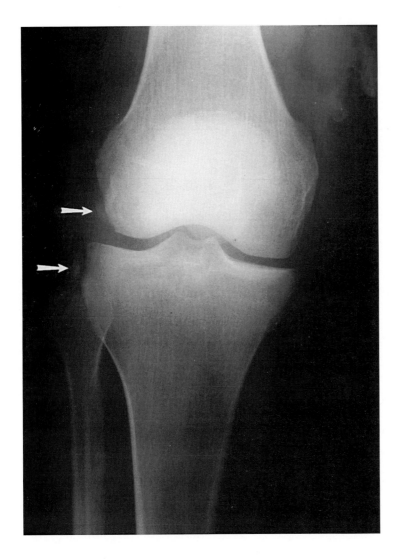

FIG. 26-3. Lateral collateral ligament (LCL) avulsion fracture. The A–P radiograph demonstrates an avulsed fragment at the insertion of the lateral capsular ligament.

luxation of the tibia. Bicompartmental osteoarthritis was also recognized with no deviation in the frontal plane. Osteoarthritis of the lateral femorotibial compartment was very uncommon (8). Incidence reports of osteoarthritis following ligament injury are presented in Tables 27-8 and 27-18.

An area of controversy involves the optimal choice of projections to assess all of these radiographic signs. Generally, although multiple views are obtained, the protocols are inconsistent from one institution to another (4,21). A comparative study of both knees must be obtained, and the two following projections are required for the examination of the femorotibial joint: (i) a frontal unipodal weight-bearing view in slight flexion and (ii) a lateral view, with the patient supine with 30° of knee flexion. The first of these, the weight-bearing view, is obtained for detecting early degenerative change of the femorotibial joints, particularly the degree of joint space narrowing (1,23,36). Biomechanical studies have demonstrated that the highest pressure about the femorotibial joint occurs with slight flexion

(walking) and that the posterior part of the articular surface is principally involved. These data explain why the weight-bearing view must be obtained in slight flexion in which the x-ray beam is tangent to this posterior critical area where osteoarthritis begins. This view can also detect (a) osteophytes along the anterior condylar portion of the femur and (b) "pointing" of the tibial spines.

Many radiographic findings associated with the ACL-deficient knee have been described (2,8,11,19): intercondylar tubercle beaking; intercondylar eminence spurring and hypertrophy; inferior patellar facet osteophyte; joint space narrowing with buttressing osteophytosis; intercondylar notch narrowing; posterior osteophyte of the medial tibial plateau; and lateral notching of the lateral femoral condyle. Intercondylar notch narrowing, well-seen on frontal examination, is characterized by proliferative changes of the tibial spine and the intercondylar area of the femoral condyle with secondary stenosis of the notch. It represents a reliable sign of chronic instability when it is observed

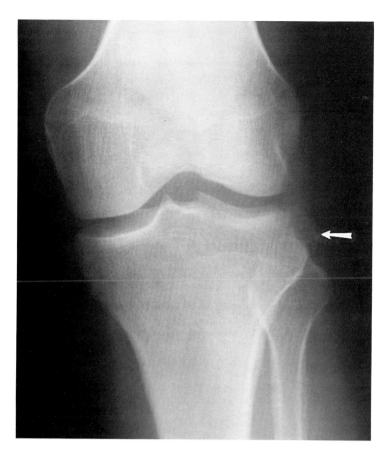

FIG. 26-4. LCL avulsion, upper arrow. Segond fracture. The typical avulsed fragment of this injury is observed just lateral to the lateral plateau (*lower arrow*) on this A–P projection.

in a knee without significant joint space narrowing, and it should be recognized by an orthopedic surgeon who is considering a notchplasty prior to an intraarticular ligamentous reconstruction (11). A posteromedial osteophyte of the medial plateau, identified on the lateral view, also is an early sign of chronic instability when the knee radiograph is otherwise normal. This osteophyte represents a response to repetitive stress at the tibial insertion of the posterior component of the MCL, and it is indicative of a deficient ACL (Fig. 26-6) (8,19).

On a lateral radiograph of the knee, a groove in the middle third of the lateral femoral condyle is a constant normal finding. In some cases, it is very large (7,14,21). This change and a less constant groove in the anterior part of the medial femoral condyle (Fig. 26-7) reflect the position of the anterior part of the corresponding tibial plateau when the knee is fully extended (14). The lateral notch sign, which has recently been described, is an exaggeration of this normal indentation and represents an abnormal finding when it is greater than 2 mm in depth on the lateral radiograph (2). This alteration may be seen in chronic or acute ACL-deficient knees, and it results from anterior subluxation of the lateral tibial plateau secondary to impingement upon the lateral or posterolateral tibial margin. These findings can be compared to the Hill–Sachs lesion affecting the posterolateral aspect of the humeral head in patients with recurrent anterior glenohumeral dislocations.

With the exception of the weight-bearing A–P view of the knee (which can be considered a stress view), stress radiography has not been widely used. Views obtained with application of varus or valgus stress or with anterior or posterior "drawer" maneuvers to evaluate the limits of knee motion are discussed in Chapter 25.

Sequelae of an old avulsion injury affecting the cruciate or collateral ligaments, as well as those of previous meniscectomy (deformity of the femoral condyle and marginal osteophytosis), may be evident on routine radiographs. A common finding is ossification in the soft tissue adjacent to the upper pole of the medial condyle (the Pelligrini–Stieda syndrome), which results from injury to the tibial collateral ligament at its femoral insertion. An associated varus deformity can be appreciated by a scanogram of the lower limbs in the standing position.

A complete evaluation of an unstable knee should include radiographic study of the patellofemoral joint for three reasons: (i) Tibiofemoral subluxation may alter patellofemoral mechanics (11,43); (ii) anterior knee pain is common after ACL reconstruction (Chapter 28); and (iii) degenerative changes are frequently observed in ligament-injured knees (Tables 27-8 and

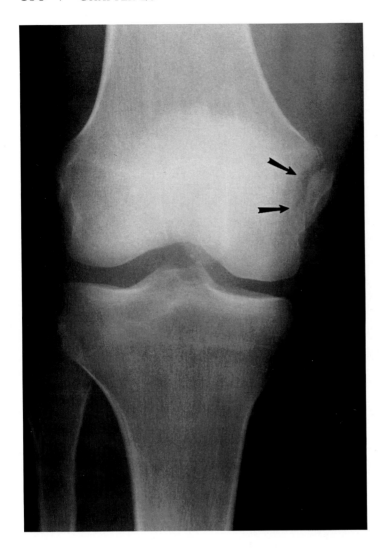

FIG. 26-5. MCL avulsion fracture. An A–P radiograph demonstrates a large avulsion fragment at the femoral insertion of the MCL (*arrows*).

27-18). Various projections have been described for the evaluation of the patellofemoral joints. In general, two views must be obtained: Both must be tangent to the joint, with no more than 30° of flexion and the cassette placed perpendicular to the beam (one in neutral position, the other with external rotation of the legs) (17,29). These projections allow the detection of joint space narrowing and patellofemoral joint instability characterized by lateral subluxation of the patella.

ARTHROGRAPHY

As a general rule, arthrography of the knee is used for the evaluation of the menisci and, to a lesser degree, the cruciate ligaments and articular cartilage (3,5,6,10,13,15,30,40,47). Arthrography of the knee is less important in the assessment of acute ligamentous injury, although arthrography is useful in evaluating whether a meniscus tear is the cause of pain lingering for 4–10 weeks after an MCL tear. Arthrography remains an appropriate tool for the diagnosis of meniscal

abnormalities (tear or degeneration) in cases of chronic instability secondary to ligamentous injury (11). Arthrography is particularly helpful when the tear is located in the peripheral undersurface of the meniscus, a site that is difficult to evaluate fully with arthroscopy (11,19). The arthrographic study can precisely define the site of abnormalities, allowing differentiation between a simple capsular separation and a capsular separation associated with an intrameniscal tear (Fig. 26-8). Arthrography allows identification of meniscus tears that are potentially reparable.

Arthrography can be used to diagnose an ACL tear if the procedure is carefully performed and interpreted (33,35). An abnormal cruciate ligament can be diagnosed when the ligament is absent or has a wavy or irregular appearance on a stress lateral view. To an inexperienced examiner, an infrapatellar plica can simulate an intact ACL on this view, leading to diagnostic error in the patient with a torn ACL. The infrapatellar plica, however, can be distinguished from the ACL by its more anterior insertion on the tibia. One further problem in arthrographic interpretation

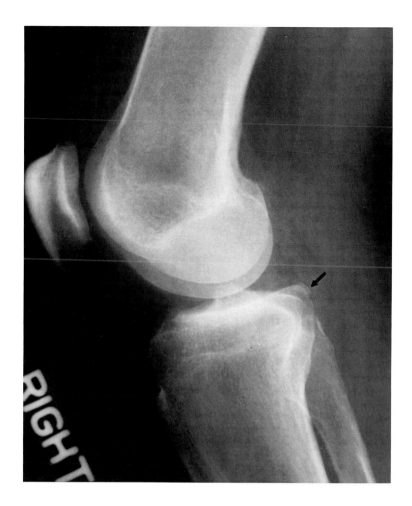

FIG. 26-6. Chronic instability related to an ACL-deficient knee. Lateral view of the knee demonstrates a posteromedial osteophyte on the tibial plateau (*arrow*), an indirect sign of old rupture of the ACL with secondary chronic stress reaction at the tibial insertion of the posterior portion of the MCL.

occurs when there is disruption of the ACL with an intact synovial sheath; the profile of the sheath may simulate that of an intact ACL (3).

An MCL tear may be diagnosed by arthrogram. Disruption of both the superficial and deep fibers of the MCL may be accompanied by a characteristic pattern of extravasation of contrast material. This finding, however, is not constant and may be absent in chronic injuries or in those limited to the superficial fibers. Because the LCL is an extracapsular structure, it cannot be evaluated by arthrography.

COMPUTED TOMOGRAPHY

Ever since the early application of CT to the musculoskeletal system, this technique has been used to evaluate many different disorders of the knee, including (a) patellofemoral malalignment and (b) damage to the menisci and the ligaments (Fig. 26-9) (16,24,31,32,34,42). If multiple planes and image reconstruction are used, all of the anatomic structures of the meniscocapsular ligamentous complex of the knee are demonstrated. Some authors have stressed the capabilities of CT in the assessment of cruciate

ligament injuries. However, these descriptions have been conflicting not only with respect to the need for intraarticular contrast material but also with respect to whether the contrast material should be radiopaque, radiolucent (air), or both radiopaque and radiolucent. Furthermore, authors disagree regarding the position that the patient should assume in the CT gantry (40). Consequently, the clinical application of CT to ligamentous injury of the knee is not clearly documented. Conversely, the diagnosis of patellofemoral malalignment by CT is not difficult.

MAGNETIC RESONANCE IMAGING

Physical Concepts

When a sample of tissue is placed in an external magnetic field, some hydrogen nuclei line up parallel or antiparallel to the lines of force. In this situation, the tissue sample exhibits magnetization. Nuclei aligned against the magnetic field are in a slightly higher energy state than those aligned parallel to the field. Nuclei can be shifted from parallel to antiparallel alignment by exposing the tissue to a pulse of radiofrequency en-

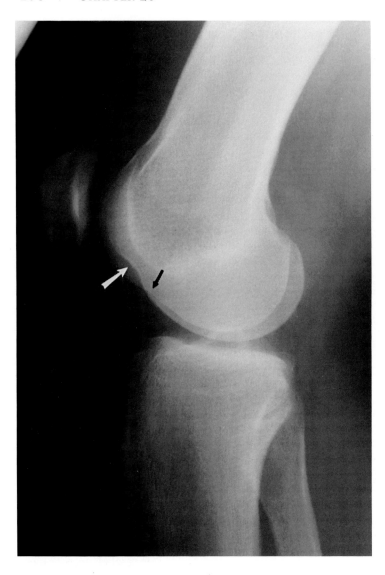

FIG. 26-7. Normal grooves of the medial and lateral femoral condyles in a patient without a history of ligamentous injury. Lateral view of the knee demonstrates the grooves of the medial (*white arrow*) and lateral (*black arrow*) femoral condyles.

ergy, with the frequency corresponding to the energy difference between the two alignment states. When the radiofrequency pulse is terminated, the nuclei return to their original alignment, giving up energy in the form of a radiowave. The signal is detected by an antenna and converted by computer to a pictorial image in a fashion similar to that of a CT scanner. The final signal obtained by the computer is related to the selected time of repetition (TR) and time to echo (TE), the total numbers of hydrogen protons contained in the tissue volume of interest, and both T1 and T2 relaxation times. T1 and T2 are inherent properties of the tissue that relate to the liquidity and chemical and molecular composition; these parameters are given and fixed, whereas TR and TE can be selected by the operator. TR is the length of time from the beginning of the sequence to the beginning of the next sequence, or the length the signal is allowed to grow. The latter phenomenon is logarithmic and is controlled by T1. TE is the length of time from the beginning of the sequence

to the time of echo, or time that the signal is received. TE can also be described as the length of time that the signal is allowed to decay. This phenomenon is also logarithmic and governed by T2. The optimal T1-weighted image has a short TR and short TE. Conversely, the best T2-weighted image has a long TR and a long TE. On T1-weighted images, subcutaneous fat and bone marrow have the brightest signal. Hyaline cartilage is intermediate in signal intensity, and muscle has even less intensity. On T2-weighted images, effusions have the brightest signal, followed in decreasing order by subcutaneous fat, bone marrow, and muscle. Ligaments, tendons, and cortical bone remain low in signal intensity.

Multiple protocols using variable pulse sequences and imaging planes can be used in the evaluation of the knee. The precise protocol that is chosen is dependent upon the specific clinical situation. In general, in the evaluation of ligamentous injury, both T1- and T2-weighted images are useful, and images in both the

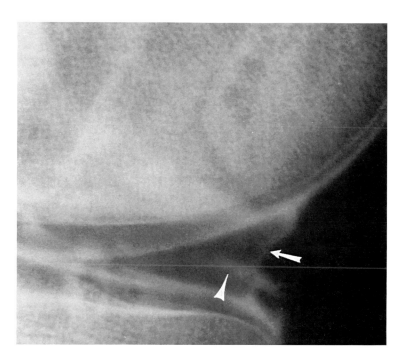

FIG. 26-8. Complex tear of the posterior aspect of the medial meniscus. An arthrogram shows both the vertical (*arrow*) and the horizontal (*arrowhead*) component of this complex tear of the medial meniscus.

coronal and sagittal planes are obtained. In order to compete with arthrography and arthroscopy in the evaluation of ligamentous injuries, MR of the knee must include complete examination of both soft tissue and osseous components. It is imperative that any pertinent conventional radiographs be made available for correlation at the time of interpretation of the MR examination.

Menisci

The normal anatomy of both menisci is well-demonstrated on coronal and sagittal MR scans. The normal internal substance of the menisci produces no significant signal on either T1- or T2-weighted images (Fig. 26-10). (39). Meniscal tears appear on MR images as focal areas of increased signal intensity that extend to an articular surface (Fig. 26-11) (22,37,38). Similar areas of increased signal intensity that do not communicate with an articular margin do not represent macroscopically evident tears and explain the negative arthroscopic findings that may be encountered in patients with abnormal MR meniscal signal (46). Histologically, intrameniscal signal is associated with myxoid change. Coronal and sagittal scans allow identification of the exact morphology of meniscal tears (Fig. 26-12). Indeed, recent studies have shown a high accuracy of MR in the diagnosis of meniscal tears. In an evaluation of 242 patients, MR had an overall accuracy for detection of meniscal abnormalities of 93% (sensitivity 95%, specificity 91%) and had a false-negative rate of 4.8% (28).

Anterior Cruciate Ligament

Sagittal MR images of the knee can be obtained with the patient supine and the leg externally rotated 10–20°, or oblique MR images can be obtained with the leg in a neutral position. In either situation, the plane of the section is parallel to the long axis of the ACL so that the ligament is identified completely on one image. In some situations, the coronal plane can also be helpful in the assessment of the ACL.

The normal ACL appears as a smooth, well-defined structure of low signal intensity on a sagittal image through the intercondylar notch (Fig. 26-13) (2,39,48). At its tibial site of attachment, two or three separate ligamentous fibers may be evident (Fig. 26-14). The T2-weighted sagittal image may also be useful, since the high signal intensity of joint fluid outlines the anterior margin of the ACL.

The most important finding in the diagnosis of a tear of the ACL by MR imaging is discontinuity of the ligament in the sagittal plane, which, in the case of an acute injury, is accompanied on T2-weighted sequences by high signal intensity within the ligamentous substance (presumably representing both edema and local hemorrhage) (Fig. 26-15). Another finding associated with a torn ACL is the loss of its normal course in the sagittal plane. A wavy irregular contour of the anterior margin of the ACL represents a third clue to the diagnosis of a torn ACL by MR imaging. Finally, anterior bowing of the PCL represents a supportive sign in cases of ACL tear when the major findings are also present. However, this sign depends, in part, on

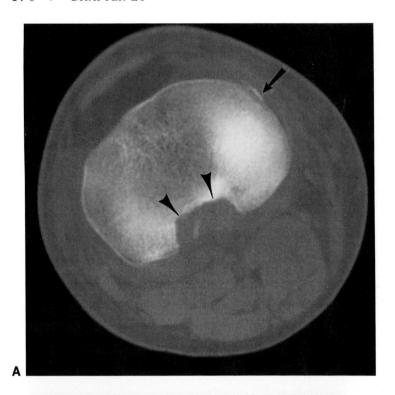

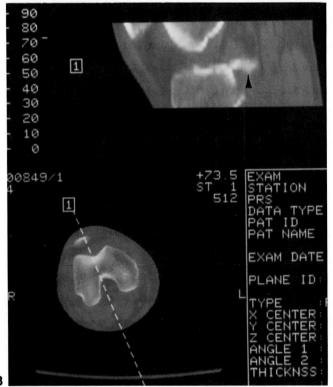

FIG. 26-9. PCL avulsion fracture demonstrated by CT. **A:** Transaxial scan at the level of the tibial plateau. Note the defect in the midportion of the posterior tibial plateau resulting from the avulsion fracture of the PCL (*arrowheads*). A small fragment of bone is also identified adjacent to the medial plateau, indicating MCL injury (*arrow*). **B:** This reconstructed image in the midsagittal plane demonstrates the avulsed fragment at the tibial insertion of the PCL (*arrowhead*).

patient positioning and is not consistently present (18,22,37,48).

Several recent studies have demonstrated the accuracy of MR imaging in the detection of complete tears of the ACL. Mink (28) studied 242 patients with MR followed by arthroscopy and found that the MR

examination allowed accurate assessment of the ACL in 95% of patients. This investigator noted that the sagittal T2-weighted image was especially helpful in this assessment.

A multitude of operative procedures for the repair of the ACL have been developed during the past dec-

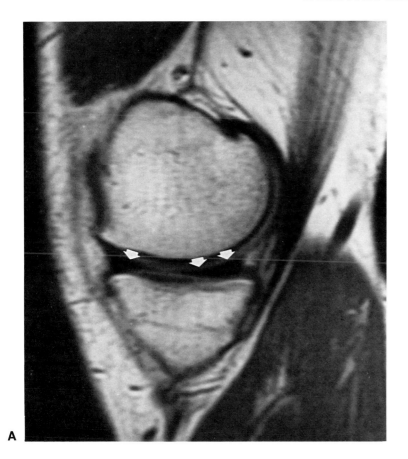

A

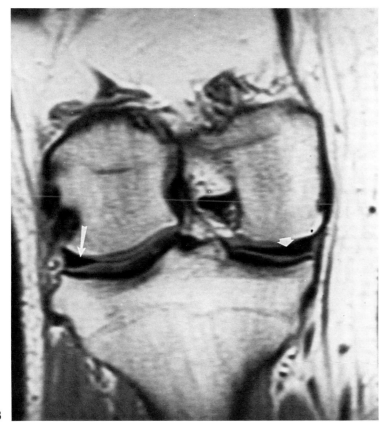

B

FIG. 26-10. Normal anatomy of the meniscal structure, demonstrated by MR imaging. **A:** Sagittal plane view. The arrows point to the meniscus. **B:** Coronal plane demonstrates the normal anatomy of the medial (*small arrow*) and lateral (*large arrow*) menisci.

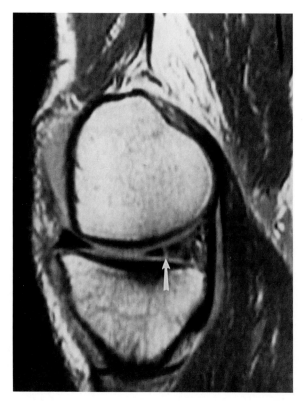

FIG. 26-11. Posterior medial meniscal tear (*arrow*). MR findings. Sagittal scan demonstrating abnormal vertical hyperintense signal in the posterior aspect of the medial meniscus.

ade. Although data are incomplete, it appears that MR can also be used in the postoperative period for the detection of ACL graft failures.

Posterior Cruciate Ligament

The entire length of the normal PCL is usually seen on a single sagittal image as a wide, low-signal-intensity structure with a slightly convex posterior curvature projecting within the intercondylar notch (Fig. 26-16) (26,39). The meniscofemoral ligaments of Humphry and Wrisberg, which are intimately associated with the PCL, also can be identified in both the sagittal and the coronal planes. In the sagittal plane, the ligament of Humphry, which emerges anterior to the PCL, can be differentiated from a torn ACL without difficulty. The diagnosis of PCL tears is based on the same criteria described previously for tears of the ACL (Fig. 26-17) (37,48).

Medial Collateral Ligament

The architectural arrangement of the collateral ligaments is presented in Chapter 4. Although MR cannot delineate all of the individual components of the MCL, it allows identification of the tibial collateral ligament on both T1- and T2-weighted images. The normal ligament is best seen in the coronal plane as a thin dark band extending from the femoral epicondyle to the medial portion of the tibia (Fig. 26-18) (39). A portion of this signal presumably originates from the capsular ligament because this structure becomes indistinguishable anatomically from the overlying oblique extension of the tibial collateral ligament in the posterior third of the capsule. The two fiber bundles of the tibial collateral ligament (vertical and oblique) cannot be differentiated with MR imaging. The ligament is often separated from the meniscus by a high-signal-intensity area that represents an intraligamentous bursa. This bursa should not be mistaken for evidence of a meniscocapsular separation. A complete tear (Grade III) of the tibial collateral ligament is diagnosed on the basis of discontinuity of the ligament on coronal images. Such a tear is associated with edema and local hemorrhage, which are best seen with T2-weighted sequences. A sprain of the tibial collateral ligament results in surrounding edema, with preservation of its continuity (Fig. 26-19) (12,26). The differentiation between Grade I and Grade II injuries of the tibial collateral ligament depends on clinical diagnosis rather than on MR findings.

Lateral Capsular Ligamentous Complex

MR imaging allows delineation of the iliotibial band, the biceps femoris tendon in layer I, and the patellar retinaculum in layer II. The fibular collateral ligament lies in the third layer and can also be identified with MR imaging (Fig. 26-20). It inserts on the fibular head along with the biceps femoris tendon as the conjoint tendon. This insertion is evident on coronal and sagittal MR images, whereas the joint capsule itself is not reliably observed (26).

The diagnostic criteria for disruption of any component of the lateral capsular ligamentous complex by MR imaging are identical to those for the medial side of the knee (26). Because isolated injury to the lateral collateral ligament is extremely rare, MR has the additional advantage of affording evaluation of the associated lesions involving the ACL and PCL.

Additional Structure and Findings

Joint effusions commonly accompany any type of ligamentous injury to the knee. Normally, acutely hemorrhagic synovial fluid yields (a) moderate signal in-

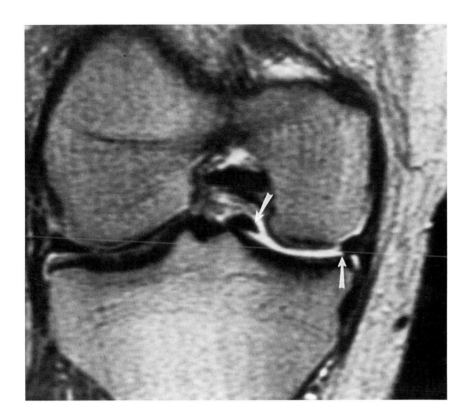

FIG. 26-12. Bucket-handle lesion of the medial meniscus. T2-weighted MR image in the coronal plane demonstrating both central and peripheral fragments of the torn medial meniscus (*arrows*).

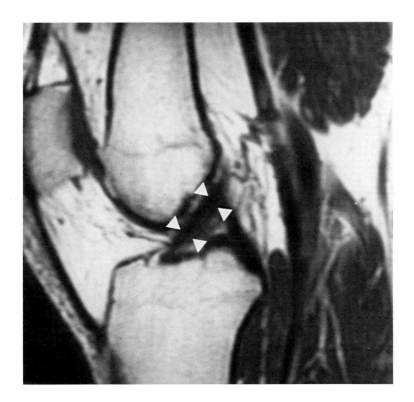

FIG. 26-13. Normal anatomy of the ACL, demonstrated by MR imaging. Sagittal T1-weighted image demonstrates the ACL as a smooth low-signal-intensity structure (*arrowheads*).

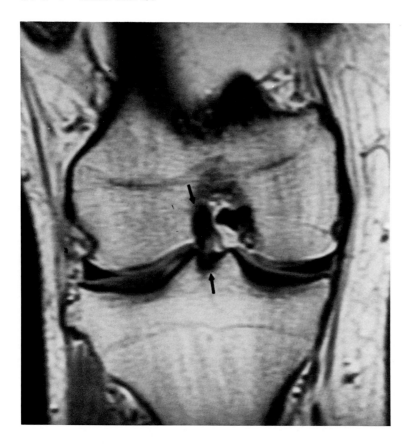

FIG. 26-14. Normal anatomy of the ACL, demonstrated by MR imaging. This coronal T1-weighted image shows multiple ligamentous bundles of the ACL at its tibial attachment (*arrows*).

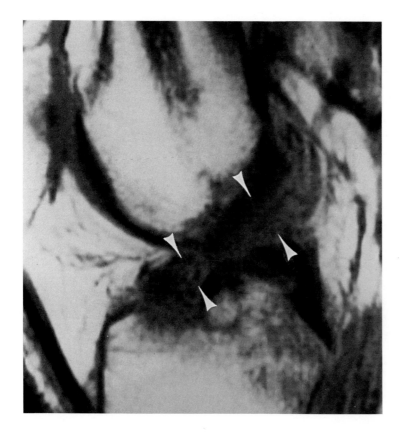

FIG. 26-15. Tear of the ACL, demonstrated by MR imaging. Sagittal T1-weighted image shows abnormal signal intensity in the intracondylar area (*arrowheads*); the normal structure of the ACL is not identified.

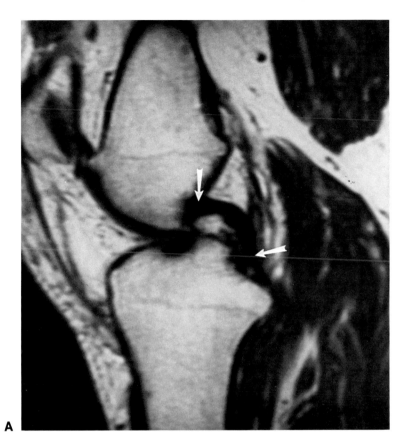

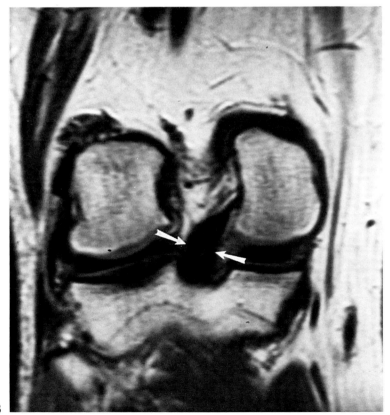

FIG. 26-16. Normal anatomy of the PCL, demonstrated by MR imaging. The normal PCL is observed on both sagittal (A) and coronal (B) T1-weighted images (arrows).

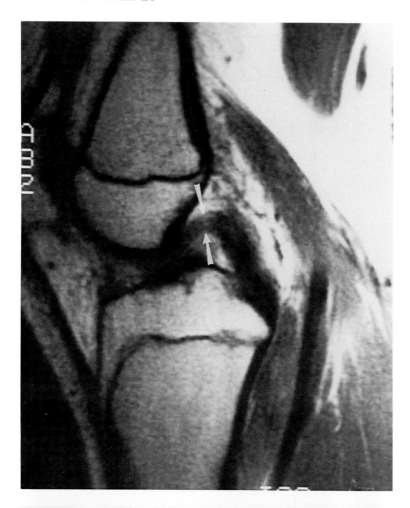

FIG. 26-17. PCL tear, demonstrated by MR imaging. Attenuated signal of the proximal portion of the PCL is noted on this sagittal T1-weighted image (*arrows*).

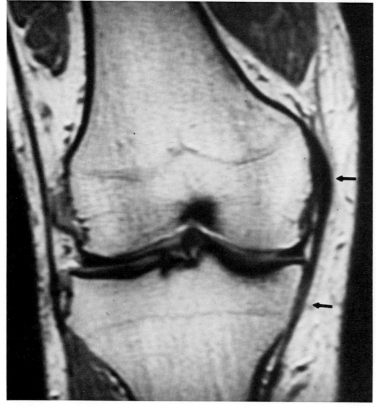

FIG. 26-18. Normal anatomy of the MCL, demonstrated by MR imaging. Coronal T1-weighted images demonstrate the normal MCL extending from the femoral epicondyle to its proximal tibial insertion (*arrows*).

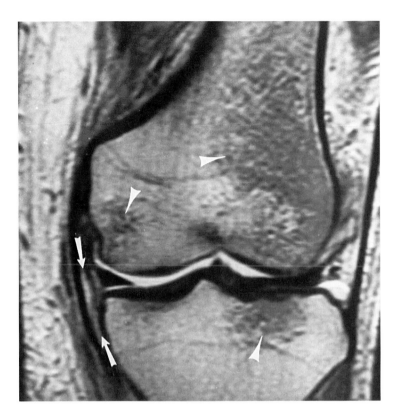

FIG. 26-19. MCL injury, demonstrated by MR imaging. Coronal T1-weighted sequence demonstrates abnormal signal intensity lateral to the MCL (*arrows*), with increased distance between the MCL and the proximal tibia. Other findings include abnormal signal intensity in the marrow of both the femur and tibia, possibly representing areas of bone contusion (*arrowheads*).

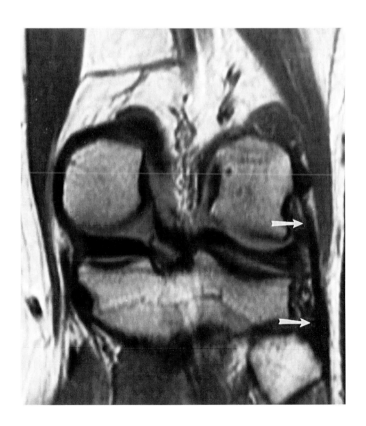

FIG. 26-20. Normal anatomy of the fibular collateral ligament, demonstrated by MR imaging. T1-weighted coronal image shows the entire ligament, indicated by arrows.

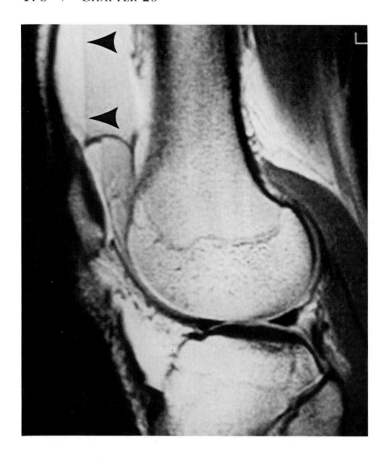

FIG. 26-21. Sagittal T1-weighted images demonstrate a fat–fluid level in the suprapatellar pouch (*arrowheads*).

tensity on T1-weighted images and (b) high signal intensity on T2-weighted images. In cases of lipohemarthrosis, a fat–fluid level (which can be observed on cross-table lateral radiographs of the knee) also can be depicted by MR imaging as high-intensity fat globules lying above less intense synovial fluid in the suprapatellar bursa (Fig. 26-21).

Plain films remain the preferred study for the evaluation of those osseous lesions that are associated with acute ligamentous injuries; however, MR allows detection of bone abnormalities prior to, or in the absence of, their appearance on conventional radiographs (27). Certain abnormal osseous findings that are associated with collateral ligamentous injury presumably represent a form of compression fracture. On T1-weighted images, these bone "bruises" produce bands of low signal that become bright on T2-weighted images (Fig. 26-22).

Current Status of MR Imaging

Four years after the initial clinical application of MR, it is premature to define its precise role in the evaluation of ligamentous injury of the knee. At some institutions, however, MR already has replaced arthrog-

raphy of the knee in the diagnosis of meniscal abnormalities. Several investigations have also established its high accuracy in the diagnosis of ligamentous injury, particularly those involving the ACL; moreover, MR imaging appears to compare favorably with arthroscopy, generally considered the gold standard in this clinical setting. The advantages of MR are numerous: superb soft tissue contrast discrimination, high spatial resolution, multiplanar imaging capability, and, in particular, lack of ionizing radiation.

Although many questions remain to be answered regarding the precise impact of MR imaging in the management of acute and chronic ligamentous injuries of the knee, the following clinical situations constitute reasonable indications for the technique. In acute knee trauma, MR can be useful, particularly in cases of collateral ligament injuries, in which it allows evaluation of associated cruciate and meniscal lesions. In Grade I and II MCL injuries, MR can influence management by affording analysis of the integrity of the medial meniscus. In chronic instability of the knee secondary to ligamentous injury, MR allows determination of status of the menisci, ligaments, and cartilage prior to operative intervention. Future improvements in the spatial resolution of MR will probably render it the method of choice in this setting.

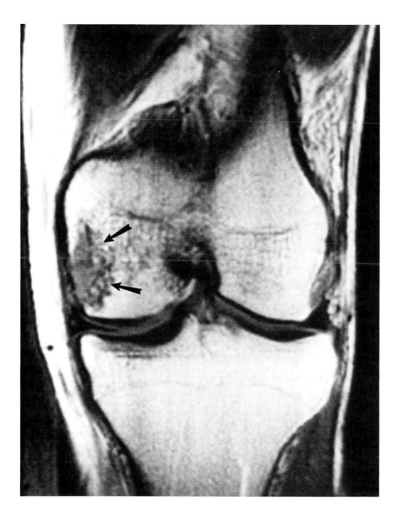

FIG. 26-22. MCL injury, demonstrated by MR imaging. The coronal T1-weighted image demonstrates abnormal low signal intensity in the medial femoral condyle adjacent to the MCL, possibly representing an avulsion fracture (*arrows*).

REFERENCES

1. Ahlback S. Osteoarthritis of the knee. *Acta Radiol (Stockh)* 1968;277:1–72.
2. Back BR, Warren RF. Radiographic indicators of the anterior cruciate ligament injury. In: Feagin JA Jr, ed. *The crucial ligaments*. New York: Churchill Livingstone, 1988;317–327.
3. Brown DW, Allman FL, Eaton SB. Knee arthrography: a comparison of radiographic and surgical findings in 295 cases. *Am J Sports Med* 1978;6:165–172.
4. Cockshott WP, Racoveanu NT, Burrows DA, Ferrier M. Use of radiographic projections of the knee. *Skeletal Radiol* 1985;13:131–133.
5. Crabtree SD, Bedford AF, Edgar MA. The value of arthrography and arthroscopy in association with a sports injuries clinic: a prospective and comparative study of 182 patients. *Injury* 1981;13:220–226.
6. Daniel D, Daniels E, Aronson D. The diagnosis of meniscus pathology. *Clin Orthop* 1982;163:218–224.
7. Danzig LA, Newell JD, Guerra J, Resnick D. Osseous landmarks of the normal knee. *Clin Orthop* 1981;156:201–206.
8. Dejour H, Walch G, Deschamps G, Chambat P. Arthrose du genou sur laxité chronique antérieure. *Rev Chir Orthop* 1987;73:157–170.
9. Dietz GW, Wilcox DM, Montgomery JB. Segond tibial condyle fracture: lateral capsular ligament avulsion. *Radiology* 1986;159:467–469.
10. Dumas J-M, Edde DJ. Meniscal abnormalities: prospective correlation of double-contrast arthrography and arthroscopy. *Radiology* 1986;160:453–456.
11. Feagin JF Jr, Cabaud HE, Curl WW. The anterior cruciate ligament: radiographic and clinical signs of successful and unsuccessful repairs. *Clin Orthop* 1982;164:54–58.
12. Gallimore GW Jr, Harms SE. Knee injuries: high resolution MR imaging. *Radiology* 1986;160:457–461.
13. Gilles H, Seligson D. Precision in the diagnosis of meniscal lesion: a comparison of clinical evaluation, arthrography, and arthroscopy. *J Bone Joint Surg [Am]* 1979;61:343–346.
14. Harison RB, Wood MB, Keats TE. The grooves of the distal articular surface of the femur. A normal variant. *AJR* 1976;126:751–754.
15. Ireland J, Trickey EL, Stoker DJ. Arthroscopy and arthrography of the knee: a critical review. *J Bone Joint Surg [Br]* 1980;62:3–6.
16. Kursunoglu S, Pate D, Resnick D, Andre M, Sartoris DJ. Computed arthrotomography with multiplanar reformation and three-dimensional image analysis in the evaluation of the cruciate ligaments: preliminary investigation. *J Can Assoc Radiol* 1986;37:153–156.
17. Laurin CA, Dussault R, Levesque HP. The tangential x-ray investigation of the patellofemoral joint: x-ray technique, diagnostic criteria and their interpretation. *Clin Orthop* 1979;144:16–26.
18. Lee JK, Yao L, Phelps CT, Wirth CR, Czajka J, Lozman J. Anterior cruciate ligament tears: MR imaging compared with arthroscopy and clinical tests. *Radiology* 1988;166:861–864.
19. Lemaire M. Les instabilités chroniques antérieures et internes du genou. Etude théorique. Diagnostic clinique et radiologique. *Rev Chir Orthop* 1983;69:3–16.
20. Lynch MA, Henning CE, Glick KG. Knee joint surface changes.

Long-term follow-up meniscus tear treatment in stable anterior cruciate ligament reconstructions. *Clin Orthop* 1983;172:148–153.

21. Malghem J, Maldague B. Le profil du genou. Anatomie radiologique différentielle des surfaces articulaires. *J Radiol* 1986;67:725–735.

22. Mandelbaum BR, Finerman GA, Reicher MA, et al. Magnetic resonance imaging as a tool for evaluation of traumatic knee injuries. *Am J Sports Med* 1986;14:361–370.

23. Marklund T, Myrnerts R. Radiographic determinations of cartilage height in the knee joint. *Acta Orthop Scand* 1974;45:752–755.

24. Martinez S, Korobkin M, Fondren FB, Hedlund LW, Goldner JL. Diagnosis of patellofemoral malalignment by computed tomography. *J Comput Assist Tomogr* 1983;7:1050–1053.

25. McDaniel WJ Jr, Dameron TB Jr. The untreated anterior cruciate ligament rupture. *Clin Orthop* 1983;172:158–163.

26. Mink JH. The ligaments of the knee. In: Mink JH, ed. *Magnetic resonance imaging of the knee*. New York: Raven Press, 1987;93–111.

27. Mink JH. Pitfalls in interpretation. In: Mink JH, ed. *Magnetic resonance imaging of the knee*. New York: Raven Press, 1987;141–155.

28. Mink JH, Levy T, Crues JH. Tears of the anterior cruciate ligament and menisci of the knee: MR evaluation. *Radiology* 1988;167:769–774.

29. Miremad C, Combelles F, Lemaire M. Articulation fémoro-patellaire. Intérêt des incidences axiales en rotation externe. *J Radiol* 1980;61:347–351.

30. Nicholas JA, Freiberger RH, Killoran PJ. Double contrast arthrography of the knee. Its value in the management of 225 knee derangements. *J Bone Joint Surg [Am]* 1970;52:203–220.

31. Passariello R, Trecco F, Depaulis F, Bonanni G, Masciocchi C, Beomonte Zobel B. Computed tomography of the knee joint: technique of study and normal anatomy. *J Comput Assist Tomogr* 1983;7:1035–1042.

32. Passariello R, Trecco F, Depaulis F, DeAmicis R, Bonanni G, Masciocchi C. Computed tomography of the knee: clinical results. *J Comput Assist Tomogr* 1983;7:1043–1049.

33. Pavlov II. The radiographic diagnosis of the anterior cruciate ligament deficient knee. *Clin Orthop* 1983;172:57–63.

34. Pavlov H, Hirschy JC, Jorg JS. Computed tomography of the cruciate ligaments. *Radiology* 1979;132:389–393.

35. Pavlov H, Warren RF, Sherman MF, Cayea PD. The accuracy of double-contrast arthrographic evaluation of the anterior cruciate ligament. A retrospective review of 163 knees with surgical confirmation. *J Bone Joint Surg [Am]* 1983;65:175–183.

36. Railhac JJ, Fournie A, Gay R, Mansat M, Putois J. Exploration radiologique du genou de face en légère flexion et en charge. Son intérêt dans le diagnostic de l'arthrose fémorotibiale. *J Radiol* 1981;62:157–166.

37. Reicher MA, Hartzman S, Bassett LW, Mandelbaum B, Duckwiler G, Gold RH. MR imaging of the knee: Part I. Traumatic disorders. *Radiology* 1987;162:547–551.

38. Reicher MA, Hartzman S, Duckwiler G, Bassett LW, Anderson LJ, Gold RH. Meniscal injuries: detection using MR imaging. *Radiology* 1986;159:753–757.

39. Reicher MA, Rauschning W, Gold RH, Bassett LW, Lufkin RB, Glen W Jr. High resolution magnetic resonance of the knee: normal anatomy. *AJR* 1985;145:895–902.

40. Resnick D. Arthrography, tenography and bursography. In: Resnick D, Niwayama G, eds. *Diagnosis of bone and joint disorders*, 2nd ed. Philadelphia: WB Saunders, 1988;303–440.

41. Resnick D, Goergen TG, Niwayama G. Physical injury. In: Resnick D, Niwayama G, eds. *Diagnosis of bone and joint disorders*, 2nd ed. Philadelphia: WB Saunders, 1988;2756–3008.

42. Rickards D, Chapman JA. Computed tomography of the anterior cruciate ligament. *Clin Radiol* 1984:35:327–329.

43. Segal P, Lallement JJ, Raguet M, Jacob M, Gerard Y. Les lésions ostéo-cartilagineuses de la laxité antéro-interne du genou. *Rev Chir Orthop* 1980;66:357–365.

44. Segond P. Recherches cliniques et expérimentales sur les épanchements sanguins du genou par entorse. *Progres Med (Paris)* 1879;7:379–381.

45. Sherman MF, Warren RF, Marshall JL, Savatshy GJ. A clinical and radiographic analysis of 127 cruciate insufficient knees. *Clin Orthop* 1986;227:229–237.

46. Stoller DW, Martin C, Crues JV, Kaplan L, Mink JH. Meniscal tears: pathologic correlation with MR imaging. *Radiology* 1987;163:731–735.

47. Thijn CJP. Accuracy of double contrast arthrography of the knee joint. *Skeletal Radiol* 1982;8:187–192.

48. Turner DA, Prodromos CC, Petasnick JP, Clark JW. Acute injury of the knee: magnetic resonance evaluation. *Radiology* 1985;154:711–722.

49. Warren RF. Acute ligament injuries. In: Insall JN, ed. *Surgery of the knee*. New York: Churchill Livingstone, 1984;261–294.

50. Woods GW, Stanley RF, Tullos HS. Lateral capsular sign: x-ray clue of a significant knee instability. *Am J Sports Med* 1979;7:27–33.

Knee Ligaments: Structure, Function, Injury, and Repair, edited by D. Daniel, et al.

CHAPTER 27

The Fate of Unoperated Knee Ligament Injuries

H. Paul Hirshman, Dale M. Daniel, and Kenji Miyasaka

INCIDENCE OF LIGAMENT INJURY

Injuries of the knee are extremely common, and their incidence has apparently been rising during the past few decades (1,3,31,49). Incidences have been calculated for certain sports, such as skiing (11,14,54,59) and professional football (60). The frequencies of various injuries have been calculated in patients presenting acutely to a hospital (26,43), in patients presenting specifically with knee ligament injuries (1,31), in patients presenting with hemarthrosis of the knee (9,40), and in patients undergoing knee surgery (32,45,49,52). There has been no study, however, to delineate the incidence of knee ligament injuries in an unselected segment of the general population at large.

The Kaiser Permanente Medical Center in San Diego, California serves the Kaiser Health Plan members in the greater San Diego area. This population represents a segment of the local population which is selected by choice of health plan only. Because of the nature of that health plan, it receives virtually all of its care at San Diego Kaiser facilities. During the study period of mid-1985 through mid-1988, the San Diego Health Plan averaged 280,000 members.

Patients who present to Kaiser emergency rooms with a soft tissue knee injury are referred to the Knee Injury Clinic of the Department of Orthopedics if they have at least one of the following: (a) effusion, (b) pathologic joint motion, or (c) disability that keeps them from working. Patients with fractures (except minor avulsions) or femorotibial dislocations, however, are not referred to the Knee Injury Clinic. They are evaluated acutely by orthopedists in the emergency room and thus are excluded from this study.

The statistics that we shall present are based on the *initial* San Diego Kaiser Knee Injury Clinic diagnosis. This diagnosis was based on standard clinical examination and radiographs. Patients suspected of having knee ligament injuries underwent instrumented measurements with the KT-1000 knee ligament arthrometer. Cruciate ligament injuries were diagnosed by KT-1000 documentation of pathologic motion. Pathologic posterior motion was defined as either (a) posterior tibial subluxation of 2 mm or more in 60–90° of knee flexion or (b) a 20-lb posterior drawer test difference of >2mm (7). Pathologic anterior motion was defined as ≥3 mm of difference between the anterior displacement of the injured and the uninjured knee

H. P. Hirshman: Department of Orthopaedics, Scripps Clinic, La Jolla, California 92037.

D. M. Daniel: Department of Orthopedic Surgery, University of California, San Diego, School of Medicine, La Jolla, California 92037; and Kaiser Permanente Medical Center, San Diego, California 92120.

K. Miyasaka: University of California, San Diego, School of Medicine, La Jolla, California 92037.

with a 20-lb, 30-lb, or manual maximum displacement force with the knee in 30° of flexion. Collateral ligament injuries were graded on a scale of I to III as follows:

I = Pain or tenderness without opening to varus or valgus stress (i.e., no pathologic motion).
II = Abnormal joint space opening, but a firm end point.
III = Abnormal joint space opening and a soft end point.

During the 3-year study, 2547 patients were evaluated in the San Diego Kaiser Knee Injury Clinic. Eighteen hundred thirty-three presented within 1 month of their injury and so were classified as *acute*. Of these, 819 had knee ligament injuries. This represents an injury rate of 98 per 100,000 population per year. Three hundred nineteen of these had isolated Grade I collateral ligament injuries (306 medial and 13 lateral). Ligament injuries with pathologic motion (i.e., Grade II or Grade III) were diagnosed in 500 patients, or 60 per 100,000 population per year. Three hundred fifty-eight (72%) of these patients were male and 142 (28%) were female. The distribution of ligaments that were injured is presented in Table 27-1.

Sixty-one percent of the acute ligament injuries with pathologic motion were sustained in sports activities (Table 27-2). The majority of the isolated anterior cruciate ligament (ACL) (70%), isolated medial collateral ligament (MCL) (54%) and combined ACL/MCL (61%) injuries were sustained in sports activities. In contrast, the majority of the isolated and combined posterior cruciate ligament (PCL) (59%) and lateral collateral ligament (LCL) (59%) injuries were not sports-related.

Football (49), baseball (51), soccer (54), and skiing (57) accounted for almost equal numbers of acute knee ligament injuries in the San Diego population, whereas basketball (30) accounted for a little more than half as many. These five sports accounted for 78% of the sports injuries and 47% of the total injuries. Interestingly, the profile of the knee ligament injuries in the different sports does not vary greatly among the sports. However, baseball seemed to produce more PCL injuries and fewer combined ACL/MCL injuries than the other sports, whereas basketball and soccer produced more ACL injuries and skiing more MCL injuries than were seen in the other sports and in the total population (Table 27-3). Vehicular accidents produced a very different profile of injuries. Isolated ACL, isolated MCL, and isolated and combined PCL injuries each accounted for about one-quarter of the vehicular total. Thus in the vehicular group, ACLs are underrepresented and PCLs are overrepresented. It is worth remembering that this group also probably produced more of the knee dislocations that were not included in this study.

Table 27-4 shows the age of patients presenting to the San Diego Kaiser Knee Injury Clinic. All of the various subtypes of injury presented approximately the same age distribution. Within each age group, the pattern of injuries was quite similar to the pattern of injuries in the entire population. Thus, while age seems to be a factor influencing the incidence of acute knee ligament injuries with pathologic motion, age does not seem to influence dramatically the specific pattern of ligament injury within the injured group.

All of the data we have discussed are based on the 500 injuries seen between 1983 and 1986. Another set of data was generated at the San Diego Kaiser Knee Injury Clinic for the 5-year period from mid-1981 through mid-1986. During that period there were 392 patients who met the following criteria:

1. acute hemarthrosis, examined within 2 weeks of injury;
2. no posterior sag and no Grade III MCL or LCL;
3. nothing by history or examination to suggest patella injury;
4. normal radiographs (except patients with minor avulsion fractures, who were included); and
5. no history of prior injury or surgery to either knee.

Of these patients, 113 were stable by KT-1000 at acute exam and later in follow-up. Thirty-three of these 113 stable knees had partial tears documented by arthroscopy. The remaining 279 were unstable by KT-1000 examination (right–left difference ≥3 mm) and were diagnosed as complete ACL tears. Two hundred thirty-two had their tears confirmed by arthroscopy, with 201 undergoing arthroscopy within 12 weeks of injury. Forty-seven had pathologic motion by KT-1000

TABLE 27-1. ***Acute ligament injuries with pathologic motion***[a]

Ligament injury				
ACL	MCL	PCL	LCL	Number
X				238 (48%)
	X			144 (29%)
		X		18 (4%)
			X	10 (2%)
X	X			64 (13%)
	X	X		8 (2%)
X			X	6 (1%)
		X	X	1
X		X		5 (1%)
X	X	X		4(1%)
X		X	X	1
X	X		X	1
Total: 319 (63%)	221 (44%)	37 (7%)	19 (4%)	500

[a] Study performed at San Diego Kaiser; n = 500; X = ligament injury with pathologic motion.

TABLE 27-2. Acute knee ligament injuries with pathologic motion: activity at time of injury[a]

Ligament injury	Activity at time of injury								Total
	Football	Baseball	Basketball	Soccer	Skiing	Other sports	Vehicle	Miscellaneous	
ACL single-ligament injury	27 (11%)	25 (11%)	19 (8%)	33 (14%)	23 (10%)	38 (16%)	15 (6%)	58 (24%)	238
MCL single-ligament injury	14 (10%)	16 (11%)	6 (4%)	10 (7%)	19 (13%)	13 (9%)	14 (10%)	52 (36%)	144
MCL–ACL combined injury	6 (9%)	1 (2%)	3 (5%)	9 (14%)	12 (19%)	8 (13%)	9 (14%)	16 (25%)	64
PCL injury (18 isolated, 19 combined)	1 (3%)	5 (14%)	2 (5%)	0	1 (3%)	6 (16%)	14 (38%)	8 (21%)	37
LCL injury (10 isolated, 7 combined)	0	3 (18%)	0	1 (6%)	1 (6%)	2 (12%)	1 (6%)	9 (53%)	17
Total:	48 (10%)	50 (10%)	30 (6%)	53 (11%)	56 (11%)	67 (13%)	53 (10%)	143 (29%)	500

[a] Study performed at San Diego Kaiser; $n = 500$.

TABLE 27-3. Acute knee ligament injuries with pathologic motion: activity-specific profile[a]

Activity	ACL	MCL	ACL–MCL	PCL isolated and combined	LCL isolated and combined	Total
Football	27 (56%)	14 (29%)	6 (13%)	1 (2%)	0	48
Baseball	25 (50%)	16 (32%)	1 (2%)	5 (10%)	3 (6%)	50
Basketball	19 (63%)	6 (20%)	3 (10%)	2 (7%)	0	30
Soccer	33 (62%)	10 (19%)	9 (17%)	0 (2%)	1	53
Skiing	23 (41%)	19 (34%)	12 (21%)	1 (2%)	1 (2%)	56
Vehicle	15 (28%)	14 (26%)	9 (17%)	14 (26%)	1 (2%)	53
Knee injury clinic	238 (48%)	144 (29%)	64 (13%)	37 (7%)	17 (3%)	500

[a] Study performed at San Diego Kaiser; $n = 500$.

TABLE 27-4. Acute knee ligament injuries with pathologic motion: age-specific profile[a]

Age (years)	ACL	MCL	ACL–MCL	PCL isolated and combined	LCL isolated and combined	Total
0–14	9 (53%)	4 (24%)	0 (0%)	3 (18%)	1 (6%)	17
15–29	135 (49%)	74 (27%)	34 (13%)	24 (9%)	7 (3%)	274
30–44	83 (47%)	55 (31%)	23 (13%)	10 (13%)	6 (3%)	177
>44	11 (34%)	11 (34%)	7 (22%)	0 (0%)	3 (9%)	32
Total:	238 (48%)	144 (29%)	64 (13%)	37 (7%)	17 (3%)	500

[a] Study performed at San Diego Kaiser; $n = 500$.

on initial examination and follow-up, but they did not undergo arthroscopy.

Of these unstable ACL injuries, 68% occurred in males and 32% occurred in females. Thus, breakdown by sex is similar to that found in the 500 total ligament injuries (72% male, 28% female) analyzed above. Fifty-five (20%) of these patients had sustained Grade II collateral ligament injuries: 47 (17%) medial and 8 (3%) lateral. The age range of the patients was 13–60. Age distribution was as follows: 12 patients were younger than age 15 (4%), 177 patients were age 15–29 (63%), 78 patients were age 30–44 (28%), and 12 patients were age 44 or above (6%). Although the criteria for inclusion in these two San Diego Kaiser studies were different, comparison of the data with that in Table 27-4 shows that the similarity of the age pattern is striking.

In the group of 279 patients with documented ACL tears, 44 (16%) were injured in football, 31 (11%) in baseball, 25 (9%) in basketball, 38 (14%) in soccer, 41 (15%) in skiing, 29 (10%) in other sports, 29 (10%) in vehicular accidents, and 42 (15%) in other ways. Again, direct comparison with the 500 patients in the 3-year study is not entirely appropriate because of the different selection criteria, but a glance at Table 27-2 reveals that the sport distribution is similar.

THE ACL-INJURED KNEE

Introduction

Having examined the incidence of knee ligament injuries with pathologic motion, let us see what we know of the outcome of these injuries. The ideal natural history study of any specific acute knee ligament injury would identify all the patients who sustained this injury within the study group. It would document definitively the presence of this injury and definitively exclude or subcategorize patients with additional injuries (including other ligament injuries, fractures, chondral injuries, and meniscal injuries). It would follow these patients over a long time without intervention and finally definitively assess the status of all these patients objectively, subjectively, and functionally at the conclusion. Of course, no such study has been done, but it may be surprising to see how far we are from the ideal, while at the same time looking to see what we can reasonably conclude from the data that we actually possess.

Interest in the outcome of ACL injuries dates back at least to Stark's paper (53) on cruciate ligament injuries treated by bracing, published in 1850. After World War II, O'Donoghue (45) emphasized study of knee ligament injuries. He pointed out poor results in patients with unrepaired ACLs and contrasted these patients with his operative results. He did not provide

systematic follow-up of an unselected group of non-operatively treated patients. O'Donoghue reported degenerative changes in the knees of dogs who underwent experimental section of the ACL. Marshall (36) reported similar results in dogs. These results are interesting but difficult to extrapolate to the human knee because gait, weight-bearing, physical activity, and physiologic aging are so different between species.

In 1965, Liljedahl (33) again gave anecdotal reports of poor results including osteoarthritis in patients where ACL lesions were untreated. Jacobsen (25) reported observing articular cartilage damage in over half of the knees of patients who had sustained ACL injuries at least 6 months before the time of arthrotomy. Of course, only symptomatic patients underwent arthrotomy. Liljedahl did point out, however, that almost half of the patients with chondral changes had intact menisci, suggesting that ligamentous laxity alone could lead to joint dysfunction. He did not, however, exclude collateral ligament injuries in his study group.

In a classic paper published in 1976, Feagin (13) reported the 5-year follow-up of 32 West Point cadets who had sustained "isolated" ACL injuries. All of the patients underwent surgical repair of the ligament. The results of surgery were so poor that Feagin regarded the data as "similar to the natural history of the unrepaired ACL," though he did not furnish any natural history data. Of the 32 patients, 17 had sustained significant reinjury within 5 years, 12 requiring reoperation. Ten of these 12 had medial meniscus tears, and one had a lateral meniscus tear. Twenty-four of the 32 were impaired in athletic endeavors, and 12 had impairment in "ordinary" activities. If this did approximate natural history data, the prognosis appeared poor, but the assertion that the prognosis of a knee with a failed operation is identical to the prognosis of an unoperated knee is open to question.

Youmans (58) made the well-known assertion about ACL injury that "in the case of a skilled athlete, it may well be the beginning of the end of his career," although he provided little data to directly substantiate it. In the same year, Chick (2) presented a much more optimistic assessment of the prognosis of ACL injury. He studied 30 patients with "minimum to mild anterior instability." His patients were competitive athletes less than 30 years old whose ACL tear was confirmed at the time of meniscectomy. Eighty-three percent returned to full activity with mean follow-up of 2.6 years, although 20% had intermittent effusion, 33% experienced occasional "slipping of the knee" during sports, and 56% had some radiographic changes on follow-up x-rays. The question of whether ACL-deficient patients who have less "instability" or pathologic motion have a better prognosis than those with more motion has never been answered by a direct prospective comparison with matched groups, but Chick's paper suggested that this might be true.

The Acute Knee Hemarthrosis

Following up on the lead of Gillquist's study (18) entitled "Arthroscopy in Acute Injuries of the Knee Joint," published in 1977, in 1980 DeHaven (9) published an article that furnished important data for the analyses of papers on the natural history of ACL injuries. De Haven reported the results of arthroscopies on 113 consecutive athletes who had sustained "significant acute trauma to the knee with immediate disability and the early onset of hemarthrosis but who did not have demonstrable clinical laxity." In many cases, standard clinical tests could not be performed because of pain and splinting. All patients were arthroscoped within 21 days of injury. ACL injuries were found in 81 (72%). In 68 cases, these ACL lesions were judged to be acute. Of these 68 cases, 44 (65%) had "significant" meniscal tears (Table 27-5).

These data suggested that in many cases, isolated ACL tears (single ligament injuries) are accompanied by acute meniscal tears. The "natural history" of the ACL-deficient knee is probably significantly influenced by the presence or absence of meniscal pathology and by the treatment of that pathology. Ideal studies would document the status of the menisci in the acute phase of the injury so that the long-term outcome could be ascribed to ACL injury alone and/or ACL injury with treated or untreated meniscal injury. Such studies could be used to counsel patients in whom the presence or absence of acute meniscal tears with the ACL tears was known from arthroscopy or magnetic resonance imaging.

In 1980 Noyes (40) also published an article on the results of arthroscopy of the knee in patients with acute hemarthrosis and "absent or negligible instability on clinical examination" in the office. As in DeHaven's study, all patients underwent arthroscopy within 3 weeks of injury. In contrast to DeHaven, however, Noyes excluded patients who were found to have chronic ACL injuries. Of 85 patients, 61 (72%) had complete or partial ACL tears. Of these 61, 38 (62%) had meniscal tears, 13 (21%) medial only, 23 (38%) lateral only, and two (3%) medial and lateral. These findings are in substantial agreement with those of DeHaven (Table 27-5). In the group with ACL injuries, Noyes noted six (12%) with femoral chondral fractures and six (10%) with "significant fibrillation" of the chondral surface, usually on the lateral side. These acute chondral lesions may affect the long-term prognosis of ACL-injured knees. The ideal natural history study would determine the presence or absence of such chondral lesions as well as meniscal injuries in the acute phase so that the specific implications of chondral lesions could be determined in the setting of isolated ACL injuries with or without meniscal tears.

Function and Arthritis After ACL Disruption

Fetto (16) published a paper in 1980 entitled "The Natural History and Diagnosis of Anterior Cruciate Ligament Insufficiency." Fetto quoted Ivar Palmer, who had stated that "the critical study still remained to be done, i.e., a prospective analysis of anterior cruciate insufficiency and its sequelae." Fetto concluded from his study that the ACL-deficient knee without surgical treatment "appears to invariably embark upon a course of progressive deterioration and dysfunction."

TABLE 27-5. *Meniscal injuries accompanying ACL tears*

Study	Knees studied	Percentage with any meniscus tear	Percentage with medial meniscus tear only	Percentage with lateral meniscus tear only	Percentage with medial and lateral meniscus tear	Total percentage with medial meniscus tear	Total percentage with lateral meniscus tear
Acute ACLS							
DeHaven (9)	68	65	13	34	18	31	52
Noyes (40)	61	62	21	38	3	24	41
Woods (57)	99	45	18	20	7	25	27
Indelicato (23)	44	68	36	9	10	46	19
Total acute ACLs							
(four studies):	272	58	21	26	11	32	37
Chronic ACLS							
Woods (57)	122	88	48	17	23	71	40
Indelicato (23)	56	91	55	11	25	80	36
Fowler (17)	51	72	35	35	2	37	37
Total chronic ACLs							
(four studies):	229	84	48	21	17	65	38

Unfortunately, Fetto's study did not closely approximate Palmer's ideal "critical study." Seventy-one percent of the patients presented for treatment more than 2 weeks after injury, strongly suggesting potential bias toward symptomatic cases. Of 223 patients with ACL tears, 148 (66%) had additional ligament injuries and an unknown number had sustained meniscal or chondral lesions. Forty-seven patients underwent early ligament surgery and 83 underwent reconstruction at an average of 32 months (6–84) post-injury. The average duration of follow-up on the nonoperative patients was only 22 months (6–132) post-injury. The criteria used to select patients for early or late surgery were not specified.

Nevertheless, it was striking that by 5 years post-injury, only 15% of the unoperated knees with isolated or combined ACL ligament injuries rated better than poor on the Hospital for Special Surgery knee score, especially when the same authors reported 82% good to excellent results and only 4% poor results in MCL injuries (Grades I–III). The results of isolated ACL injuries were alleged to be "approximately equal in end-stage total scores" to the results of combined ligament injuries. Details of the follow-up evaluations, however, were scantily reported in this paper.

Also in 1980, McDaniel (37) reported a more favorable prognosis in "Untreated Ruptures of the Anterior Cruciate Ligament. A Follow-up Study." McDaniel sought to remedy some of the deficiencies of earlier studies such as short follow-up, inclusion of associated ligament injuries, and extrapolations from animal or cadaver studies. His data, however, were still based on a retrospective review and were therefore subject to unintended case selection and bias. ACL lesions were noted at arthrotomy, which was usually performed for meniscectomy. Thus, 43 of the 53 knees studied underwent meniscectomy when they entered the study, and only patients with symptoms severe enough to warrant arthrotomy could enter the study. The majority of patients entered the study more than 3 months after the index injury.

One of the main points of this paper was that 72% of the patients returned to strenuous sports "at levels ranging from weekend recreational sports to college football and professional baseball." The positive impression that this gives, however, is qualified by the fact that few details were provided. McDaniel did not give details about which sports the patients played, level of participation, or the level of symptoms the patients experienced while they played. The average follow-up score on the Hospital for Special Surgery knee score was 37.8, rating a fair-plus. There was one excellent result (2%), 10 good (19%), 24 fair-plus (45%), 16 fair-minus (30%), and two poor (4%). Seventy-three percent had a sense of discomfort, 58% had swelling, 56% experienced weakness, and 43% had giv-

ing way with unspecified activity; moreover, 68% had x-ray abnormalities, although only 6% had "frank osteoarthritis." This suggests that the results were not as drastically different from Fetto's as the papers' abstracts might suggest.

Many of McDaniel's patients entered the study at the time of meniscectomy, but eight additional meniscectomies were performed at subsequent surgeries and only eight patients (15%) had both menisci at follow-up. The series clearly reported primarily on the long-term results of ACL-deficient knees that had undergone meniscectomy. In 1983, McDaniel (38) reported further follow-up on all but one of the patients he presented in 1980. The average age of the patients was now 33, with follow-up averaging 14 years after injury and 11 years after index arthrotomy. There had been little change in symptoms, sports participation, or function, but x-ray changes had progressed, especially in the compartments that had undergone meniscectomy.

In 1983 Giove (19) reported the results obtained by treating 24 patients with ACL tears by a rehabilitation program emphasizing the hamstrings. "All patients returned to some sports participation, with 14 (59%) returning to their full preinjury level of participation." The patients were selected randomly from a retrospective analysis of hospital records, follow-up averaging 44 months. The instabilities were apparently mild in comparison to most ACL studies in that only five patients (21%) had a positive pivot shift test. Giove suggested that involuntary guarding augmented by hamstring training may have reduced the percentage with positive pivot shifts. Of the 14 patients who returned to preinjury sports participation, only three had no symptoms, whereas 11 had occasional or recurring mild discomfort, swelling, or instability. Eight patients had to reduce sports participation, whereas two returned to only "minimum participation." In this analysis, all sports were treated as a group, but Giove noted that patients who participated in sports such as football, volleyball, basketball, and racquetball did not do nearly as well as those who participated in swimming, golf, bicycling, and running. Thus a more detailed look at Giove's results shows that ACL tears often caused significant signs and symptoms in patients who play cutting and jumping sports.

Noyes published two papers in 1983 dealing with the ACL-deficient knee. The first paper (41) reported on functional disability in 103 *symptomatic* patients with ACL injuries who were evaluated an average of 5.5 years after injury. Patients with significant collateral ligament injuries were excluded. Most patients had continued to participate in vigorous sports, but none "had proper initial treatment, rehabilitation, or counseling." Noyes pointed out that this group of ACL-injured patients would be expected to have the poorest prognosis. Eighty-five patients (83%) returned to sports after injury, but 53 of these subjects (62%) sustained a significant reinjury within 1 year of the index injury. Only 36 patients (35% of the total group) were participating in strenuous sports at 5-year follow-up, and only 11 had no limitations. These numbers are not much worse than Giove's, despite the fact that Noyes stressed the ominous prognosis while Giove emphasized positive outcomes. This contrast illustrates the importance that the author's perspective plays in his assessment of his results. As in all areas of science, especially controversial ones, the reader must analyze the data carefully himself instead of relying entirely on the author's conclusions.

Of Noyes' patients, 32 (31%) reported moderate to severe disability in walking, 45 (44%) in activities of daily living, and 77 (75%) in turning and twisting sports. Of 103 patients, 51 (50%) had undergone meniscectomy, 41 (40%) having had both medial and lateral menisci removed. These meniscectomized patients had a two- to fourfold increase of symptoms of pain and swelling with activity. Of the patients followed more than 5 years after injury, 43% showed moderate to severe osteoarthritic changes on x-ray. Surprisingly, no statistically significant correlation could be demonstrated between x-ray findings and the presence or absence of meniscectomy, although many of the changes "by Fairbank criteria could be ascribed to meniscectomy." Noyes speculated that some of the patients with pain and swelling may have had meniscal tears that had not come to meniscectomy. These meniscal tears themselves may have contributed to Fairbank changes, making it more difficult to establish a statistically significant effect of meniscectomy.

In the second paper (42) of this series, Noyes reported the results of placing 84 patients with symptomatic ACL-deficient knees on a program of rehabilitation, bracing, and activity modification. About one-third of these patients improved so that they had minimal or no symptoms with activities of daily living or light recreational activities. Most of these patients still had symptoms, especially during strenuous sports. Only 9% returned to full competitive athletics. About one-third of the patients were unchanged despite the program, and one-third worsened during it. Noyes could not predict which patients would improve on his program. He reported that statistical analysis showed that those who had giving way, even only two or three times per year, were at significant risk of developing arthritic changes, although he did not furnish the data that substantiated this assertion. He also enunciated his famous "rule of thirds" for ACL injuries: "One-third of the patients with this injury will compensate adequately and be able to pursue recreational activities, one-third will be able to compensate but will have to give up significant activities, and one-third will do poorly and will probably require future reconstructive surgery." A tabulation of papers reporting sports function after nonoperative treatment of ACL tears is presented in Table 27-6, and symptoms in chronic ACL patients during activities of daily living are presented in Table 27-7.

Lynch (35) published a paper in 1983 which had interesting implications regarding the significance of meniscal injuries in the prognosis of ACL-injured patients. Unfortunately for our purposes, her study group consisted of patients who had undergone successful surgical stabilization of ACL injuries. She analyzed pain and Fairbank's changes at a mean follow-up of 3.8 years after surgery. Patients were divided into groups consisting of those with no meniscal tear, those with a tear that had been "left alone," those with a tear that had been repaired, and those who had undergone partial or total meniscectomy. In this group of

TABLE 27-6. *Sports activity in patients with nonoperative treatment of isolated ACL injuries*

Author	Sports participation	Remarks
Chick (2)	83% "full athletic activity"	Excluded patients with moderate or severe anterior instability
McDaniel (37)	73% in some "strenuous sports"; in 42%, the knee did not restrict or limit any sports activity	Little detail on sports functions
Giove (19)	59% returned to "full preinjury level of participation, but only 13% had "no significant signs or symptoms"	Patients involved in "heavy participation" sports did less well
Noyes (41)	35% in strenuous sports, but only 11% without limitation	Only symptomatic patients were included in this study
Walla (56)	42% in high-intensity sports with limitations; 14% in same sports at same level	
Satku (50)	46% play preinjury sports	Few details about sports
Fowler (17)	22% in pivoting sports activity moderation; 17% uninhibited in pivoting sports	All patients were symptomatic
San Diego Kaiser	53% playing reinjury sport; 31% playing the sport without hindrance	

TABLE 27-7. *Pain, swelling, and giving way in chronic ACL patients during activities of daily living*

Author	Number of patients	Pain—more than mild or infrequent	Swelling—more than infrequent	Giving way	Years of average follow-up	Remarks
McDaniel (37)	49	38%	10%	Not reported for ACL	14	
Noyes (41)	103	30%	14%	21%	5.5	Selected population of "worst cases"
Hawkins (20)	40	18%	18%	11%	4	30% who underwent reconstruction not included
San Diego Kaiser	34	0%	0%	9%	5	

stabilized patients, pain and Fairbank's changes were very infrequent in those who had not injured their menisci. The patients who had undergone meniscal repair did almost as well. Those with tears that had been "left alone" had a high incidence of pain but only a moderate incidence of Fairbanks's changes, whereas those who had undergone partial or total meniscectomy had much less pain but a much higher incidence of Fairbank's changes. No similar study of patients with unreconstructed ACLs has been done, although such a study would allow us to differentiate more clearly between the long-term prognosis of an "isolated" ACL injury without meniscal damage and the "isolated" ACL injury with meniscal pathology.

Table 27-8 presents data on radiographic changes in chronic ACL patients. Papers with follow-up of 5 years or more report that a high percentage of ACL patients show radiographic changes. Changes judged to be of at least moderate severity are not uncommon. Authors such as Satku (50) and Fowler (17) reported that x-ray changes correlate with meniscal injury or meniscal surgery, but others such as Giove (19) and Noyes (41) did not corroborate this. Several authors, such as Satku (50) and Walla (56), showed that changes were more severe in those patients who were followed for longer intervals. No study provided the 30- or 40-year follow-up desirable in studying potential degenerative changes caused by injuries in young patients.

In 1984, Jokl (27) reported on the results of nonoperative treatment of 28 patients with combined severe ACL and MCL injuries. His study reported better outcomes after the combined injury than most other studies report after isolated ACL injury. The follow-up in this paper was particularly short, averaging 3

TABLE 27-8. *Radiographic changes in patients with nonoperative treatment of isolated ACL injuries*

Author	X-ray changes	Years of average follow-up	Remarks
Chick (2)	50% mild changes	2.6	All patients had index meniscectomy
McDaniel (37)	56% flattening or squaring of femoral condyles; 24% joint space narrowing; 10% "frank osteoarthritis"; 14% normal	14	When they entered study, all had arthrotomy and most had meniscectomy
Giove (19)	59% "variable degenerative changes" vs. 32% changes in uninvolved knee; meniscectomized knees no worse than others	3.7	41% had meniscectomy
Noyes (41)	25% minimum arthritis; 21% moderate or severe arthritis; 54% normal (44% of patients followed more than 5 years had moderate or severe changes)	5.5	Only symptomatic patients included; all athletes; 50% had meniscectomy
Walla (56)	39% moderate or severe changes; 26% normal (66% with more than 5 years follow-up showed moderate or severe changes)	5.6	All former athletes; 61% had meniscectomy
Hawkins (20)	43% mild to moderate changes	4	20% had meniscectomy
Satku (50)	44% mild changes; 38% moderate to severe changes; 18% normal	6	58% had meniscectomy
Fowler (17)	21% degenerative changes	5.8	72% had meniscectomy

years, with 13 patients (46%) having follow-up of less than 2 years. Previous papers, such as those of Noyes, suggest that results may deteriorate with a few years more follow-up.

Nevertheless, the reported results are striking. Eleven of 15 (73%) patients returned to contact sports, although Jokl did not give details about any signs or symptoms that might accompany participation. Nineteen of 28 (68%) returned to preinjury sports activity. Twenty (71%) rated good or excellent on the Hospital for Special Surgery knee assessment, 5 (18%) rated fair-plus, and 3 (11%) rated fair-minus. Although the authors stated that "our study revealed results much the same as those of McDaniel," McDaniel reported only 21% good to excellent, 45% fair-plus, 30% fair-minus, and 4% poor results. This difference is even more striking because MCL instability can cause a loss of up to five points on the 50-point assessment. While McDaniel excluded patients with collateral ligament injuries, all of Jokl's patients had acute Grade III MCL sprains. Part of the difference between the results of Jokl's series and those of McDaniel's series may be due to the fact that all of Jokl's patients were seen on the day of injury, so that there was no bias toward selecting symptomatic patients. In addition, Jokl excluded patients with "mechanical locking of the knee because of torn meniscus," so that he had no initial meniscectomies and only four (14%) during follow-up; in McDaniel's series, however, 43 meniscectomies were performed on 53 patients at the index operation, and still eight more (15%) were required during the study.

In 1985, Walla (56) reported a retrospective study of 38 former athletes who had torn their ACLs at least 2 years prior to evaluation (mean 5.6 years). All had positive Lachman and pivot shift tests. None had medial or lateral laxity, and none had undergone ligament reconstruction, although 61% had undergone a meniscectomy. Walla felt that the patients had "progressed quite well," but, as we have previously seen, that is a subjective evaluation. Thirty-one (82%) had sustained a significant reinjury, most within a year of the index injury. Only 12 (32%) could participate in vigorous sports without pain, swelling, or instability. Moderate or severe radiographic changes were present in five (22%) of 23 patients injured less than 5 years prior to study and in 10 (67%) of 15 injured more than 5 years prior. These radiographic changes were reported to be more frequent in patients who had undergone meniscectomy, but data on patients who had not undergone meniscectomy were not provided.

In 1986, Hawkins (20) reported a retrospective analysis of 40 patients with isolated ACL injuries. The mean age at the time of injury was 22, and 17 of the 40 patients were less than 20 years old. Follow-up was greater than 2 years for all patients and averaged 4

years. All patients were seen because of the initial injury, not because of continued symptoms, and all were seen within 4 weeks of injury. Twenty-five patients had arthroscopically proven complete ACL tears, whereas 15 were considered to have tears on the basis of positive pivot shift tests. Four (16%) of the 25 patients who underwent arthroscopy also had meniscal tears and underwent meniscectomy. The ACL injuries were treated with physical therapy and bracing, although most patients did not use their braces.

The follow-up picture was "somewhat grim." Twelve (30%) required late reconstruction because of "giving way." Of the 28 patients who did not undergo ACL reconstruction, 24 (86%) experienced "giving way" and restricted their activities to minimize their symptoms. Only four patients (10%) were able to resume the same level of sports without reconstructive surgery. Hawkins developed and described an "arbitrary rating system" incorporating objective and subjective factors. On this scale, there were no excellent ACL-injured knees, five (12.5%) good knees, 23 (57.5%) fair knees, and 12 (30%) poor knees.

In 1986, Satku (50) followed a group of ACL-injured patients for 6 years with the aim of trying to define "patients in whom current and potential disability outweighed the risks of surgery." In these patients, rupture of the ACL was said to be their "predominant injury," but other pathology was not specifically excluded. Satku reported that 55 patients (63%) were able to return to preinjury sports after injury, including four of the patients with bilateral ACL deficiency. By the time of follow-up (2–11 years, average 6 years), however, only 40 of these 55 were still able to participate in sports. Sixteen of 38 knees (42%) examined less than 5 years after injury had undergone meniscectomy, while 40 of 59 knees (68%) examined more than 5 years after injury had undergone meniscectomy. He thus implied significant ongoing risks of meniscal injury even several years after ACL injury.

Satku obtained follow-up radiographs of 49 of the 59 knees he followed for more than 5 years. Thirty-five of these knees had undergone meniscectomy and five others were said to have clinical signs and symptoms of meniscal injury. Of these 40 knees, 19 (48%) had moderate or severe radiographic "deterioration," whereas none of the nine patients without evidence of meniscal pathology showed such changes. The "signs and symptoms" said to imply meniscal injury are not specified and could overlap those of post-traumatic arthritis. Nevertheless, there is a strong implication, as in Lynch's paper (35), that much of the degenerative effect of ACL injury is mediated by meniscal injury. Lynch correlated degenerative changes in patients who had undergone successful ACL reconstruction with meniscal injury and surgery. Satku suggested a similar correlation in patients whose ACLs had not

TABLE 27-9. *Percentage of meniscus lesions that were judged to be reparable in ACL-injured knees*

Author	Number of acute ACL patients	Percentage of meniscal tears reparable	Number of chronic ACL patients	Percentage of meniscal tears reparable
Woods (57)	99	50	122	27
Indelicato (23)	44	65	56	57
San Diego Kaiser	68[a]	17	73[b]	56

[a] An additional 27 meniscus lesions "left alone."
[b] An additional 18 meniscus lesions "left alone."

been reconstructed. In addition, Satku hypothesized that much of the functional deterioration in terms of sports participation which he observed could have been due to meniscal injuries and their long-term degenerative effects.

In 1987, Fowler (17) reported the results of meniscal arthroscopic surgery and rehabilitation in the treatment of patients with symptomatic chronic ACL insufficiency. He stressed that all the patients were symptomatic, so that this paper did not attempt to define the natural history of *all* ACL-injured patients. He excluded patients with "associated primary collateral or PCL damage." All patients underwent arthroscopic treatment at an average of 4.26 years after injury (range 6 months to 37 years). He found 37 of 51 knees (73%) had meniscal damage. Nine patients (18%) had a "full, uninhibited return to pivoting sports, though only five returned to their preinjury level of competition." Eleven (22%) returned to "pivoting sports" with some modification of activity and awareness of their pathology. Thirteen (25%) returned to athletics, excluding pivoting sports; 18 (35%) stopped all athletics. Four chose to undergo ACL reconstruction, and four others were considering surgery.

The Incidence of Meniscus Tears and Chondral Lesions

Woods (57) reported a prospective study of 234 consecutive patients with positive Lachman tests and "either an acute hemarthrosis or continued complaints of pain, effusion, or giving way following an acute injury. All were examined under anesthesia and by arthroscopy. Patients with collateral ligament injuries were *not* excluded. Meniscus tears were found in 44 of 99 acute cases (45%), 11 of 13 subacute cases and 107 of 122 chronic cases (88%). Table 27-5 presents the results obtained by pooling the series of acute ACL injuries reported by DeHaven (9), Noyes (40), Woods (57), and Indelicato (24), although the criteria each author used to select eligible patients were slightly different. Of the combined total of 272 patients, 58% had meniscal tears. At the time of the acute arthroscopy,

roughly one-third of the patients had torn lateral menisci. One-ninth had torn both menisci. Comparing the chronic to the acute knees we can see that 84% of the chronic cases had meniscal tears, while 58% of the acute cases had tears. Sixty-three percent of the chronic cases had torn medial menisci as compared to 32% of the acute cases, whereas the percentage with torn lateral menisci was just less than 40% in both chronic and acute cases. All suspected acute ACL tears underwent arthroscopy, but patients with chronic ACL tears underwent arthroscopy only if they were symptomatic. Therefore we can say that patients with chronic ACL tears who are symptomatic appear to have medial meniscal tears much more often than do patients with acute tears. These additional meniscal tears could contribute to the degenerative changes seen in some knees with chronic ACL injuries.

Both Indelicato and Woods emphasized that many of the meniscal tears in the ACL-injured knees were potentially reparable. Woods reported 50% of acute tears, whereas Indelicato reported 65%. The incidence of surgically repaired acute meniscus tears in the San Diego Kaiser series was less than that reported by Woods and Indelicato, whereas the rate of repair in chronics was higher (Table 27-9). More of the medial meniscus tears were judged to be reparable than lateral meniscus tears (Table 27-10).

Chondral changes in the ACL-disrupted knee are presented in Table 27-11. Indelicato noted that 10 (23%) of the acute cases demonstrated chondral fractures of the femoral condyles with "free fragments of articular cartilage." Noyes had reported 20%. Indelicato noted "significant articular changes" in 30 (54%) of his chronic cases, whereas DeHaven used the same

TABLE 27-10. *Meniscal tears judged to be reparable in chronic ACL-injured knees*

Author	Medial	Lateral	Total
Woods (57)	31/86 (36%)	6/49 (12%)	37/135 (27%)
Indelicato (23)	31/45 (69%)	6/20 (30%)	37/65 (57%)
San Diego Kaiser	41/71 (58%)	0/2 (0%)	41/73 (56%)

TABLE 27-11. *Chondral changes in ACL-injured knees noted at arthroscopy*

Author	Number of acute ACL patients	Chondral changes (%)	Number of chronic ACL patients	Chondral changes (%)
Noyes (40)	61	20	—	—
DeHaven (9)	—	—	13	69
Indelicato (23)	44	23	56	54
Fowler (17)	—	—	51	22
San Diego Kaiser	201	18	145	54
Total:	306	19	252	47

phrase to describe 9 (69%) of the 13 cases of chronic ACL tears with acute hemarthrosis which he arthroscoped. Again it must be noted that only symptomatic chronic ACL cases underwent arthroscopy, so that the numbers we have for the incidence of "significant articular changes" in chronic ACL cases probably are higher than they would be if all chronic ACL cases were arthroscoped in a prospective, randomized study. The pooled data indicate that the incidence of chondral changes in the chronic population was more than twice the incidence in the acute population. Table 27-12 presents the incidence of chondral lesions by compartment in two studies. Lateral compartment damage was less frequent than damage in the medial and patellofemoral compartments. In examining all the data, however, it is essential to remember that we only have data on those chronic patients whose symptoms were felt to justify arthroscopy or ACL reconstruction.

There are two patient populations from the San Diego Kaiser study that include the incidence of associated meniscal and chondral damage associated with an ACL injury. The first is the study of 279 acute ACL disruptions cited earlier in this chapter. Two hundred one of those patients underwent arthroscopic examination within 12 weeks of injury. Fifty-three percent of the patients in that group had meniscus pathology (Table 27-13). Longitudinal tears greater than 1 cm in length within 4 mm of the periphery were repaired. Other meniscus tears that were judged unstable were excised. Tears that were felt to be stable were left alone. The incidence of meniscus tears is similar to those reported by other authors cited in Table 27-5. Other authors do not report the number of meniscus

tears that were left alone. In the San Diego Kaiser study, 22% of patients had tears that were left alone, while 31% with tears underwent excision or repair. In other words, only 58% of the tears required surgery. Chondral lesions were noted in 18% of patients.

Of the 279 patients with an acute ACL tear in the San Diego Kaiser study, 55 had an acute ACL reconstruction. Fifty-nine of the remaining 224 patients had at least one operation for care of their chronic condition. The follow-up of this group was 2–7 years, with a mean of 4 years. Fifty of the 59 patients had a late surgery within 24 months of injury. The surgical procedures they underwent are listed in Table 27-14. Note that 41 of the 59 patients had meniscus surgery. The incidence of patients requiring later surgery was twice as great for patients who were initially injured as a teenager when compared to those who were 20 or older at the time of their initial injury. Fifty of the 59 patients who had late surgery had been arthroscoped at the time of the initial injury. Twenty of the 41 patients who had meniscus surgery at the later operation had no meniscus pathology at the time of the acute arthroscopy.

The second San Diego Kaiser population for which data are available regarding meniscal and chondral lesions in ACL patients is derived from a separate review of 346 ACL reconstructions performed between 1982 and 1988. One hundred two reconstructions were performed within 3 months of injury, 99 were performed between 4 and 12 months of injury, and 145 were performed more than 12 months after injury (mean 3 years, range 1–19 years). The findings in the patients operated on more than 12 months after injury are presented in Table 27-11 as chronic cases. The incidence of meniscus tears, meniscus repairs, and chondral changes is higher in those undergoing ACL reconstruction than in those with an acute ACL disruption. Forty-seven of the 145 patients had surgery greater than 2 years after injury. In this group of patients, 87% had meniscus pathology and 64% had chondral lesions. This sample of chronic ACL patients is clearly biased, since all of these patients had symptoms warranting reconstruction.

San Diego Kaiser ACL Follow-up Study

The San Diego Kaiser study also provides information about the long-term outcome of ACL injury in a small

TABLE 27-12. *Chondral damage in chronic ACL-injured knees*

Author	Cases	Percentage of Chondromalacia patellae	Percentage of Medial compartment damage	Percentage of Lateral compartment damage
Fowler (17)	51	24	16	7
San Diego Kaiser	145	24	37	16
Total:	196	24	32	14

TABLE 27-13. *San Diego Kaiser Review*

	Acute ACL[a]		Chronic ACL[b]	
	n	Percent	n	Percent
Number evaluated	201		145	
Any meniscus pathology	107	53	108	76
Medial meniscus pathology	50	25	107	75
Lateral meniscus pathology	77	38	12	8
Medial and lateral meniscus pathology	20	10	10	7
Meniscus pathology, no surgery	45	22	37	12
Prior medial meniscus surgery	0	0	22	14
Prior lateral meniscus surgery	0	0	4	3
Medial meniscus tear, no surgery	27	13	14	8
Lateral meniscus tear, no surgery	32	16	6	4
Any meniscus surgery	62	31	71	49
Medial meniscus repair	9	5	41	29
Medial meniscus partial excision	14	7	26	18
Medial meniscus complete excision	0	0	4	3
Lateral meniscus repair	2	1	0	0
Lateral meniscus partial excision	42	21	2	2
Lateral meniscus complete excision	1	0.5	0	0
Any chondral changes	37	18	68	47
Patellar change	15	8	32	22
Medial compartment changes	14	7	52	36
Lateral compartment changes	10	5	23	16
Prior meniscus surgery		0		17
Prior medial meniscus surgery		0		14
Prior lateral meniscus surgery		0		3

[a] Clinical examination within 14 days of injury. Arthroscopy within 12 weeks of injury.
[b] Arthroscopic examination at the time of ACL reconstruction surgery, which was more than 12 months after injury.

group of nonrandomly selected patients. Of the 279 patients with "isolated" ACL injury which we have discussed several times, 55 (20%) underwent acute reconstruction at the discretion of the patient and surgeon. Of the remaining 224 patients, 41 (18%) subsequently underwent reconstruction because of chronic symptoms. Of the remaining 183 patients, 51 were 5

or more years post-injury at the time of evaluation in 1988. Thirty-four (67%) of these 51 were available for study. None of these patients had chosen to undergo reconstruction, so on the average they presumably represent a group with less-than-average disability. Although braces were prescribed for all, 29 (85%) never used them. Thirteen (38%) reported that they never

TABLE 27-14. *Acute ACL injuries not reconstructed within 3 months of injury[a]*

	Age (years)						Total	
	<20		20–29		>29			
	n	Percent	n	Percent	n	Percent	n	Percent
Patients								
Cohort	69		78		77		224	
Patients having surgery	28	41	16	21	15	19	59[b]	26
ACL reconstructions	24	35	9	12	8	10	41	18
Without meniscus surgery	4	6	6	8	2	3	12	5
With meniscus repair	9	13	1	1	1	1	11	5
With meniscus excision	11	16	2	3	5	6	18	8
Meniscus surgery	21	30	8	10	12	16	41	18
Repair	12	17	6	8	11	14	29	13
Excision	9	13	2	3	1	1	12	5
Diagnostic arthroscopy only	3	4	2	3	1	1	6	3

[a] San Diego Kaiser follow-up study; follow-up period 2–7 years, mean 4 years. Surgical procedures were performed more than 3 months after injury; 50 of the procedures were performed within 24 months of injury.
[b] Fifty of the 59 patients had a previous arthroscopy within 3 months of injury.

TABLE 27-15. *Specific task performance (percentage) in ACL-disrupted patients, 5 years since injury*[a]

Task	No problem	Mild impair-ment	Moderate impair-ment	Unable to do
Getting out of chair	100	0	0	0
Prolonged standing	76	21	3	0
Walking	94	6	0	0
Walking on uneven ground	65	35	0	0
Ascending stairs	85	15	0	0
Descending stairs	88	12	0	0
Climbing	71	29	0	0
Kneeling or squatting	56	44	0	0
Jogging	71	23	0	6
Running fast	63	19	6	12
Jumping	66	22	3	9
Twisting or pivoting	53	35	3	9
Cutting	50	29	3	18

[a] Study performed at San Diego Kaiser; $n = 34$.

had knee pain, 21 (62%) had occasional pain, and none had continuous pain. Pain was mild in 14, moderate in six, and severe in one. Twenty-eight (82%) never had swelling, whereas six had infrequent swelling. Three (9%) had reported giving way with activities of daily living, whereas five (15%) had giving way with sports. Their ability to perform 13 specific tasks is listed in Table 27-15. Clearly, many of these patients experienced significant disability. Nine (26%) of the San Diego Kaiser patients reinjured the ACL-deficient knee.

Five (15%) had a negative pivot shift, 15 (44%) were 1+, 12 (35%) were 2+, and none were 3+. In two patients (6%), guarding made the test impossible to evaluate. Thirty-one patients (91%) had no effusion at the time of examination, three (9%) had a slight effusion, and none had a larger effusion. The mean side-to-side difference on the 20-lb pull with the KT-1000 was 2.9 mm. On the manual maximum, the side-to-side difference averaged 5.9 mm. In terms of objective function, utilizing the tests described in Chapter 29, 26 of 34 (76%) had a hop index of ≥90, while 27 (93%) of 29 tested had a quadriceps index of ≥80%.

The sports participation of these patients was documented in detail. Patients were asked to report their hours of sports participation by sport prior to injury and at the time of follow-up. The two sports to which they devoted the most time were ranked by hours of participation as first sport and second sport. Participation of less than 50 hours per year was considered

nonparticipation. Sports were classified as low, moderate, or high risk (see Chapter 29).

Prior to injury, 20 (59%) of the patients participated in a high-risk sport as their first sport, and only six (18%) did not participate in any sport at least 50 hours per year. At follow-up, only eight (24%) patients participated in a high-risk sport as their first sport, and 13 (38%) did not participate in any sport. Mean total hours of participation in their two favorite sports dropped from 279 hours per year prior to injury to 166 hours per year at follow-up.

Of the 32 patients who participated in sports, 17 (53%) still participated in their first sport. Five (16%) were afraid to compete, and eight (25%) had given up the sport because they no longer had the desire or time. When follow-up is long, many patients decrease their sports participation for reasons unrelated to knee disability. Many papers in the literature on sports participation after ACL injury do not explicitly address this fact. Of the 17 patients who still participated in their first sport, 15 participated more than 50 hours per year. Of these 15, 10 felt their performance was the same as before injury. Thus, for whatever reason, only 10 of 32 (31%) patients participated in their first sport without any hindrance from the injured knee 5 years after injury.

A review of several studies reporting on athletic participation after ACL injury is presented along with other data in Table 27-6. With the exception of Chick's paper (2), which specifically excluded patients with moderate or severe instability, the results are more uniform than might be expected. While some authors, such as Giove (19), chose to stress the fact that most patients can participate in some form of sports after injury, the bulk of the data shows that many patients cannot return to sports that require cutting. Only a small percentage can return to those cutting sports with no limitation.

Partial ACL Tears

The extent of ACL tears is difficult to ascertain even by arthroscopy. Some authors report that patients with partial ACL tears have no significant instability (44). Others report that the instability and prognosis of patients with partial tears are similar to those of patients with complete tears.

A recent analysis of 30 patients with arthroscopically diagnosed partial ACL tears in the San Diego Kaiser series led to the conclusion that patients can be divided into two groups at the time of initial injury. In the San Diego Kaiser study, one group consisted of 14 patients who were stable by KT-1000 measurement at the initial evaluation. The other group consisted of 16 patients who met the KT criteria of complete ACL disruption at the initial examination. When retested 1 year later, one of the 14 stable patients was found to be unstable. All of the 16 unstable patients remained unstable. Patients with partial ACL tears who were stable by KT criteria did well on subjective, objective, and functional evaluations performed 1 year after injury. On the other hand, patients who were unstable by KT criteria reduced their hours of sports participation and rated themselves lower on a task evaluation questionnaire. The difference between the stable and unstable knees was statistically significant. It appears, therefore, that patients with partial tears can be classified as stable or unstable shortly after injury. The prognosis of the stable patients may approximate that of patients without ACL tears, whereas the unstable group may approximate patients with complete ACL tears. Longer follow-up and more studies are necessary to corroborate or refute the existence of these two subgroups and to provide more data on the prognosis of each.

Summary

A review of the data presented reveals several points of consensus. Acute ACL tears are accompanied by meniscal tears in a little over 50% of cases (Tables 27-5 and 27-12). The incidence of lateral tears is slightly greater than that of medial tears. In chronic ACL-injured patients who have enough symptoms to warrant arthroscopy (and that is a major qualification), four of five patients have meniscal tears; moreover, medial tears are much more common than lateral tears. About 40% of surgical meniscus tears are reparable. Studies by Noyes (41), Walla (56), and Satku (50) present information on the number of nonreconstructed ACL-injured patients who came to meniscectomy within 5 years of injury—50%, 61%, and 58%, respectively. Their patients were not specifically preselected, since chronic symptoms warranted arthroscopy. On the other hand, some meniscal tears were undoubtedly missed in these studies because some patients did not undergo arthrotomy or arthroscopy.

Less data are available regarding chondral changes in ACL patients. Indelicato (23) and the Kaiser study both document the fact that chondral changes are more than twice as frequent in chronic patients who come to arthroscopy than in acute patients. In those chronic patients, medial and patellar chondral damage is more common than lateral damage.

McDaniel (37,38), Hawkins (20), and the San Diego Kaiser study all point out that most patients with chronic ACL-deficient knees do not have more than mild or infrequent pain with activities of daily living (Table 27-7). These authors also agree that during activities of daily living, few patients have giving way or

more than occasional swelling. Noyes (41), in his study of symptomatic, athletically active patients, found more frequent problems during activities of daily living. In Hawkin's paper and in the San Diego Kaiser study, however, some patients left the study group to undergo ACL reconstruction. These were presumably the most symptomatic patients. In Hawkins' study, all patients were initially treated nonoperatively, but 30% came to ACL reconstruction. In the San Diego Kaiser study, 20% of the patients underwent acute reconstruction, and 18% of the remainder underwent delayed reconstruction. Although the need for reconstruction is a matter of judgment, these figures are consistent with Noyes' famous "rule of thirds," according to which one-third of patients will need ACL reconstruction.

Each of the studies we have discussed has its own special biases. We have pointed out some of them in the course of this review. Pooling such disparate data represents an interesting (but potentially misleading) oversimplification. Many of the selection biases (e.g., toward symptomatic patients) are common to most of the papers. Pooling the data does not eliminate such biases and obscures some of the information available to the careful reader of the individual studies.

From the data we now possess, it certainly appears that most patients with ACL injuries do well with activities of daily living even after follow-up in the range of 5 years. Most can participate in some sports activity if they are inclined to do so, but most will have some limitations in vigorous sports and only a few will be entirely asymptomatic. Approximately half the patients will tear their menisci at the time of ACL rupture. Some of those tears may heal and others will develop. There are more medial tears in the chronic group than in the acute group. Chondral damage is found in 20% of the patients who undergo acute arthroscopy when their ACL is torn, and it is also found in more than 40% of those who undergo arthroscopy later. Degenerative changes are seen by x-ray in a substantial number of cases. Although there is some very strong evidence linking these changes to meniscal pathology, this causal relationship has not been established directly. A long-term follow-up of patients with ACL tears whose menisci were specifically documented to be intact at the time of injury and at follow-up would be of great value. Magnetic resonance imaging (MRI) may make such a study more practical.

THE PCL-INJURED KNEE

Literature Review

Our review of the information available on the natural history of the isolated ACL tear has revealed that good data are available, although no study is ideal. Information on the natural history of the isolated PCL tear, however, is a good deal more meager, partly because such tears are less frequent. In the San Diego Kaiser study of 500 ligament tears with pathologic motion, ACL tears represented 63% of all ligament injuries, whereas PCL tears represented 7%. The San Diego Kaiser data also demonstrated that "isolated" ACL injuries represent a greater proportion of total ACL injuries than "isolated" PCL injuries do of total PCL injuries (Table 27-1). Of 319 ACL injuries, 238 (75%) were isolated. Of 37 PCL injuries, only 18 (49%) were isolated. Thus, isolated ACL injuries represented 48% of the total, whereas isolated PCL injuries were only 4%. There were 238 isolated ACLs and 18 isolated PCLs, a ratio of over 13 to one.

In early papers on ligament injuries, Palmer (47) and O'Donoghue (45) remarked that the results of non-operative treatment of PCL injuries are unsatisfactory, although no detailed information was given. In 1968, Trickey (55) reported on the results of treatment of 17 patients whose "predominant" injury was rupture of the PCL. He pointed out that in his experience, most injuries were the result of vehicular trauma and involved bony avulsion from the tibia.

In 1980, Hughston (21) reported follow-up on 29 patients with PCL tears that he repaired. He cited the opinions of Palmer and Abbott that "failure to repair the PCL usually results in a poorly functioning knee," but he did not attempt to substantiate this opinion. In Hughston's report, associated ligament pathology was present in all 29 cases. There were 22 ACL tears, 26 MCL tears, two lateral ligament injuries, and one combined medial and lateral injury. In addition, 24 patients (83%) had medial meniscal tears, nine of which were reparable, and three (10%) had lateral meniscus tears, one of which was reparable. Because of the high incidence of ACL tears associated with these PCL injuries, however, it is impossible to attribute these meniscal tears to PCL injury per se. Twenty-two of the 29 injuries were sustained in sports. All the tears were in substance, often near the femoral attachment. In contrast, in other series in which motor vehicle trauma predominated, a high incidence of tibial avulsion injuries was reported.

In 1981, Loos (34) reported on 102 cases of PCL injury from a registry of knee surgeries in the United States and Australia. All of these cases underwent surgery. Fifty-nine were operated upon acutely (within 3 weeks of injury), whereas 43 were operated upon chronically. Of the 59 acute cases, 26 (44%) had tears of the ACL, 27 (46%) had tears of the MCL, and 18 (31%) had tears of the lateral complex. In addition, there were 17 meniscal tears (29%). Loos also reviewed five previously reported series of PCL tears and concluded that when all the data were pooled, ACL tears were present in greater than 65%, MCL

tears in greater than 50%, and meniscal tears in greater than 30%. Loos reported 22% "isolated" PCL tears in his series; however, he noted that in many of these cases, operative treatment was unsuccessful. Loos felt that this may have been due to failure to diagnose associated ligament injuries, and he advised caution in making the diagnosis of "isolated" PCL injury.

In comparing Loos' data to the San Diego Kaiser Knee Injury Clinic data, it is important to note that knee dislocations were excluded from the Kaiser series. PCL-injured patients with dislocations have associated ligament injuries. Many isolated PCL injuries were undoubtedly missed in the early literature (Table 27-16). The recent emphasis on accurate diagnoses of PCL injuries and the use of KT-1000 to make examination more sensitive (7) may be responsible for the detection of isolated PCL injuries that could have been missed when Loos compiled his series. Finally, different series of PCL injuries include patients collected from very different populations. Loos also pointed out the fact that some series include mainly patients whose PCLs were injured in motor vehicle accidents while others include mainly sports injuries. These populations differed in the average age of the patients, the type of trauma, and even the site and type of the PCL injury, as we have noted. There may also be a difference in the pattern of associated ligament injuries. In the San Diego Kaiser series, 15 (41%) of the 37 PCL injuries were sports-related, 14 (38%) were caused by motor vehicle trauma, and eight (22%) were in the miscellaneous category, including falls.

In 1983, Clancy (3) made important observations on the status of 48 PCL-injured knees in the context of reporting on PCL reconstruction. In 15 acute cases, there was no sign of articular cartilage damage and no meniscal injuries were reported. In 33 cases who came to PCL reconstruction at least 1 month after injury (mean 3 years after injury), 48% had meniscus pathology and 52% had associated ligament injuries. There were preoperative radiographic degenerative changes in 12 (36%) of the 33 patients: mild in seven, moderate in three, and severe in two. At arthrotomy, however, articular damage was far more common, and Clancy found that x-ray was not a sensitive test for chondral damage. Twenty-one (64%) patients had articular damage in the medial compartment. In 16 (48%) the damage was graded moderate or severe. Furthermore, only two (13%) of 16 patients with an interval of less than 2 years between injury and surgery had such changes, whereas 14 (82%) of 17 with an interval of 2 years or longer demonstrated moderate or severe damage. Clancy inferred that significant medial chondral damage becomes more frequent over time.

Interpretation of these data with respect to the natural history of isolated PCL injuries is complicated by the inclusion of patients with associated ligamentous

TABLE 27-16. Meniscal injuries in PCL-injured patients

Author	Number of patients	Percentage of medial meniscal tears	Percentage of lateral meniscal tears	Percentage of associated ligament injuries	Percentage undergoing arthrotomy/ arthroscopy	Acute (A) or chronic (C)	Remarks
Moore (39)	18	55	28	100	100	A	
Hughston (21)	29	72	10	100	100	A	
Loos (34)	59	25	3	78	100	A	34% with bony avulsion
Hughston (22)	29	66	52	100	100	C	
Clancy (4)	33	48	29	52	100	C	The 16 isolated cases
	16	38	25	0	100	C	are a subset of the
	10	0	0	20	100	A	33 chronic cases
Cross (5)	116	40	21	16	56	97% C	No specific comments on ACL injuries
Parolie (48)	25	12	4	0	20	56% C	16% had locking at time of study
Fowler (17)	13	8	8	0	100	A	38% partial tears
San Diego Kaiser	17	6	12	0	71	Mixed	

and meniscal injuries in this series. Note that from Table 27-16 the three series reporting isolated PCL tears had an incidence of meniscus injury of less than 20%, whereas those series with 100% associated ligament injuries had an incidence of greater than 50% meniscus tears. Analyzing Clancy's data reveals that 10 of his 33 patients had isolated PCL tears and no meniscal damage. Six of these were operated upon within 2 years of injury. Five had no articular damage, whereas one had mild changes. On the other hand, of the four patients who were operated upon more than 2 years after injury, one showed mild changes, one showed moderate changes, and two showed severe changes. This suggests that Clancy's hypothesis may hold even for isolated PCL injuries, at least in those patients who are symptomatic enough to warrant surgery. Clancy also remarked that only three (9%) of his patients had moderate or severe *lateral* changes, and his data show that all had undergone lateral meniscectomy. Six patients (18%) had mild patellofemoral changes, and six had moderate or severe patellofemoral changes. Clancy's data appeared to show a much higher incidence of medial compartment chondral changes in patients with isolated or combined PCL injuries than were seen in roughly comparable series of isolated ACL injuries (Table 27-12), whereas the incidence of lateral and patellofemoral changes was similar to that in the ACL patients.

Clancy only reported the preoperative symptoms of 13 of the 33 patients who underwent PCL reconstruction. Instability was a more common complaint among the six patients with combined ligament injuries than among the seven patients with isolated PCL injuries, but even the latter group apparently experienced instability while descending stairs and walking on uneven ground. Clancy concluded that "functional instability is not the major symptom of isolated insufficiency of the posterior cruciate. The symptoms of pain, aching after activity, and effusion caused by changes in the articular cartilage are the main disabling features."

Follow-up studies by Degenhardt (8) and Hughston (22) conclude that PCL injury alone in the patient with good quadriceps strength is compatible with "many years of good function" (Degenhardt). The prognosis is poor if there has been a meniscectomy or if there are multiple instabilities.

Cross (5) corroborated Degenhardt's observation that good results correlated strongly with good quadriceps strength. He documented better results in patients who sustained their injuries in sports as opposed to motor vehicle accidents. He attributed this, in part, to their greater readiness to participate in vigorous quadriceps rehabilitation, although the severity of injury and associated injuries may have played a role. Cross also stated that he found a "poor" correlation between the degrees of posterior drawer and the functional result. His data on 89 patients who did not undergo reconstruction show, however, that poor or fair results were achieved by 10 of 23 (43%) patients with a "3+" posterior drawer, nine of 47 (19%) with a "2+", one of 17 (6%) with a "1+," and none of two with a "0." This seems to indicate a strong correlation between degree of posterior drawer and functional result, in agreement with Degenhardt. Finally, Cross observed that of the 67 patients who underwent neither meniscal nor PCL surgery, 32 (48%) achieved excellent results, 22 (33%) good results, four (6%) fair results, and only nine (13%) poor results. Of course, these were the patients who did not have symptoms warranting surgery, and so they represent a selected group.

In 1986, Parolie (48) published a paper entitled "Long-Term Results of Nonoperative Treatment of

Isolated Posterior Cruciate Ligament Injuries in the Athlete." Patients with "significant concurrent ligamentous injuries" were excluded. Along with 11 acute injuries, the authors reported on 14 chronic injuries from two distinct groups. One group consisted of patients whose injuries were detected on preseason athletic physicals. The patients would be expected to have a better-than-average function. The other group consisted of patients presenting for second opinions "concerning the instability of the knee." These patients would be expected to be more symptomatic than a randomly selected group. Neither group would be expected to be a fair sample of chronic PCL injuries. Parolie did not specify the number in each of these subgroups. Twenty-three of the total group of 25 patients had been injured playing sports, and all patients were "athletes," which, according to Cross, would give them a better-than-average prognosis. Twenty patients (80%) were "satisfied" with their knees at follow-up averaging 6.2 years. Seventeen (68%) had "full return to their previous athletic functions without disability," four patients (16%) returned to their previous sports at a decreased level of function, and four (16%) were not participating in their previous sports but were involved in "less vigorous physical activities." Parolie found that patients who achieved mean Cybex II torques on the involved sides greater than those on the uninvolved sides were more likely to have satisfactory results than those who did not. This corroborates Cross' findings based on quadriceps bulk and force.

Knee pain was reported in 13 patients (52%), but no patient felt that this pain was "more than a nuisance." None had consistent pain, and the majority "could not localize the pain within one compartment." Three (12%) had pain with stair climbing, and 12 (48%) had stiffness following prolonged sitting; this suggests possible patellofemoral disease. Three (12%) complained of giving way with exercise, and two (8%) had giving way with activities of daily living (Table 27-17).

There was radiographic evidence of arthritis in nine patients (36%), all having medial involvement, but in eight the changes were classified as mild (i.e., without joint space-narrowing). Two (8%) had lateral changes, one of whom had undergone lateral meniscectomy, and four (16%) had patellofemoral changes, one of whom had undergone internal fixation of a fractured patella. Parolie implied some contrast to the findings of Clancy, but Clancy reported that only 36% of his patients had radiographic degenerative changes, with only 15% having moderate or severe changes. Clancy stressed the poor correlation between radiographic changes and the articular damage seen at operation which concerned him. In contrast to Clancy, Parolie stated that he did not find any relationship between length of follow-up and severity of arthritic changes, but he did note that mean follow-up in the patients who showed radiographic degenerative changes was 8.4 years, whereas for those who did not, follow-up averaged 5.5 years. The contrasts between the data of Parolie and Clancy are not as dramatic as they might seem from the conclusions that the authors reach (Table 27-18).

In 1987, Fowler (17) published a report entitled "Isolated Posterior Cruciate Ligament Injuries in Athletes." In this study, unlike all others, all 13 patients were seen acutely. They presumably represent an unselected series of isolated PCL injuries in athletes. In 12 of 13 patients the PCL tear was confirmed arthroscopically. There were five partial tears by arthroscopy, but all patients demonstrated posterior sag and posterior drawer. In seven patients, midsubstance tears were visualized arthroscopically; in one patient,

TABLE 27-17. *Pain, swelling, and giving way in chronic PCL patients*

Author	Number of patients	Pain	Swelling	Giving way	Isolated tears (%)	Average years of follow-up
Dandy (6)	20	70% had aches with prolonged walking; 55% had pain while descending stairs	20% of cases swell with walking	45% of cases give way on uneven ground 30% of cases give way while descending stairs	100	7.2
Cross (5)	116	34%; no details	No comment	38%; no details	83	>5
Parolie (48)	25	52% had occasional pain, none of which was consistent or more than "nuisance"	16%	20% of cases gave way, including 12% with exercise and 8% with activities of daily living	100	6.2
San Diego Kaiser	17	71% had infrequent pain, only 6% of which was more than mild	18% of cases swell, only 6% of which are frequent	0%	100	2.3

TABLE 27-18. *Degenerative radiographic changes in patients with chronic PCL injury*

Author	Number of patients	Degenerative change on x-ray (%)	Years between injury and evaluation	Isolated PCL injuries (%)	Remarks
Degenhardt (8)	22	23	7.5	70	
Hughston (22)	29	31	Unknown	0	7 medial; 1 lateral; 1 medial and lateral
Clancy (4)	3	36	3	48	7 mild; 3 moderate; 2 severe
Parolie (48)	25	36	6.2	100	7 medial; 2 medial and lateral; 8 mild; 1 moderate

however, "direct visualization of the PCL was not obtained." Patients with bony avulsion injury of the PCL were specifically excluded, as were patients who did not sustain their injury during athletic events.

Associated arthroscopic findings included one medial meniscal tear in a degenerative medial compartment, one lateral meniscal tear in a degenerative lateral compartment, one hemorrhagic but intact ACL, and two intact but hemorrhagic posterolateral capsules. Patients with anterior or collateral ligament instability were excluded. All patients were placed on a vigorous physical therapy program. Average follow-up was 2.6 years. All patients returned to previous activity with no limitations, and Cybex testing revealed no significant difference in strength or fatigue between the normal and injured knee in any patient.

With respect to chondral damage in the isolated PCL-injured knee, Fowler reported on "degenerative change" in one medial compartment (7%) and one lateral compartment (7%) in his 13 patients who underwent arthroscopy after acute injury. Clancy stated explicitly that he saw no chondral injuries in the 15 acute PCL injuries on which he operated. This suggests a lower incidence of acute chondral damage than that seen in ACL-injured patients (Table 27-11). Only Clancy provided any data based on direct inspection of the articular cartilage in chronic patients with isolated PCL injuries. He operated upon 16 such patients, all of whom were, of course, symptomatic. Only six (38%) had no articular changes. Two had changes involving only the patellofemoral joint, whereas eight (50%) had medial or lateral changes, with four (25%) having severe changes in the medial compartment. Clancy's data suggest an incidence of chondral damage as high as that seen in chronic ACL-injured patients (Table 27-11). His series is very small, however, and his findings have not been directly supported or refuted in the literature. Others have looked at the issue of degenerative changes in the PCL-injured knee by radiographic technique (Table 27-18), although Clancy's

work demonstrated that this is a less sensitive method of evaluation. The incidence of x-ray changes is not dissimilar to that in isolated ACL-injured knees (Table 27-8), but the number of patients who had isolated PCL injuries is much smaller.

San Diego Kaiser PCL Follow-up Study

At San Diego Kaiser there is a current ongoing study of PCL-injured patients. Between 1984 and 1987, 35 patients were seen who had PCL injuries confirmed by arthroscopy and/or KT-1000 measurements and who had no ACL injury and no Grade III collateral injury. In contrast to the results of the San Diego Kaiser ACL study, none of these patients underwent acute or chronic reconstruction. At present, 17 (49%) of these patients have been reevaluated at a mean follow-up of 27 months (range 11–45 months) with the same protocol used for 34 nonreconstructed ACL-injured patients 5 years since injury.

Of the 17 patients in the study, 12 underwent arthroscopy prior to the follow-up examination. One (6%) had a torn medial meniscus, and two (12%) had torn lateral menisci. This low incidence of meniscal pathology is in agreement with most other studies of isolated PCL-injured knees (Table 27-16) and is in marked contrast with isolated ACL-injured knees (Table 27-13).

In the 17 San Diego Kaiser patients with average follow-up of 27 months, it was found that pain was the predominant symptom as Clancy had noted. Only five (29%) of the patients had no pain. Other authors with longer follow-up found pain to be a frequent complaint (Table 27-17), but usually not a severe one. ACL-injured patients seem to have a greater incidence of more than mild knee discomfort during activities of daily living (Table 27-7). In the San Diego Kaiser series, 14 patients (82%) had no swelling. This was in general agreement with other authors (Table 27-17). Patients

TABLE 27-19. *Specific task performance (percentage) in PCL-disrupted patients*[a]

Task	No problem	Mild impair-ment	Moderate impair-ment	Unable to do
Getting out of chair	100	0	0	0
Prolonged standing	88	12	0	0
Walking	100	0	0	0
Walking on uneven ground	100	0	0	0
Ascending stairs	88	12	0	0
Descending stairs	88	12	0	0
Climbing	71	29	0	0
Kneeling or squatting	65	29	6	0
Jogging	71	0	0	29
Running fast	65	24	0	12
Jumping	71	12	0	18
Twisting or pivoting	47	29	0	24
Cutting	35	29	6	29

[a] Study performed at San Diego Kaiser; *n* = 17; mean follow-up period 27 months.

with isolated ACL injuries may have had more frequent swelling with activities of daily living (Table 27-7), but the data are equivocal.

In the San Diego Kaiser series, no patient reported "giving way." This is in contrast to the results of other reports (Table 27-17). Cross (5), for example, reported that 44 patients complained of "straight instability of the knee which lacked the precipitancy of anterior cruciate insufficiency." Cross' remark points out one of the difficulties of this analysis, since this complaint of "instability" may or may not be classified as "giving way," depending on the author's interpretation. In Parolie's paper (48), five patients had "giving way," but four had locking and presumably had torn menisci or loose bodies. If these patients were classified as "giving way," their symptoms may have been due to secondary internal derangements, and not to the torn PCL per se. It appears from Table 27-17 that "giving way" with activities of daily living is as common or more common among PCL-injured patients than among ACL-injured patients (cf. Table 27-7). As Cross points out, however, the subjective nature of the instability symptom is certainly different in the two groups. One may question whether it is wise to use the term "giving way" to apply to both.

Table 27-19 presents the data on the specific task performance in the San Diego Kaiser PCL patients. In contrast to Dandy's report (6), none of the San Diego Kaiser patients had any difficulty walking on uneven ground. Sixty-five percent of the PCL patients had no difficulty kneeling or squatting (versus 56% of the ACL patients; cf. Table 27-15), despite the special concern about patellofemoral problems in PCL patients. On the other hand, only 35% of the San Diego Kaiser PCL patients had no difficulty cutting, whereas 50% of the ACL patients had no difficulty. In other vigorous activities such as jogging, running fast, jumping, and twisting or pivoting, the PCL patients did no better than the ACL patients. It should be recalled that none of the PCL patients had been reconstructed, whereas the most symptomatic ACL patients had been reconstructed and were thus removed from the series under analysis.

In terms of objective function (utilizing the tests described in Chapter 29), 13 of 17 (76%) had a normal hop index of >90, while 15 of 17 (88%) had a normal quadriceps index of ≥80%. These results are similar to those of the ACL patients. The mean corrected 90° passive posterior side-to-side displacement difference on KT-1000 examination was 6.2 mm, with sixteen (94%) showing a difference of >2.5 mm and 77% showing a difference of >5 mm.

The sports participation of the PCL patients was documented, as had been done for the ACL patients. Prior to injury, nine (53%) of the patients participated in a high-risk activity as their first sport, and all participated in some sport. At follow-up, eight (47%) participated in a high-risk activity as their first sport, but three (18%) no longer participated in any sport more than 50 hours per year. In contrast to the specific task performance, the PCL patients did better by this criterion than the ACL patients. Mean total hours of participation in the two favorite sports, however, fell from 361 hours per year to 141 hours per year at follow-up, a drop similar to that seen in ACL patients. Twelve (71%) still participated in their first sport, two (12%) were afraid to compete, and three (18%) no longer had the desire or time. Of the 12 who participated, however, only four participated over 50 hours per year and only one of these felt that his performance was the same as before the injury. Three felt they were at 90% of their preinjury level. These results are about the same as, or poorer than, the results of the ACL patients. Table 27-20 shows that other authors generally found that the sports prognoses for PCL-injured patients is better than that for ACL-injured patients (cf. Table 27-6).

THE COLLATERAL-LIGAMENT-INJURED KNEE

It is refreshing to turn from the controversies surrounding the outcome of unreconstructed cruciate ligament injuries to the clearer topic of isolated MCL injuries. As previously noted, Palmer (47), dissatisfied

TABLE 27-20. *Sports activity in patients with chronic PCL injury*

Author	Number of patients	Quality of activity	Isolated PCL injury (%)	Years between injury and evaluation	Remarks
Savatsky (51)	64	Over 50% could not participate in any recreational sports	Not stated	Not stated	85% had instability and probably many associated ligament injuries
Degenhardt (8)	23	78% were able to participate in sports with running and cutting; 13% were more limited by age than by knee	70	7.5	
Parolie (48)	25	68% had full return to previous sport; 16% returned to previous sport but were not as good; 16% became involved in less vigorous activity	100	6.2	All 11 were seen acutely and were rehabilitated; all returned to full sports
Fowler (17)	13	100% returned to previous activity with no limitations	100	2.6	All were seen acutely and were rehabilitated

with the results of plaster cast treatment of all ligament injuries, recommended surgical treatment. O'Donoghue (46) popularized this approach to MCL injuries.

In 1974, however, Ellsasser (12) reported excellent results in nonoperative treatment of isolated Grade II MCL and LCL injuries in professional football players. Seventy-four injuries were treated (64 MCL, 10 LCL). Crutches and physical therapy were used, but no braces or casts. In 69 cases (93%) the players returned to sports within 8 weeks, and 73 (99%) ultimately did well without ligament surgery. Ellsasser felt that "a well-muscled thigh is a prerequisite to the early mobilization program" and that "for the individual with inadequate muscles, use of cylinder cast for three or four weeks is advisable," but he gave no data to support this suggestion. He also felt that Grade III injuries required surgery but that "surgeons who advocate surgical repair for every injury to the knee in which some degree of instability is demonstrable will be operating on many knees that would have an excellent result without operation."

In 1978, Fetto (15) presented a retrospective analysis of 265 MCL injuries, with 6-month follow-up on 222. Nonoperative treatment of Grade II and III injuries consisted of cylinder casts for 4–6 and 6–10 weeks, respectively. At the discretion of the patient and surgeon, 150 cases (57%) underwent surgery. In terms of valgus stability and total "knee score" on the Hospital for Special Surgery (HSS) system, nonoperative treatment of Grade II patients yielded results that were as good as those obtained using operative treatment, with 86% good to excellent results. Isolated Grade III injuries also did as well under nonoperative as operative

treatment with 64% good to excellent results. They did not do as well, however, as isolated Grade II MCL lesion.

"Mixed lesions" were defined as lesions that had "clinically evident concurrent compromise of two or more ligament structures." In terms of valgus instability and total score, patients with "mixed lesions" did not do as well as patients with isolated MCL lesions. Grade II MCL lesions had a 53% incidence of "mixed lesions," whereas Grade III MCL lesions had a 78% incidence. Over 95% of the mixed lesions involved the ACL. Fetto observed that a good to excellent result in mixed injuries was more closely correlated with recovery of ACL stability than of MCL stability.

In 1983, Indelicato (23) published his classic paper, entitled "Non-operative Treatment of Complete Tears of the Medial Collateral Ligament of the Knee." This was a prospective study designed to compare the results of operative and nonoperative treatment of isolated Grade III injuries of the MCL. For 18 months, all patients suspected of having this injury were examined under anesthesia to confirm the diagnosis. Arthroscopy was performed to rule out meniscal, chondral, and cruciate ligament injuries. These patients, who comprise "Group I," underwent surgical repair of the MCL by suture or stapling and were then placed in toe-to-groin casts with minimum weight-bearing for 6 weeks. After the casts were removed, the patients were enrolled in a well-defined, supervised rehabilitation program.

During the next 18 months, all patients with this suspected injury were again examined under anesthesia and by arthroscopy. These patients, who comprised "Group II," were casted without open surgery. After 2 weeks, the patients in Group II were converted to ankle-to-groin cast braces allowing motion from 30° to 80° of flexion for 4 weeks and were allowed to bear weight as tolerated. They were then placed on the same rehabilitation program as the patients in Group I. Group I consisted of 16 patients who were followed an average of 3.1 years. Group II consisted of 20 patients who were followed an average of 2.4 years.

The accuracy of clinical examination in making the diagnosis of Grade III MCL tears was confirmed in this study, since all the patients in Group I with the preoperative diagnosis of Grade III tear were found to have complete tears at their open surgical procedures. Fifteen (94%) of the 16 patients in Group I, as well as 17 (85%) of the 20 patients in Group II, had good or excellent objective results. Fourteen (88%) of the 16 in Group I had good to excellent knee scores, and 18 (90%) of 20 in Group II had good to excellent scores. Thus, patients who had nonoperative care fared as well as those who underwent surgery. In addition, they regained strength (as measured by Cybex II) more rapidly than the surgical patients. In no patient in either group, however, was absolutely normal stability of the MCL reestablished, when measured against the contralateral knee. A firm, abrupt end point was achieved, and small degrees of laxity "appeared to have no functional significance," at least within the period of follow-up reported.

In 1986, Jones (28) published a report entitled "Nonoperative Management of Isolated Grade III Collateral Ligament Injury in High School Football Players." His study group was similar to Group II in Indelicato's paper. Jones followed 24 patients: 22 had MCL injuries, and two had LCL injuries. He did not arthroscope the patients when they entered the study, but he relied on clinical criteria to rule out cruciate and meniscal injuries. He found during his study that he had missed one ACL injury and bucket-handle meniscus tear.

In this study, the nonoperative management protocol was a little more aggressive than in Indelicato's. The patients were immobilized for only 1 week, and an off-the-shelf rehabilitation knee brace was used for this. The range of motion in the brace was then increased weekly from 30° to 60° up to 30° to 110°. Weight-bearing was permitted as tolerated, and early exercises were performed under a trainer's supervision. The knees were stress-tested out of the brace weekly, and the braces were removed when "stability was achieved." When full range of motion, strength, and running and cutting ability returned to normal, the athletes were permitted to return to full contact drills. All knees regained stability in the coronal plane (mean time 29 days). The athletes returned to contact drills at a mean time of 34 days after injury (range 30–46

days). There were no reinjuries, but mean follow-up was only 6 months.

In contrast, in 1988 Kannus (29) reported a very poor prognosis for nonoperative treatment of Grade III MCL injuries. He had a 9-year follow-up on 27 patients. He attributed his results to the fact that his patients were not athletes and the fact that he had much longer follow-up than other authors. While both of these points are interesting, the crucial fact is that in his series, all of the Grade III MCL patients had some anterior "instability:" Grade 1+ in three (11%), 2+ in eight (30%), 3+ in eight (30%), and 4+ in eight (30%). This strongly suggests that many, if not most, of these patients had ACL tears as well, despite the fact that these tears were not diagnosed at the time of injury. Thus many of her patients had mixed lesions, and these patients are known to have a much poorer prognosis. It appears that patients with true isolated MCL tears, even those with Grade III tears, can do as well with nonoperative care as with operative repair. The type and amount of bracing and rehabilitation required remain to be determined.

There is much less written about isolated lateral injuries of the knee. Ellsasser (12) reported 10 cases in his series of Grade II collateral ligament injuries, whereas Jones (28) reported two cases. These authors imply that lateral injuries have the same prognosis as medial injuries, if the cruciates are intact. They give little specific attention to lateral injuries. The San Diego Kaiser study on the incidence of knee ligament injuries found the incidence of isolated MCL injuries to be more than 14 times that of isolated LCL injuries (Table 27-1). DeLee (10) stated that severe straight lateral instability with >10 mm of joint opening more than the contralateral knee usually implies ACL and PCL injury. The little information that we do possess suggests that truly isolated lateral injuries probably have prognoses that are as good as those of medial injuries.

THE MULTIPLE-LIGAMENT-INJURED KNEE

If we try to study the outcome of nonreconstructed combined or "mixed" knee ligament injuries, we find that our data is even more inadequate than when we studied cruciate injuries. This is hardly surprising, since the difficulties in performing such a study must be even greater than those in performing studies of isolated cruciate injuries. As the San Diego Kaiser study demonstrates (Table 27-1), isolated ACL injuries are more common than combined injuries. Even though isolated PCL injuries comprise only 48% of all PCL injuries, the remaining 52% of combined injuries must then be subfractionated into smaller groups for meaningful study. The largest such subgroup of PCL injuries, that of combined PCL–MCL injuries, consisted of only eight patients in the entire San Diego Kaiser experience of 500 patients. This group was half the size of the isolated PCL group, and even this group probably has to be broken into Grade II and Grade III MCL injuries for meaningful analysis.

The largest group of combined injuries is the group of combined ACL–MCL injuries. This group comprised 64 patients in the San Diego Kaiser study and was larger than the entire PCL-injured group. Nevertheless, there are no papers on the combined injury which meet the standards of our best recent papers on isolated ACL injuries. It is often believed that the combined ACL–MCL injury has a far worse prognosis than the isolated ACL injury. In 1980, however, Fetto (16) concluded that "the isolated anterior cruciate injury, although initially less impressive, if unresolved, resulted in a relatively greater total amount of dysfunction and deterioration with time than did the mixed lesions." Fetto's data, however, suggest a very similar prognosis, with the mixed lesions, if anything, doing slightly worse than the isolated ACLs. In 1984, Jokl (27), as we have noted, reported a better prognosis in his series of Grade III MCL and ACL injuries than most authors report for isolated ACL injuries. Kannus (29), on the other hand, reported a poor prognosis in his series on MCL injuries, the majority of whom had associated ACL injuries. He did not separate the combined injuries from the isolated injuries in his analysis of results. There is, at present, no paper that employs modern diagnostic techniques to define combined ACL–MCL injuries and that directly compares the prognosis of these patients treated nonoperatively with the prognosis of patients with isolated ACL injuries treated nonoperatively.

This review of the outcome of unreconstructed knee ligament injuries shows us how far we have come in defining that outcome. It also suggests how much further we should be able to go in the near future.

ACKNOWLEDGMENTS

This work was supported by the Southern California Kaiser Permanente Research Program, San Diego, California 92120 and NIH Grant AR39359-01.

REFERENCES

1. Balkfors B. The course of knee-ligament injuries. *Acta Orthop Scand [Suppl]* 1982;198:1–99.
2. Chick RR, Jackson DW. Tears of the anterior cruciate ligament in young athletes. *J Bone Joint Surg* 1978;60A:970–973.
3. Clancy WG Jr. Knee ligamentous injury in sports: the past, present and future. *Med Sci Sports* 1983;15:9–14.
4. Clancy WG Jr, Shelbourne KD, Zoellner GB, Keene JS, Reider B, Rosenberg TD. Treatment of knee joint instability secondary to rupture of the posterior cruciate ligament. Report of a new procedure. *J Bone Joint Surg* 1983;65A:310–322.
5. Cross MJ, Powell JF. Long-term followup of posterior cruciate ligament rupture: a study of 116 cases. *Am J Sports Med* 1984;12:292–297.
6. Dandy DJ, Pusey RJ. The long-term results of unrepaired tears of the posterior cruciate ligament. *J Bone Joint Surg* 1982;64B:92–94.
7. Daniel DM, Stone ML, Barnett P, Sachs R. Use of the quadriceps active test to diagnose posterior cruciate-ligament disruption and measure posterior laxity of the knee. *J Bone Joint Surg* 1988;70A:386–391.
8. Degenhardt TC, Hughston JC. Chronic posterior cruciate instability: non-operative management. *Orthop Trans* 1981;5:486–487.
9. DeHaven KE. Diagnosis of acute knee injuries with hemarthrosis. *Am J Sports Med* 1980;8:9–14.
10. DeLee JC, Riley MB, Rockwood CA Jr. Acute posterolateral rotatory instability of the knee. *Am J Sports Med* 1983;11:199–207.
11. Ellison AE. Skiing injuries. *JAMA* 1973;223:917–919.
12. Ellsasser JC, Reynolds FC, Omohundro JR. The non-operative treatment of collateral ligament injuries of the knee in professional football players. An analysis of seventy-four injuries treated non-operatively and twenty-four injuries treated surgically. *J Bone Joint Surg* 1974;56A:1185–1190.
13. Feagin JA, Curl WW. Isolated tear of the anterior cruciate ligament: 5-year follow-up study. *Am J Sports Med* 1976;4:95–100.
14. Feagin JA Jr, Lambert KL, Cunningham RR, Anderson LM, Riegel J, King PH, VanGenderen L. Consideration of the anterior cruciate ligament injury in skiing. *Clin Orthop* 1987;216:13–18.
15. Fetto JF, Marshall JL. Medial collateral ligament injuries of the knee: a rationale for treatment. *Clin Orthop* 1978;132:206–218.
16. Fetto JF, Marshall JL. The natural history and diagnosis of anterior cruciate ligament insufficiency. *Clin Orthop* 1980;147:29–38.
17. Fowler PJ, Messieh SS. Isolated posterior cruciate ligament injuries in athletes. *Am J Sports Med* 1987;15:553–557.
18. Gillquist J, Hagberg G, Oretorp N. Arthroscopy in acute injuries of the knee joint. *Acta Orthop Scand* 1977;48:190–196.
19. Giove TP, Miller SJ 3d, Kent BE, Sanford TL, Garrick JG. Non-operative treatment of the torn anterior cruciate ligament. *J Bone Joint Surg* 1983;65A:184–192.
20. Hawkins RJ, Misamore GW, Merritt TR. Followup of the acute nonoperated isolated anterior cruciate ligament tear. *Am J Sports Med* 1986;14:205–210.
21. Hughston JC, Bowden JA, Andrews JR, Norwood LA. Acute tears of the posterior cruciate ligament. Results of operative treatment. *J Bone Joint Surg* 1980;62A:438–450.
22. Hughston JC, Degenhardt TC. Reconstruction of the posterior cruciate ligament. *Clin Orthop* 1982;164:59–77.
23. Indelicato PA. Non-operative treatment of complete tears of the medial collateral ligament of the knee. *J Bone Joint Surg* 1983;65A:323–329.
24. Indelicato PA, Bittar ES. A perspective of lesions associated with ACL insufficiency of the knee. *Clin Orthop* 1985;198:77–80.
25. Jacobsen K. Osteoarthrosis following insufficiency of the cruciate ligaments in man. A clinical study. *Acta Orthop Scand* 1977;48:520–526.
26. Jensen JE, Conn RR, Hazelrigg G, Hewett JE. Systematic evaluation of acute knee injuries. *Clin Sports Med* 1985;4:295–312.
27. Jokl P, Kaplan N, Stovell P, Keggi K. Non-operative treatment of severe injuries to the medial and anterior cruciate ligaments of the knee. *J Bone Joint Surg* 1984;66A:741–744.
28. Jones RE, Henley MB, Francis P. Nonoperative management of isolated grade III collateral ligament injury in high school football players. *Clin Orthop* 1986;213:137–140.
29. Kannus P. Long-term results of conservatively treated medial collateral ligament injuries of the knee joint. *Clin Orthop* 1988;226:103–112.
30. Kannus P, Jarvinen M. Conservatively treated tears of the anterior cruciate ligament. Long term results. *J Bone Joint Surg* 1987;69A:1007–1012.
31. Kannus P, Jarvinen M. Long-term prognosis of conservatively

treated acute knee ligament injuries in competitive and spare time sportsmen. *Int J Sports Med* 1987;8:348–351.

32. Liljedahl S-O, Nordstrand A. Injuries to the ligaments of the knee: diagnosis and results of operation. *Injury* 1969;1:17–24.

33. Liljedahl S-O, Lindvall N, Wetterfors J. Early diagnosis and treatment of acute ruptures of the anterior cruciate ligament. A clinical and arthrographic study of forty-eight cases. *J Bone Joint Surg* 1965;47A:1503–1513.

34. Loos WC, Fox JM, Blazina ME, Del Pizzo W, Friedman MJ. Acute posterior cruciate ligament injuries. *Am J Sports Med* 1981;9:86–92.

35. Lynch MA, Henning CE, Glick KR Jr. Knee joint surface changes. Long-term follow-up meniscus tear treatment in stable anterior cruciate ligament reconstructions. *Clin Orthop* 1983;172:148–153.

36. Marshall JL, Olsson SE. Instability of the knee. A long-term experimental study in dogs. *J Bone Joint Surg* 1971;53A:1561–1570.

37. McDaniel WJ Jr, Dameron TB Jr. Untreated ruptures of the anterior cruciate ligament. A follow-up study. *J Bone Joint Surg* 1980;62A:696–705.

38. McDaniel WJ Jr, Dameron TB Jr. The untreated anterior cruciate ligament rupture. *Clin Orthop* 1983;172:158–163.

39. Moore HA, Larsen RL. Posterior cruciate ligament injuries. Results of early surgical repair. *Am J Sports Med* 1980;8:68–78.

40. Noyes FR, Bassett RW, Grood ES, Butler DL. Arthroscopy in acute traumatic hemarthrosis of the knee. Incidence of anterior cruciate tears and other injuries. *J Bone Joint Surg* 1980;62A:687–695,757.

41. Noyes FR, Mooar PA, Matthews DS, Butler DL. The symptomatic anterior cruciate deficient knee. Part I: the long-term functional disability in athletically active individuals. *J Bone Joint Surg* 1983;65A:154–162.

42. Noyes FR, Matthews DS, Mooar PA, Grood ES. The symptomatic anterior cruciate deficient knee. Part II: the results of rehabilitation, activity modification, and counseling on functional disability. *J Bone Joint Surg* 1983;65A:163–174.

43. O'Beirne J, O'Dwyer T, O'Rourke JS, Quinlan W. The diagnosis of knee injuries in causalty—a prospective study. *Injury* 1984;15:232–235.

44. Odensten M, Lysholm J, Gillquist J. The course of partial anterior cruciate ligament ruptures. *Am J Sports Med* 1985;13:183–186.

45. O'Donoghue DH. An analysis of end results of surgical treatment of major injuries to the ligaments of the knee. *J Bone Joint Surg* 1955;37A:1–13,124.

46. O'Donoghue DH. Surgical treatment of injuries to ligaments of the knee. *JAMA* 1959;169:1423–1431.

47. Palmer I. On the injuries to the ligaments of the knee joint; clinical study. *Acta Chir Scand [Suppl]* 1938;81:3–282.

48. Parolie JM, Bergfeld JA. Long-term results of nonoperative treatment of isolated posterior cruciate ligament injuries in the athlete. *Am J Sports Med* 1986;14:35–38.

49. Pickett JC, Altizer TJ. Injuries of the ligaments of the knee. A study of types of injury and treatment in 129 patients. *Clin Orthop* 1971;76:27–32.

50. Satku K, Kumar VP, Ngoi SS. Anterior cruciate ligament injuries. To counsel or to operate? *J Bone Joint Surg* 1986;68B:458–461.

51. Savatsky GJ, Marshall JL, Warren RF, Baugher WH. Posterior cruciate ligament injury. *Orthop Trans* 1980;4:293.

52. Solonen KA, Rokkanen P. Operative treatment of torn ligaments in injuries of the knee joint. *Acta Orthop Scand* 1967;38:67–80.

53. Stark J. Two cases of rupture of the crucial ligaments of the knee-joint. *Edinb Med Surg J* 1850;74:267–271.

54. Tapper EM. Ski injuries from 1939 to 1976: the Sun Valley experience. *Am J Sports Med* 1978;6:114–121.

55. Trickey EL. Rupture of the posterior cruciate ligament of the knee. *J Bone Joint Surg* 1968;50B:334–341.

56. Walla DJ, Albright JP, McAuley E, Martin RK, Eldridge V, El-Khoury G. Hamstring control and the unstable anterior cruciate ligament deficient knee. *Am J Sports Med* 1985;13:34–39.

57. Woods GW, Chapman DR. Repairable posterior menisco-capsular disruption in anterior cruciate ligament injuries. *Am J Sports Med* 1984;12:381–385.

58. Youmans WT. The so-called 'isolated' anterior cruciate ligament tear or anterior cruciate ligament syndrome: a report of 32 cases with some observation on treatment and its effect on results. *Am J Sports Med* 1978;6:26–30.

59. Young LR, Oman CM, Crane H, Emerton A, Heide R. The etiology of ski injuries: an eight year study of the skier and his equipment. *Orthop Clin North Am* 1976;7:13–29.

60. Zarins B, Adams M. Knee injuries in sports. *N Engl J Med* 1988;318:950–961.

Knee Ligaments: Structure, Function, Injury,
and Repair, edited by D. Daniel, et al.
© 1990 by Raven Press, Ltd. All rights reserved.

CHAPTER 28

Complications of Knee Ligament Surgery

Raymond A. Sachs, Alan Reznik, Dale M. Daniel, and Mary Lou Stone

Knee ligament surgery is high-risk surgery. There are few common elective orthopedic procedures that have as many complications and marginal results as knee ligament surgery. However, for the athlete participating in high-risk sports, joint instability will result in repeated injury, progressive impairment, and joint damage; therefore, knee ligament surgery is indicated. Table 28-1 presents the incidence of complications associated with knee ligament surgery from three sources: (i) Knee ligament surgery reported in the English literature prior to 1988 was reviewed, and the incidence of reported complications were compiled. (ii) In 1986 a ligament surgery complications questionnaire was sent to 50 North American orthopedic surgeons who had presented knee studies to major medical meetings and/or participated in the ACL[1] Study

Group (Convener John Feagin, Jackson, Wyoming). Thirty-three physicians completed the form. The surgeons were asked to record the complications in their last 100 cases. Their collective experience is listed in Table 28-1. (iii) The clinic records and follow-up evaluations of ligament surgery performed at the San Diego Kaiser Hospital between 1983 and 1988 was reviewed ($n = 390$). There were 329 single-ligament procedures and 61 multiple-ligament procedures. The single-ligament cases were all ACL surgeries. The multiple ligament procedures consisted of 43 ACL/MCL cases, 5 ACL/LCL cases, and 13 PCL operations combined with other ligament repairs. Forty percent of the ACL single-ligament procedures and 90% of the multiple-ligament procedures were performed within 6 weeks of injury. The mean patient age for the ACL single-ligament procedures was 25.0 years, and that for the multiple-ligament procedures was 26.3 years. Intraoperative and postoperative complications within 12 months of surgery are reviewed for the entire group. Longer follow-up data on various subsets of the group will be presented. Many of the complications associated with knee ligament surgery are discussed below.

R. A. Sachs: Department of Orthopedic Surgery, Kaiser Permanente Medical Center, San Diego, California 92120.
A. Reznik: Department of Orthopedics and Rehabilitation, Yale University School of Medicine, New Haven, Connecticut 06511.
D. M. Daniel: Department of Orthopedic Surgery, University of California, San Diego, School of Medicine, La Jolla, California 92037; and Kaiser Permanente Medical Center, San Diego, California 92120.
M. L. Stone: Department of Orthopedics, Kaiser Permanente Medical Center, San Diego, California 92120.
[1]ACL, anterior cruciate ligament; PCL, posterior cruciate ligament; MCL, medial collateral ligament; LCL, lateral collateral ligament.

ANESTHETIC MORTALITY

Anesthetic mortality in knee ligament surgery has been reported in the literature (Table 28-1). This was not

TABLE 28-1. *Complications of knee ligament surgery*

Complication (references)	Incidence		San Diego Kaiser	
	Literature[a]	Surgeon poll[b]	Percent	Case reviewed
Anesthetic mortality (14,65)	.01%		0%	390
Vascular injury (19,33,35,44,45,69,102,113,115)	.01%	0%	0%	390
Cutaneous nerve injury (9,10,47,57,96,120)	50%			
Major nerve injury (4,19,73,77,113,121)	0%	.005%	0%	390
Tourniquet palsy (20,28,85,101,109,126)	22–100%[c]			
Deep-vein thrombosis (12,34,39,46,50,52,70,71,78,82,89,115,119,125)	3.5%	1%	.75%	390
Skin necrosis (42,46,121)	2%	.5%	.75%	390
Superficial infection (46,54,63,121)	4%	1%	0.75%	390
Deep infection (46,121)	1.6%	.5%	.75%	390
Reflex sympathetic dystrophy (21,25,26,51,56,58,62,87,96,97,99,111,112,122)	0%	.75%	0%	390
Manipulation (1,23,38,41,42,46,49,80,81,83,90,93,98,117,118)	4%	4%	7%	390
Flexion contracture (5,10,30,42,46,92,121)	32%	24%	20%[d]	180
Patello femoral pain (30,46,63,121)	32%	12%	19%	126
Quadriceps weakness (5,46,63,121)	47%	23%	62%[e]	180
Effusion (10,13,17,42,43,46,48,54,72,86,104,106,110,116,129)	13%	2.5%	12%	205
Knee pain—location unspecified (6,10,30,42,46,48,54)	15–65%[f]	10%		
Extensor mechanism disruption (6,10,29,30,46,48,68)	1%	.75%	0%	390
Growth-plate disturbance (11,16,60,61,78,100,105,108)	8%			
Secondary procedure within 1 year[g]			10%	390

[a] Estimates are based only on articles that mention either the presence or absence of the listed complications.

[b] Mean incidence reported by 33 surgeons in 1986 who each estimated complications in their last 100 cases.

[c] Estimates based on reports in patients undergoing arthrotomy for nonligamentous surgery.

[d] Prone heel height difference ≥ 5 cm (Fig. 3-1).

[e] Quadriceps strength $<80\%$ of that of contralateral normal knee.

[f] Represents knee pain from all sources combined. Few literature reports differentiate joint pain from patellofemoral pain, pain, stiffness, neuroma, impingement, and so on.

[g] See Table 28-2.

included in the surgeon poll. There were no cases in the San Diego Kaiser series. Lunn (65) reviewed anesthetic complications in all types of surgery in Cardiff, Wales between 1972 and 1977 ($n = 108,878$). Lunn constructed five overall risk categories based on the subjective assessment of the patient's degree of overall illness. The categories were nearly identical to the American Society of Anesthesiologists (ASA) classification (74). There were 197 deaths. The results of this study can be summarized as follows:

Anesthesia believed causative of death: 1 per 10,000.
Anesthesia partly or totally causative of death: 2 per 10,000.
Deaths related at all to anesthesia: 5 per 10,000.

These figures are probably applicable to a general orthopedic surgery practice. However, patients undergoing knee ligament surgery are the youngest and healthiest segment of the population (ASA Class I or II). ASA Class I and II patients make up more than 80% of all patients (66,124) but suffer less than 40% of anesthetic deaths (32). Therefore, in this special subgroup, mortality due to anesthesia is no greater than 0.5 per 10,000.

The major cause of anesthetic death is thought to be human error. Most studies (14,32,53,65,74,123) have concluded that 65–89% of anesthetic deaths involve some error. In Lunn's report, 27 of 32 (84%) probable anesthetic deaths were classified as avoidable. Cooper (14) reported on "critical incidents" in the operating room. Critical incidents included such things as airway, intravenous (I.V.), or arterial-line disconnections, equipment failure, and human error. It was concluded that 70% of critical incidents were due to human error and that approximately 50% of overall anesthesia-related morbidity and mortality was preventable.

VASCULAR INJURIES

There were no cases of vascular injuries in the San Diego Kaiser review or from the surgeon poll. Hohf's survey of vascular injuries in orthopedic operations reported 352 cases in 1163 responses (35). Sixty-one were associated with knee injury. Knee surgery vascular injuries resulted in 21 amputations, which represented 34% of reported vascular injuries to the knee. Arthrotomy represented more than half of the cases (32 patients), and tourniquet-induced thrombosis was responsible for two cases. The popliteal artery was injured in 85% of the cases. The remaining 15% of the injuries around the knee were divided among the anterior tibial, posterior tibial, genicular, and recurring collateral arteries.

There are several reports of vascular injury associated with knee dislocation (33,69). McCoy (69) reported four cases of low-velocity knee dislocations with vascular injuries, only one of which had overt signs of vascular disruption. Three of the four cases were sports injuries. This study points out that intimal tears may be present with distal pulses intact. The author recommends an arteriogram in all cases of knee dislocation, regardless of the presence of peripheral pulses. The possibility of a knee dislocation should be considered when dealing with multiple-ligament injuries.

Green (33) evaluated 245 knee dislocations with a 32% incidence of popliteal artery injury. In those knees with either straight anterior or posterior dislocation, 40% were associated with a vascular lesion. When the artery was not explored (19 cases), 89% of these injuries resulted in amputation. There were uniformly poor results and an 85% amputation rate if exploration and repair was performed after 8 hours. On the other hand, when repair was done within 8 hours, there was an 87% limb salvage rate. They attributed these findings to irreversible changes occurring after 6–8 hours of ischemia. Thus, the author recommended early exploration and repair along with prophylactic fasciotomy in all cases of vascular injury after dislocation.

There are several reports of vascular injury after arthroscopic surgery. DeLee's survey of 118,590 revealed nine cases of vascular injury representing approximately 1% of all complications (19). These nine cases resulted in four amputations. Jeffries (44) reported two cases of popliteal artery injury after partial lateral meniscectomy. He cautions the reader about the cavalier use of power suction shavers in the posterior lateral compartment of the knee. Popliteal artery aneurysm has been reported after meniscectomy (45). Meniscal repairs are also associated with vascular injury when the posterior lateral meniscus is involved (69).

Roth (102) reported a vascular complication secondary to placing an artificial ligament in the over-the-top position. An arteriogram revealed a sharp cutoff of the popliteal artery. The artery was found trapped between the ligament graft and bone when the popliteal fossa was explored. The limb's vascularity was restored by bypassing the entrapment with a saphenous vein graft.

FLUID EXTRAVASATION AND COMPARTMENT SYNDROME

Fruengaard (31) reported compartment syndrome as a complication of arthroscopy. Noyes (84) studied fluid dissection that can occur with flexion of a knee distended for the purpose of arthroscopy. In 300 clinical cases he saw this on four occasions with rapid resolution after tourniquet release. He reported that fluid can dissect via the path of the semimembranous bursa, beneath the pes anserinus and into the calf muscles even with an intact knee capsule. In cadaveric specimens he demonstrated that extravasation of fluid can cause an elevation of pressure in the calf compartments high enough to initiate a compartment syndrome. Cadaveric studies by Peek (95) revealed that the presence of a capsular defect elevated compartment pressures 80 mm above normal. In his *in vivo* model, using swine hind limbs, the side without a capsular defect demonstrated that the pressure elevation caused by saline extravasation had returned to normal within 15 minutes after the tourniquet was released. In contrast, in the swine experiment with a capsular defect, the pressure remained above 40 mm mercury for at least 8 hours after the tourniquet was released. Histologic studies of the limbs tested 8 days following pressurization revealed fibrous replacement of intracompartmental muscles on the capsular defect side but revealed no changes in the limb without a capsular defect. His results imply that extravasation with a capsular tear can cause compartment syndrome and tissue death. This experimental result is analogous to compartment syndrome in humans, since pressures within a compartment greater than 30–40 mm of mercury is considered diagnostic of compartment syndrome in the clinical setting (67,79,127).

Compartment syndrome has not been reported as a result of ligament reconstruction in the literature or in the surgeon poll. There have been no cases in the San Diego Kaiser review. However, arthroscopic-assisted ligament reconstruction may result in fluid extravasation, especially if a capsular defect is present, and could result in a compartment syndrome. The clinician should be aware of the possible complication and should monitor the size, swelling, and circulatory status of the limb both intraoperatively and postoperatively. When the diagnosis is entertained, prompt compartment pressure measurements should be made and fasciotomy performed when indicated.

NEUROLOGIC INJURY IN KNEE LIGAMENT SURGERY

Incision Nerve Injury

Probably no aspect of knee ligament surgery receives less attention than the simple act of making a skin incision. Yet, the occurrence of postoperative numbness, dysesthesia, or painful neuromas following a median parapatellar incision is common. Kummel (57) stated the following: "The current management of the infrapatellar branch of the saphenous nerve in knee surgery resembles the old saying about the weather: Everybody talks about it but nobody does anything." The incidence of sensory nerve injury was not included in our poll of surgeons and has not been included in our patient review.

The saphenous nerve becomes subcutaneous above the medial side of the knee, where it emerges behind the tendon of the sartorius muscle. It gives off one or more infrapatellar branches that curve forward to supply the anteromedial part of the leg below the knee and runs downward with the great saphenous vein to give off a series of medial cutaneous branches (36). The infrapatellar nerve is rarely a single nerve and usually consists of a plexus or multiple rami that extend both above and below the joint line on the medial aspect of the knee, frequently crossing over extensively into the lateral side of the knee (59). Thus, no incision on the medial side of the knee can be assured of avoiding the nerve (9,57). Swanson (120) reported that 63% of 87 patients undergoing medial meniscectomy showed immediate dysesthesia following the operation, with persistence of this dysesthesia occurring in 44.4% at 6 months. Johnson (47) reported on (a) 76 patients who had medial arthrotomies and (b) 18 patients who had lateral arthrotomies. Of the patients with medial incisions, 54% had sensory loss, which in 30% was irritating and disabling to some extent. Of patients with lateral incisions, 33% had sensory loss, but only 11% complained of irritation or hypersensitivity. The problem of damage to the infrapatellar branch of the saphenous nerve may extend beyond numbness or dysesthesia. Poehling (96), in an examination of 35 patients with clinically significant reflex sympathetic dystrophy of the knee, found evidence of insult to the infrapatellar branch of the saphenous nerve in all patients. He stated that patients with persistent nonmechanical pain syndromes in the knee often have had trauma to the infrapatellar branch of the saphenous nerve and that vasomotor abnormalities can be demonstrated in a high percentage of these patients.

Damage to superficial nervous structures is most likely to occur at two points during knee ligament surgery. Damage to the infrapatellar branch of the saphenous nerve may occur during a medial arthrotomy incision, particularly if no attempt is made to isolate rami during the superficial dissection. Secondly, cutaneous branches of the saphenous nerve proceeding distally in the leg may be damaged during repair of the tibial insertion of the MCL or during harvesting of the sartorius or gracilis tendons. It is likely that a certain incidence of damage to superficial nerves on the medial side of the knee is unavoidable during complex knee ligament surgery. However, use of laterally based skin incisions whenever possible, along with careful dissection in the region of the sartorius tendon and muscle, can limit morbidity.

Nerve Injury in Arthroscopic Procedures

In a nationwide review commissioned by the Arthroscopy Association of North America, DeLee (19) reported 63 neurologic injuries in 118,590 arthroscopies. In a review of 2640 arthroscopic procedures done in a large, experienced group of arthroscopists, neurologic injury was reported in 0.7% of patients (115). Reports of injury to the saphenous nerve during arthroscopic meniscus repair varies from 1% to 22% of cases (4,73,77). Injury to the peroneal nerve has been reported less often but was damaged in one of 96 meniscal repairs performed by Miller (73). Avoidance of neurologic injury during arthroscopic meniscus repair may be accomplished by adopting a "semi-open" technique, always inserting a retractor in a posterolateral or posteromedial incision of the knee so as to protect the respective neurovascular structures at risk (113).

Nerve Injury from Tourniquet Use

In 1904, Cushing (15) described the pneumatic tourniquet. Its use in knee ligament surgery is now taken for granted. The sparsity of reports of adverse effects from tourniquet usage have no doubt fostered the impression that tourniquet usage is without risk. In fact, it is likely that large numbers of patients incur transient nerve injury during knee ligament surgery, but complete recovery occurs within a few days to a few weeks.

Ochoa (85) reported that the delayed recovery of peripheral nerves post-surgery is the result of a slowly resolving axonal compression syndrome caused by the pneumatic tourniquet. His studies revealed a conduction block or reduced conduction velocity at the site of the tourniquet, with normal conduction velocities being maintained in nerve fibers distal to the tourniquet. Histological studies showed local demyelination under the tourniquet with preservation of axonal continuity. He concluded that the nerve lesion associated with tourniquet use occurs at the edge of the cuff and consists of a longitudinal shearing of the axon in relation to the Schwann cell as a result of the pressure gradient caused by the tourniquet. In most cases, this lesion is reversible.

Fowler (28) produced confirmatory data. By maintaining a cuff pressure of 1000 mm of mercury in baboons for 1–3 hours, he produced a consistent paralysis of distal muscles lasting up to 3 months. There was a significant correlation between the duration of compression and subsequent conduction block. When cuff pressure was reduced to 500 mm of mercury, similar but lesser changes were noted. Rorabeck (101) performed an experimental study in dogs, varying pneumatic tourniquet pressure from 250 mm to 500 mm of mercury and varying time of application from 1 to 2 hours. Impairment of sciatic nerve conduction velocity occurred with every tourniquet application regardless of pressure and duration of application. In all cases, recovery occurred following release of the tourniquet. The rate of recovery was related to both pressure and time.

In a prospective investigation, Dobner (20) studied 24 patients undergoing meniscectomy with the use of a tourniquet and compared them to 24 patients undergoing meniscectomy done without the usage of the tourniquet. His results showed that 71% of patients in the tourniquet group had electromyogram (EMG) evidence of denervation and a functional capacity of 39% of the normal leg when tested 6 weeks postoperatively. In the control group, there was no evidence of denervation in any patient, and at 6 weeks an average functional capacity of 79% was measured. In a similar study, Saunders (109) observed 48 patients after meniscectomy. Thirty patients (62) demonstrated EMG abnormalities following arthrotomy. Abnormal EMGs were found in 85% of the patients with tourniquet times of greater than 60 minutes, in 71% with times of 30–60 minutes, in 58% with times of 15–30 minutes, and in 22% with times of less than 15 minutes.

Postoperative weakness of quadriceps function following knee arthrotomy has usually been attributed to pain inhibition or lack of motivation. However, the delayed recovery may be the result of a slowly resolving axonal compression syndrome caused by the pneumatic tourniquet or may be due to direct muscle injury induced by muscle compression (91,94,109). Clinical studies have shown that the degree of conduction block is related to both increased pressure and increased duration of tourniquet application. It is likely that with the prolonged tourniquet applications commonly used in knee ligament surgery, virtually all patients are affected by an incomplete postoperative tourniquet palsy. Surgeons should minimize the tourniquet pressure and period of time that the tourniquet is used. The use of wider tourniquets may allow lower cuff inflation pressures and decrease muscle and nerve injury (76).

DEEP-VEIN THROMBOSIS

Venous thromboembolic disease is the leading cause of death among patients who survive at least 7 days following trauma (27). While the incidence of venous thromboembolic disease has been studied following meniscectomy and following total knee replacement, to date there are no in-depth studies of the incidence of either thrombotic or embolic complications following knee ligament surgery. One case was observed in the Kaiser review, and cases are reported in the literature and in the surgeon poll (Table 28-1). Clinical risk factors for the development of venous thrombosis include advanced age, previous venous thromboembolism, the presence of malignant disease, cardiac failure, prolonged immobilization, obesity, and varicose veins (50). However, the subject of risk factors remains controversial. In a review of 638 total knee replacements, Stulberg (119) found no high-risk population. Cohen (12) found no significant differences in venous thrombosis with patient age, sex, corticosteroid therapy, spinal versus general anesthesia, or tourniquet time. Only previous venous thromboembolic disease was predictive of increased risk. McKenna (71) noted that patients who had taken preoperative aspirin or other nonsteroidal anti-inflammatory medications had a significantly lower incidence of thromboembolism following total knee arthroplasty than their unmedicated counterparts. However, he noted no other significant differences between the two groups.

An overview of the literature indicates that with increasing complexity of the operation and with increasing age, the incidence of deep-vein thrombosis increases. The incidence of deep-vein thrombosis following arthroscopic surgery ranges from 0.1% to 1.6% (19,89,125). With knee arthrotomy an incidence as low as 8% was reported by Nilsen (82) in his study of patients 20–35 years old, whereas an incidence of 57% was reported by Cohen (12) in older patients undergoing knee arthrotomy for degenerative disease. In patients undergoing total knee arthroplasty, there is general agreement that the incidence of deep-vein thrombosis is high, with rates of 46–72% being reported (52,64,71,119).

Patients undergoing knee ligament surgery are usually young, athletic, and healthy. They have none of the risk factors identified by Kakkar (50) and Hull (39) except for the possible adverse effect of postoperative immobilization. Thus it is not surprising that thromboembolic disease following knee ligament surgery is rarely reported. However, the preponderance of research would indicate that even in this most favored population, at least 10% of patients develop silent postoperative deep-vein thrombosis. It is likely that the majority of these thrombi are small and localized in the calf. Yet, while rare, a sudden, fatal, pulmonary embolus originating from the lower extremity and occurring without premonitory clinical signs may be the most common cause of mortality following knee ligament surgery.

KNEE INFECTION

The San Diego Kaiser review of 390 cases revealed six infections. Three infections were superficial. All superficial infections centered around a screw with spiked washer used to attach a hamstring graft to the proximal tibia. Two presented as failure to heal the distal end of the tibia wound. The infection resolved with the use of oral antibiotics and removal of the fixation device which was performed 7 and 12 weeks after surgery. One knee remained stable, whereas the other knee exhibited recurring instability. The third superficial infection followed a blow to the anterior aspect of the knee 6 months after surgery, with resulting wound breakdown over the screw and soft tissue washer. After the fixation device was removed and the patient was placed on oral antibiotics, the infection resolved and the knee remained stable.

Three infections were deep. None occurred within 8 weeks of the ligament surgery. All occurred after a secondary arthrotomy procedure. In the 390-patient Kaiser review, there were a total of 61 secondary procedures performed in 40 patients within 12 months of ligament surgery (Table 28-2). Arthrotomies were performed in four patients to gain range of motion. Two of those patients developed a deep infection. Surgery was performed for fixation failure in three patients, one of whom developed an infection.

In one case the infection followed an open procedure with lateral release performed to gain joint motion 2 months after an acute patellar tendon ACL reconstruction. Two weeks after the secondary open procedure the patient presented with chills, fever, and a pyarthrosis that cultured *Staphylococcus aureus*. The patient was treated with open débridement, I.V. antibiotics, a rotation flap for secondary wound closure, and a split-thickness skin graft to the donor site. The patient's infection resolved, and she regained good knee function.

The second case developed following an arthroscopic procedure to gain range of motion performed 7 months after an acute MCL repair and hamstring graft ACL reconstruction. This was the patient's fourth secondary procedure performed to gain joint motion, including an arthrotomy 6 months after the ligament surgery. Three days after the arthroscopy the patient presented with a pyarthrosis that cultured *Bacteroides fragilis* and *Staphylococcus aureus*. An open-wound débridement was performed, and I.V. antibiotics were given. The infection resolved, but the patient developed a painful arthrofibrosis in 20° of flexion.

The third deep infection developed following a procedure to retension an over-the-top 8-mm polypropylene–patellar tendon composite graft 6 months after the index procedure. Two weeks after the secondary procedure the patient presented with chills and fever.

TABLE 28-2. *Secondary procedures within 12 months of ligament surgery*

Indication	Patients	Manipulation closed	Arthroscopy	Other operative procedures
Single-ligament ACL surgery (n = 329)				
Limited range of motion	16	20	2	2
Fixation failure	3			3
Chronic effusion	4		4	1
Metal removal	2			2
Graft impingement	3		3	
Skin graft	2			2
Infection	2		1	1
Total	32 (10%)	20	10	11
Multiple-ligament surgery (n = 61)				
Limited range of motion	11	11	5	2
Infection				1
Total	11 (18%)			

Joint aspiration grew *Staphylococcus epidermidis*. The composite graft was removed. An iliotibial band procedure was performed (3) at the time of the graft removal. The patient was placed on I.V. antibiotics, and the infection resolved.

REFLEX SYMPATHETIC DYSTROPHY

"Reflex sympathetic dystrophy" (RSD) is a term that is currently accepted for a disorder that includes a constellation of symptoms with a wide array of causes (26,62,97). Classically, it presents in any extremity as hypersensitivity to painful stimuli associated with cool mottled skin, limb atrophy, osteoporosis, increased vascularity of the limb, and restricted range of motion. Clinical situations associated with RSD include: injuries involving soft tissues, fractures, treatment of fractures (particularly cast immobilization), surgical procedures of any type, and nerve trauma. The incidence of classical RSD after trauma to the hand or foot is 0.9% (97). An examination of 3000 knee injuries (most without surgical pathology) yielded 14 cases of RSD, a 0.5% incidence rate (122). Our literature review of knee ligament reconstruction literature did not discover reports of RSD. The surgeon poll tabulated an incidence of 0.75% after ACL reconstruction. There were no cases diagnosed in the San Diego Kaiser review of 390 patients. However, 27 (7%) patients had procedures performed under anesthesia as treatment for limited range of motion. Perhaps some of these patients represented a form of reflex sympathetic dystrophy resulting in decreased motion of the knee.

GRAFT DONOR SITE COMPLICATIONS

The most common autograft tissue used for ACL are the distal portion of the iliotibial tract, one or two hamstring tendons, or one-third of the patellar tendon. Graft donor site morbidity should be considered when planning ligament graft surgery.

Numerous authors have reported on reconstructions using the iliotibial band (2,3,22,54,63). While the efficacy of iliotibial band reconstruction has been questioned, few reports are present in the literature which comment on the adverse effects of the sacrifice of a portion of this tendon. Teitge (121) reported increased varus laxity in 91% of patients with iliotibial band reconstructions; however, no patient had symptomatic varus instability. Losee (63) reported on the use of the iliotibial band in the "sling and reef" procedure. Postoperatively, 19 of 50 patients (38%) had a hernia of the vastus lateralis through a defect in the remaining iliotibial band. None of the patients were symptomatic. The San Diego Kaiser review included 38 patients with an Insall iliotibial band intraarticular ACL graft (42).

Two patients demonstrated postoperative herniation of the vastus lateralis through a defect in the iliotibial band. This herniation was cosmetically objectionable and mildly symptomatic on exertion. No patient requested reconstruction of the fascial defect.

Complications of patellar tendon reconstruction have been reported. McCarroll (68) reported an isolated case of patellar fracture that occurred 6 months after bone–patellar tendon–bone reconstruction. He postulated it was a stress fracture due to the decreased vascularization of the patella following the surgery. Bonamo (6) reported avulsion of the patellar tendon from the inferior pole of the patella in two patients at 4 months and 8 months after reconstruction of the ACL using the central third of the patellar tendon. In both of these patients, repair of the patellar tendon resulted in an uneventful recovery. This same complication was reported by the Kennedy LAD research group (18). In their series of 148 patients with a Marshal McIntosh ACL reconstruction augmented by a polypropylene braid, rupture of the patellar tendon occurred in four cases (2.7%). All occurred within the first 6 months after surgery. In each case the rupture was related to a traumatic event involving hyperflexion of the knee. At the time of surgical repair of the patellar tendon rupture, in all cases the ACL graft was observed to be intact. All four patients went on to uneventful recovery. In the San Diego Kaiser review there were no cases of patellar fracture or tendon rupture.

Cabaud (8) evaluated the patellar tendon in dogs after using the middle third for ACL reconstruction. He reported no loss of strength at 4 months after reconstruction, and he noted increased strength at 8 months. However, in a similar study utilizing dogs (n = 22), Burks (7) reported the patellar tendon strength after harvesting the middle third to be 70% of the control side at 3 months and 60% at 6 months. The cross-sectional area of the tendon was greater than the control side at both 3 and 6 months and histologically revealed poor collagen organization. Burks harvested the middle third of the patellar tendon, and he closed the prepatellar fascia but not the defect. At 3 and 6 months the mean tendon lengths were 10% shorter than the control side. Paulos (93) reported symptomatic patella baja secondary to patellar tendon graft harvest for ACL surgery.

The effect of harvesting the patellar tendon on patellofemoral morbidity was discussed by Huegel (37) in a 6-month comparison of allograft versus autograft. In the allograft group, 68% (15/22) were asymptomatic with 80% quadriceps strength. By comparison, only 20% (5/25) in the autograft group had 80% quadriceps strength, and 60% had either donor site or patellofemoral discomfort.

Patellar tendon and hamstring tendon were the usual graft sources in the San Diego Kaiser series. Table 28-3 presents data 1 year after surgery on 180 patients who have been sorted into four groups based on graft source and postoperative rehabilitation program. The graft source used in surgery was selected by the surgeon. The hamstring was often selected as the graft source in the less athletic patient having a ACL reconstruction in association with a meniscus repair. The patellar tendon was usually selected for patients involved in high-risk sport or in patients with greater joint instability. Despite the fact that the patient groups are dissimilar, the data are of interest. In the patellar tendon patients there was a higher percentage of patients with flexion contracture, quadriceps weakness, and poor hop function. Using a hamstring tendon graft source did result in decreased knee flexion strength, but overall it appeared to result in less morbidity. However, KT-1000 measurements indicated that better stability was obtained with the patellar tendon graft.

POSTOPERATIVE GRAFT IMPINGEMENT

Postoperative impingement of the ACL graft in the intercondylar notch may block full extension and/or may produce a chafing of the graft which can weaken it with resulting disruption. Graft impingement is predominantly affected by placement of the tibial tunnel. Anterior or lateral placement of the tibial tunnel may result in graft impingement unless a notchplasty is performed (Chapter 2). Yaru (128) observed that anterior tibial translation produced by active extension of the knee caused graft impingement in a greater flexion arc than could be produced with passive knee extension. He recommended that with passive motion there should be a 2-mm clearance between the anterior portion of the intercondylar notch and the ligament graft to avoid impingement when the patient actively extends.

In the San Diego Kaiser series of 390 ACL reconstructions, there were 12 cases (3%) that postopera-

TABLE 28-3. *Evaluation 1 year after ACL reconstruction (n = 180)*

	Graft source			
	Patellar tendon		Hamstring tendon(s)	
Post-op flexion	30[a]	0[b]	30[a]	0[b]
Number	60	56	45	19
Age (mean)	25	26	23	26
Surgery within 6 weeks of injury	7 (12%)	15 (27%)	21 (47%)	5 (26%)
Flexion contracture[c]				
Mean	4	2	4	1
>5°	19 (32%)	6 (11%)	11 (24%)	0
Flexion loss				
>10°	4 (7%)	0	4 (9%)	0
Patellar irritability				
>1[d]	5 (8%)	0	3 (7%)	0
Quadriceps index[e]				
Mean	61	74	75	81
<80	49 (82%)	30 (54%)	25 (56%)	7 (37%)
Flexion index[e]				
Mean	75	97	88	88
<90	27 (45%)	15 (27%)	22 (49%)	10 (53%)
Hop index[e]				
Mean	75	81	83	84
<90	45 (75%)	36 (64%)	28 (62%)	7 (37%)
KT-1000 30° ($I - N$)				
20-lb anterior				
Mean mm	1.5	1.8	2.7	2.2
>2.5 mm	20 (33%)	17 (30%)	23 (51%)	10 (53%)
Manual maximum				
Mean mm	2.9	3.2	2.8	3.6
>2.5 mm	29 (48%)	35 (63%)	25 (56%)	12 (63%)
>5.0 mm	8 (13%)	8 (14%)	9 (20%)	3 (16%)

[a] Postoperative immobilization in 20–30° of flexion for 3 weeks, followed with a range-of-motion brace or hinged cast for an additional 3–4 weeks with a range of motion of 20–100°.

[b] Postoperative immobilization in 0° of flexion; postoperative program is presented in Fig. 3-2.

[c] Flexion contracture measured as prone heel height difference (1 cm = 1°) (Fig. 3-1 and Table 3-1).

[d] There were no contralateral knees with patellar irritability >1.

[e] Quadriceps, flexion, and hop index are expressed in relation to the contralateral normal knee (injured/normal × 100).

tively demonstrated an audible and palpable "thunk" as the patient extended his/her knee. The "thunk" was rarely painful, but in the more severe cases it was annoying. In no patient could the "thunk" be produced by passively extending the leg. In six of the cases the "thunk" was annoying enough that the patients consented to arthroscopic surgery. The patients were arthroscoped under local anesthesia so the knee could be actively extended to produce the "thunk." In all six patients, arthroscopy revealed impingement of the graft on the anterior and/or lateral walls of the intercondylar notch which was reduced or eliminated by excising bone to open the anterior portal of the intercondylar notch.

JOINT STIFFNESS

The goal of ligament reconstruction is to restore normal knee kinematics. A knee with a 10° flexion contracture is probably a greater impairment than is the usual knee with an ACL disruption. During the past 5 years, surgeons have shortened the period of postoperative immobilization and have reduced the incidence of postoperative joint stiffness (24,83).

Nonphysiologic motion restriction after surgery may be secondary to (a) nonisometric graft placement and improper graft tensioning (Chapter 10), (b) adhesions and intraarticular soft tissue proliferation (Chapter 15), and (c) soft tissue mechanical changes resulting from injury (Chapters 15, 18, and 19) and/or joint immobilization (Chapters 15, 16, and 17). Laboratory studies on the response of knee ligaments to injury are discussed in detail in Chapters 18 and 19.

After properly performed ligament surgery followed by short periods of immobilization, mobilization of the limb with passive stretching and active range of motion usually restores joint motion. On occasion, the following are necessary: manipulation under anesthesia, arthroscopic release of adhesions (90,118), and open surgery (81,93). We have found the modified bicycle to be a useful range-of-motion device (Fig. 3-8).

In the San Diego Kaiser review of 390 ligament procedures, a range-of-motion procedure under anesthesia was performed on 27 patients (7%) within 12 months of the ligament surgery. There were a total of 329 patients who had single-ligament ACL reconstruction surgery. Sixteen of those patients (5%) had a postoperative manipulation under anesthesia. There were 61 patients with multiple-ligament repairs; 11 of these patients (18%) had a manipulation. This rate was significantly higher than that of the patients who underwent single-ligament surgery ($p < 0.005$). Nine percent of patients (12 of 132) who had an ACL reconstruction within 6 weeks of injury had a manipulation, whereas only 2% (4 of 197) who had an ACL reconstruction at

greater than 6 weeks after injury had a manipulation ($p < 0.005$).

Mohtadi (75) reviewed 527 ACL reconstructions and reported that 37 patients (7%) were manipulated because they failed to gain a satisfactory range of motion. A satisfactory range of motion was defined as 10–120° by 3 months after surgery. In a comparison between the manipulated and nonmanipulated patients, the author reported no statistically significant differences between the two groups in relation to age, sex, knee, meniscal repair, or performance of a concomitant MCL repair. He reported that the need for manipulation, if surgery was done at less than 6 weeks after injury, was 11% (25 of 228 cases) compared to 4% (12 of 299) if the surgery was done at 6 or more weeks after injury. These statistics are similar to those of the San Diego Kaiser study.

Paulos (93) reported stiffness of the knee following surgery secondary to (a) fibrous hyperplasia of the anterior soft tissues of the knee (including the anterior fat pad) and (b) shortening of the patellar tendon. Paulos emphasizes the importance of early patellar mobilization to prevent development of the condition. In the San Diego Kaiser review there is one case of infrapatellar contracture syndrome which is presented as Case 8 in Chapter 3.

To improve our understanding of the postoperative course after ligament surgery, we developed a postoperative evaluation protocol in 1986. Some additional observations were added to the protocol in 1987. Table 28-4 presents early postoperative data on 141 consecutive ACL reconstructions to document the course of thigh atrophy, joint effusion, range of motion, and joint stability measurements. The rehabilitation program of all patients followed the protocol presented in Fig. 3-1. Thirty-one percent of the patients were reconstructed within 6 weeks of injury. All measurements were performed by author MLS. Because of the addition of some observations to the evaluation in 1987 and the inability of patients to come for all scheduled clinic visits, the number of observations for each data point ranges from 64 to 141 (mean 90, S.D. 31). One hundred thirty-three patients were evaluated at the 24-week follow-up visit.

All patients were immobilized 10–14 days in a cast applied to immobilize the knee in 0° of flexion. After the cast was removed, the patient was placed on a continuous passive motion (CPM) machine for 1 hour and was then examined. Note that 27% had a flexion contracture on that initial examination after 1 hour of CPM. The patients were then placed in a range-of-motion brace with a 50° extension stop and no flexion stop. At night the brace was removed and the patient was placed in a splint with the knee in extension. At 6 weeks, 66% of the patients had flexion of greater than 90°. If the patient did not have flexion of greater than

90° by 8 weeks after surgery, we considered manipulation under anesthesia. Because of a lack of progress in recovering the flexion arc in these patients, some manipulations were performed 6 weeks after surgery. With this postoperative program in 141 ACL reconstructions within 6 months of surgery we have performed nine secondary procedures on seven patients (5%) to improve flexion (eight closed manipulations, one arthroscopic procedure, and no arthrotomies). This is in comparison to our prior postoperative program in 188 ACL reconstructions; 14 procedures were performed in nine patients (5%) to improve flexion and/or extension (12 closed manipulations, one arthroscopic procedure, and one arthrotomy).

WEAKNESS, PAIN, AND FLEXION CONTRACTURE

Flexion contracture, patellofemoral pain, and quadriceps weakness are the three most common complications of knee ligament surgery. They are implicated in suboptimal results following ACL reconstruction and are causes for patient dissatisfaction.

Flexion Contracture

Flexion contracture was noted in 32% of the cases reported in the literature and was found in 24% of cases included in our surgeon poll (Table 28-1). Prior to 1986, the knees of the patients in the San Diego Kaiser series were immobilized in 30° of flexion for 3 weeks after surgery and were then placed in a hinged cast or brace with a 30° extension stop for another 3–5 weeks. Evaluation 1 year after surgery revealed that 30 of 105 patients (29%) had a flexion contracture of greater than 5°, measured as prone heel height difference of greater than 5 cm. [Referenced to 0° of extension, 16 patients (15%) had a flexion contracture of greater than 5°.] There was a positive correlation between flexion contracture, patellar irritability, quadriceps weakness, and impairment on the same one-leg hop for distance (Fig. 28-1). There was a positive correlation between flexion contracture and age (107). Since 1986 the operated knee has been immobilized in extension for 10–14 days after surgery (Fig. 3-1). In patellar tendon graft patients the incidence of flexion contracture of greater than 5° has dropped from 32% to 11% ($p < 0.005$), and in hamstring graft patients it has dropped from 24% to 0% ($p < 0.01$) (Table 28-3). In the 75 patients immobilized after surgery in full extension we have not observed a correlation between age and flexion contracture.

Patellofemoral Pain

A 1982 San Diego Kaiser retrospective review of 36 patients with normal patellofemoral joints at the time of surgery revealed that only one-third had a normal patellofemoral clinical examination 1 year after surgery. Of the remaining patients, one-third had anterior knee crepitus but no pain, while the other one-third not only had anterior knee crepitus but also had anterior knee pain. In a later review of 126 postoperative patients, a 19% incidence of patellofemoral pain was noted (107). Correlations between patellar symptoms and other factors are presented in Fig. 28-1. The effects of patellar irritability and knee flexion contracture were found to be additive in relation to their effect on quadriceps strength. One year after surgery, 17 of 18 patients (94%) with both a flexion contracture of greater than 5° and an irritable patella had quadriceps strength of less than 80% of the contralateral knee as compared to 18 of 33 patients (55%) with a flexion contracture of less than 6° and no patella irritability. As noted in Table 28-3, 8% of knees immobilized after surgery in 30° of flexion had moderate to severe patellar irritability (discomfort with patellar manipulation), whereas none of the 75 patients immobilized in 0° of flexion had moderate or severe patellar irritability. In no patient did the contralateral knee have moderate or severe patellar irritability.

Quadriceps Weakness

Quadriceps weakness is the single most common complication reported post-ACL reconstruction. It is reported in 47% of patients in our literature review and in 23% of patients in the surgeon's poll. In the San Diego Kaiser review presented in Table 28-1, peak extension torque at 60°/sec was measured 1 year after surgery and was compared to each patient's normal contralateral knee ($n = 180$). One hundred eleven patients (62%) had quadriceps strength which was less than 80% of that of the contralateral normal knee. An additional test used to compare limb function was the one-leg hop for distance. This test evaluates strength and confidence in the tested leg (Chapter 29). One hundred sixteen patients' (64%) hop for distance on the operated knee was less than 90% of that of the contralateral normal knee. As noted in Fig. 28-1, there is a positive correlation between quadriceps weakness and a flexion contracture. As recorded in Table 28-3, patients immobilized postoperatively at 0° of flexion had less flexion contracture and greater quadriceps strength 1 year after surgery than did those immobilized at 30° of flexion.

Effusion

Joint effusion occurs after all knee ligament surgery. In most patients there is a persistent effusion for 3–9 months (Table 28-4). Like many observations, the re-

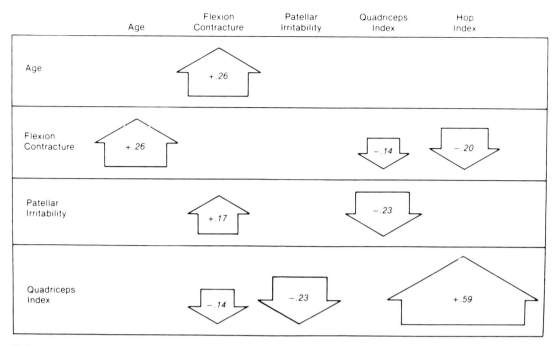

FIG. 28-1. Evaluation of 126 patients 1 year after ACL reconstruction. Patients were treated by postoperative cast immobilization in 30° of flexion for 3 weeks followed by a range-of-motion brace with a 30° extension stop for 3–5 weeks. Arrows indicate a statistically significant ($p <$ 0.05) correlation. The value within the arrow indicates the extent of the correlation. Positive correlations are indicated as arrows pointing up, and negative correlations are denoted by arrows pointing down. Flexion contracture is defined as prone heel height difference of greater than 5 cm.

ported incidence of effusion is largely dependent on the evaluation system of the examiner (Chapter 29). The incidence of joint surface injury in the acute ACL-injured knee is about 20%, and the incidence in the chronic ACL-injured knee is about 50% (Fig. 27-11). Therefore, it is likely that on follow-up examination, many patients would have an effusion secondary to the joint surface pathology. In the literature the reported incidence of chronic effusion following ligament surgery is 13% (Table 28-1), whereas in our surgeon poll it is 2.5%. One year after ACL surgery in the San Diego Kaiser Group B, 25 of 205 patients (12%) had an effusion. Twenty patients were evaluated to have a 1+ effusion, and five had a 2+ effusion. It is of interest that four of the five patients with a 2+ effusion had their autogenous graft augmented with a 3M Kennedy ligament augmentation device (LAD). The incidence of effusion may increase when synthetic ligaments are used. Olsen (88) reported that synthetic-ligament wear particles induced elevated levels of neutral proteinases in tissue culture. *In vivo* studies revealed that wear particles accumulated in the synovial and subsynovial tissue, resulting in a mild to moderate synovial hypertrophy. Effusions have been reported associated with a number of synthetic ligaments: carbon fiber (104), Dacron (55), GORE-TEX (40), and LAD (103).

Young (129) reviewed studies of nerve pathways and quadriceps function which reflected changes that occurred as a response to effusion. He observed that when saline was injected into the normal knees, the amount of quadriceps inhibition was related to the amount of fluid injected. As low as 40 mm of saline may inhibit more than 50% of the nerve activity in the quadriceps. Based on these studies and the work of others, the author suggested a network of factors that contribute to quadriceps inhibition and flexion contracture (Fig. 28-1).

Ogilvie-Harris (86) examined the effect of prostaglandin inhibition and the subsequent decrease in periarticular inflammation on the rate of recovery after arthroscopic meniscectomy. This double-blind study of 139 patients showed that the use of a prostaglandin inhibitor (naproxen sodium) resulted in significantly less pain, less synovitis, and less effusion. There was a significantly more rapid return of quadriceps function, range of motion, sports participation, and gainful employment in patients who were given nonsteroidal anti-inflammatory drugs than in those who were not given that drug. Review of the ACL San Diego Kaiser 1-year postoperative data suggests a relationship between effusion and a decrease in quadriceps strength. The quadriceps index in the 25 patients with an effusion was 60%, while it was 71% for the 180 patients without an effusion.

TABLE 28-4. *Recovery after ligament surgery*

	Postoperative week			
	2	6	12	24
Effusion				
0	0	0	8%	57%
1	36%	62%	80%	38%
2	64%	28%	12%	5%
3	0	0	0	0
Knee circumference (N − I)				
<1 cm	8%	12%	13%	30%
1–3 cm	69%	84%	83%	69%
>3 cm	22%	4%	4%	1%
Mean cm	2.9	1.8	1.4	1.0
Thigh circumference (N − I)				
<1 cm	8%	3%	3%	21%
1–3 cm	70%	28%	57%	67%
>3 cm	22%	68%	40%	12%
Mean cm	2.3	4.2	3.3	1.6
Flexion contracture[a]				
<1 cm	30%	11%	35%	57%
1–5 cm	42%	39%	45%	39%
6–10 cm	22%	41%	16%	4%
>10 cm	5%	10%	4%	0%
Mean cm	3.9	5.9	3.3	1.3
Flexion (degrees)				
0–40	26%	2%	0%	0%
41–90	70%	32%	4%	0%
91–120	4%	53%	35%	12%
>120	0%	13%	62%	88%
Mean	52	101	123	130
KT-1000 (N − I)				
20-lb anterior				
>2.5 mm		13%	31%	37%
Mean mm		−0.5	1.9	1.9
Manual maximum				
>2.5			41%	51%
>5 mm			9%	13%
Mean			2.2	2.7
Quadriceps active				
>2.5		16%	24%	40%
Mean		−0.2	1.0	2.0
Pivot shift				
0				89%
1				10%
2				1%
3				0%

[a] Measured as prone heel height difference (1 cm = 1°).

GROWTH-PLATE INJURY

Growth disturbance, angular deformity, and loss of joint congruity are sequelae of injury (fractures) of the growth-plate and, therefore, are concerns of surgeons attempting to reconstruct the ACL in a patient with significant growth potential (11,16,108). Studies on growth and leg-length discrepancy yield some data to assess the risk in patients with paraphyseal or transphyseal surgery. If 1 cm is an acceptable leg-length discrepancy (105), then growth-plate disturbance is not an issue after the age of 15.5 years for the average male and after the age of 14 years for the average female (using 50 percentile of growth as a guide) (78,108). It is our approach to calculate the bone age from wrist radiographs and estimate the remaining distal femoral and proximal tibia growth in any patient with open growth plates considered for ACL reconstruction surgery. There were nine patients under age 15 in the San Diego Kaiser review of 500 ACL-injured patients (Chapter 23). Ligament surgery was not performed acutely in any of the nine youngsters.

In the only large series of ACL reconstructions in adolescent athletes, Libscomb (61) addressed the possibility of growth arrest. He examined both knee stability and complications in 24 patients seen after reconstructions using semitendinosus and gracilis tendons intraarticularly and Ellison or Losse extraarticular supplementation. His population consisted of (a) 11 patients with completely open physes and (b) 13 patients with partially open physes. In this series an 8-mm drill hole was placed in the femoral epiphysis (avoiding the femoral physis) and a 6.4-mm drill hole was placed across the tibial physis. Preoperative leg-length discrepancy measurements were not made. Postoperative measurements after skeletal maturity revealed a less-than-5-mm difference in 17 patients. Of the five patients with a 6- to 10-mm difference, the injured limb was shorter in two and longer in three. An average limb-length discrepancy of 7–8 mm is seen in 77% of the normal population (105). The two remaining reconstructions resulted in one limb 2 cm shorter and one limb 1.3 cm longer than the uninjured side. The 2-cm difference was attributed to the use of staples for ligament fixation, which spanned the epiphysis. No explanation for the 1.3-cm leg lengthening was given.

SUMMARY

There are a number of major complications that may result from knee surgery: anesthetic death, vascular injury, major nerve injury, deep-vein thrombosis with pulmonary embolism, deep infection, and reflex sympathetic dystrophy. Fortunately, the incidence of these complications is low. In the San Diego Kaiser review of 390 patients, the only major complications were three deep-wound infections. Interestingly, none of the infections occurred after the initial ligament surgery. One occurred 3 days after an arthroscopy procedure that had been preceded 1 month earlier by an open procedure to gain joint motion. A second occurred 2 weeks after an open procedure to gain range of motion. In the third patient the infection occurred after an open procedure to explore a loose graft.

While the incidence of major complications is low, the incidence of joint morbidity following knee ligament surgery is high, including: flexion contracture, patellofemoral pain, quadriceps weakness, and joint stiffness requiring manipulation under anesthesia. These complications are secondary to the trauma of graft implantation, the morbidity of graft harvest, and the postoperative immobilization program. Arthroscopic graft implantation may decrease the trauma of graft implantation but does not affect the morbidity of graft harvest. The hamstring graft appears to be a less morbid graft source than the patellar tendon graft, but the patellar tendon is a stronger graft that provides a greater opportunity for strong fixation (Chapter 2). In the future, perhaps allografts or prosthetic grafts will provide an alternative to autografts and reduce surgical morbidity of graft harvest.

Surgical timing and the postoperative rehabilitation program will affect (a) the incidence of joint stiffness requiring manipulation and (b) the incidence of flexion contracture. The incidence of joint stiffness is higher in patients with an acute injury than in patients with a chronic injury. To minimize the incidence of flexion contracture and joint stiffness, the knee should have a full range of motion and not be inflamed at the time of surgery. The patient who has undergone multiple-ligament repairs is at higher risk of joint stiffness than the patient with a single-ligament reconstruction. In a prospective randomized study of 50 ACL reconstructions using intermittent passive motion beginning the day after surgery, we did not demonstrate an improved range of motion at 6 months after surgery in the early passive motion group compared to our standard treatment group (Fig. 3-1). Therefore, we are not using passive motion routinely in single-ligament ACL surgery. We do, however, use passive motion after multiple-ligament surgery.

There is a correlation between knee flexion contracture, quadriceps weakness, and patellofemoral pain. By immobilizing our patients at 0° of flexion for 10–14 days after surgery and then beginning an active motion program, we have decreased the incidence of flexion contracture and patellofemoral pain 1 year after surgery and improved the quadriceps strength (Table 28-3). This change in our rehabilitation program from immobilization in 30° of flexion for 3 weeks has not resulted in a higher incidence of joint instability.

To minimize joint stiffness and muscle wasting after surgery, some surgeons are advocating an earlier motion and exercise program than is presented in Fig. 3-1 (24,59,83,114). We are concerned that the large forces placed on the ACL by quadriceps contraction from 0° to 50° of flexion may result in graft disruption (Chapter 11). We limit quadriceps contraction to 50–120° of flexion during the first 6 weeks. The 6-week period of maximum graft protection is to allow graft fixation site healing (Chapters 2 and 21). Further laboratory studies on muscle–ligament interaction, graft fixation site strength, and graft healing, as well as carefully monitored clinical studies, will better clarify this issue.

The stability of most patients' knees is improved by ligament surgery, but about half of our patients have persistent pathologic motion. The evaluation of joint motion after surgery is further discussed in Chapters 24 and 29.

REFERENCES

1. Akeson WH, Amiel D, Abel MF, Garfin SR, Woo SL-Y. Effects of immobilization of joints. *Clin Orthop* 1987;219:28–37.
2. Andrews JR, Sanders R. A "mini-reconstruction" technique in treating anterolateral rotatory instability (ALRI). *Clin Orthop* 1983;172:93–96.
3. Arnold JA. A lateral extra-articular tenodesis for anterior cruciate ligament deficiency of the knee. *Orthop Clin North Am* 1985;16:213–222.
4. Barber FA, Stone RG. Meniscal repair: an arthroscopic technique. *J Bone Joint Surg* 1985;67B:39–41.
5. Bertoia JT, Urovitz EP, Richards RR, et al. Anterior cruciate reconstruction using the MacIntosh lateral-substitution over-the-top repair. *J Bone Joint Surg* 1985;67A:1183–1188.
6. Bonamo JJ, Krinick RM, Sporn AA. Rupture of the patellar ligament after use of its central third for anterior cruciate reconstruction. A report of two cases. *J Bone Joint Surg* 1984;66A:1294–1297.
7. Burks RT, Haut RC, Lancaster RL. Biomechanical and histological observations on the dog patellar tendon after removal of its central one-third; Personal Communication.
8. Cabaud HE, Feagin JA, Rodkey WG. Acute anterior cruciate ligament injury and augmented repair. Experimental studies. *Am J Sports Med* 1980;8:395–401.
9. Chambers GH. The prepatellar nerve. A cause of suboptimal results in knee arthrotomy. *Clin Orthop* 1972;82:157–159.
10. Clancy WG Jr, Nelson DA, Reider B, et al. Anterior cruciate ligament reconstruction using one-third of the patellar ligament, augmented by extra-articular tendon transfers. *J Bone Joint Surg* 1982;64A:352–359.
11. Clanton TO, DeLee JC, Sanders B, et al. Knee ligament injuries in children. *J Bone Joint Surg* 1979;61A:1195–1201.
12. Cohen SH, Ehrlich GE, Kauffman MS, Cope C. Thrombophlebitis following knee surgery. *J Bone Joint Surg* 1973;55A:106–112.
13. Collins HR. U.S. experience with GORE-TEX reconstruction of the anterior cruciate ligament. In: Friedman MJ, Ferkel RD, eds. *Prosthetic ligament reconstruction of the knee.* Philadelphia: WB Saunders, 1988;165–179.
14. Cooper JB, Newbower RS, Kitz RJ. An analysis of major errors and equipment failures in anesthesia management: considerations for prevention and detection. *Anesthesiology* 1984;60:34–42.
15. Cushing H. Pneumatic tourniquets: with especial reference to their use in craniotomies. *Med News (NY)* 1904;84:577–580.
16. Czitrom AA, Salter RB, Willis RB. Fractures involving the distal epiphyseal plate of the femur. *Int Orthop* 1981;4:269–277.
17. Daniel DM, Van Kempen CL. Synthetic augmentation of the biological anterior cruciate ligament substitution. In: Friedman MJ, Ferkel RD, eds. *Prosthetic ligament reconstruction of the knee.* Philadelphia: WB Saunders, 1988;65–70.
18. Daniel DM, Woodward EP, Losse GM, Stone ML. The Marshall/MacIntosh anterior cruciate ligament reconstruction with the Kennedy ligament augmentation device: report of the United States clinical trials. In: Friedman MJ, Ferkel RD, eds. *Prosthetic ligament reconstruction of the knee.* Philadelphia: WB Saunders, 1988;71–78.
19. DeLee JC. Complications of arthroscopy and arthroscopic surgery: results of a national survey. *Arthroscopy* 1985;1:214–220.

20. Dobner JJ, Nitz AJ. Postmeniscectomy tourniquet palsy and functional sequelae. *Am J Sports Med* 1982;10:211–214.
21. Doupe J, Cullen CH, Chance GQ. Post-traumatic pain and the causalgia syndrome. *J Neurol Neurosurg Psychiatry* 1944;7:33–48.
22. Ellison AE. Distal iliotibial-band transfer for anterolateral rotatory instability of the knee. *J Bone Joint Surg* 1979;61A:330–337.
23. Enneking WF, Horowitz M. The intra-articular effects of immobilization on the human knee. *J Bone Joint Surg* 1972;54A:973–985.
24. Epstein RM. Morbidity and mortality from anesthesia: a continuing problem. *Anesthesiology* 1978;49:388–389.
25. Fermaglich DR. Reflex sympathetic dystrophy in children. *Pediatrics* 1977;60:881–883.
26. Ficat RP, Hungerford DS. Disorders of the patellofemoral joint. *Reflex sympathetic dystrophy*. Baltimore: Williams & Wilkins, 1977;149–169.
27. Fitts WH Jr. Thromboembolism: the clinical picture. *J Trauma* 1969;9(8):661–667.
28. Fowler TJ, Danta G, Gilliatt RW. Recovery of nerve conduction after a pneumatic tourniquet: observations on the hindlimb of the baboon. *J Neurol Neurosurg Psychiatry* 1972;35:638–647.
29. Friedman MJ, Ferkel RD. *Prosthetic ligament reconstruction of the knee*. Philadelphia: WB Saunders, 1988.
30. Friedman MJ, Sherman OH, Fox JM, et al. Autogenic anterior cruciate ligament (ACL) anterior reconstruction of the knee. A review. *Clin Orthop* 1985;196:9–14.
31. Fruengaard S, Holm A. Compartment syndrome complications arthroscopic surgery. Brief report. *J Bone Joint Surg* 1988;70B:146–147.
32. Goldstein A Jr, Keats AS. The risk of anesthesia. *Anesthesiology* 1970;33:130–141.
33. Green NE, Allen BL. Vascular injuries associated with dislocation of the knee. *J Bone Joint Surg* 1977;59A:236–239.
34. Harris WH, Athanasoulis C, Waltman AC, Saltzman EW. Cuff-impedance phlebography and ^{125}I fibrinogen scanning versus roentgenographic phlebography for diagnosis of thrombophlebitis following hip surgery. A preliminary report. *J Bone Joint Surg* 1976;58A:939–944.
35. Hohf RP. Arterial injuries occurring during orthopedic operations. *Clin Orthop* 1963;28:21–37.
36. Hollinshead WH. *Anatomy for surgeons*, 2nd ed. New York: Harper and Row, 1969.
37. Huegel M, Indelicato P. Trends in rehabilitation following anterior cruciate ligament reconstruction. *Clin Sports Med* 1988;7:801–811.
38. Hughston JC. Complications of anterior cruciate ligament surgery. *Orthop Clin North Am* 1985;16:237–240.
39. Hull RD, Raskob GE. Prophylaxis of venous thromboembolic disease following hip and knee surgery. *J Bone Joint Surg* 1986;68A:146–150.
40. Indelicato PA, Pascale MS, Huegel MO. Early experience with the GORE-TEX polytetrafluoroethylene anterior cruciate ligament prosthesis. *Am J Sports Med* 1989;17:55–62.
41. Insall JM. Disorders of the patella. In: Insall JM, ed. *Surgery of the knee*. New York: Churchill Livingstone, 1984;191–260.
42. Insall J, Joseph DM, Aglietti P, et al. Bone-block iliotibial-band transfer for anterior cruciate insufficiency. *J Bone Joint Surg* 1981;63A:560–569.
43. Jackson DW, Wondler G, Simon TM. Intraarticular reaction associated with the use of freeze-dried, ethylene oxide sterilized bone–patellar tendon bone allografts in the reconstruction of the anterior cruciate ligament. Paper presented at the AOSSM Annual Meeting, February 1989.
44. Jeffries JT, Gainor BJ, Allen WC, Cikrit D. Injury to the popliteal artery as a complication of arthroscopic surgery. A report of two cases. *J Bone Joint Surg* 1987;69A:783–785.
45. Jimenez F, Utrilla A, Cuesta C, et al. Popliteal artery and venous aneurysm as a complication of arthroscopic meniscectomy. *J Trauma* 1988;28:1404–1405.
46. Johnson RJ, Eriksson E, Haggmark T, et al. Five- to ten-year follow-up evaluation after reconstruction of the anterior cruciate ligament. *Clin Orthop* 1984;183:122–140.
47. Johnson RJ, Kettelkamp DB, Clark W, Leaverton P. Factors affecting late results after meniscectomy. *J Bone Joint Surg* 1974;56A:719–729.
48. Jones KG. Reconstruction of the anterior cruciate ligament using the central one-third of the patellar ligament. *J Bone Joint Surg* 1970;52B:838–839.
49. Judet R. Mobilization of the stiff knee. *J Bone Joint Surg* 1959;41B:856–857.
50. Kakkar VV, Howe CT, Nicolaires AN, Renney JTG, Clark MB. Deep vein thrombosis of the leg. Is there a "high risk" group? *Am J Surg* 1970;120:527–530.
51. Katz MM, Hungerford DS. Reflex sympathetic dystrophy affecting the knee. *J Bone Joint Surg* 1987;69B:797–803.
52. Kaushal SP, Galante JO, McKenna R, Bachmann F. Complications following total knee replacement. *Clin Orthop* 1976;121:181–187.
53. Keats AS. Role of anesthesia in surgical mortality. In: Orkin FK, Cooperman LH, eds. *Complications in anesthesiology*. Philadelphia: JB Lippincott, 1983;3–13.
54. Kennedy JC, Stewart R, Walker DM. Anterolateral rotatory instability of the knee joint. An early analysis of the Ellison procedure. *J Bone Joint Surg* 1978;60A:1031–1039.
55. Klein W, Jensen K. Arthritis in artificial ACL ligaments. Presented at the 6th Congress of the International Society of the Knee, Rome, Italy, May 1989.
56. Kozin R, Ryan LM, Carerra GF, Soin JS, Wortmann RH. The reflex sympathetic dystrophy syndrome (RSDS). III. Scientific studies, further evidence for the therapeutic efficacy of systemic cortical steroids, and proposed diagnostic criteria. *Am J Sports Med* 1981;70:23–30.
57. Kummell BM, Zazanis GA. Preservation of infrapatellar branch of saphenous nerve during knee surgery. *Orthop Rev* 1974;August:43–45.
58. Lankford LL, Thompson JE. Reflex sympathetic dystrophy, upper and lower extremity: diagnosis and management. *Instructional Course Lectures AAOS* 1977;26:163–178.
59. Lanz T, Wachsmuth W. *Praktisch Anatomie, Bank 1, Tiel 4: Bein und statik*. Berlin: Springer-Verlag, 1938.
60. Largenskiold A. Surgical treatment of partial closure of the growth plate. *J Pediatr Orthop* 1981;1:3–11.
61. Libscomb AB, Anderson AF. Tears of the anterior cruciate ligament in adolescents. *J Bone Joint Surg* 1986;68A:19–28.
62. Livingston WK. *Pain mechanisms: a physiologic interpretation of causalgia and its related states*, 1st ed. New York: Macmillan, 1943.
63. Losee RE, Johnson TR, Southwick WO. Anterior subluxation of the lateral tibial plateau. *J Bone Joint Surg* 1978;60A:1015–1030.
64. Lotke PA, Ecker ML, Alavi A, Berkowitz H. Indications for the treatment of deep venous thrombosis following total knee replacement. *J Bone Joint Surg* 1984;66A:202–208.
65. Lunn JN, Hunter AR, Scott DB. Anaesthesia-related surgical mortality. *Anaesthesia* 1983;38:1090–1096.
66. Marx GF, Mateo CV, Orkin LR. Computer analysis of postanesthetic deaths. *Anesthesiology* 1973;34:54–58.
67. Matsen FA 3d. Compartmental syndrome. An unified concept. *Clin Orthop* 1975;113:8–14.
68. McCarroll JR. Fracture of the patella during a golf swing following reconstruction of the anterior cruciate ligament. A case report. *Am J Sports Med* 1983;11:26–27.
69. McCoy GF, Hannon DG, Barr RJ, Templeton J. Vascular injury associated with low velocity dislocations of the knee. *J Bone Joint Surg* 1987;69B:285–287.
70. McGinty JB, Gevss LF, Marvin RA. Partial or total meniscectomy. *J Bone Joint Surg* 1977;59A:763–766.
71. McKenna R, Bachmann F, Kaushal SP, Galante JO. Thromboembolic disease in patients undergoing total knee replacement. *J Bone Joint Surg* 1976;58A:928–932.
72. McMaster WC. Open anterior cruciate ligament reconstruction with procol bioprosthesis: results at 24 months—U.S. series. In: Friedman MJ, Ferkel RD, eds. *Prosthetic ligament reconstruction of the knee*. Philadelphia: WB Saunders, 1988;97–100.

73. Miller DB. Arthroscopic meniscus repair. *Am J Sports Med* 1988;16:315–320.
74. Miller RD. *Anesthesia,* 2nd ed. New York: Churchill Livingstone, 1986.
75. Mohtadi NHG, Webster-Bogaert S, Fowler PJ. Limitation of motion following ACL reconstruction. Presented at the annual meeting of the AOSSM, Traverse City, 1989.
76. Moore MR, Garfin SR, Hargens AR. Wide tourniquets eliminate blood flow at low inflation pressures. *J Hand Surg* 1987;12A:1006–1011.
77. Morgan CD, Casscells SW. Arthroscopic meniscus repair: a safe approach to the posterior horns. *Arthroscopy* 1986;2:3–12.
78. Moseley CF. A straight-line graph for leg-length discrepancies. *J Bone Joint Surg* 1977;59A:174–179.
79. Mubarak SJ. Diagnosis, in Chapter 5 "A practical approach to compartment syndromes." *AAOS* 1982;Instructional Course Lectures:92–102.
80. Müller W, Biedert R, Hefti F, Jakob RP, Munzinger U, Stäubli HU. OAK knee evaluation. A new way to assess knee ligament injuries. *Clin Orthop* 1988;232:37–50.
81. Nicoll EA. Quadricepsplasty. *J Bone Joint Surg* 1963;45B:483–490.
82. Nilsen DW, Westre B, Jaer O, et al. A clinical and phlebographic study of postoperative deep vein thrombosis following knee meniscus extirpation. *Thromb Haemost* 1982;47:291–292.
83. Noyes FR, Mangine RE, Barber S. Early knee motion after open and arthroscopic anterior cruciate ligament reconstruction. *Am J Sports Med* 1987;15:149–160.
84. Noyes FR, Spievack ES. Extraarticular fluid dissection in tissues during arthroscopy. A report of clinical cases and a study of intraarticular and thigh pressure in cadavers. *Am J Sports Med* 1982;10:464–468.
85. Ochoa J, Danta G, Fowler TJ, Gilliatt RW. Nature of the nerve lesion caused by a pneumatic tourniquet. *Nature* 1971;233:265–266.
86. Ogilvie-Harris DJ, Bauer M, Corey P. Prostaglandin inhibition and the rate of recovery after arthroscopic meniscectomy. A randomized double-blind prospective study. *J Bone Joint Surg* 1985;67B:567–571.
87. Ogilvie-Harris DJ, Roscoe M. Reflex sympathetic dystrophy of the knee. *J Bone Joint Surg* 1987;69B:804–806.
88. Olson EJ, Kang JD, Fu FH, Georgescu HI, Mason GC, Evans CH. The biochemical and histological effects of artificial ligament wear particles: *in vitro* and *in vivo* studies. *Am J Sports Med* 1988;16:558–570.
89. Orbon RJ, Poehling GG. Arthroscopic meniscectomy. *South Med J* 1981;74:1238–1242.
90. Parisien JS. The role of arthroscopy in the treatment of postoperative fibroarthrosis of the knee joint. *Clin Orthop* 1988;229:185–192.
91. Patterson S, Klenerman L. Effect of pneumatic tourniquets on the ultrastructure of skeletal muscle. *J Bone Joint Surg* 1979;61B:178–183.
92. Paulos LE, Butler DL, Noyes FR, Grood ES. Intra-articular cruciate reconstruction. II. Replacement with vascularized patellar tendon. *Clin Orthop* 1983;172:78–84.
93. Paulos LE, Rosenberg TD, Drawbert J, Manning J, Abbott P. Infrapatellar contracture syndrome. An unrecognized cause of knee stiffness with patella entrapment and patella infera. *Am J Sports Med* 1987;15:331–341.
94. Pedowitz RA, Schmidt A, Hargens AR, Gershuni DH, Rydevik BL. Muscle injury induced by the pneumatic tourniquet: a quantitative assessment. *Orthop Trans* 1989;12(3):549.
95. Peek RD, Haynes DW. Compartment syndrome as a complication of arthroscopy. A case report and a study of interstitial pressures. *Am J Sports Med* 1984;12:464–468.
96. Poehling GG, Pollock FE Jr, Koman LA. Reflex sympathetic dystrophy of the knee after sensory nerve injury. *Arthroscopy* 1988;4:31–35.
97. Poplawski ZJ, Wiley AM, Murray JF. Post-traumatic dystrophy of the extremities. *J Bone Joint Surg* 1983;65A:642–655.
98. Reid HS, Camp RA, Jacob WH. Tourniquet hemostasis. A clinical study. *Clin Orthop* 1983;177:230–234.
99. Rico H, Merono E, Gomez-Castresana F, Torrubiano J, Espinos D, Diaz P. Scintigraphic evaluation of reflex sympathetic dystrophy: comparative study of the course of the disease under two therapeutic regimes. *Clin Rheumatol* 1987;6:233–237.
100. Riseborough EJ, Barrett IR, Shapiro F. Growth disturbances following distal femoral physeal fracture-separations. *J Bone Joint Surg* 1983;65A:885–893.
101. Rorabeck CH, Kennedy JC. Tourniquet-induced nerve ischemia complicating knee ligament surgery. *Am J Sports Med* 1980;8:98–102.
102. Roth JH, Bray RC. Popliteal artery injury during anterior cruciate ligament reconstruction. Brief report. *J Bone Joint Surg* 1988;70B:840.
103. Roth JH, Shkrum MJ, Bray RC. Synovial reaction associated with disruption of polypropylene braid-augmented intraarticular anterior cruciate ligament reconstruction. A case report. *Am J Sports Med* 1988;16:301–305.
104. Rusch RM. Integraft anterior cruciate ligament reconstruction. In: Friedman MJ, Ferkel RD, eds. *Prosthetic reconstruction of the knee.* Philadelphia: WB Saunders, 1988;52–58.
105. Rush WA, Steiner HA. A study of lower extremity length inequality. *AJR* 1945;(89)56:616–623.
106. Rushton N, Dandy DJ, Naylor CP. The clinical, arthroscopic and histological findings after replacement of the anterior cruciate ligament with carbon-fibre. *J Bone Joint Surg* 1983;65B:308–309.
107. Sachs RA, Daniel DM, Stone ML, Garfein RF. Patellofemoral problems after ACL reconstruction. *Am J Sports Med* 1989;17(6):in press.
108. Salter RB, Harris WR. Injuries involving the epiphyseal plate. *J Bone Joint Surg* 1963;45A:587–622.
109. Saunders KC, Louis DL, Weingarden SI, Waylonis G. Effect of tourniquet time on postoperative quadriceps function. *Clin Orthop* 1979;143:194–199.
110. Schmidt SA, Kjaersgaard-Anderson P, Pedersen NW, Kristensen SS, Pedersen P, Nielsen JB. The use of indomethacin to prevent the formation of heterotopic bone after total hip replacement. A randomized, double-bind clinical trail. *J Bone Joint Surg* 1988;70A:834–838.
111. Schutzer SF, Gossling HR. The treatment of reflex sympathetic dystrophy syndrome. *J Bone Joint Surg* 1984;66A:625–629.
112. Schwartzman RJ, McLellan TL. Reflex sympathetic dystrophy. A review. *Arch Neurol* 1987;44:555–561.
113. Scott GA, Jolly BL, Henning CE. Combined posterior incision and arthroscopic intra-articular repair of the meniscus. An examination of factors affecting healing. *J Bone Joint Surg* 1986;68A:847–861.
114. Shelbourne DK, Nitz PA. Accelerated rehabilitation following ACL reconstruction. Presented at the annual meeting of the AOSSM, Traverse City, 1989.
115. Sherman OH, Fox JM, Snyder SJ, et al. Arthroscopy—"no problem surgery". An analysis of complications in 2640 cases. *J Bone Joint Surg* 1986;68A:256–265.
116. Sodemann B, Persson P-E, Nilsson OS. Prevention of heterotopic ossification by nonsteroid antiinflammatory drugs after total hip arthroplasty. *Clin Orthop* 1988;237:158–163.
117. Somerville EW. Flexion contracture of the knee. *J Bone Joint Surg* 1959;41B:857.
118. Sprague NF III, O'Connor RL, Fox JM. Arthroscopic treatment of postoperative knee fibroarthrosis. *Clin Orthop* 1982;166:165–172.
119. Stulberg BN, Insall JN, Williams GW, Ghelman B. Deep-vein thrombosis following total knee replacement. An analysis of 638 arthroplasties. *J Bone Joint Surg* 1984;66A:194–201.
120. Swanson AJ. The incidence of prepatellar neuropathy following medial meniscectomy. *Clin Orthop* 1983;181:151–153.
121. Teitge RA, Indelicato PA, Kerlan RK, et al. Iliotibial band transfer for anterolateral rotatory instability of the knee: summary of 54 cases. *Am J Sports Med* 1980;8:223–227.
122. Tietjen R. Reflex sympathetic dystrophy of the knee. *Clin Orthop* 1986;209:234–243.
123. Tinker JH. Anesthetic risk. In: Rogers MC, ed. *Current practice in anesthesiology.* Toronto: BC Decker, 1988;1–5.

124. Vacanti CJ, VanHouten RJ, Hill RC. A statistical analysis of the relationship of physical status to postoperative mortality in 68,388 cases. *Anesth Analg* 1970;49:564–566.

125. Walker RH, Dillingham M. Thrombophlebitis following arthroscopic surgery of the knee, *Contemp Orthop* 1983;6:29–33.

126. Weingarden SI, Louis DL, Waylonis GW. Electromyographic changes in postmeniscectomy patients. Role of the pneumatic tourniquet. *JAMA* 1979;241:1248–1250.

127. Whitesides TE, Haney TC, Morimoto K, Haradat H. Tissue pressure measurements as a determinant for the need of fasciotomy. *Clin Orthop* 1975;113:43–51.

128. Yaru NC, Daniel DM, Penner D, Farhoumand I. The effect of tibial attachment site on graft impingement in an anterior cruciate ligament reconstruction. Personal Communication.

129. Young A, Stokes M, Iles JF. Effects of joint pathology on muscle. *Clin Orthop* 1987;219:21–27.

Knee Ligaments: Structure, Function, Injury, and Repair, edited by D. Daniel, et al.
© 1990 by Raven Press, Ltd. All rights reserved.

CHAPTER 29

Ligament Surgery

The Evaluation of Results

Dale M. Daniel, Mary Lou Stone, and Barbara Riehl

The results of knee ligament surgery are dependent on the patient, knee pathology, surgical procedure, and postoperative care. The reported results are dependent on the "true results," the testing protocol, the tester's precision and accuracy, and the interpretation of the test data. Reports of knee ligament surgery should define the population (43), the joint pathology, the treatment program, and the evaluation methodology. This chapter will discuss designing a clinical study to evaluate knee ligament surgery and will present data on a patient population pre- and post-ACL reconstruction. Many of the ideas presented in this chapter have evolved from the International Knee Documentation Committee (conveners John Feagin, M.D. and Werner Müller, M.D.). The *American Journal of Sports Medicine's Supplement on Sports Injury Research* has been a primary reference for this chapter (36).

PATIENT POPULATION

A *cohort* is a designated group of patients (43). The patients are selected from a specific population. Ad-

D. Daniel: Department of Orthopedic Surgery, University of California, San Diego, School of Medicine, La Jolla, California 92037; and Kaiser Permanente Medical Center, San Diego, California 92120.
M. L. Stone: Department of Orthopedics, Kaiser Hospital of San Diego, San Diego, California 92120.
B. Riehl: Kaiser Permanente Medical Center, San Diego, California 92120.

mission criteria are established to define who will be entered into a study. Admission criteria consist of (a) eligibility criteria, which give the conditions that a participant must have in order to enter the study, and (b) exclusion criteria, which specify the conditions that preclude one from participating in the study (43).

A cohort study follows a defined group of patients over a period of time. The study may be either retrospective or prospective. A study is retrospective if the outcome or events of interest have occurred before the study is initiated (43). In this chapter, data on a prospective cohort study of ACL surgery (SDK79) will be presented. The population source for SDK79 was members of the San Diego Kaiser Permanente Health Plan having ACL surgery between 1983 and 1986. Seventy-nine patients fulfilled the admission criteria that are presented in Table 29-1. Study reports should include (a) cohort demographics, (b) other medical conditions that might affect knee function, (c) prior treatment, (d) patient activity prior to injury and after injury prior to surgery, (e) symptoms, (f) impairments, and (g) knee pathology.

Three components have been used to characterize patient activity: functional level, intensity level, and frequency of participation (exposure). Some investigators have combined two or more of these components into one scale (38,46,47). We have chosen to record each item separately (Table 29-2). The patient's overall functional level is the highest level that is per-

TABLE 29-1. *Admission criteria, SDK79*

Inclusion criteria
1. Anterior cruciate ligament disruption.
2. Injury to index surgery interval >6 months.
3. Ligament surgery confined to intraarticular ACL reconstruction.
4. Evaluation pre- and postoperatively performed by authors MLS and BR.

Exclusion criteria
1. Posterior cruciate ligament disruption.
2. Systemic disease impairing patient for sports activities.
3. Lower-limb pathology other than in the index knee.

---

formed a minimum of 50 hours a year. The functional levels are listed in Table 29-2. Heavy labor is listed under functional level II; work that involves agility activities, such as those of a fireman, is listed under functional level III.

STUDY DESIGN

Treatment results are compared to a *control* population, which may be the normal population, an untreated patient population, or a similar population treated in an alternative manner (12,43,44,52,53). When evaluating a patient with a stable chronic condition, the patient's posttreatment evaluation may be compared to the pretreatment evaluation as is done with cohort SDK79. It is imperative that the same evaluation system be utilized before treatment and after treatment (44). Optimally, the same tester, who is not the treating physician, will perform the pretreatment and posttreatment evaluation to minimize tester bias and variability (*detection bias*) (44).

Suppose we wish to evaluate the results of two sur-

TABLE 29-2. *Patient activity*

Functional levels
Level I:	Activity of daily living.
Level II:	Straight running; sports that do not involve lower-limb agility activities; occupations involving heavy lifting.
Level III:	Activities that require lower-limb agility but not involving jumping, hard cutting, or pivoting.
Level IV:	Activities involving jumping, hard cutting, or pivoting.

Intensity
W:	Work-related or occupational
LR:	Light recreational
VR:	Vigorous recreational
C:	Competitive

Exposure
Number of hours per year of participation at any given functional level and intensity.

---

gical treatment procedures (e.g., patellar tendon ACL reconstruction with and without a prosthetic ligament augmentation device). If the outcome of the study is to be interpreted as an evaluation of the augmentation device, the augmentation device must be the only independent variable. All other aspects of patient selection and care that will influence the treatment outcome would ideally be evenly distributed between the experimental group (augmented patients) and the control group (nonaugmented patients). The greatest probability of minimizing the nonequal distribution of the many other variables that will influence the patients' outcome is to prospectively randomize patients into an augmented and nonaugmented group (Fig. 29-1) (43–45). If an initial feature occurring in participants is a major prognostic factor for determining outcome, the investigator may use *stratified randomization* for that particular feature to reduce the chances of dissimilarity at the initial-state evaluation. For example, stratified randomization might be done for athletes of different levels of participation (44). The use of historic controls or a concurrent nonrandomized control group will probably result in two groups that are significantly different with respect to a number of recognized and unrecognized patient and treatment variables (12,43–45).

TREATMENT PROGRAM

The treatment consists of the surgical procedure and the postoperative care program. If a study is designed to compare two surgical procedures, it is essential that surgeons for Procedure A are equally as skilled as the surgeons for Procedure B, to avoid *performance bias* (Fig. 29-1) (44). Surgical procedures in addition to the ligament procedures should be documented (e.g., meniscus repair or excision, joint surface débridement, loose body removal, osteophyte excision, and lateral release). The details of the ligament procedure should be recorded, including graft harvest, implantation technique, orientation, tensioning, and fixation. We routinely evaluate the knee flexion arc and KT-1000 measurements after the wound is closed prior to applying the postoperative dressing (Fig. 2-16). Postoperative radiographs document the tunnel placement (Fig. 3-4).

Both patient groups should follow the same postoperative care program. Documentation of the postoperative care program should include (a) an immobilization and protection program, (b) exercise regimens, and (c) time to return to stressful work and sports. An example of a postoperative care program is presented in Fig. 3-2.

SDK79 represents a number of surgical techniques and postoperative programs. Data from this study are not presented as a report on a specific treatment pro-

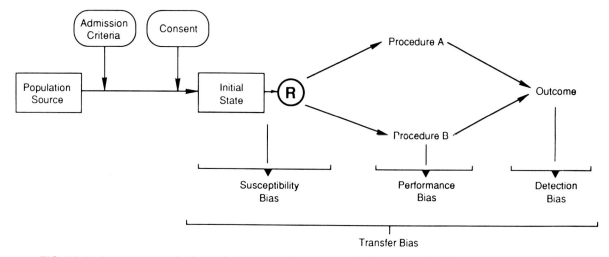

FIG. 29-1. A summary of where, in a randomized clinical trial, potential biases may occur. *Susceptibility bias:* bias that occurs from contrasting the results of therapy for two prognostically dissimilar groups. *Performance bias:* bias resulting from dissimilar levels of skill in performing the procedures. *Detection bias:* outcomes are not measured in a comparable manner. *Transfer bias:* differential loss to follow-up occurs in the two treatment groups. R indicates the point when patients are randomized. (From ref. 44.)

gram. The data are presented as an example of pre- and post-ACL-reconstruction data.

PATIENT EVALUATION

The knee evaluation is divided into four parts: (i) historic record of patient activity, symptoms, and impairments; (ii) tests of patient function; (iii) documentation of the knee motion limits, as well as clinical assessment of joint inflammation; and (iv) ancillary evaluation of joint pathology (radiographs, bone scan, magnetic resonance imaging, arthroscopy). The same evaluation system should be used for the experimental and control population. It is preferable that the knee evaluation not be performed by the treating surgeon. To minimize detection bias, pre- and posttreatment measurements of the control group and experimental group should be performed by the same evaluator (Fig. 29-1). This is especially true in reporting the clinical instability examination. To minimize detection bias, all patients in SDK79 were evaluated preoperatively and postoperatively by authors BR and MLS. BR interviewed the patient, filled out the questionnaire, and performed the function tests; MLS performed the clinical examination and the arthrometer measurements. Demographic data for SDK79 cohort are presented in Table 29-3.

Functional Level

The functional levels for the cohort prior to injury, after injury prior to repair, and at the follow-up ex-

amination are presented in Table 29-4. In only two cases, both at the postinjury prerepair evaluation, the level of function at work (carpenter and fireman) was higher than the level of function in sports. The number of patients participating in specific sports for more than 50 hours a year is presented in Table 29-5. The average number of hours of participation in sports is presented for each evaluation interval in Table 29-6. For many patients the decrease in sports participation is not knee-related. As the patients grow older and change their lifestyle, the availability of sports participation and their interests may change (38). Prior to injury, most SDK79 patients were recreational athletes. There were no patients in SDK79 participating in competitive sports prior to injury beyond the high-school level. Since injury no patient has participated in competitive sports.

TABLE 29-3. Patient population, SDK79

Sex	
Male:	50 (63%)
Female:	29 (37%)
Age	
Mean:	25
Range:	15–39
Prior ligament surgery	
Five patients (6%)	
Interval, injury to index surgery	
Mean:	2.5 years
Range:	7 months to 19 years
[52 patients (66%) <24 months after injury]	
Interval, index surgery to postsurgery evaluation	
Mean:	3.2 years
Range:	2–5 years

TABLE 29-4. Functional levels, SDK79[a]

Level	Prior to injury		After injury, prior to surgery		Post-surgery	
	N	Percent	N	Percent	N	Percent
I	3	4	53	67	23	29
II	3	4	11	14	19	24
III	26	33	10	13	26	24
IV	47	59	5	6	10	13
Mean level	3.5		1.6		2.3	

[a] Each patient is placed in the highest functional level of participation for 50 or more hours per year. In only two cases was the patients' functional level at work higher than their functional level in sports.

TABLE 29-5. Sports participation greater than 50 hours per week, SDK79

Level	Sport	Prior to injury	After injury prior to surgery	Post-surgery
II	Biking	10	5	11
	Bowling	2	2	2
	Boxing	1		
	Golfing	3	2	4
	Hiking	1		3
	Jogging	10		2
	Aerobics—low impact			1
	Rollerskating	1		2
	Scuba diving			3
	Swimming	6	4	3
	Weightlifting	2		7
III	Aerobics	3	1	2
	Badminton	1		
	Baseball/softball	23	2	7
	Dancing	1	1	2
	Motorcycle racing	2		1
	Orienteering	1		
	Racketball	12	1	2
	Skateboarding	1	1	1
	Snow skiing	5		2
	Surfing	5	1	2
	Tennis	9		7
	Track	4		
	Waterskiing	2	2	3
	Wrestling	2		
IV	Basketball	16		7
	Figure skating	1		
	Football	12	2	
	Gymnastics	10	1	1
	Martial arts	3	1	2
	Rugby	3		
	Soccer	10		1
	Volleyball	4	1	

TABLE 29-6. Average hours of sports participation SDK79

Level	Prior to injury	After injury prior to surgery	Post-surgery
II	114	36	124
III	272	31	70
IV	234	11	30
Total	620	78	224

Impairments and Symptoms

An inventory of impairments for SDK79 and for 50 normal subjects is presented in Table 29-7. Noyes (38) has recommended that symptoms and impairments be related to specific activities. An example format being field tested by the International Knee Documentation Committee is presented in Fig. 29-2. If the patient does not perform or has not attempted a specific task, the impairment is graded as unknown. A subject must participate at a functional level for a minimum of 50 hours a year before it can be stated the patient has no symptoms or impairments at that level.

Knee *giving way* with sports activities is a major complaint of patients with an anterior cruciate ligament (ACL) tear. Prior to surgery, 96% of SDK79 patients complained of giving way and at follow-up examination 4% complained of giving way. Noyes (37) has suggested that the symptom *giving way* be classified as either *full giving way* or *partial giving way*. We are now dividing giving way into (a) full giving way, defined as a giving way event that results in the patient

TABLE 29-7. Specific task performance (Percent of subjects reporting no impairment)

	Normal[a]	Unilateral ACL-injured patients, SDK79	
		Prior to surgery	Post-surgery
Number:	50	79	79
Standing:	100	52	72
Walking:	100	50	90
Climbing:	96	17	78
Stairs:	96	34	83
Kneeling or squatting:	80	7	43
Jogging:	80	15	63
Running:	94	17	75
Jumping:	94	11	68
Twisting or pivoting:	96	3	70
Cutting:	98	3	70

[a] Subjects between age 15 and 30 with no history of knee injury.

Functional Levels

	I	II	III	IV
Swelling				
Pain				
Giving Way (Partial)				
Giving Way (Full)				
Walking				
Squatting				
Stairs				
Limited Motion				
Running				
Cutting				
Jumping				

FIG. 29-2. Symptoms and impairments are related to functional level. Symptoms and impairments are recorded on a scale of 0 to 3 (0 = none, 1 = mild, 2 = moderate, and 3 = severe). This format is being tested by the International Knee Documentation Committee. Entries are made for every category and functional level. An "X" is placed in the appropriate box if the question is not applicable or if there are no data to record.

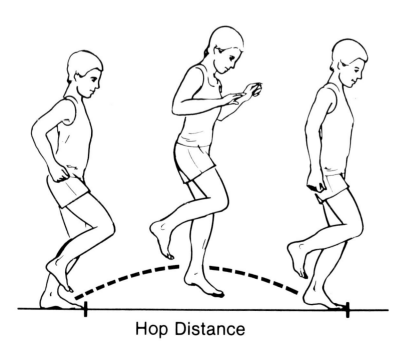

Hop Distance

FIG. 29-3. The one-leg hop. This test is performed by having the patient stand on only the test leg, hop for distance, and land on only the test leg. The distance hopped is measured. (From ref. 11.)

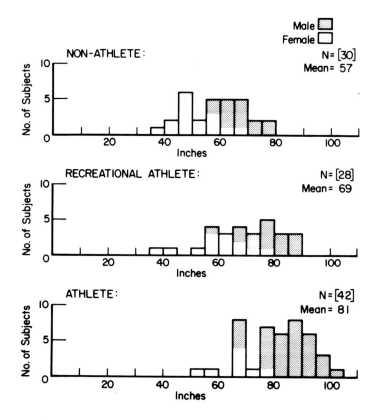

FIG. 29-4. The one-leg-hop distance for 100 normal subjects aged 15 to 45. Subjects were classified with respect to athletic activity. The classifications were as follows: competitive athlete (member of an extramural high-school or college team); recreational athlete (participation in a sport for 4 hours or more a week but not training for competition); and nonathlete.

falling down and/or developing swelling after the event, and (b) partial giving way, defined as an episode when the knee gave way but the patient did not fall to the ground or develop swelling after the event.

Functional Tests

A number of investigators have utilized functional tests in their evaluation system. Reported tests have included strength tests (5,9,10,16–18,21,29,35,40,49,54), hop tests (9,10,47,48), agility tests (9,10,22,47,48), and gait analysis studies (3,6,31,51). The San Diego Kaiser evaluation system includes two functional tests: (i) the one-leg hop for distance and (ii) Cybex strength testing. For both the one-leg hop for distance and strength testing, the injured knee is compared to the patient's contralateral normal knee and the result is expressed as a percentage of normal knee function (index = injured divided by normal, multiplied by 100).

The one-leg hop for distance is a useful lower-limb function test that requires a minimum of space, equipment, and time. The test may be performed in the hallway of a clinic. The distance jumped is measured with a tape measure. The test is performed by having the patient stand on only the test leg, hop for distance, and land on only the test leg (Fig. 29-3) (11). Each leg is tested three times, alternating between the normal leg

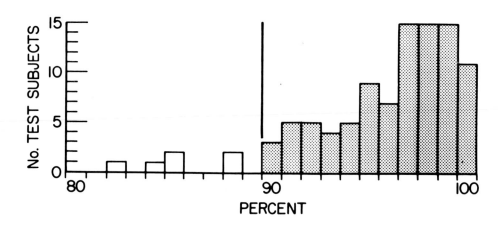

FIG. 29-5. Hop index in normal subjects (limb with lesser hop distance divided by limb with greater hop distance, multiplied by 100). N = 100; mean = 96%; range = 82–100%.

TABLE 29-8. The one-leg hop for distance, SDK79

	Pre-repair	Post-repair
Unable to hop	25 (32%)	6 (6%)
Able to hop	54 (68%)	73 (94%)
Index		
<70	17 (22%)	2 (3%)
70–79	8 (10%)	7 (9%)
80–89	16 (20%)	20 (25%)
>89	13 (15%)	44 (56%)

TABLE 29-10. SDK79 joint surface grading system

Cartilage—classification of pathology
0 = Normal
1 = Fibrillation/fissuring $<\frac{1}{2}$ inch
2 = Fibrillation/fissuring $\geq\frac{1}{2}$ inch or cartilage erosion to bone $<\frac{1}{2}$ inch
3 = Cartilage erosion to bone $\geq\frac{1}{2}$ inch or diffuse fibrillation/fissuring

and the injured leg. Hop distance for normal subjects is presented in Fig. 29-4, and the hop index in the normal subjects (greater/lesser × 100) is presented in Fig. 29-5. The mean dominant-limb hop distance in the normal group was 2% greater than the nondominant-limb hop distance. The left/right limb ratio was >0.9 in 95% of subjects. There was not a significant effect of sex or athletic participation on the left/right limb ratio (two-way ANOVA; $p > 0.1$). Based on these data, we have classified a hop index (mean hop of an injured limb divided by the mean hop distance of the patient's normal limb, multiplied by 100) of >89 to be satisfactory. Pre- and postoperative data for SDK79 patients are presented in Table 29-8.

Isokinetic strength tests at 60° per second with a Cybex II isokinetic dynamometer (Lumex, Inc., Bay

TABLE 29-9. Isokinetic strength tests (60° per second)

	Normal subjects[a]	SDK79[b] Pre-repair	SDK79[b] Post-repair
Number	100	58	58
Quadriceps index			
>89	78	14 (24%)	25 (43%)
80–89	11	7 (12%)	15 (26%)
70–79	6	7 (12%)	10 (17%)
<70	5	30 (52%)	8 (14%)
Mean	98	67	86
Hamstring index			
>89	76	22 (38%)	45 (78%)
80–89	14	15 (26%)	9 (16%)
70–79	5	7 (12%)	2 (3%)
<70	5	14 (24%)	2 (3%)
Mean	97	80	99
Thigh circumference[c]			
≤1 cm		31 (53%)	31 (53%)
1.5–2 cm		9 (16%)	15 (26%)
>2 cm		18 (31%)	12 (21%)
Mean (cm)		1.6	1.3

[a] Data on normal subjects were recorded as nondominant/dominant × 100. Data on normal subjects are courtesy of Marilynn Wyatt (54).
[b] SDK79 data were recorded as injured/noninjured × 100.
[c] Normal limb minus injured limb 10 cm proximal to patella.

Shore, New York) has been included in our evaluation. Wyatt (54) reported quadriceps and hamstring torque values during isokinetic exercise in 100 normal subjects (50 females and 50 males) at 60°, 180°, and 300° per second on the Cybex II isokinetic dynamometer. She reported that the mean ratios of nondominant to dominant knee torque values were equal to or greater than 97% in all the tests performed in her study. She noted that the torque values decreased as speeds of exercise increased and that the ratio of hamstring torque values to quadriceps torque values increased as the test speed increased. Normal data from Wyatt's study, as well as data from SDK79, are presented in Table 29-9.

Joint Pathology

Joint surface and meniscus pathology should be documented at the time of surgery. In SDK79 there were only six patients with normal joint surfaces and menisci. Sixteen patients had a normal medial meniscus, and 47 patients had a normal lateral meniscus. Also reported were the following: meniscus repairs—23 medial and 0 lateral; meniscus excision—16 medial and 11 lateral; prior meniscus excision—21 medial and 11 lateral. The remaining menisci had some meniscus pathology (3 medial and 10 lateral), but no meniscus surgery was performed. Joint surface pathology was graded in SDK79 using the system presented in Table 29-10. The data are presented in Table 29-11. A number of cartilage grading systems have been reported (4,7,14,15,19,24,25,42). Noyes (39) has reported a system using four separate and distinct variables: (i) description of the articular cartilage, (ii) the extent (depth) of the involvement, (iii) the diameter of the lesion, and (iv) the location of the lesion (Table 29-12).

TABLE 29-11. Hyaline surface pathology SDK79

Grade	Compartment Medial	Compartment Lateral	Compartment Patellofemoral
0	43 (54%)	65 (82%)	60 (76%)
1	28 (35%)	10 (13%)	14 (18%)
2	8 (10%)	4 (5%)	4 (5%)
3	0	0	0

TABLE 29-12. *Grading system for articular cartilage lesions*[a]

Surface description	Extent of involvement	Diameter (mm)	Location	Degree of knee flexion

1. Cartilage surface intact	A. Definite softening with some resilience remaining
	B. Extensive softening with loss of resilience (deformation)
		<10
		≤15
		≤20
		≤25
		>25
			Patella
			A. Proximal third
			  Middle third
			  Distal third
			B. Odd facet
			  Middle facet
			  Lateral facet
				Degree of knee flexion where the lesion is in weight-bearing contact (e.g., 20–45°)

2. Cartilage surface damaged: cracks, fissures, fibrillation, or fragmentation	A. < half of the thickness
	B. ≥ half of the thickness
			Trochlea
			Medial femoral condyle
			  a. anterior third
			  b. middle third
			  c. posterior third
			Lateral femoral condyle
			  a. anterior third
			  b. middle third
			  c. posterior third	

3. Bone exposed	A. Bone surface intact
	B. Bone surface cavitation
			Medial tibial condyle
			  a. anterior third
			  b. middle third
			  c. posterior third
			Lateral tibial condyle
			  a. anterior third
			  b. middle third
			  c. posterior third	

[a] From ref. 39.

Joint pathology should also be documented radiographically (2,13) and may be documented with bone scans (9,34,50).

We have used joint effusion, joint line tenderness, and patellofemoral irritability as our clinical indicators of joint inflammation. These observations have taken on new importance as studies are done to evaluate (a) the safety of allografts and prosthetic ligaments and (b) the inflammation resulting from graft wear (41). In 1985, two centers in San Diego were studying a polypropylene braid (3M LAD) to augment a patellar tendon autograft. The two centers reported a different incidence of joint effusion. The question was posed: Was the difference the result of tester evaluation (detection bias), or was there a *true* effusion difference. To evaluate the variability of the clinical examination, one evening a group of examiners from the two centers examined the same 21 postoperative ligament reconstruction patients with a patellar tendon–3M LAD reconstruction. The number of patients with effusions was recorded as follows by the five different examiners: 4, 3, 2, 1, and 0. Analysis of the data revealed that the difference between the incidence of effusion between the two centers may have been due to *detection bias* and not be a true difference in incidence.

The patellofemoral irritability and joint effusion for the SDK79 patients are presented in Table 29-13. We currently also record knee circumference right–left

(R–L) difference, an objective measurement of joint inflammation.

Motion Limits

The clinical limits of motion examination is performed as described in Chapter 1. The flexion arc is measured with the patients prone. The thighs are supported by the examining table (Fig. 3-1). Beginning flexion is measured with a goniometer, and heel height difference is also recorded (Fig. 3-1). Active knee flexion is measured with a goniometer. The flexion arc data are presented in Table 29-14.

The clinical evaluation of the ACL-reconstructed

TABLE 29-13. *Joint inflammation SDK79*

	Pre-repair	Post-repair
Effusion grade		
0	45 (57%)	70 (89%)
1	19 (24%)	9 (11%)
2	14 (18%)	0
3	1 (1%)	0
Patella irritability grade		
0	57 (72%)	71 (90%)
1	17 (22%)	7 (9%)
2	4 (5%)	1 (1%)
3	1 (1%)	0

TABLE 29-14. *Flexion arc, SDK79*

Beginning flexion

Degrees of flexion	Non-injured knee	Injured knee Pre-repair	Injured knee Post-repair
<−5	15 (19%)	16 (20%)	12 (15%)
−5 to +5	64 (81%)	58 (73%)	63 (80%)
6 to 10	0	4 (5%)	4 (5%)
>10	0	1 (1%)	0

Heal height difference	Injured minus normal Pre-repair	Post-repair
<−5 cm	3	0
−5 cm to +5 cm	69 (87%)	74 (94%)
6 cm to 10 cm	4 (5%)	5 (6%)
>10 cm	3 (4%)	0

Prone maximum active flexion

Degrees of flexion	Injured knee Pre-repair	Post-repair
<100	4 (5%)	0
100 to 120	9 (11%)	3 (4%)
121 to 134	23 (29%)	26 (33%)
≥135	43 (54%)	50 (63%)

Degrees of flexion	Normal minus injured Pre-repair	Post-repair
0 to 5	56 (71%)	73 (92%)
6 to 10	4 (5%)	3 (4%)
11 to 20	4 (5%)	2 (3%)
>20	14 (19%)	1 (1%)

patient centers on the evaluation of anterior tibial displacement with the Lachman test and the pivot shift test. The International Knee Documentation Committee conducted a study to evaluate the reproducibility of the clinical examination. Eleven members of the committee each evaluated the same 10 patients. One patient had no ligament injuries. Nine patients had sustained an ACL and/or PCL (posterior cruciate ligament) tear. Seven of the patients had been reconstructed. The examiners were blinded to patient histories. In a round-robin fashion, each of the examiners examined the 11 patients. Joint displacements were estimated as millimeters of displacement from the anatomic resting position. All patients were also evaluated by three instrumented testing systems: Genucom (Faro, Champlain, New York), KSS (Acufex MicroSurgical, Norwood, Massachusetts), and KT-1000 (MEDMetric, San Diego, California). Each company provided an examiner skilled with their device to test the patients. Figure 29-6A presents the clini-

cians' estimates of anterior tibial displacement at 25° of flexion in the normal knees, and Fig. 29-6B presents data from the three testing instruments. Figure 29-7 presents data from tests performed on a knee model.

Because many of the patients had sustained PCL injuries, there was a great deal of inconsistency between examiners in judging if joint motion was anterior or posterior from the anatomic resting position. Therefore, injured minus contralateral normal knee data are presented as total anterior–posterior (A–P) displacement in Figs. 29-8 and 29-9. In this study of total A–P displacement, a side-to-side difference of greater than 3 mm A–P is classified as pathologic. The mean clinical displacement, the KSS, and the KT-1000 were in agreement as to displacement classification in all patients measured at 25° and 90° of flexion. There was a great discrepancy between examiners. For example, at 25° of flexion, examiner F stated that only two patients had a side-to-side difference of greater than 3 mm, whereas examiners A and E reported that eight of the patients had a side-to-side difference of greater than 3 mm. It would greatly affect the reported results of a study if examiner A did all the preoperative examinations and examiner F did all the postoperative examinations. The clinical evaluation performed by different examiners may introduce a significant level of detection bias.

Previous investigators have compared the results of instrumented testing and the clinical examination (1,21,32). Arthrometer test reproducibility is discussed in Chapters 23 and 24. We use the KT-1000 arthrometer to measure anterior tibial displacement. As the displacement force increases, the R–L difference in a pathologic population increases. We routinely perform the following tests at 25° of flexion: 20 lb posterior; 15, 20, and 30 lb anterior; manual maximum anterior; and quadriceps active test (Chapter 24). Data for SDK79 group are presented in Table 29-15. An R–L difference of less than 3 mm is considered normal (Chapter 24). Note that there is a greater number of patients classified as pathologic (R–L difference > 2.5) when the limb is tested at higher forces. The test prior to repair, without anesthesia, was performed by author MLS, who also performed the postrepair follow-up tests. The examinations under anesthesia were performed by the operating surgeon.

The pivot shift test has been a mainstay of the ACL evaluation (8,12,23,26–28,33,46). As part of the International Knee Documentation Committee study referred to above, the pivot shift test was performed by each examiner on all patients with the tibia held in internal rotation, neutral position, and external rotation as reported by Jakob (26). The patients appeared to remain relaxed during the entire examination period. The mean pivot shift grade of the last three examinations of the day were the same as that of the first

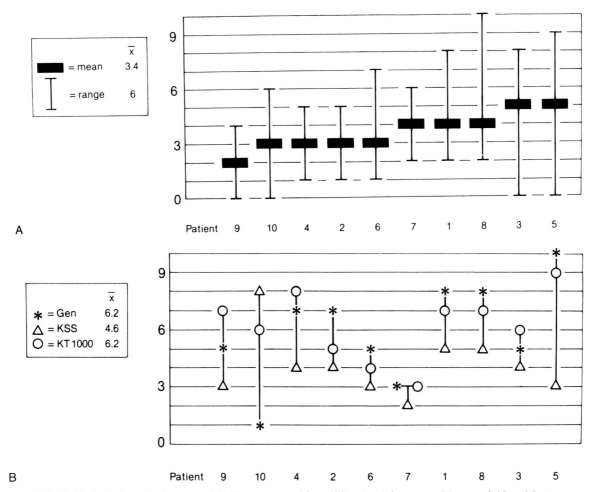

FIG. 29-6. Anterior displacement (25°; expressed in millimeters) in normal knee of 10 subjects. **A:** Displacement mean and range by manual examination, estimated by 11 examiners. **B:** Displacement measured by three instrumented testing devices.

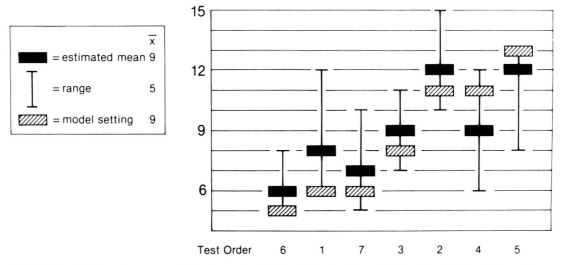

FIG. 29-7. Tests on knee model designed by Roland Jakob, (Bern, Switzerland). Model is set for a measured anterior–posterior displacement (25°; expressed in millimeters). Eleven examiners estimated the amount of displacement allowed at each setting.

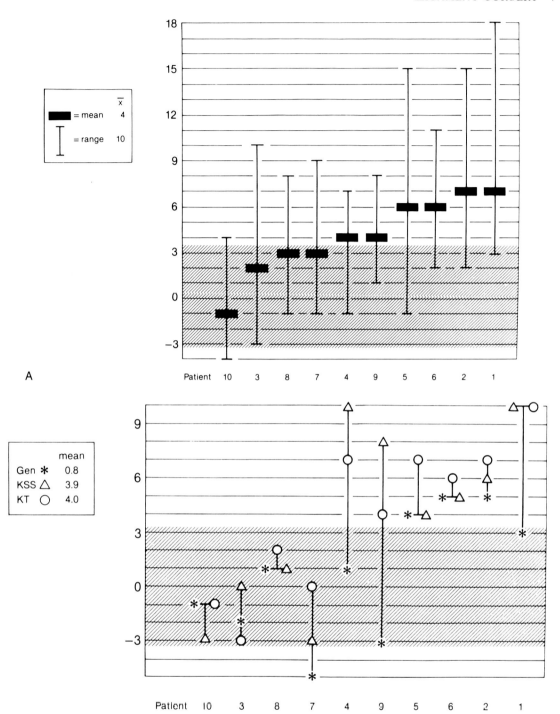

FIG. 29-8. Anterior–posterior displacement (25°; injured minus contralateral normal knee data, expressed in millimeters) in knee-injured patients. **A:** Mean and range of measurements estimated for each patient by 10 examiners. **B:** Measurements recorded by testing devices.

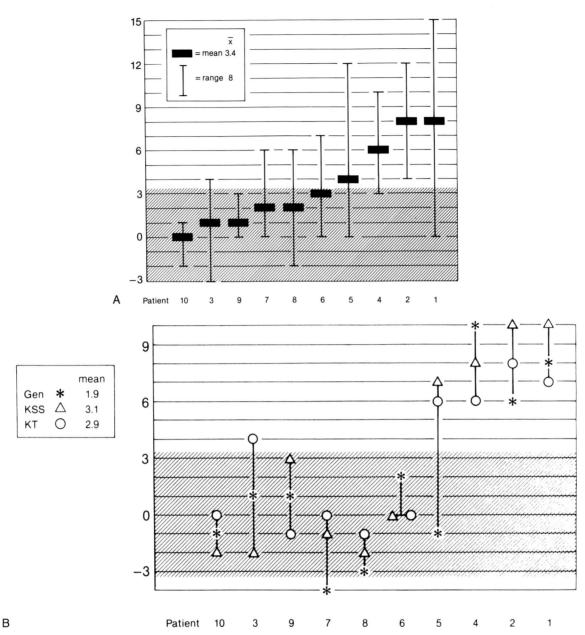

FIG. 29-9. Anterior–posterior displacement (90°; injured minus contralateral normal knee data, expressed in millimeters) in knee-injured patients. **A:** Mean and range of measurements estimated for each patient by 11 examiners. **B:** Measurements recorded by testing devices.

three examinations of the morning. The mean pivot shift grade in internal rotation, neutral position, and external rotation was 0.8. Therefore, the position of the limb while the pivot shift was being performed did not appear to affect how the clinicians graded the pivot shift. There was a great difference between the examiners' pivot shift grading. Examiner F recorded that only one patient had a positive pivot shift, while examiner J recorded that seven of the 10 patients had a positive pivot shift. The pivot shift grading for the SDK79 patients is presented in Table 29-16. The test prior to repair, without anesthesia, was performed by author MLS, who also performed the postrepair fol-

low-up tests. The examination prior to repair, with anesthesia, was performed by the operating surgeon.

RATING RESULTS

It is a simple matter to classify an excellent result: no knee-related impairments, normal functional tests, and normal motion limits. It is a simple matter to classify a failure following a reconstruction for chronic instability: no decrease in impairments, no improvement in functional tests, and persistent pathologic motion. But where should we draw the line between excellent and good, good and fair, and fair and failure? Are there certain aspects of the evaluation that are more impor-

TABLE 29-15. *KT-1000 anterior displacement (injured minus contralateral normal knee data, expressed in millimeters), SDK79*

| | Pre-repair | | Post-repair | |
	Without anesthesia	With anesthesia	With anesthesia	Follow-up
		20 lb		
N	78	77	76	79
<3	3 (4%)	9 (12%)	72 (95%)	45 (57%)
3–5	22 (28%)	18 (23%)	3 (4%)	26 (33%)
5.5–7.5	33 (42%)	25 (33%)	1 (1%)	7 (9%)
>7.5	20 (25%)	25 (32%)	0	1 (1%)
Mean	6.3 mm	6.3 mm	0.0 mm	2.3 mm
		Manual maximum		
N	77	77	59	79
<3	0	2 (3%)	52 (88%)	20 (25%)
3–5	5 (7%)	4 (5%)	7 (12%)	29 (37%)
5.5–7.5	19 (25%)	20 (26%)	0	23 (29%)
8–10	18 (23%)	15 (20%)	0	4 (5%)
>10	35 (45%)	36 (47%)	0	3 (4%)
Mean	9.6 mm	9.6 mm	−1.1 mm	4.0 mm
		Quadriceps active		
N	77			79
<3	15 (20%)			44 (56%)
3–5	26 (35%)			23 (29%)
5.5–7.5	20 (27%)			9 (11%)
>7.5	14 (18%)			3 (4%)
Mean	4.9 mm			2.3 mm

tant? If the patient is a failure in one category of the evaluation, should the overall evaluation be classified as a failure? Arbitrary judgments need to be made. A number of investigators have made these judgments and have devised grading systems to rate the surgical results (8,23,27,28,30,33,38,46). There is significant variation between the different point systems. A need exists for a standardized evaluation system or at least a standardized core of measurement parameters that may be incorporated into specialized evaluation systems. The International Knee Documentation Committee, under the auspices of The American Orthopedic Society for Sports Medicine and the European Society of Knee Surgery and Arthroscopy, is developing a core knee evaluation protocol.

TABLE 29-16. *Pivot shift grade, SDK79*

| | Pre-repair | | |
Grade	Without anesthesia	With anesthesia	Post-repair
0	1 (1%)	1 (1%)	44 (56%)
1	16 (20%)	6 (8%)	18 (23%)
2	30 (38%)	37 (47%)	10 (13%)
3	5 (6%)	23 (29%)	0
Unknown	27 (34%)[a]	12 (15%)[b]	7 (9%)[a]

[a] Patient guarding, could not test.
[b] Not recorded.

REPORTING RESULTS

Reports on knee surgery, except in rare instances, require a follow-up of 2 years duration (20). We have found that most graft failures are revealed by 6 months after surgery (12). However, vigorous return to sporting activity does not usually occur until the second year after injury. A 2-year follow-up provides evaluation of the motion limits and patient function. A 5-year follow-up is probably needed in order to evaluate the success of the ligament surgery to prevent late meniscus tears. Though intercondylar radiographic changes following an ACL injury may be seen as early as 6 months after injury (13), a follow-up of 10 years is probably required in order to evaluate the efficacy of ligament surgery to reduce the incidence of degenerative arthritis. Perhaps the bone scan will provide an earlier measure of joint degeneration. The changes on scan secondary to joint arthrosis will need to be distinguished from changes secondary to bone tunnels.

REFERENCES

1. Anderson AF, Lipscomb AB. Preoperative instrumented testing of anterior and posterior knee laxity. *Am J Sports Med* 1989;17:387–392.
2. Bach BR, Warren RF. Imaging: radiographic indicators of an-

terior cruciate ligament injury. In: Feagin JA, ed. *The crucial ligaments,* vol 1. New York: Churchill Livingstone, 1988;317–327.

3. Belcher MK, Reider B, Andriacchi TP. Alterations in stair-climbing function associated with an anterior cruciate deficient knee. *Orthop Res Soc, Trans 31st Annu Meeting, Atlanta.* 1984;9:134.

4. Bentley G, Dowd, G. Current concepts of etiology and treatment of chondromalacia patellae. *Clin Orthop* 1984;189:209–228.

5. Campbell DE, Glenn W. Rehabilitation of knee flexor and knee extensor muscle strength in patients with meniscectomies, ligamentous repairs, and chondromalacia. *Phys Ther* 1982;62:10–15.

6. Carlson S, Nordstrand A. The coordination of the knee muscles in some voluntary movements and in the gait in cases with and without knee injuries. *Acta Chir Scand* 1968;134:423.

7. Casscells SW. Gross pathological changes in the knee joint of the aged individual: a study of 300 cases. *Clin Orthop* 1978;132:225–232.

8. Clancy WG, Ray JM, Zoltan DJ. Acute tears of the anterior cruciate ligament. *J Bone Joint Surg* 1988;70A:1483–1488.

9. Collier BD, Johnson RP, Carerra GF, Isitman AT, Veluvolu P, Knobel J, et al. Chronic knee pain assessed by SPECT: comparison with other modalities. *Radiology* 1985;157:795–802.

10. Daniel D, Malcom L, Stone ML, Peth H, Morgan J, Riehl B. Quantification of knee stability and function. *Contemp Orthop* 1982;5:83–91.

11. Daniel DM, Stone ML, Riehl B, Moore MR. The one leg hop for distance. *Am J Knee Surg* 1988;1:212–213.

12. Daniel DM, Woodward EP, Losse GM, Stone ML. The Marshall/Macintosh anterior cruciate ligament reconstruction with the Kennedy ligament augmentation device: report of the United States Clinical Trials. In: Friedman MJ, Ferkel RD, eds. *Prosthetic ligament reconstruction of the knee.* Philadelphia: WB Saunders, 1988;71–78.

13. Feagin JA, Cabaud HE, Curl WW. The anterior cruciate ligament: radiographic and clinical signs of successful and unsuccessful repairs. *Clin Orthop* 1982;164:54–58.

14. Ficat RP, Hungerford DS. Chondrosis and arthrosis, a hypothesis. In: Ficat RP, Hungerford, eds. *Disorders of the patellofemoral joint.* Baltimore: Williams & Wilkins, 1977;194–243.

15. Ficat RP, Philippe J, Hungerford DS. Chondromalacia patellae: a system of classification. *Clin Orthop* 1979;144:55–62.

16. Garrick JG. Determinants of return to athletic activity. *Orthop Clin North Am* 1983;14:317–321.

17. Giove TP, Miller SJ III, Kent BE, Sanford TL, Garrick JG. Nonoperative treatment of the torn anterior cruciate ligament. *J Bone Joint Surg* 1983;65A:184–192.

18. Gleim W, Nicholas JA, Webb JN. Isokinetic evaluation following leg injuries. *Phys Sportsmed* 1978;6:75–82.

19. Goodfellow J, Hungerford DS, Woods C. Patello-femoral joint mechanics and pathology, part 2: chondromalacia patellae. *J Bone Joint Surg* 1976;58B:291–299.

20. Guidelines for Authors. *Am J Sports Med* 1988;16(2). (Appearing at the front of issue.)

21. Gurtler RA, Stine R, Torg JS. Lachman test evaluated. *Clin Orthop* 1987;216:141–150.

22. Hamberg P, Gillquist J. Knee function after arthroscopic meniscectomy. *Acta Orthop Scand* 1984;55:172–175.

23. Harter RA, Osternig LR, Singer KM, James SL, Larson RL, Jones DC. Long-term evaluation of knee stability and function following surgical reconstruction for anterior cruciate ligament insufficiency. *Am J of Sports Med* 1988;16:434–443.

24. Insall JN. Disorders of the patella. In: Insall JN, ed. *Surgery of the knee.* New York: Churchill Livingstone, 1984;191–260.

25. Insall JN, Faluo KA, Wise DW. Chondromalacia patellae—a prospective study. *J Bone Joint Surg* 1976;58A:1–8.

26. Jakob RP, Stäubli HU, Deland JT. Grading the pivot shift: objective tests with implications for treatment. *J Bone Joint Surg* 1987;69B:294–299.

27. Jensen JE, Slocum DB, Larson RL, James SL, Singer KM. Reconstruction procedures for anterior cruciate ligament insufficiency: a computer analysis of clinical results. *Am J Sports Med* 1983;11:240–248.

28. Lukianov AV, Gillquist J, Grana WA, DeHaven KE. An anterior cruciate ligament (ACL) evaluation format for assessment of artificial or autologous anterior cruciate reconstruction results. *Clin Orthop* 1987;218:167–180.

29. Lysholm J. The relation between pain and torque in an isokinetic strength test of knee extension. *Arthroscopy* 1987;3:182–184.

30. Lysholm J, Gillquist J. Evaluation of knee ligament surgery results with special emphasis on use of a scoring scale. *Am J Sports Med* 1982;10:150–154.

31. Marans HJ, Jackson RW, Glossop ND, Young MC. Anterior cruciate ligament insufficiency: a dynamic three-dimensional motion analysis. *Am J Sports Med* 1989;17:325–332.

32. Markolf KL, Pattee GA, Strum GM, Gallick GS, Sherman OH, Dorey FJ. Instrumented measurements of laxity in patients who have a Gore-Tex anterior cruciate-ligament substitute. *J Bone Joint Surg* 1989;71A:887–893.

33. Marshall JL, Fetto JF, Botero PM. Section II, general orthopaedics—Knee ligament injuries: a standardized evaluation method. *Clin Orthop* 1977;123:115–129.

34. Mooar P, Gregg J, Jacobstein J. Radionuclide imaging in internal derangements of the knee. *Am J Sports Med* 1987;15:132.

35. Murray SM, Warren RF, Otis JC, Kroll M, Wickiewicz TL. Torque–velocity relationships of the knee extensor and flexor muscles in individuals sustaining injuries of the anterior cruciate ligament. *Am J Sports Med* 1984;12:436.

36. Noyes FR, Albright JP, eds. "Sports Injury Research." *Am J Sports Med* 1988;16(Suppl 1). [Special issue.]

37. Noyes FR, Barber SD, Mooar S. A rational for assessing sports activity levels and limitations in knee disorders. *Clin Orthop* 1989;246:238–249.

38. Noyes FR, McGinniss GH, Mooar LA. Functional disability in the anterior cruciate insufficient knee syndrome: review of knee rating systems and projected risk factors in determining treatment. *Sports Med* 1984;1:278–302.

39. Noyes FR, Stabler CL. A system for grading articular cartilage lesions at arthroscopy. *Am J Sports Med* 1989;17:505–513.

40. Odensten M, Tegner Y, Lysholm J, Gillquist J. Knee function and muscle strength following distal iliotibial band transfer for anterolateral rotatory instability. *Acta Orthop Scand* 1983;54:924–928.

41. Olson EJ, Kang JD, Fu FH, Georgescu HI, Mason GC, Evans CH. *Am J Sports Med* 1988;16:558–570.

42. Outerbridge RE. The etiology of chondromalacia patellae. *J Bone Joint Surg* 1961;43B:752–757.

43. Rudicel S. How to choose a study design. *Am J Sports Med [Suppl]* 1988;16(1):43–47.

44. Rudicel S. How to avoid bias. *Am J Sports Med Suppl* 1988;16(1):48–52.

45. Rudicel S, Esdaile J. The randomized clinical trial in orthopedics. Obligation or option? *J Bone Joint Surg* 1985;67A:1284–1293.

46. Straub T, Hunter RE. Acute anterior cruciate ligament repair. *Clin Orthop* 1988;227:238–250.

47. Tegner Y, Lysholm J. Rating systems in the evaluation of knee ligament injuries. *Clin Orthop* 1985;198:43–49.

48. Tegner Y, Lysholm J, Lysholm M, Gillquist J. A performance test to monitor rehabilitation and evaluate anterior cruciate ligament injuries. *Am J Sports Med* 1986;14:156–159.

49. Tegner Y, Lysholm J, Lysholm M, Gillquist J. Strengthening exercise for old cruciate ligament tears. *Acta Orthop Scand* 1986;57:130–134.

50. Thomas RH, Resnick D, Alazraki NP, Daniel DM, Greenfield R. Compartmental evaluation of osteoarthritis of the knee. *Radiology* 1975;116:585–594.

51. Tibone JE, Antich TJ, Fanton GS, Moynes DR, Perry J. Functional analysis of anterior cruciate ligament instability. *Am J Sports Med* 1986;14:276–284.

52. Wade CE. What is the question? *Am J Sports Med [Suppl]* 1988;16(1):38–42.

53. Wade CE. What is the value of the case-control study? *Am J Sports Med [Suppl]* 1988;16(1):53–54.

54. Wyatt M, Edwardo A. Comparison of quadriceps and hamstring torque values during isokinetic exercise. *J Orthop Sports Phys Ther* 1981;3:48–56.

Knee Ligaments: Structure, Function, Injury, and Repair, edited by D. Daniel, et al.
© 1990 by Raven Press, Ltd. All rights reserved.

CHAPTER 30

Experimental Design and Statistical Analysis

Richard L. Lieber

The major purpose for proper experimental design and statistical analysis is the extraction of the "truth" in an experimental setting. The benefits of proper planning and analysis cannot be overstated. Many potentially superb ideas have not been realized because of poor experimental design. The significance of numerous excellent experiments has not been extracted because of shoddy or qualitative analysis. Interestingly, while many scientists and clinicians are trained in their specialty, very few are explicitly tutored in experimental design and statistical analysis.

The purpose of this chapter is to briefly describe, by example, the steps in planning, executing, and analyzing experimental data. The proper experimental execution consists of a number of discrete steps: (a) planning and designing the experiment, (b) executing the experiment, and (c) analyzing and interpreting the data from the experiment. Emphasis will be placed on steps a and b. If these suggestions are followed, costs are decreased, direction is maintained, and the project retains continuity. Most importantly, the data ultimately have more impact because results are concisely and accurately presented.

R. L. Lieber: Department of Surgery, University of California, San Diego, School of Medicine, La Jolla, California 92093; and Division of Orthopedics and Rehabilitation, Veterans Administration Medical Center, La Jolla, California 92161.

PLANNING AND DESIGNING THE EXPERIMENT

Stating the Hypothesis

It is preferable to perform an experiment when a clearly stated hypothesis is to be tested. All too frequently, investigators who possess a great deal of intellectual capacity and use highly sophisticated experimental methods do not make a significant contribution to their field because their research lacks direction and design. By clearly stating the hypothesis, the attention of the research team is focused on the central issue. Other ancillary issues arising during the course of the investigation are seen as ancillary, and the direction of the research is not sidetracked.

The Null Hypothesis

The hypothesis to be tested statistically is stated in terms of the null hypothesis. The null hypothesis states that there is no (null) effect of experimental treatment. In one of the most common embodiments, this type of experiment is designed with a control group (receiving no treatment) and one or more experimental groups receiving treatment. Ultimately, the null hypothesis will be tested and a *p* value will be obtained. Let us propose the following null hypothesis: Surgical reconstruction of the ACL has no effect on knee laxity. In

TABLE 30-1. Statistical errors related to the null hypothesis

		Null hypothesis	
		Accepted	Rejected
Null	True	Correct decision	Type I error
hypothesis	False	Type II error	Correct decision

order to test this hypothesis, a control group (receiving no surgery) and an experimental group (receiving surgical reconstruction) are both tested for laxity.

We have a number of choices related to the null hypothesis (Table 30-1). Obviously, the null hypothesis can be either true or false. Additionally, we can choose to accept or reject the null hypothesis. This results in four potential decisions, two of which are correct and two of which are incorrect (Table 30-1). Suppose, for example, that the null hypothesis is true. That is, there is no difference in laxity between experimental and control groups. If we accept the null hypothesis, we have made the correct decision. If we reject the null hypothesis, we have made an incorrect decision. We have committed what is known in statistics as type I error, rejecting a true null hypothesis. This can be viewed in more clinical terms as a "false positive" (Table 30-2). Thus, in our experiment, type I error concludes that there is a significant effect of surgical reconstruction when, in fact, there is not. The alternate possibility is that the null hypothesis is false. That is, surgical reconstruction has a significant effect on knee laxity. If we reject the null hypothesis, we have again made the correct decision. If we accept the null hypothesis, we have made an incorrect decision, committing what is known as type II error, accepting a false null hypothesis. This can be viewed in clinical terms as a "false negative" (Table 30-2). We concluded that there was no effect of surgery when, in fact, there was.

Of course, we would like to commit as few errors as possible. We prefer not to commit either type I or type II error, but it should be clearly pointed out that the p value is directly related only to type I error. That is, the p value is simply the probability (denoted α) of committing type I error in a given experiment (Table

TABLE 30-2. Interpretation and control of statistical error

Condition	Greek symbol	Meaning	Controlled using
Type I error	α	False positive	Significance level
Type II error	β	False negative	Statistical power

30-2). When we state that "the results are significant ($p < 0.05$) . . .," we are saying that we are potentially committing type I error less than 5% of the time. The problem with this automatic use of $p < 0.05$ as the level for statistical significance is that many times (especially in clinical situations) it is not acceptable to commit type I error 5% of the time (see below), whereas in other cases we might be willing to commit type I error a greater percentage of the time. The significance level should actually be determined based on its meaning in the context of the experiment performed.

In order to decrease the probability of committing type II error (denoted β), we must design our experiment with sufficient statistical power.

Statistical Power and the Choice of Sample Size

Although we are familiar with setting limits for type I error (by choosing a critical p value), we are not as familiar with limiting type II error. However, as discussed below, controlling type II error can be equally or more important than type I error. Many of us have observed presentations where a small sample size was used (e.g., $n = 3$), statistical analysis was performed, and a p value was obtained which was greater than 0.05. The speaker concluded that the treatment had no effect. Immediately, a protester stated that the sample size was not large enough to demonstrate the difference. We may also have observed the situation where an individual performed an experiment with, say, 10 individuals per sample, obtained a p value of around 0.07, and was then encouraged to add a few more individuals to the sample in order to achieve statistical significance! In yet another setting, we may have observed a surgeon performing an experiment with a small sample size comparing a new surgical technique to the standard technique. Based on a high p value, the surgeon concluded that there was no significant difference between the new and standard methods and that the new method should be used. All of these situations can arise when one has not considered statistical power in the experimental design. [Interestingly, a recent review of 71 "negative" randomized clinical trials (6) concluded that over half of the "negative" results were simply a result of lack of sufficient statistical power.]

Statistical power is simply $1 - \beta$, the logical negative of type II error. If type II error is analogous to a false negative (i.e., accepting a false null hypothesis), then power is the probability of not committing a false negative. In other words, we want to be sure that if we obtain a p value greater than 0.05, we are not incorrectly accepting a false null hypothesis. We want to be sure we are not committing type II error. In the example stated above, we may wish to design the experiment with a power of 95%. In that case, we would be 95% sure that if anterior cruciate ligament (ACL) reconstruction had an effect on knee laxity (the null hypothesis were false), we would not falsely conclude that it did not.

Designing an Experiment of a Given Power

Several methods (graphs, tables, equations) have been developed which allow the experimenter to set the significance level (the critical p value) and the statistical power and then to determine the sample size required to achieve that design (2,9,11). Using these methods, the experimenter chooses α and β, estimates the sample variance, anticipates the magnitude of the treatment effect, and calculates (or observes on a graph) the required sample size.

For example, in an unpublished study of ACL reconstruction by Daniel, the 30°/20-lb KT-1000 anterior displacement was measured in 118 patients. Presurgical reconstruction and 1 year postsurgical reconstruction difference between the injured and normal leg was 5.4 ± 2.9 mm preoperatively and 2.4 ± 2.2 mm postoperatively. Suppose that a new operation were developed which we thought would decrease laxity by another 1 mm. How many subjects would need to be evaluated to demonstrate a 1-mm decrease in laxity? As mentioned above, the important considerations are the sample variability (here, the standard deviation of the sample, which is 2.2 mm), the magnitude of the treatment effect (in this case 1.0 mm, which is 1 mm "better" than the standard procedure), the significance level ($\alpha = 0.05$), and the statistical power (95%). Using standard procedures (7), it is calculated that approximately 130 individuals would be needed to demonstrate such a difference. It would require fewer subjects to demonstrate a large treatment difference. For example, if the new surgical procedure improved laxity by 2 mm, only about 35 subjects would be needed. In other words, because the treatment effect is large, it is easier to demonstrate. Of course, this example only holds true for this combination of significance, power, treatment magnitude, and sample variability. Changes in any parameter will change the required sample size.

Graphs of the relationship between statistical power, significance level, and sample size are shown in Fig. 30-1. Note that as either power increases or significance level decreases, sample size increases (Fig. 30-1A and B). Note also that if a relatively small treatment effect is anticipated ($\delta = 1$ mm, Fig. 30-1A), a larger sample size is required than if the anticipated treatment effect is large ($\delta = 2$ mm, Fig. 30-1B).

Nonstandard p Values

A survey of the scientific literature, especially the literature related to biology and medicine, reveals that an overwhelming majority of investigators set the critical p value to 0.05. It should be obvious based on the previous discussion that there is nothing "magic" about a p value of 0.05. The p value of 0.05 simply indicates that we are willing to commit type I error 5% of the time. However, there may be situations where the investigator is not willing to commit type I error 5% of the time or even 1% of the time. In such cases, the critical p value should be adjusted accordingly.

An understanding of the basis for selection of a critical p value and statistical power is especially important in clinical science. For example, in an experiment that attempts to demonstrate a significant decrease in knee laxity using a new surgical procedure as opposed to using an established procedure, if the critical p value is 0.05 the investigator is willing to incorrectly conclude 5% of the time that the new surgical procedure is more effective even if it actually is not. If the new procedure represents an increased risk to the patient or a significant increase in expense or rehabilitation time, the surgeon may only be willing to commit type I error 1% of the time or a fraction of a percent of the time. In such a case, a critical p value of 0.05 may be too high.

It should also be noted that, at times, type II error may be more important to an investigator than type I error. For example, suppose that a safe experimental drug were administered to prevent thrombophlebitis after knee surgery. In this case, type I error would indicate that the drug had an effect when in fact it did not. The detriment to the patient is that he or she would take a drug that had no effect. While this could represent an expense, it may not represent a medical or scientific problem. However, suppose type II error were committed in the same study. Type II error would indicate that the drug had no effect when in fact it had an effect. In this case, an effective drug would be withheld from the patient, which could represent a large problem. It may be that in this example, the power of the test should be 99.9%, while the critical p value should only be 0.1. The interpretation of the meaning of the p value is therefore paramount in selecting its value and in guarding against cookbook application of statistical methods (12,13).

Designing the Experiment

If only one treatment is tested (and, therefore, only one control and experimental group used), design and analysis are very simple. In fact, one should clearly focus on a specific hypothesis and avoid the use of

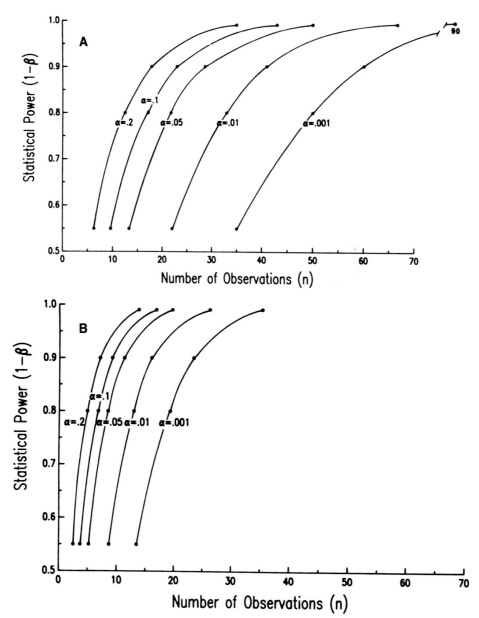

FIG. 30-1. Graphical relationship between statistical power, significance level, and sample size. In this example, δ refers to the magnitude of the anticipated treatment difference. **A:** Calculations for δ = 1 mm represent the case where the anticipated treatment effect is relatively small. **B:** Calculations for δ = 2 mm represent the case where the anticipated treatment effect is relatively large. Note that, in general, for a large treatment effect, the required sample size is smaller.

numerous groups to test ancillary factors. The use of numerous groups to test the main and secondary effects is counterproductive. With more experimental groups, statistical tests are less powerful and the main treatment effect may be confounded simply to enable a qualitative statement about a lesser issue. If multiple treatment effects are desired, they should be addressed serially rather than with a single, multifaceted experiment. Again, the experimental groups should be designed to specifically test the main hypothesis. If this

requires narrowing the scope of the experimental hypothesis, so be it.

Analysis of Variance (ANOVA)

The most common experimental design involving more than two groups usually involves analysis using analysis of variance (ANOVA) (3). The null hypothesis for ANOVA is that the mean of all groups is the same.

That is, if we have n groups, the null hypothesis for ANOVA states that

$$\mu_1 = \mu_2 = \mu_3 = 1 \cdots = \mu_n \qquad [1]$$

where μ_i represents the mean of the ith group. If we obtain a significant p value following analysis, this indicates that all of the group means are not identical. It should be emphasized that we do not know *which* means are different from the others. When performing an ANOVA on multiple groups, if any *one* mean value is significantly different from any other *one* mean, the overall ANOVA p value will be significant. In order to determine precisely *which* means are different from the others, multiple paired comparisons must be performed.

Multiple Paired Comparisons

Multiple paired comparisons are not simply performed as a series of simple t-tests. The important point to consider in multiple paired comparisons is that *the number of paired comparisons affects the experimental significance level*. This is based on the idea that, if we performed a large number of paired comparisons, there would be a certain probability that we would obtain a significant difference simply by chance. Thus, the more paired comparisons made, the "harder" it must be to determine a significant difference. A number of methods for making such a correction to the significance level have been developed (4,7,10). One of the simplest of these correction methods is known as the "Bonferroni approximation" (see Appendix C of ref. 4 for a comparison of the relative merits of the different approximations). Simply stated, the Bonferroni approximation requires that the significance level of the single paired comparison be reduced by dividing the experimental significance level by the number of paired comparisons made. In effect, this "adjustment" makes it more difficult to demonstrate statistical significance as more comparisons are made. This is due to the fact that if a sufficient number of paired comparisons is made, significant differences may be achieved based on chance alone. Importantly, the comparisons to be made must be decided *before* the data are observed in order to satisfy the assumptions of random sampling. It is therefore not justified to perform a simple t-test between two groups that "look" different based on observation of the results after performing the experiment.

Linear Regression

In addition to hypotheses that center on comparisons of group means, it is often of interest to investigate the correlation or covariance between two parameters (5).

The null hypothesis in linear regression is that there is no significant correlation between the independent and dependent variables. The analysis yields two important parameters: the correlation coefficient (r) and the significance of the correlation (p). Both parameters are important and must be considered simultaneously in order to correctly interpret the results.

The p value obtained from linear regression directly tests whether there is a significant correlation between the two variables. Mathematically, the statistic tests whether the slope of the linear equation is significantly different from zero. If the p value is not significant (e.g., $p > 0.05$), then the resulting equation should be ignored. Many errors in data interpretation have been made as a result of overinterpretation of equations obtained in nonsignificant statistical tests.

The correlation coefficient (r) represents the "goodness of fit" of the experimental data to the linear equation. Note that any experimental data can be "fit" to a line by using the method of least squares (5). How well these data are described by a line is indicated by the correlation coefficient. The correlation coefficient can vary between $+1$ and -1 (a plus sign indicates a positive slope, and a minus sign indicates a negative slope). A correlation coefficient of 1 indicates a perfect fit to a line.

It is difficult to state the "limits" of an acceptable correlation coefficient. Relatively low r values (0.3–0.5) can be highly significant and should be strongly regarded by the experimentalist. However, relatively high correlation coefficients (0.8–0.95) can be obtained easily with very few data points or with only two values of the independent variable. Thus, correct interpretation of the regression statistics is dependent on an understanding of the meaning and relative importance of the two values.

EXECUTING THE EXPERIMENT

The most rudimentary requirement for any experiment is to determine the *accuracy* and *resolution* of the measuring system. "Accuracy" refers to the closeness of an observed value to the true (standard) value. "Resolution" refers to the precision with which a measurement can be made. For example, with the advent of the new digital scales (and other digital devices), a sample mass can easily be indicated as 12.324120 g. Thus, the mass can be resolved to 0.000001 g. However, the balance must be calibrated against a standard mass and may be accurate only to about 0.01 g. How precise should the experimental values be reported? The most conservative answer would be to limit the number of significant figures to the device accuracy. It is certainly allowable to retain all figures during intermediate calculations. However, when the data are presented, the number of significant figures should be trimmed according to device accuracy.

Based on the discussion on sample size, it should be apparent that minimizing experimental variability is tantamount to increasing statistical power. By decreasing unwanted random error, the amount of information obtained from each observation is increased. In short, sloppy experimental technique *causes* more work for the investigator who has to unnecessarily increase sample size to offset the increased variance. This particular point refers to *random* experimental variability—that is, variability which can tend to increase or decrease an experimental value with equal probability. Another type of shoddy experimental technique can result in *systematic* experimental bias. That is, the poor technique always tends to change the result in the same direction. The classic example is the case of dry weight measurements where, if the samples are not fully dried, an artificially increased mass is recorded.

Sometimes it is impossible to avoid systematic experimental variability. For example, in repeated recordings of skeletal muscle tetanic tension, the muscle tends to deteriorate over time. In such a case, *randomizing the order of experimentation* can be of use. In this case, the increased experimental error due to specimen deterioration is still present. However, the deterioration does not *systematically* affect the results. Randomizing such variables as order of experimentation, sides on which surgery is performed, time of day the measurements are made, or specimen testing sequence can all help to avoid systematic experimental variability.

Another method for decreasing experimental variability is to establish a specific protocol (in writing) and make sure that everyone adheres to it. This is especially useful to ensure that experimental protocols do not "evolve" during the course of experimentation performed by different individuals. In any case, all technicians should be encouraged to write down every observation, along with times of day, to enable retrospective answering of questions that often arise during data analysis. If such observations are not recorded in writing, it is often impossible to diagnose causes for observed data variations.

ANALYZING AND INTERPRETING THE EXPERIMENT

Data Screening

First, data must be screened to ensure that no transcription errors occurred (if appropriate) and to test the sample distribution. A convenient method to perform this task, especially with large data sets, is to investigate the sample summary descriptive statistics. Of greatest interest are the statistics referring to sample variability. Specifically, sample standard deviation, coefficient of variation, range, and Z-scores can quickly locate experimental values that are orders of magnitude away from the mean. Be sure that if large variabilities are present, they are not due to simple errors in data manipulation, conversion, or transcription.

Sample Outliers

A second reason for large variabilities is the presence of outliers—data that are much different than the rest of the data set. Under what conditions is it justifiable to omit data? The easiest decision, which, by the way, is not a statistical decision, is the case when the scientist knows that something went wrong *during* the experiment. For example, if a very low contractile tension was observed when testing a muscle specimen, and the surgeons suspected that they may have damaged the motor nerve during surgical isolation, the expert decision might be to omit the data. This observation should be recorded on the data sheet during the dissection so that it is possible to objectively and retrospectively evaluate data quality. It should be emphasized that this is not a statistical decision at all but is, instead, an expert decision.

The more difficult decision arises when one has a data point that is very far from the mean and yet the experiment seemed to go fine. A number of criteria have been developed to address such a case (4). One of the most common is to omit data points that are more than two standard deviations away from the mean. However, this method has been criticized (8). If sample sizes are large enough, it is difficult for a single outlier to bias the results. A second method involves statistical analysis based on a "trimmed" mean in order to compensate for data at the "tails" of the sample. These analyses are available using Biomedical Data Processing (BMDP) program P7D (4).

Normality of Sample Distribution

Most parametric statistical tests (i.e., statistical tests that evaluate a *parameter* such as a mean or a variance) require that the data be normally distributed and that the variance between groups be equal. Standard screening programs, such as BMDP P2D, are available to evaluate two important sample parameters: skew and kurtosis. "Skew" refers to the symmetry of the sample distribution, which can be to the left or to the right. "Kurtosis" refers to the proportion of the sample in the "tails" versus the central "bell" portion of the sample distribution. Thus, just because a frequency distribution appears to be a "bell-shaped" curve does not ensure that the distribution is normal. The most common skew and kurtosis indices are the so-called g_1 and g_2 parameters. When these parameters are greatly different from zero, they suggest skew or kurtosis. A negative value of g_1 (skew) indicates left skew, whereas a positive value of g_1 suggests right skew. Similarly, a negative value of g_2 (kurtosis) suggests platykurtosis (too much "weight" in the tails), whereas a positive value of g_2 suggests leptokurtosis (too much "weight" in the center of the curve).

The most common example of samples that are virtually certain *not* to be normally distributed are ratios and percentages. In such cases, the use of ordinary parametric statistical tests is not appropriate without appropriate data transformation.

Arithmetic Transformations

Data transformations are simply mathematical functions that are used to cause a sample to conform to the mathematical requirements of a statistical test—usually normality or equality of variance between groups (1). A useful statistical program that can be used to investigate the need for transformation is BMDP program P7D. In this program, a diagnostic plot of the data can be obtained to suggest whether no transformation, a log transformation, an arc sine transformation, or a square root transformation is required. After just a few experiences with this program, an investigator can become very adept at making data fulfill requirements of parametric tests. If no transformation improves the condition of the data set, nonparametric statistics may be required. Details of these methods can be found elsewhere (1,4).

Upon initial exposure to transformation functions, most investigators respond with skepticism. It seems "fishy" to simply apply a mathematical function to a data set and then perform the same statistical analysis that was previously inappropriate. However, the purpose of the transformation is to cause the data set to satisfy the *mathematical* requirements of the statistical test. This is simply a mathematical adjustment of the data which does not affect the values themselves. Some statisticians actually claim that the investigator should provide good reasons for *not* transforming their data!

Testing the Hypothesis

After having designed an excellent experiment, having performed it carefully, and having performed the appropriate analysis, one often finds that obtaining the actual p value obtained from the statistical test is almost anticlimatic. Having chosen the significance level (see above), a p value less than that indicates a significant effect of treatment. If the p value is close but not quite significant, the investigator should not panic but should, instead, simply report the p value. Some statisticians have even questioned the use of p values at all, since the choosing of a significance level is an arbitrary decision.

Multivariate Analysis

This class of analysis can be extremely useful in clinical settings. One of the most pressing needs in clinical medicine (as well as experimental settings) is the evaluation of the quality of the subjective impression based on objective data. For example, if the outcome of a surgical procedure were scored as "poor," "fair," "good," or "excellent," based on the expert opinion of the investigator, *and* numerous objective measurements were made, these two classes of data could be compared using multivariate analysis. The most common method for performing such an analysis is stepwise discriminant analysis. This method is extremely powerful, but it is so rarely used in clinical studies that it will be described in some detail here.

The simple purpose of discriminant analysis is to determine the most powerful objective discriminators between groups which are determined based on expert opinion. This opinion may be as simple as determining the various groups of data (control, experimental #1, experimental #2, etc.) or may be a subjective rating of an outcome as described above. The power of the method is that only the *unique* discriminators are entered into the discriminating equations. Thus, if two objective values are actually measures of the same thing, only one will enter as a discriminator.

After the discriminating equation is obtained, the data from which it was obtained are retrospectively classified based on the discriminating function. In this way, the power of the function can be evaluated.

Perhaps more important than retrospective classification is the predictive potential for discriminant analysis. For example, suppose that a good preoperative discriminator for the quality of a surgical outcome was the laxity of the nonoperative leg. This would indicate that if one had information regarding the control leg laxity, one could predict the success of the surgical procedure.

SUMMARY

A well-planned and well-executed experiment can provide important information to the body of scientific and clinical knowledge. Proper planning and analysis not only saves time and energy but also increases the amount of information extracted from all experiments.

The null hypothesis tested by a specific statistical method (ANOVA, multivariate analysis, linear regression, etc.) should be understood to avoid being "fooled" by simple conclusions based only on p values. If just a few of these techniques can be used for each project, in just a few short years the investigators will have greatly improved their ability to answer scientific questions.

REFERENCES

1. Box GEP, Cox DR. Analysis of transformations. *J R Stat Soc [B]* 1964;26:211–252.
2. Dixon WJ, Massey FJ Jr. *Introduction to statistical analysis*, 4th ed. New York: McGraw–Hill, 1983.
3. Dixon WJ. *BMDP statistical software*. Los Angeles: University of California Press, 1983.
4. Draper NR, John JA. *Applied regression analysis*, 2nd ed. New York: John Wiley & Sons, 1981.
5. Freiman JA, Chalmers TC, Smith H Jr, Kuebler RR. The importance of beta, the type II error and sample size in the design and interpretation of the randomized control trial. Survey of 71 "negative" trials. *N Engl J Med* 1978;299:690–695.
6. Lieber RL. Invited opinion: statistical significance and statistical power in hypothesis testing. *J Orthop Res* 1990; in press.
7. Miller RG Jr. *Simultaneous statistical inference*. New York: McGraw–Hill, 1981.
8. Poole C. Beyond the confidence interval. *Am J Public Health* 1987;77:195–199.
9. Rohlf FJ, Sokal RR. *Statistical tables*, 2nd ed. San Francisco: WH Freeman, 1981.
10. Scheffe H. *The analysis of variance*. New York: John Wiley & Sons, 1959.
11. Sokal RR, Rohlf FJ. *Biometry*, 2nd ed. San Francisco: WH Freeman, 1981.
12. Thompson WD. Statistical criteria in the interpretation of epidemiologic data. *Am J Public Health* 1987;77:191–194.
13. Thompson WD. On the comparison of effects. *Am J Public Health* 1987;77:491–193.

Subject Index

Note: A *t* following a page number indicates tabular material and an *f* following a page number indicates an illustration. Drugs are listed under their generic names. When a drug trade name is listed, the reader is referred to the generic name.

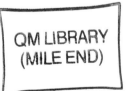